MW01484678

CORE CURRICULUM FOR
RHEUMATOLOGY NURSING

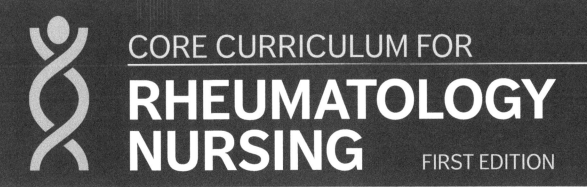

CORE CURRICULUM FOR
RHEUMATOLOGY NURSING
FIRST EDITION

EDITORIAL BOARD

Sheree C. Carter, PhD, RN
Assistant Professor
The University of Alabama
Capstone College of Nursing
Tuscaloosa, Alabama

Cathy Patty-Resk, MSN, RN, CPNP
Pediatric Nurse Practitioner
Children's Hospital of Michigan
Detroit, Michigan

Victoria Ruffing, RN, CCRP
Nurse Manager
Johns Hopkins Arthritis Center
Baltimore, Maryland

Deborah Hicks, RN
Clinical Coordinator / Infusion Nurse
Greenwood Regional Rheumatology Center
Greenwood, South Carolina

Published by

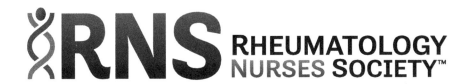

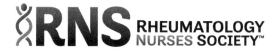

2131 Woodruff Rd Suite 2100#200, Greenville, SC 29607
http://RNSnurse.org

CORE CURRICULUM FOR RHEUMATOLOGY NURSING - First Edition
ISBN: 978-0-615-90131-2

Copyright © 2015 by Rheumatology Nurses Society, Inc. as Publisher

Bulk quantity discounts are available to corporations, professional associations, academic institutions, and other qualified organizations. For details and specific discount information, contact the RNS National Headquarters via the above contact information or send an email to Publishing@RNSnurse.org

NOTICES

Knowledge, medical litature, and best practices in Rheumatology Nursing are constantly changing. As new research, findings, and experience broaden our understanding, changes in methods, professional practices, or medical treatment may become necessary. Readers must always rely on their own experience and knowledge in evaluating and using any information, methods, compounds, or experiments described herein. In using such information or methods they should be mindful of their own safety and the safety of others, including parties for whom they have a professional responsibility.

Regarding any drug or pharmaceutical products mentioned in this book, readers are urged to check the package insert for each drug for indications, dosage, and for added warnings and precautions; and are advised to check the most current information provided on procedures featured, or by the manufacturer of each product to be administered. It is the responsibility of practitioners, relying on their own experience and knowledge of their patients, to make diagnoses, determine dosages, and provide the best treatment for each individual patient while taking all appropriate safety precautions.

Care has been taken to confirm the accuracy of the information presented and to describe generally accepted practices. However, neither the Publisher nor the authors, contributors, editors, consultants, or contractors assume any liability and are not responsible for errors or omissions or for any consequences from application, including but not limited to any injury and/or damage to persons or property as a matter of product liability, negligence or otherwise; or from any use or operation of any methods, products, instructions, or ideas contained in the material in this book; and make no warranty, express or implied, with respect to the content of the publication to the fullest extent of the law.

Publishing Services Coordinator: Lyons Den Solutions, LLC (LyonsDS.com)
Project Manager: Kevin D. Lyons
Layout and Design: Lyons Den Solutions, LLC
Printing Partner: Documation, Inc.
Printed in the United States of America
Last digit is the print number: 9 8 7 6 5 4 3 2 1

CONTRIBUTORS

EDITORIAL BOARD

Sheree C. Carter, PhD, RN
Assistant Professor
The University of Alabama
Capstone College of Nursing
Tuscaloosa, Alabama

Cathy Patty-Resk, MSN, RN, CPNP
Pediatric Nurse Practitioner
Children's Hospital of Michigan
Detroit, Michigan

Victoria Ruffing, RN, CCRP
Nurse Manager
Johns Hopkins Arthritis Center
Baltimore, Maryland

Deborah Hicks, RN
Clinical Coordinator / Infusion Nurse
Greenwood Regional Rheumatology Center
Greenwood, South Carolina

CHAPTER AUTHORS

Jenny de la Torre Aboki, RN, BSc, MSc, PGdipRheum
Rheumatology Nurse Specialist
Rheumatology Department
Alicante General and University Hospital
Alicante, Spain

Jill Bernhardt, RN, FNP
Nurse Practitioner
Optum Healthcare
Rochester, New York

Ruth Busch, MSN, APRN, BC
Advanced Practice Registered Nurse
Arthritis and Rheumatology Clinics of Kansas
Wichita, Kansas

Sheree C. Carter, PhD, RN
Assistant Professor
The University of Alabama
Capstone College of Nursing
Tuscaloosa, Alabama

Linda Cowden, RN
Research Nurse Coordinator in Rheumatology
University of Alabama at Birmingham
Birmingham, Alabama

Janice L. Cuzzell, MSN, RN
Senior Rheumatology Clinical Coordinator
Immunology & Ophthalmology
Genentech, Inc.
San Francisco, California

Theresa R. Evans, RN
Registered (Primary) Nurse
Allergy, Asthma, Immunology of Rochester, P.C.
Rochester, New York

Vivian A. Gaits, RN, MSN, ACNS-BC, AOCN, CRNI
Sr. Rheumatology Clinical Coordinator
Genentech, Inc.
San Francisco, California

Rebecca L. Gamble, BA, RN
Infusion Nurse
Greenwood Regional Rheumatology Center
Greenwood, South Carolina

Diane Gilbert, BSN, RN, CRNI
Staff Nurse IV
Infusion Center
Kaiser Permanente
Fresno, California

CHAPTER AUTHORS (continued)

Deborah Hicks, RN
Clinical Coordinator / Infusion Nurse
Greenwood Regional Rheumatology Center
Greenwood, South Carolina

Vanessa K. Hill, MSN, NP-C
Family Nurse Practitioner
Division of Immunology and Rheumatology
University of Alabama at Birmingham
Birmingham, Alabama

Yvonne van Eijk-Hustings, RN, PhD
Health Care Scientist and Rheumatology Nurse
Department of Patient and Care /
Department of Rheumatology
Maastricht University Medical Centre
Maastricht, the Netherlands

Dawn E. Isherwood, MSIR, BSN, RN
National Health Educator
Lupus Foundation of America, Inc.
Washington, District of Columbia

Samantha R. Judd, MSN, RN, CPNP
Pediatric Nurse Practitioner
Children's Hospital of Michigan
Detroit, Michigan

Elizabeth Kirchner, CNP
Certified Nurse Practitioner
Rheumatologic and Immunologic Disease
Cleveland Clinic
Cleveland, Ohio

Victor Mo, MSN, RN
Practice Manager
Rheumatology
Barry Shibuya, MD, Inc.
Fremont, California

Deanna L. Owens, MSN, RN
Director of Infusion & Clinical Services
Low Country Rheumatology
North Charleston, South Carolina

Ina Radziunas, MEd, BScN, RN
Clinical Nurse Specialist
The Centre for Osteoporosis & Bone Health
Women's College Hospital
Toronto, Ontario, Canada

Cathy Patty-Resk, MSN, RN, CPNP
Pediatric Nurse Practitioner
Children's Hospital of Michigan
Detroit, Michigan

Victoria Ruffing, RN, CCRP
Nurse Manager
Johns Hopkins Arthritis Center
Baltimore, Maryland

Maria Cusano-Sanzo, MSN, RN, CPN
Rheumatology Clinical Coordinator,
Genentech, Inc.
San Francisco, California
Formerly Program Clinical Care Coordinator
Connecticut Children's Medical Center
Hartford, Connecticut

Christine A. Stamatos, DNP, ANP-C
Nurse Practitioner Research Associate
Stony Brook University Medical Center and
Rheumatology Associates of Long Island
Nurse Practitioner
L.I. Regional Arthritis and Osteoporosis Care
Babylon, New York

Pamela M. Vath, MS, FNP-BC
Senior Rheumatology Clinical Coordinator
Genentech, Inc.
San Francisco, California

Patricia Weinstein, PhD, ARNP, NP-C, CNE
Adjunct Faculty, College of Nursing
University of Central Florida
Orlando, Florida

Iris Zink, MSN, RN, ANP-BC
Nurse Practitioner
Beals Institute Center for Arthritis, Osteoporosis,
and Autoimmune Disorders
Lansing, Michigan

CONTRIBUTORS (continued)

SECTION EDITORS

Ruth Busch, MSN, APRN, BC
Advanced Practice Registered Nurse
Arthritis and Rheumatology Clinics of Kansas
Wichita, Kansas

Sheree C. Carter, PhD, RN
Assistant Professor
The University of Alabama
Capstone College of Nursing
Tuscaloosa, Alabama

Deanna S. Harris, MSN, RN
Multi-Specialty Infusion Nurse Manager
ARC-KC Allergy Rheumatology Clinic of Kansas City
Overland Park, Kansas

Deborah Hicks, RN
Clinical Coordinator / Infusion Nurse
Greenwood Regional Rheumatology Center
Greenwood, South Carolina

Betty B. Loflin, FNP-BC
Senior Rheumatology Clinical Coordinator
Genentech, Inc.
San Francisco, California
Formerly Nurse Practitioner
Arthritis Associates of Mississippi
Jackson, Mississippi

PRINCIPLE REVIEWERS

Iris Zink, MSN, RN, ANP-BC
Nurse Practitioner
Beals Institute Center for Arthritis,
Osteoporosis, and Autoimmune Disorders
Lansing, Michigan

Elizabeth Kirchner, CNP
Certified Nurse Practitioner
Rheumatologic and Immunologic Disease
Cleveland Clinic
Cleveland, Ohio

PRODUCTION REVIEWERS

Ruth Busch, MSN, APRN, BC

Vicki L. Lyons

Linda Grinnell-Merrick, MS, NP-BC

Deanna L. Owens, MSN, RN

Claire M. Ruffing, PhD

Maria Cusano-Sanzo, MSN, RN, CPN

Timothy Ray Walker, RN

CHAPTER CONTRIBUTORS

Nancy Crigger, PhD, FNP-BC

Sylvia Nobles, MSN, FNP

Luis Oquendo, MSN, MBA, HCA, RN

Lourdes Sejismundo, BSN, RN

Karen Towner, BSN, RN, AE-C

Barbara Voshall, DNP, RN

Acknowledgments

Project Management & Publishing Services

Kevin D. Lyons
Executive Director
Rheumatology Nurses Society, Inc.

Chief Executive Officer and President
Lyons Den Solutions, LLC
Sarasota, Florida

Cover Design: Derek Cole

Editorial Services

Keleita L. (Shay) Stephens
Pensacola, Florida

Rheumatology Nurses Society
would like to thank and recognize the following
for their generous financial support:

AbbVie, Inc.

Horizon Pharma

CONTENTS

CONTENTS (continued)

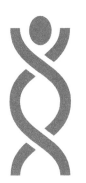

Introduction
Core Curriculum
for Rheumatology Nursing

Victoria Ruffing, RN, CCRP

> *The trained nurse has become one of the great blessings of humanity, taking a place beside the physician and the priest, and not inferior to either in her mission.* Sir William Osler, 1897

The complexities of rheumatic diseases and the treatments for them are a challenge for rheumatology nurses. Translating the knowledge nurses acquire into the appropriate care and education for patients can be equally as challenging. The information presented in this *Core Curriculum* is designed for all nurses in rheumatology. This *Core Curriculum* will be invaluable for orienting nurses to rheumatology, furthering professional development, providing continuing education, and developing individual care plans for patients with rheumatic conditions.

Before the advent of biologic therapy, patients with rheumatic conditions had few treatment options. Rheumatology nurses were few in number, and their roles were often limited. When biologic therapies became available, a great need for nurses in rheumatology practices emerged. Who else could administer infusions and educate patients on self-injection? The nurses in rheumatology practices also could help with getting medications authorized and keeping track of inventory and supplies. Of course, these were not the thoughts of the nurses entering the specialty or those already working in rheumatology practices...we knew we could do more, much more.

In 2007, three nurses, Therese Dexter, Elizabeth Grace, and Victoria Ruffing, started the Rheumatology Nurses Society (RNS). These nurse leaders recognized the need for education of nurses in rheumatology, a component of nursing practice lacking in nursing education curricula. The founders of RNS questioned how nurses in rheumatology could educate themselves and their peers, and thus, improve patients' quality of life. Starting with a website and membership drive, RNS then held its first conference with 80 attendees. The most striking realization of that first meeting was that this was a passionate group of nurses, eager for more information. The founders were tasked with expanding opportunities to educate nurses about rheumatology nursing and moving toward certification in the specialty.

On November 9, 2012, the American Nurses Association Board of Directors announced its recognition of rheumatology nursing as a nursing specialty, approval of the rheumatology nursing scope of practice statement, and acknowledgment of the standards of practice for rheumatology registered nurses (RNs) and Advanced Practice Registered Nurses (APRNs) in rheumatology. These accomplishments were the first step in moving toward a certification program for rheumatology nurses. This *Core Curriculum* is another component of reaching that goal. However, it is also much more. This is *your* reference on rheumatic diseases and treatments and the nursing implications related to both.

The authors, section editors, and reviewers involved in producing this text have not been rewarded in any way other than that they may take personal satisfaction in creating the first *Core Curriculum for Rheumatology Nursing*. The countless hours devoted to this endeavor are so that nurses interested in rheumatology nursing may be equipped with the knowledge needed to practice in the specialty.

Although the quote by Sir William Osler was written over 100 years ago, how apt it is for the specialty of rheumatology nursing. As Sir Osler so eloquently stated, nurses are equals with other healthcare professionals in the care of patients, and none more so than rheumatology nurses.

Victoria Ruffing, RN, CCRP
Co-Founder
Rheumatology Nurses Society

1
1.1
1.2
1.3
1.4
1.5
1.6
1.7
1.8
1.9

SECTION 1

RHEUMATOLOGY NURSING:
A SPECIALTY

Contents of Section 1

1
1.1
1.2
1.3
1.4
1.5
1.6
1.7
1.8
1.9

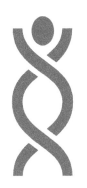

Section 1.1
Evolution of Rheumatology Nursing

Yvonne van Eijk-Hustings, RN, PhD

Introduction

In today's clinical rheumatology practice, nurses are accessible members of multidisciplinary teams, and they often act as the interface between the patient and other members of the team. However, the role of rheumatology nurses differs between countries and areas. In some countries, rheumatology nursing has developed to become a recognized specialty with nurses undertaking advanced and extended roles (Carr, 2001), but in others, rheumatology as a nursing specialty does not exist. Consequently, care given by rheumatology nurses is not equally available for all individuals with rheumatic diseases.

In order to reduce these unwanted differences and to emphasize rheumatology nursing, several initiatives have been taken. In Europe, the European League Against Rheumatism (EULAR) developed recommendations for the role of the nurse in the management of chronic inflammatory arthritis (van Eijk-Hustings et al., 2012).

The evolution of rheumatology nursing has been influenced by a variety of developments that cannot be considered separately; all should be taken into account. Insight into these developments is pivotal in order to understand the value of rheumatology nursing and the obstacles to implement rheumatology nursing care. This chapter, therefore, will provide an historic overview of important issues in the evolution of rheumatology nursing.

Learning Objectives

Upon completion of this chapter, the nurse will be able to:

1. Discuss an historic overview of rheumatology.

2. Describe an historic overview of rheumatology-related nursing care.

3. Identify the major determinants of the evolution of rheumatology nursing.

4. Identify obstacles to implementation of rheumatology nursing care.

1
1.1
1.2
1.3
1.4
1.5
1.6
1.7
1.8
1.9

Content Outline

I. History.

A. History of rheumatology.

1. Rheumatology is a relatively young field in medicine.

   a. Jan van Breemen, a Dutch physician, was one of the first to emphasize special attention for rheumatic diseases.

   b. The first international society for rheumatology was founded in 1927 (Maltbee, n.d.).

   c. The American Rheumatism Association was founded in the early 1930s.

2. Treatment options with regard to medications were limited.

   a. Treatment was focused on pain control and suppression of inflammation.

   b. Inflammation could be influenced by the use of corticosteroids (in use since the 1950s) and some slowly working disease-modifying antirheumatic drugs (DMARDs) such as sulfasalazine (in use since the 1930s), antimalarials (in use since the 1940s), and chrysotherapy (gold salts, in use since about 1915).

   c. Rehabilitation medicine and rheumatology collaborate in comprehensive care for patients with disabling arthritis. Interdisciplinary care for patients with rheumatoid arthritis by several medical specialists and social workers is described, but nurses are not considered a "discipline" yet (Jacox et al., 1963).

3. In case of exacerbations, patients were hospitalized, where traditionally, nursing care had been provided (Pigg, 1990).

B. Care for patients with rheumatic diseases.

1. The main aim of care during hospitalization was to maintain mobility (Peasnell, 1984).

   a. In the acute phase, the patient with rheumatoid arthritis was nursed at rest (Wright, 1977).

   b. Care comprised support in daily activities (personal hygiene), prevention of contractures, and skin care in case of corticosteroid use (Hosking, 1984).

   c. Patient education as important with regard to adherence to treatment was recognized early on (Hosking, 1984; Miale & Plotz, 1953; Wright, 1977).

   d. The role of nurses was often limited to care of seriously disabled persons.

   e. Nurses' roles were taken for granted (Pigg, 1990).

2. Permanent disability was the most common course of rheumatic diseases.

   a. In their homes, patients received support from community nurses (Rhodes, 1977).

   b. Besides professional support, patients often depended on help from friends or relatives to be able to function in their homes (Rhodes, 1977).

   c. If this support was not available or sufficient, care was administered in nursing homes.

II. The 70s and 80s.

A. New professionals in health care appeared in the U.S.

1. Physician assistants (PAs) and nurse practitioners (NPs) appeared to assist the busy physician (Hooker, 2008).

   a. A Physician Assistant (PA) is a healthcare professional who is licensed to practice medicine as part of a team with physicians.

   b. NPs are trained in nursing school; their role is considered an extension of nursing responsibility; and they provide advanced care under the Nurse Practice Act in the state in which they practice (Hooker, 2008).

   c. NPs can deliver a broader range of services than nurses, and by doing so, they are cost-effective and contribute to accessibility of care (Hooker, 2008).

2. PAs and NPs in rheumatology.

   a. The expansion of rheumatology services with specialized nurses and NPs began in the late 60s (Hooker, 2008).

   b. In the U.S., NPs first developed their expertise to manage patients with rheumatoid arthritis in primary care (Brown-Skeers, 1979).

B. Development of rheumatology nursing.

1
1.1
1.2
1.3
1.4
1.5
1.6
1.7
1.8
1.9

1. The rheumatology nursing specialty developed alongside the development of rheumatology as a distinct medical specialty (Hale & Hill, 2006).

    a. Rheumatology nursing as a sub-specialty was recognized in the UK in 1981 and in the U.S. in 1983 (Hale & Hill, 2006).

    b. Nursing interest in the field of rheumatology increased (Pigg, 1990).

2. Development was triggered by the use of specialized nurses as clinical metrologists: Nurses responsible for the conduct and recording of clinical trials on effects of drug treatments (Bird, Wright, & Galloway, 1980).

    a. In the clinical trials, the nurses were responsible for the measurements according to the study protocol. In doing so, they had regular contacts with patients.

    b. As the therapies became more complicated, patient education and reassurance was incorporated in the measurements. This service was valued by patients (Hill, 1985).

    c. Patient education, resulting in a knowledgeable patient, was considered an important component in treatment (Christman, 1987).

3. The first nurse-led arthritis clinics in the UK were developed in the 1980s.

    a. An increasing outpatient workload, a shortage of medical staff, a reduction in hours of work for junior physicians, and government pressure all contributed to the establishment of these clinics.

    b. Willingness of nurses to innovate and advance their practice also was a contributing factor (Hill, 2006).

4. Increasingly, a collaborative approach of rheumatologists' and nurses' consultations was implemented.

    a. Nurses began to take responsibility for a wider area of patient management.

    b. The role of nurses changed, incorporating technical and patient-management skills that were previously the physician's domain (Hill, 2005).

    c. Evaluation of the service among patients showed acceptability and satisfaction with the service provided (Hill, 1986).

III. The 90s.

A. Developments in rheumatology.

1. Increased knowledge became available about the nature of inflammatory diseases.

    a. Abnormal reactions of the immune system are essential in the etiology of inflammatory disorders.

    b. Therefore, treatment increasingly focused on interfering with the immune system.

2. A change in treatment strategies followed.

    a. Of importance was the use of methotrexate (MTX), which had been introduced in the 1980s (Weinblatt et al., 1985).

    b. There also was a tendency toward intensive and combined therapy (Boers et al., 1997). There was a growing insight into the advantages of a multidisciplinary approach as a more holistic approach in order to reduce disability and to restore function (Madigan & FitzGerald, 1999; Vliet Vlieland & Hazes, 1997).

    c. Treatment and care increasingly moved toward outpatient care.

B. Developments in rheumatology nursing.

1. Roles and tasks for rheumatology nurses became more illuminated.

    a. It became clear that nurses provided physical care combined with education and counseling as well as assessing problems and coordinating services (Pigg, 1995).

    b. The insight increased that nursing care should not only focus on managing exacerbations but also on health promotion and empowering patients toward self-management (Madigan & FitzGerald, 1999).

    c. Also support and education for family was considered an essential role of the nurse (Arthur, 1994).

    d. The aim of nursing care was defined as helping patients manage themselves (Willis, 1999) and supporting patients' ability to cope with the disease (Newbold, 1996).

2. Nurse-led care was considered increasingly important in rheumatology, but formal evaluation was needed for several reasons.

    a. There was a lack of clear definition about content of care and the role and competencies of nurses.

1
1.1
1.2
1.3
1.4
1.5
1.6
1.7
1.8
1.9

b. There was a lack of sufficient support and a large administrative burden for nurses.

3. A growing number of studies resulted in growing evidence for the role of the nurse (van Eijk-Hustings et al., 2012).

   a. Studies showed the value of nurses with regard to patient education, satisfaction with care, accessibility of care, disease monitoring, psychosocial support, and self-management support.

   b. The literature also showed that nurses can contribute to cost-effective care.

IV. Developments in this era.

A. Rheumatology.

1. There is growing insight into the nature of rheumatic diseases resulting in a new treatment paradigm.

   a. Early, intensive treatment of inflammatory arthritis (Agarwal, 2011).

   b. Treat to target (Smolen et al., 2010), including tight control (Grigor et al., 2004).

   c. Evidence that biologic therapies are beneficial, resulting in increased use in practice (Furst et al., 2004). .

2. There is an increased need for redesign of health care in the management of chronic diseases, including rheumatic diseases.

   a. In general, a proactive, patient-centered and evidence-based approach with nurses fulfilling extended roles is promoted (Laurant et al., 2004; Loveman, Royle, & Waugh, 2003).

   b. With regard to rheumatology, practice redesign should be a priority in order to improve and guarantee care delivery (Deal et al., 2007).

   c. Increasingly, patients are involved in treatment decisions (shared decision making) as full understanding and agreement enhance compliance (Joosten et al., 2008).

B. Rheumatology nursing.

1. New treatment strategies demand more and intensive nursing care.

   a. With regard to early, intensive treatment, patients increasingly need support from nurses in understanding treatment choices (Ruffing, 2007).

   b. As the use of biologics increased, rheumatology infusion nurses have become vital to safe delivery and care (Dexter, 2008).

2. The demands on knowledge and skills of nurses increase accordingly.

   a. Knowledge about disease state, clinical expertise in administration, and monitoring of adverse events is required (Dexter, 2008).

   b. Skills with regard to patient-centered support, patient education, information sharing, and coordination of care are also required (Oliver, 2011).

   c. Self-management support is crucial in order to ensure patients are capable of participating in treatment decisions, managing their own symptoms, and understanding risks of treatment (Dexter, 2008; Oliver, 2011).

3. The recognition of rheumatology nursing as a nursing specialty.

   a. The American Nursing Association (ANA) Board of Directors recognized rheumatology nursing as a nursing specialty on November 9, 2012.

   b. The ANA Board of Directors also approved the rheumatology nursing scope of practice statement provided by Rheumatology Nurses Society (RNS), and acknowledged the rheumatology nursing standards of practice for a period of five years, commencing with the publication date of *Rheumatology Nursing: Scope and Standards of Practice* (ANA & RNS, 2013).

4. Defining the scope and standards of practice for rheumatology nursing through the publishing of *Rheumatology Nursing: Scope and Standards of Practice* (ANA & RNS, 2013).

   a. To protect and preserve the healthcare consumer's right to quality care and to protect the nurse who is administrating the care.

   b. To assist in developing policy and procedures in all practices and settings involving the care of patients with a rheumatic condition.

   c. To provide a tool to orient new nurses entering the specialty and to assist the lifelong education of nurses practicing in rheumatology.

1
1.1
1.2
1.3
1.4
1.5
1.6
1.7
1.8
1.9

Summary

Rheumatology is a young field in medicine.

» In the past, treatment options with regard to medications were limited.

» In case of exacerbations, patients were hospitalized.

» Rheumatic diseases often resulted in disability.

» Care was focused on physical support.

Nurses' role in care for patients with rheumatic diseases has changed because of:

» Developments within health care (e.g., redesign).

» Professional developments (e.g., nurse practitioners; recognition of rheumatology nursing as a specialty by the American Nurses Association in 2012).

» Developments within rheumatology (e.g., complicated treatment regimens).

Evidence for the advantages of rheumatology nursing care is increasingly available.

References

Agarwal, S.K. (2011). Core management principles in rheumatoid arthritis to help guide managed care professionals. *Journal of Managed Care Pharmacy, 17*(9b), S3-S8.

American Nurses Association and Rheumatology Nurses Society. (2013). *Rheumatology nursing: Scope and standards of practice.* Silver Spring, MD: Nursesbooks.org

Arthur, V. (1994). Nursing care of patients with rheumatoid arthritis. *British Journal of Nursing, 3*(7), 325-327.

Bird, H.A., Wright, V., & Galloway, D. (1980). Clinical metrology—a future career grade? [Clinical Trial]. *Lancet, 2*(8186), 138-140.

Boers, M., Verhoeven, A.C., Markusse, H.M., van de Laar, M.A., Westhovens, R., van Denderen, J.C., ... Van der Linden, S. (1997). Randomised comparison of combined step-down prednisolone, methotrexate and sulphasalizine with sulphasalizine alone in early rheumatoid arthritis. *Lancet, 350*(9074), 309-318.

Brown-Skeers, V. (1979). How the nurse practitioner manages the rheumatoid arthritis patient. *Nursing, 9*(6), 26-35.

Carr, A. (2001). Defining the extended clinical role for allied health professionals in rheumatology. *ARC Conference Proceedings No. 12.* Chesterfield, UK: Arthritis Research Campaign.

Christman, C. (1987). Protocol for administration and management of chrysotherapy (gold therapy). *Nurse Practitioner, 12*(10), 30.

Deal, C.L., Hooker, R.S., Harrington, T.M., Birnbaum, N., Hogan, P., Bouchery, E., ... Bar, W. (2007). The United States Rheumatology Workforce. *Arthritis & Rhematism, 56*(3), 722-729.

Dexter, T.R. (2008). Role of the rheumatology infusion nurse...including discussion with A. Saleh, J.A. Dilliard, T.R. Dexter, V. Ruffing, P.M. Daul, D.G. Dolan, G.B. Neuberger, E. Grace. *Johns Hopkins Advanced Studies in Nursing, 6*(2), 39-44.

Furst, D.E., Breedveld, F.C., Kalden, J.R., Smolen, J.S., Burmester, G.R., Bijlsma, J.W., ... Mease, P.J. (2004). Updated consensus statement on biological agents, specifically tumour necrosis factor alpha (TNFalpha) blocking agents and interleukin-1 receptor antagonist (IL-1ra), for the treatment of rheumatic diseases, 2004. *Annals of Rheumatic Diseases* (Suppl. 2), ii2-ii12.

Grigor, C., Capell, H., Stirling, A., McMahon, A.D., Lock, P., Vallance, R., & Porter, D. (2004). Effect of a treatment strategy of tight control for RA (the TICORA study). A single blind randomised controlled trial. *Lancet, 363*, 263-269.

Hale, C., & Hill, J. (2006). Locating the evidence base for musculoskeletal nursing: An overview of the rheumatology nursing literature. *International Journal of Nursing Studies, 43*, 507-518.

Hill, J. (1985). Nursing clinics for arthritis. *Nursing Times, 81*(38), 33-34.

Hill, J. (1986). Patient evaluation of a rheumatology nursing clinic. *Nursing Times, 82*(27), 42-43.

Hill, J. (2005). Development and effectiveness of nurse-led arthritis clinics. [Review]. *Drug Benefit Trends, 17*(6), 262-270.

1
1.1
1.2
1.3
1.4
1.5
1.6
1.7
1.8
1.9

References (continued)

Hill, J. (2006). *Rheumatology nursing: A creative approach.* London: Whurr Publishers Ltd.

Hooker, R.S. (2008). The extension of rheumatology services with physician assistants and nurse practitioners. [Review]. *Best Practice & Research. Clinical Rheumatology, 22*(3), 523-533.

Hosking, S. (1984). Rheumatoid arthritis—fundamental nursing care. *Nursing, 2*(31), 900-901.

Jacox, R.F., Morgan, E.S., Vaughn, J.H., Atwater, E.C., Meyerowitz, S., & Duthie. R.B. (1963). An interdisciplinary approach to the care of patients with rheumatoid arthritis. *New York State Journal of Medicine, 1,* 1639-1651.

Joosten, E.A., DeFuentes-Merillas, L., de Weert, G.H., Sensky, T., van der Staak, C.P., & de Jong, C.A. (2008). Systematic review of the effects of shared decision-making on patient satisfaction, treatment adherence and health status. *Psychotherapy and Psychosomatics, 77*(4), 219-226.

Laurant, M., Reeves, D., Hermens, R., Braspenning, J., Grol, R., & Sibbald, B. (2004). Substitution of doctors by nurses in primary care. *Cochrane Database of Systematic Review, 4*(Art. No.: CD001271). doi: 10.1002/14651858.CD001271.pub 2

Loveman, E., Royle, P., & Waugh, N. (2003). Specialist nurses in diabetes mellitus. *Cochrane Database of Systematic Review, 2*(Art No.: CD003286). doi: 10.1002/14651858.CD003286.

Madigan, A., & FitzGerald, O. (1999). Multidisciplinary patient care in rheumatoid arthritis: Evolving concepts in nursing practice. [Review]. *Baillieres Best Practice & Research in Clinical Rheumatology, 13*(4), 661-674.

Maltbee, K. n.d. The History of Rheumatology. Retrieved from http://www.ehow.com/about_5401639_history-rheumatology.html

Miale, J.E., & Plotz, C.M. (1953). Nursing care of patients with rheumatoid arthritis during therapy with cortisone. *American Journal of Nursing, 53*(3), 290-293.

Newbold, D. (1996). Coping with rheumatoid arthritis. How can specialist nurses influence it and promote better outcomes? [Review]. *Journal of Clinical Nursing, 5*(6), 373-380.

Oliver, S. (2011). The role of the clinical nurse specialist in the assessment and management of biologic therapies. *Musculoskeletal Care, 9*(1), 54-62.

Peasnell, I.M. (1984). Maintaining mobility and independence. *Nursing, 2*(31), 919-920.

Pigg, J.S. (1990). Rheumatology nursing: Evolution of the role and functions of a subspecialty. [Editorial]. *Arthritis Care and Research, 3*(3), 109-115.

Pigg, J.S. (1995). Rheumatoid arthritis: How allied health professionals can help. *Journal of Musculoskeletal Medicine, 12*(2), 27.

Rhodes, H. (1977). Community nursing care study: Rheumatoid arthritis. [Case reports]. *Nursing Times, 73*(42), 1624-1626.

Ruffing, V. (2007). Pharmacologic management of patients with rheumatoid arthritis. [Review]. *Johns Hopkins Advanced Studies in Nursing, 5*(1), 15-22.

Smolen, J., Aletaha, D., Bijlsma, J., Breedveld, F., Boumpas, D., Burmester, G., ... van der Heijde, D. (2010). Treating rheumatoid arthritis to target: Recommendations of an international task force. *Annals of the Rheumatic Diseases, 69,* 631-637.

van Eijk-Hustings, Y., van Tubergen, A., Bostrom, C., Braychenko, E., Buss, B., Felix, J., ... Hill, J. (2012). EULAR recommendations for the role of the nurse in the management of chronic inflammatory arthritis. *Annals of the Rheumatic Diseases, 7*(1), 13-19.

Vliet Vlieland, T.P.M., & Hazes, J.M.W. (1997). Efficacy of multidisciplinary team care programs in rheumatoid arthritis. *Seminars in Arthritis and Rheumatism, 27*(2), 110-122.

Weinblatt, M.E., Coblyn, J.S., Fox, D.A., Fraser, P.A., Holdsworth, D.E., Glass, D.N., & Trentham, D.E., (1985). Efficacy of low-dose methotrexate (MTX) in rheumatoid arthritis. *New England Journal of Medicine, 312*(13), 818-822.

Willis, J. (1999). Joint initiative...how an award-winning rheumatology nurse gets patients involved in treatment. *Nursing Times, 95*(23), 34-35.

Wright, V. (1977). Rheumatoid arthritis-2. Nursing care of the patient at home and in hospital. *Nursing Times, 73*(47), 1832-1835.

1
1.1
1.2
1.3
1.4
1.5
1.6
1.7
1.8
1.9

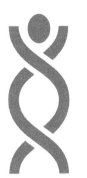

Section 1.2
Global Roles of the Rheumatology Nurse

Jenny de la Torre Aboki, RN, BSc, MSc, PGdipRheum

Introduction

This chapter focuses on the role of basic to advanced practice rheumatology nurses, taking into account the different settings in which rheumatology nurses provide care for patients with a variety of rheumatic conditions.

Dramatic changes have occurred over the past 50 years in rheumatology practice and management (Brady, 2006).

In the 1960s, the rehabilitation approach to rheumatoid arthritis was an emphasis on controlled rest (both general and local joint rest with careful positioning to avoid joint deformity) and careful exercise (specified as 5-10 minutes of bed exercise increasing to 30 minutes once or twice a day). Admission to the hospital for bed rest was recommended, and weight bearing was not permitted until the patient could do so without pain (Harris, 1968).

This point of view differs substantially from "tight control" management for rheumatic diseases. Tight control means follow-up examinations (every 3 months) and appropriate change in therapy after a maximum of 3 to 6 months in patients who do not achieve low disease activity or remission (Smolen & Aletaha, 2009). Moreover, tight control is guided by a "treat-to-target" (T2T) strategy. Treating to target is an established concept in the management of diabetes, hypertension, and hyperlipidemia. This approach embodies setting measurable targets, formulating evidence-based recommendations for assessment criteria, and adjusting drug therapy in accordance with these targets. So then, tight control leads not only to improved outcomes but also to longer survival (Firth, 2012). Recommendations for achieving optimal therapeutic outcomes in inflammatory arthritis are very common; these recommendations have recently been developed for rheumatoid arthritis as well (Smolen et al., 2010).

Rheumatology nursing has been evolving over many years, but because of the absence of a formal group or network through which nurses working with patients with rheumatic conditions could share and increase their knowledge and skills, its progress remained unappreciated until the early 1980s (Ryan & Hill, 2006).

During the 1970s and 1980s in some countries, such as in the United Kingdom, mainland Europe, Australia, and the United States, a major development was the expansion in nurse specialist and advanced practice nurse roles and the advent of the consultant nurse role. As early as 1974, however, nurses were assuming specialized roles, such as taking clinical measurements during drug trials. These responsibilities evolved into operating drug-monitoring clinics and, eventually, supervising the day-to-day management of patients with rheumatic diseases (Ryan & Hill, 2006).

Yet there is a lack of clarity about what skills make up the role of the rheumatology nurse. According to Pigg (1990), "the contribution of rheumatology nursing to the care of rheumatic disease patients has not been well understood

Learning Objectives

Upon completion of this chapter, the nurse will be able to:

1. Outline the roles experienced globally of the rheumatology nurse.
2. Discuss the potential barriers to rheumatology nurses' practice.

1
1.1
1.2
1.3
1.4
1.5
1.6
1.7
1.8
1.9

or clearly defined" (p. 114). Evidence is needed to outline which aspects of the role are essential to provide in different care settings.

Although Florence Nightingale defined nursing initially, the most cited definition of nursing is that of Henderson (1966) who stated that "the unique function of the nurse is to assist the individual sick or well in the performance of those activities contributing to health or its recovery (or to a peaceful death) that he would perform unaided if he had the necessary strength, will or knowledge, and to do this in such a way as to help him gain independence as rapidly as possible" (p. 15).

Henderson's definition contains the elements relevant to today's health care with its emphasis on empowerment, rehabilitation, education, and self-management, in addition to mentioning the evolution from a task-oriented to an inter-collaborative approach.

The International Council of Nurses (ICN) (1987) based its definition of nursing on Henderson's and expanded the definition by stressing the management role of the nurse. In 2002, ICN published a shortened version of the definition of nursing: "Nursing encompasses autonomous and collaborative care of individuals of all ages, families, groups, and communities, sick or well, and in all settings. Nursing includes the promotion of health, prevention of illness, and the care of ill, disabled, and dying people. Advocacy, promotion of a safe environment, research, participation in shaping health policy and in patient and health systems management and education are also key nursing roles" (2002).

The American Nurses Association (2008) defined nursing as "the protection, promotion, and optimization of health and abilities, prevention of illness and injury, alleviation of suffering through the diagnosis and treatment of human response, and advocacy in the care of individuals, families, communities, and populations" (American Nurses Association [ANA] 2008).

The rheumatology nurse's roles have developed at different rates and stages throughout the world. Perhaps because of its very ubiquitousness, the role of nursing in rheumatology has not been well documented (Ryan & Hill, 2006). In those countries in which the rheumatology nursing specialty does not exist, nurses practice as general nurses and might care for patients with rheumatic conditions in different settings during their careers. In addition, lack of public recognition of the nature of nurses' knowledge causes nurses' clinical learning to be neglected in some local practice settings (Benner, 1981).

In those countries in which rheumatology nursing is recognized, such as in the United States, where rheumatology nursing was recognized as a specialty area of practice by the ANA in 2012, most rheumatology nurses work in a collaborative manner and are included in interdisciplinary healthcare teams.

It has been widely acknowledged that an interdisciplinary approach is required to provide effective care for the diverse needs of patients with chronic rheumatic conditions. Over the past decade, there has been an expansion in the number and roles and responsibilities of nurses and allied health professionals working in rheumatology (Royal College of Nursing, 2009). For instance, in rheumatology nursing, the monitoring of patients taking disease-modifying antirheumatic drugs (DMARDs) has been common since the 1970s; currently the nurse's role in the monitoring of patients on biologic therapies is quite usual in daily practice.

Patients with rheumatic diseases face a plethora of problems such as physical, psychological, social, and/or family related so that members of a single profession cannot fully help the patient cope (Hill & Reay, 2002). The rheumatology community has accepted that inter-professional collaboration (Schmitt, Blue, Aschenbrener & Viggiano, 2011), meaning healthcare professionals working in a coordinated manner, can provide a better outcome for the patient (Davis, Wagner, & Groves, 2000). Although each member of the interdisciplinary team has a specific role and responsibilities, those roles and boundaries can overlap. To work successfully in an interdisciplinary team, members have to be aware of each other's role and how they can act and collaborate in a complementary manner, considering the term "collaboration" as working with others in a way that promotes/encourages each person's contributions toward achieving optimal/realistic patient/family goals. This involves intra- and interdisciplinary work with colleagues and community; in equal measure, all members of the team have to respect, cultivate, and promote professional autonomy and recognize when it is appropriate to refer issues and concerns to other team members. Communication between members of the team and the patient is vitally important. Making the interdisciplinary team work is associated with joint decision making, adaptation of care to the patient's needs, and changes in allocation of tasks between professionals. This approach can improve the quality of patient care and result in a reduced hospital stay for patients (Zwarenstein & Bryant, 2003). Nurses play a pivotal role in the interdisciplinary team that includes 1) acting as the patient's advocate; 2) ensuring individualized plans of care reflect the patient's goals; 3) coordinating the work of the team; and 4) serving as liaison with other disciplines (Fitzgerald, 2006), among others such as evaluating the patient's condition and making appropriate referrals and communicating effectively with the patient and family.

Nursing care reflects an integration of knowledge, skills, experience, attitudes, and expertise needed to meet the needs of patients and families. Thus, characteristics of a nurse's role are derived from patients' needs (Hardin & Kaplow, 2004). The nursing role consists of a combination of skills including caring, helping, supporting, teaching, comforting, and guiding.

Caring is one of the most important values of the nursing profession. Although caring often is referred to as a basic requirement of nursing practice, there is nothing basic about high quality nursing care.

Nursing care includes direct clinical practice, defined as direct interaction with patients, families, and groups of patients to promote health or well-being and improve quality of life. Direct clinical practice is characterized by a holistic perspective in the advanced nursing management of health, illness, and disease states (Tracy, 2008). Indirect clinical practice includes the provision of care through activities that influence the care of patients but do not involve direct engagement with patients. Examples include not only administrative activities such as dealing with insurance matters, effective communication with health services in the patient's community, and assessment of the need for and procurement of technical devices but also developing evidence-based guidelines or protocols for care, participating in clinical trials, conducting research, and planning, implementing, and evaluating staff development activities (Tracy, 2008).

Therefore, caring practices are nursing activities that create a compassionate, supportive, and therapeutic environment for patients and staff, with the aim of promoting comfort and healing and preventing unnecessary suffering, which includes, but is not limited to, vigilance, engagement, and responsiveness of caregivers to patients, family, and other healthcare personnel (Hardin & Kaplow, 2004).

Advanced nursing care is the application of an expanded range of practical ("knowing how") and theoretical ("knowing that") knowledge (Benner, 1981) and research-based competencies to phenomena experienced by patients within a specialized clinical area of the larger discipline of nursing (Hamric, 2008).

An advanced practice nurse has been defined as "a registered nurse who has command of an expert knowledge base and clinical competence; is able to make complex decisions using expert clinical judgement; is an essential member of an interdependent health care team and whose role is determined by the context in which s/he practices" (Nursing and Midwifery Council, 2004, p. 8).

The challenge exists to relate this definition and the competencies (considering that "competency" is an expected level of performance that integrates knowledge, skills, abilities, and judgment [American Nurses Association, 2008]) for advanced nursing practice (Nursing and Midwifery Council, 2006) into specific nursing specialties such as rheumatology nursing.

Rheumatology nurse specialists can provide education in self-management skills and in communication to patients with rheumatic conditions, provide counseling

to enhance empowerment of patients with rheumatic conditions, and enable these patients to gain rapid access to review, if needed, thus, improving the quality and continuity of care (Voyce, 1999). Nurse-led clinics are a feature of many rheumatology units and are essential for reviewing and monitoring medication efficacy and safety, controlling physical symptoms, referring patients with rheumatic conditions to the appropriate members of the interdisciplinary team, and often performing procedures such as joint injection or initiation of new medication therapies (Hehir et al., 2008). Some of these roles might be considered as extended or expanded roles. Some discussions have been reported about the different meanings of the terms "extended" and "expanded." In addition, discussion has been reported about why nurses have to undertake these roles (Hunt & Wainwright, 1994).

Hunt and Wainwright (1994) stated that there are ways the increasing responsibilities of nurses could have been recognized. One way was growth by mechanical addition of parts (extension); the other way was an organic growth of the whole (expansion). These authors describe "extension" as mechanistic; other terms used in connection with "extension" include "task-based" and "physician substitute." For instance, "Extending practice...is seen to be a task oriented activity undertaken for the convenience of other professionals and at their discretion" (Tye & Ross, 2000, p. 1091).

Terms used in "expansion" such as "an enlargement of scale or scope, or an increase in area of control" (Hunt & Wainwright, 1994, p. 14) also apply to nursing. However, if nurses continue to accept additional roles that are more focused on enabling management to comply with directives or meet targets rather than enhancing the care of patients, then that expansion may result in damage to individual nurses through "burnout" and, ultimately, may damage the profession and the patients for whom the nurses care (Read, 2011).

Role expansion is about nurses taking initiative, doing their own thinking, and making decisions based on their experience and education to improve practice for the benefit of patients and their families. The real test of the development of nursing as a profession will be the extent to which nurses do not just take on responsibility for additional tasks but the extent to which they achieve authority over the nature of their practice. Over the last 10-15 years, a plethora of articles has been published (Bernhaut & Mackay, 2002; Cox & Farmer, 2003; Jones, 2003; Munro, 2002; Nielsen, 2003; Parish, 2003) that described these and other issues related to the role of advanced practice nurses.

The term "role expansion" and "role development" are, however, acceptable and are often used interchangeably, frequently in the context of advanced nursing practice. "Advanced practice is seen by some to center on the

1
1.1
1.2
1.3
1.4
1.5
1.6
1.7
1.8
1.9

1
1.1
1.2
1.3
1.4
1.5
1.6
1.7
1.8
1.9

core therapeutic nursing role of nurturing and caring and is focused on the delivery of holistic patient care," according to Frost (1998, p. 59), or a movement toward "nurse-led care."

Read and Graves (1994) concluded that "When nursing knowledge and experience continuously informs a practitioner's decision making, even though some parts of her or his role may overlap the medical role, then that may be said to be advanced nursing practice. Conversely, when a nurse is expected to perform routine technical tasks with no opportunity to exercise nursing knowledge or make autonomous decisions, then that is when a nurse becomes an assistant to the physician" (p. 26). There is a difference between a nurse's carrying out a succession of technical tasks on a whole list of patients, and an individual nurse carrying out the specific technical tasks for those patients to whom the nurse is assigned based on those patients' needs. The former could be described as "an extended role" or serving as an assistant to a physician; the latter may be advanced practice and be classified as role development which includes expansion.

The term "role development" covers a range of meaning. The most easily understood and identified are discrete roles such as those for nurse practitioners (NPs) and clinical nurse specialists (CNSs). The creation of such roles is sometimes part of a movement toward "nurse-led care."

Over the years, a number of descriptive articles have been published that outline the care rheumatology nurses provide (Cornell, 2007; Oliver & Mooney, 2002; Ryan, 1996; Ryan & Oliver, 2002).

Throughout Europe nurse-led clinics are usually the domain of clinical nurse specialists, and these nurses normally practice in rheumatology outpatient clinics alongside their medical colleagues. In these settings, rheumatology CNSs use their knowledge and communication skills to take a holistic approach to provide care to patients with rheumatic conditions. Authentic engagement is referred to as a relationship between nurse and patient that is characterized by genuineness, honesty, trust, and being fully present (Parse, 1988). Coaching, meaning skillful guidance, and teaching to advance the care of patients, families, groups of patients, and the profession of nursing (Hamric, Spross, & Hanson, 2008) are essential characteristics in nurse-led clinics.

Nurse-led clinics exist in a number of areas: Multidisciplinary care shared medical appointment (Watts et al., 2009), nurse-led care related to acute pain services (Layzell, 2005, 2009), nurse-led care related to chronic pain services (Courtenay & Carey, 2008), breast care (Kimman et al., 2011), anticoagulation clinics (Brown et al., 1998), tissue viability (Flanagan, 1998), dysphagia (Werner, 2005), and surgical pre-admission clinics (Newton, 1996; Whiteley, Wilmott & Offland, 1997).

Significant issues commonly highlighted are the nurse's focus on patient education and providing psychological support. Moreover, improvements are often seen in administrative efficiency such as measured for nurses in pre-admission clinics by reduced number of last minute cancellations for surgery leading to significant cost savings. Reduction in patients' waiting times is another benefit, particularly in minor injury units and outpatient clinic settings, leading to improved patient satisfaction. Nurse-led care of the elderly in a day hospital was demonstrated in a small study by Booth and Waters (1995), who focused on the nurse's central coordinating role. Edwards et al., (2001) demonstrated that when patients are cared for on specialist rheumatology units they report increased confidence in nurses' ability and knowledge, while patients cared for on non-specialist units reported a lack of understanding regarding their arthritis. Although some studies have been performed to document outcomes of nurse-led care of patients with rheumatic conditions, much more research is needed in this area.

It was not until the 1980s that rheumatology nurse-led clinics began to emerge in Europe. The first clinics began when nurses working on clinical drug trials in Leeds began taking on responsibility for more patient-centered care (Bird, Wright, & Galloway, 1980). These nurses monitored disease progress and provided education and support to patients and their families. Once the clinical trial was completed, normal practice was for the nurse to return the patient to the medical clinics. However, many of these patients began to request referrals for nursing consultations because they appreciated the supportive, educational approach provided by these nurses. In 1981, the first publication about nurse-led rheumatology clinics in the United Kingdom appeared (Bird, 1983; Bird, Leathum, & LeGallez, 1981; Hill, 1986), followed by the first descriptive research on patients' evaluations of the care they received from nurses (Hill, 1986). During the following two decades, nurse-led care in all specialities, including rheumatology, has grown exponentially. Indeed, sub-specialization nurse-led clinics have been started (e.g., lupus nurse-led clinic, biologics nurse-led clinic, scleroderma nurse-led clinic). There are a number of reasons for this and they include 1) an ever-increasing outpatient workload; 2) reduction in the working hours of junior hospital physicians; 3) pressure from government; 4) and the willingness of nurses to innovate and advance their practice (Ryan & Hill, 2006).

Research has also begun to emerge demonstrating the efficacy of care from nurse-led clinics and finding nurses' extended roles to be safe and effective (Hill, 1986; Hill et al., 1994; Hill, Thorpe, & Bird, 2003; Ryan, Hassell, Lewis, & Farrell, 2006); some of these results have been replicated in mainland Europe (Temmink et al., 2001; Tijhuis et al., 2002). As roles evolve, research is slowly progressing, although much work remains to be done. For instance,

1
1.1
1.2
1.3
1.4
1.5
1.6
1.7
1.8
1.9

the efficacy of the consultant nurse in rheumatology has yet to be evaluated, as has the role of the biologics nurse specialist (Oliver, 2011).

In Europe, the most advanced clinical role to be achieved is the nurse consultant. This role provides the nurse with the opportunity to define and expand the career pathway, while allowing the experienced nurse to remain in clinical care settings. Nurse consultant roles have defined criteria: 1) expert practice; 2) professional leadership and consultancy; 3) education, training, and development; and 4) research. The only component that has a stated time allocation is that of expert practice, where it is specified that 50% of time must involve clinical care. The distribution of time spent on the other role functions is determined by the needs of the local population, the knowledge and skills of the individual nurse, and the environment in which the nurse consultant practices. One of the entry criteria for these posts is a master's-level preparation; this was the first time in Europe that a nursing role has been equated with an academic level.

Regional differences in nurse roles can be instructive; for example, a defined career pathway and nurse-led-clinics are being established in the United Kingdom, mainland Europe, Australia, and the United States, but are not being established in other countries, showing that there is a great gap in clinical and legal practice within rheumatology nursing as well as many areas where research is needed.

Content Outline

In an effort to emphasize the role of the rheumatology nurse throughout Europe, the first recommendations by the European League Against Rheumatism (EULAR) for the role of the nurse in the management of chronic inflammatory arthritis were recently published (van Eijk-Hustings et al., 2012). Based on a review of the literature involving 54 studies, 10 recommendations were formulated (see Table 1).

As also reflected in the EULAR recommendations, the roles of rheumatology nurses can be summed up in the following five domains:

I. The teaching/coaching function.

A. Applies principles of evidence-based practice and quality improvement to all patient care.

B. Provides ongoing education.

C. Designs health information and patient education appropriate to the patient's developmental level, health literacy level, learning needs, readiness to learn, and cultural values and beliefs.

Table 1

EULAR Recommendations for the Role of the Nurse in the Management of Chronic Inflammatory Arthritis (IA)

Patients should have access to nurses:

» For education to improve knowledge of IA and its management throughout the course of their disease.

» For improved communication, continuity, and satisfaction with their care.

» For nurse-led telephone services to provide ongoing support.

Nurses should:

» Participate in comprehensive disease management to control disease activity, reduce symptoms, and improve patient outcomes.

» Identity, access, and address psychosocial issues to minimize patients' anxiety and depression.

» Promote self-management skills so patients experience a greater sense of control, self-efficacy, and empowerment.

» Provide care based on protocols and guidelines according to national and local contexts.

» Have access to and participate in continuing education to maintain knowledge and skills.

» Assume extended roles after specialized education and according to national regulations.

» Implement interventions and monitoring as part of comprehensive disease management in order to achieve cost-effectiveness.

Adapted from: van Eijk-Hustings, Y., van Tubergen, A., Böström, C., Braychenko, E., Buss, B., Felix, J., Firth, J., . . . Hill, J. (2012). EULAR recommendations for the role of the nurse in the management of chronic inflammatory arthritis. *Annals of the Rheumatic Diseases, 71*(1), 13-19.

1
1.1
1.2
1.3
1.4
1.5
1.6
1.7
1.8
1.9

D. Assesses system barriers and facilitators to adoption of evidence-based practices.

E. Participates in pre-professional, graduate, and continuing education of nurses and other healthcare providers:

1. Completes a needs assessment as appropriate to guide interventions with staff.

2. Promotes professional development of staff nurses and continuing education activities.

3. Implements professional development and continuing education activities.

4. Mentors nurses to translate education into practice.

II. The patient-monitoring function.

A. Conducts comprehensive, holistic, wellness, and illness assessments using known or innovative evidence-based techniques, tools (Visual Analogue Scales [Wewers & Lowe, 1990]; Disease Activity Score in 28 joints [http://www.das-score.nl/das28/en/]), and direct and indirect methods.

1. Administers soft tissue or intra-articular joint injections.

B. Implements patient-focused plan to address problems identified. Provides direct care to selected patients based on the needs of patient and the nurse's specialty knowledge and skills.

C. Reduces the need for emergency admissions.

D. Provides additional support through a telephone advice line service.

E. Participates in musculoskeletal ultrasonography assessment.

III. Administering and monitoring therapeutic interventions and regimens.

A. Prescribes nursing therapeutics, pharmacologic and non-pharmacologic interventions, diagnostic measures, equipment, procedures, and treatments to meet the needs of patients, families, and groups, in accordance with professional preparation, institutional privileges, and local laws.

B. Monitors medication efficacy and side effects.

C. Supports patients with changes in treatment and offers advice.

D. Facilitates patient's and family's understanding of the risks, benefits, and outcomes of proposed healthcare regimens to promote informed decision making.

IV. Organizational and management roles.

A. Provides consultation to staff nurses, medical staff, and interdisciplinary colleagues.

1. Consultation: Patient, staff, or system-focused interaction between professionals in which the consultant is recognized as having specialized expertise and assists consultee with problem solving (Hamric, 2008).

B. Initiates consultation to obtain resources as necessary to facilitate progress toward achieving identified outcomes.

C. Provides leadership in promoting interdisciplinary collaboration to implement outcomes-focused patient care programs meeting the clinical needs of patients, families, population, and communities.

D. Leads system change to improve health outcomes through evidence-based practice.

E. Considers fiscal and budgetary implications in decision making regarding practice and system modifications:

1. Evaluates use of products and services for appropriateness and cost/benefit in meeting care needs.

2. Conducts cost/benefit analysis of new clinical technologies.

3. Evaluates effect of introduction or withdrawal of products, services, and technologies.

F. Provides leadership for establishing, improving, and sustaining collaborative relationships to meet clinical needs.

G. Establishes collaborative relationship within and across departments that promote patient safety, competent care, and clinical excellence.

H. Works with other healthcare professionals, including primary healthcare teams.

I. Engages in a formal self-evaluation process, seeking feedback regarding own practice, from patients, peers, professional colleagues, and others.

V. The research role.

A. Participates in conduct of or implementation of research projects, development of guidelines and protocols.

B. Adheres to Food and Drug Administration regulations, protection of human subjects.

Summary

It is essential that the role of the rheumatology nurse remain firmly rooted in patient needs and education. Unless this happens, there is a danger that rheumatology nurses could be viewed as "mini-physicians" or medical assistants instead of being at the forefront of developing the specialty and the nursing profession in the interest of the patients to whom they provide care (Read, 2011). The nursing profession needs to be about what constitutes nursing and the necessity for both a physical and emotional element in nursing practice.

Rheumatology nursing roles vary across countries from a registered nurse in clinical practice to nurse consultant introduced in England in 1998 (Department of Health, 1999).

Since 2001, there have been significant changes in rheumatology treatment strategies and health policy. The emphasis is now on managing long-term rheumatic conditions based on the treat-to-target strategies and enhancing patient empowerment and self-management. There have also been significant challenges in demonstrating the cost effectiveness of nurse activity. There are limited data available on basic issues such as number of patients seen, length of appointments, activity related to enhancing self-management, and reducing the need for additional healthcare resources. Questions remain about how to define activities, roles, and responsibilities and the prerequisite qualifications for rheumatology nurses. This is a particular problem when there are many different nursing titles used in different care settings and countries.

Nurses experience barriers to performing extended roles, so the use of innovative models of care may be limited. The main barriers include legal constraints; the attitudes of rheumatologists, patients, and, in some cases, nurses themselves because of a lack of confidence and career development; knowledge; and educational opportunities. The potential use of innovative models of care may depend on the professional and educational status of non-physician healthcare professionals in a certain country. Innovative models of care include multi/interdisciplinary teams in which all healthcare professionals participating have equal professional status, so that either a physician or a non-physician can be the team leader, compared with traditional settings, in which physicians always are team leaders (Stamm & Hill., 2011).

Although the risk of early specialization could limit the nurses' career flexibility (Benner, 1981), in the most distressed economic and staffing times, the need for maintaining a vision of excellent nursing practice is greater.

Evidence is needed to outline which aspects of the role of rheumatology nurses are essential to provide in different care settings.

References

American Nurses Association. (2008). *Professional role competence.* Retrieved from http://nursingworld.org/especiallyforyou/studentnurses.aspx

Benner, P.E. (1981). *From novice to expert: Excellence and power in clinical nursing practice.* Menlo Park, CA: Addison Wesley.

Bernhaut, J., & Mackay, K. (2002). Extended nursing roles in intermediate care: A cost benefit evaluation. *Nursing Times, 98*(21), 37-39.

Bird, H.A. (1983). Divided rheumatology care: The advent of the nurse practitioner? *Annals of the Rheumatic Diseases, 42*, 354-355.

Bird, H.A., Leatham, P., & Le Gallez, P. (1981). Clinical metrology. *Nursing Times, 77*, 1926-1927.

Bird, H.A., Wright, V., & Galloway, D. (1980). Clinical metrology – future career grade? *Lancet, 2*, 138-140.

Booth, J., & Waters, K. (1995). The multifaceted role of the nurse in the day hospital. *Journal of Advanced Nursing, 22*, 700-706.

1
1.1
1.2
1.3
1.4
1.5
1.6
1.7
1.8
1.9

References (continued)

Brady, T. (2006). Forty years of advances in the rheumatology health professions. In S.J. Bartlett (Ed.), *Clinical care in the rheumatic diseases* (3rd ed., pp. 1-3). Atlanta: Association of Rheumatology Health Professionals.

Brown, R., Taylor, F.C., Cohen, H., Ramsey, M., Miller, D.L., & Gaminar, L. (1998). Setting up a nurse-led anticoagulant clinic. *Professional Nurse, 14*(1), 21-23.

Cornell, P. (2007). Management of patients with rheumatoid arthritis. *Nursing Standard, 22*(4), 51-57.

Courtenay, M., & Carey, N. (2008). The impact and effectiveness of nurse-led care in the management of acute and chronic pain: A review of the literature. *Journal of Clinical Nursing, 17*(15), 2001-2013.

Cox, C., & Farmer, B. (2003). *Nursing Times* debate: Can nurse practitioners replace junior doctors? *Nursing Times, 99*(3), 18-19.

Davis, R.M., Wagner, E.G., & Groves, T. (2000). Advances in managing chronic disease. Research, performance measurement, and quality improvement are key. *British Medical Journal, 302*, 525-526.

Department of Health. (1999). Nurse, midwives and health visitor consultants: Establishing posts and making appointments. *Health Service Circular 1999/217.* London: Author.

Edwards, J., Mulherin, D., Ryan, S., & Jester, R. (2001). The experience of patients with rheumatoid arthritis admitted to hospital. *Arthritis Care & Research, 45*, 1-7.

Firth, J. (2012). Treating to target in rheumatoid arthritis. *Nurse Prescribing, 10*(6), 293-302.

Fitzgerald, P. (2006). Multidisciplinary team care of the rheumatic patient. In J. Hill (Ed.), *Rheumatology nursing: A creative approach* (2nd ed., pp. 312-335). London: Whurr Publishers.

Flanagan, M., (1998). The impact of change on the tissue viability nurse specialist. *British Journal of Nursing, 7*(11), 648-657.

Frost, S. (1998). Perspective on advanced practice: An educationalist's view. In G. Rolfe & P. Fulbrook (Eds.), *Advanced nursing practice* (pp. 53-77). Oxford: Butterworth and Heinemann.

Hamric, A.B. (2008). A definition of advanced nursing practice. In A.B. Hamric, J.A. Spros, & C.M. Hanson (Eds.), *Advanced practice nursing: An integrative approach* (pp. 85-108) St. Louis, MO: Saunders Elsevier.

Hamric, A.B., Spross, J.A., & Hanson, C.M. (Eds.) (2008). *Advanced practice nursing: An integrative approach* (4th Edition). St. Louis, MO: Saunders Elsevier.

Hardin, S., & Kaplow, R. (2004). *Synergy for clinical excellence: The AACN synergy model for patient care.* Aliso Viejo, CA: American Association of Critical Care Nurses.

Harris, R. (1968). Physical methods in the management of rheumatoid arthritis. *Medical Clinics of North America, 52*, 707-716.

Hehir, M., Carr, M., Davis B., Radford, S., Robertson, L., Tipler, S., & Hewlett, S. (2008). Nursing support at the onset of rheumatoid arthritis: Time and space for emotions, practicalities and self-management. *Musculoskeletal Care, 6*(2), 124-134.

Henderson, V. (1966). *The nature of nursing.* London: Collier-MacMillan.

Hill, J. (1986). Patient evaluation of a rheumatology nursing clinic. *Nursing Times, 82*, 42-43.

Hill, J., Bird, H., Harmer, R., Wright, V., & Lawton, C. (1994). An evaluation of the effectiveness, safety and acceptability of a nurse practitioner in a rheumatology outpatient clinic. *British Journal of Rheumatology, 33*, 283-288.

Hill, J., & Reay, N. (2002). The diagnosis, assessment and management of complex rheumatic diseases. *Nursing Times, 98*(9), 41-44.

Hill, J., Thorpe, R., & Bird, H. (2003). Outcomes for patients with RA – A rheumatology nurse practitioner clinic compared to standard outpatient care. *Musculoskeletal Care, 1*(1), 5-20.

Hunt, G., & Wainwright, P. (Eds.). (1994). *Expanding the role of the nurse.* Oxford: Blackwell.

International Council of Nurses. (1987). *The ICN definition of nursing.* Retrieved from http://www.icn.ch/about-icn/icn-definition-of-nursing/

International Council of Nurses. (2002). *The ICN definition of nursing.* Retrieved from http://www.icn.ch/about-icn/icn-definition-of-nursing/

Jones, A.M. (2003). Changes in practice at the nurse/doctor interface. *Journal of Clinical Nursing, 12*(1), 124-131.

Kimman, M.L., Dirksen, C.D., Voogd, A.C., Falger, P., Gijsen, B.C., Thuring, M., Lenssen, A., . . . Boersma, L.J. (2011). Economic evaluation of four follow-up strategies after curative treatment for breast cancer: Results of an RCT. *European Journal of Cancer, 47*(8), 1175-1185.

Layzell, M. (2005). Improving the management of postoperative pain. *Nursing Times, 101*(26), 34-36.

Layzell, M. (2009). A nurse-led service for pre-operative pain management in hip fracture. *Nursing Times, 105*(3), 16-18.

1
1.1
1.2
1.3
1.4
1.5
1.6
1.7
1.8
1.9

Munro, R. (2002). Crossing the pain threshold. *Nursing Times, 98*(21), 12-13.

Newton, V. (1996). Care in pre-admission clinics. *Nursing Times, 92*(1), 27-28.

Nielsen, L. (2003). A cost benefit analysis of training nurses for extended roles. *Nursing Times, 99*(28), 34-37.

Nursing and Midwifery Council. (2004). *Consultation on a framework of the standard for post-registration nursing.* London: Author.

Nursing and Midwifery Council. (2006). *Mapping of NMC competencies against KSF.* London: Author.

Oliver, S.M. (2011). The role of the clinical nurse specialist in the assessment and management of biologic therapies. *Musculoskeletal Care, 9,* 54-62.

Oliver, S., & Mooney, J. (2002). Targeted therapies for patients with rheumatoid arthritis. *Professional Nurse, 17 (12),* 716-720.

Parish, C. (2003). The future is bright. *Nursing Standard, 17*(41), 17-19.

Parse, R.R. (1988). Caring from a human science perspective. In M.M. Leininger (Ed.), *Caring: An essential human need* (pp. 129-132). Detroit, MI: Wayne State University Press.

Pigg, J.S. (1990). Rheumatology nursing: Evolution of a role and function of a subspecialty. *Arthritis Care & Research, 3,* 109-115.

Read, S.M., & Graves, K. (1994). *Reduction of junior doctors' hours in Trent region: The nursing contribution.* Sheffield: Trent Regional Health Authority.

Read, S. (2011, April 6). *New nursing roles: Deciding the future for Scotland.* Speech for the Scottish Government. Edinburgh.

Royal College of Nursing. (2009). *Rheumatology nursing: Results of a survey exploring the performance and activity of rheumatology nurses.* London: Author.

Ryan, S. (1996). Defining the role of the specialist nurse. *Nursing Standard, 10,* 27-29.

Ryan, S., & Oliver, S. (2002). Rheumatoid arthritis. *Nursing Standard, 16*(20), 45-52.

Ryan, S., Hassell, A.B., Lewis, M., & Farrell, A. (2006). Impact of a rheumatology expert nurse on the wellbeing of patients attending a drug monitoring clinic. *Journal of Advanced Nursing, 53,* 277-286.

Ryan, S., & Hill, J. (2006). The principles, practice and evolution of rheumatology nursing. In J. Hill (Ed.), *Rheumatology nursing: A creative approach* (2nd ed., pp. 3-24). London: Whurr Publishers.

Schmitt, M., Blue, A., Aschenbrener, C.A., & Viggiano, T.R. (2011). Core competencies for interprofessional collaborative practice: Reforming health care by transforming health professionals' education. *Academic Medicine, 86*(11), 1351.

Smolen, J.S., & Aletaha, D. (2009). Developments in the clinical understanding of rheumatoid arthritis. *Arthritis Research and Therapy, 11*(1), 204-209.

Smolen, J.S., Aletaha, D., Bijlsma, J.W., Breedveld, F.C., Boumpas, D., Burmester, G., Combe, B., ... van der Heijde, D. (2010). Treating rheumatoid arthritis to target: Recommendations of an international task force. *Annals of the Rheumatic Diseases, 69*(4), 631-637.

Stamm, T., & Hill, J. (2011). Extended roles of non-physician health professionals and innovative models of care within Europe: Results from a web-based survey. *Musculoskeletal Care, 9*(2), 93-101.

Temmink, D., Hutten, J.B.F., Francke, A.L., Rasker, J.J, Abu-Saad, H.H, & van der Zee, J. (2001). Rheumatology outpatient nurse clinics: A valuable addition? *Arthritis Care & Research, 45,* 280-286.

Tijhuis, G.T., Zwinderman, A.H., Hazes, J.M.W., Van Den Hout, W.B., Breedveld, F.C., & Vliet Vlieland, T.P. (2002). A randomized comparison of care provided by a clinical nurse specialist, an inpatient team, and a day patient team in rheumatoid arthritis. *Arthritis Care & Research, 47,* 525-531.

Tracy, M.F. (2008). Direct clinical practice. In A.B. Hamric, J.A. Spross, & C.M. Hanson (Eds.), *Advanced practice nursing: An integrative approach* (4th ed., p. 123-158). St. Louis, MD: Saunders Elsevier.

Tye, C., & Ross, F. (2000). Blurring boundaries: Professional perspectives of the ENP role in a major A&E department. *Journal of Advanced Nursing, 31*(5), 1089-1096.

van Eijk-Hustings, Y., van Tubergen, A., Böström, C., Braychenko, E., Buss, B., Felix, J., Firth, J., . . . Hill, J. (2012). EULAR recommendations for the role of the nurse in the management of chronic inflammatory arthritis. *Annals of Rheumatic Diseases, 71*(1), 13-19.

Voyce, M.A. (1999). The rheumatology nurse practitioner's role. *Professional Nurse, 14,* 267-270.

Watts, S.A., Gee, J., O'Day, M.E., Schaub, K., Lawrence, R., Aron, D., & Kirsh, S. (2009). Nurse practitioner-led multidisciplinary teams to improve chronic illness care: The unique strengths of nurse practitioners applied to shared medical appointments/group visits. *Journal of the American Academy of Nurse Practitioners, 21*(3), 167-172.

Werner, H. (2005). The benefits of the dysphagia clinical nurse specialist role. *Journal of Neuroscience Nursing, 37*(4), 212-215.

1
1.1
1.2
1.3
1.4
1.5
1.6
1.7
1.8
1.9

References (continued)

Wewers, M.E., & Lowe, N.K. (1990). A critical review of visual analogue scales in the measurement of clinical phenomena. *Research in Nursing and Health, 13*(4), 227-236.

Whiteley, M.S., Wilmott, K., & Offland, R.B. (1997). A specialist nurse can replace pre-registration house officers in the surgical pre-admission clinic. *Annals of the Royal College of Surgeons of England, 79*(6 Suppl), 257-260.

Zwarenstein, M., & Bryant, W. (2003). Interventions to promote collaboration between nurses and doctors (Cochrane Review). In *The Cochrane Library*. Chichester: John Wiley and Sons Ltd.

Suggested Readings

Haraoui, B., Smolen, J.S., Aletaha, D., Breedveld, F.C., Burmester, G., Codreanu, C., Da Silva, J.P., ...van der Heijde, D. (2011). Treating rheumatoid arthritis to target: A multinational recommendations assessment questionnaire. *Annals of the Rheumatic Diseases, 70*(11), 1999-2002.

Leary, A., & Oliver, S. (2010). *Clinical nurse specialists: Adding value to care - An executive summary*. London: Royal College of Nursing.

1
1.1
1.2
1.3
1.4
1.5
1.6
1.7
1.8
1.9

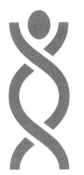

Section 1.3
Scope and Standards of Rheumatology Nursing Practice

Deborah Hicks, RN

Introduction

The scope and standards of practice for rheumatology nursing were approved by the American Nurses Association (ANA) in 2012. The document was published by ANA and the Rheumatology Nurses Society (RNS) in 2013. The document defines rheumatology nursing, the healthcare consumers to whom rheumatology registered nurses provide care, the areas in which these nurses work, and the distinct knowledge base that provides rheumatology registered nurses with a unique skill set to care for individuals who have complex, painful, chronic, deforming, debilitating, and sometimes life-threatening diseases (ANA & RNS, 2013).

Between 0.3 and 1 percent of the world's population has rheumatoid arthritis, and an even higher percentage has other rheumatic conditions. Rheumatoid arthritis and other rheumatic conditions are the leading cause of disability in the United States (Klippel, Stone, Crofford, & White, 2008). Individuals with rheumatic conditions range from infants to the elderly, all genders, all socioeconomic levels, all races, and all cultures. Expanding knowledge of the immune system has produced pharmaceutical development of targeted complex biologic therapies that have provided greater ability to treat to remission or target (T2T). The development of these new therapies, the biologic response modifiers (BRMs), has offered individuals with rheumatic diseases better treatment options that are leading to less morbidity and mortality

and a better quality of life. The pipeline of agents with other targets will continue to expand the therapeutic options for treating rheumatic conditions. Challenges remain, for not all treatments benefit all patients; financial impediments affect care; and not all healthcare consumers with rheumatic conditions receive specialized care. Rheumatology registered nurses play a significant role for these healthcare consumers by planning and implementing care, engaging outside resources, and communicating with others involved in the care of these healthcare consumers with painful, multi-organ diseases often complicated by chronic underlying conditions.

The scope and standards provide the framework for rheumatology nursing and define a competent level of rheumatology nursing care. Stakeholders and others will look to this document as the established level of competency that healthcare professionals, the public, and others can expect of the rheumatology registered nurse. The Institute of Medicine (2010) report on the Future of Nursing includes recommendations to a variety of stakeholders to ensure that nurses can practice to the full extent of their license. The Scope and Standards should provide evidence to policy makers that rheumatology registered nurses have the knowledge and skills to meet this goal (ANA & RNS, 2013).

This chapter reviews the scope of rheumatology nursing and the standards of practice expected of rheumatology registered nurses.

Learning Objectives

Upon completion of this chapter, the nurse will be able to:

1. Identify rheumatology nurse practice areas.
2. List the types of healthcare consumers to which rheumatology registered nurses provide care.
3. Describe the educational preparation of rheumatology registered nurses.
4. Identify the purpose and use of the Scope and Standards of Rheumatology Nursing Practice.
5. Identify the 16 standards of nursing practice in general terms.
6. Distinguish between the roles of the rheumatology registered nurse and the advanced practice registered nurse (APRN) in rheumatology.

1
1.1
1.2
1.3
1.4
1.5
1.6
1.7
1.8
1.9

Content Outline

I. Scope of practice.

A. Rheumatology nurses are:

1. Registered nurses and advanced practice registered nurses licensed by their respective state boards of nursing.

2. Registered nurses who care for healthcare consumers with immune mediated, systemic inflammatory musculoskeletal rheumatic diseases/conditions.

3. Registered nurses who have knowledge of the immune system and the abnormal functioning of the immune system leading to rheumatic conditions.

4. Registered nurses who understand rheumatic disease processes, targeted therapies, interaction of medications, implications of multi-drug therapy, concurrent disease states, and inter-professional collaborative relationships.

B. Rheumatology nurse practice areas and responsibilities:

1. In adult and pediatric outpatient clinics and private practices, the rheumatology registered nurse:

   a. Performs physical assessments.

   b. Teaches healthcare consumers and families about disease states and treatment options.

   c. Infuses targeted BRMs, bisphosphonates, steroids.

   d. Administers biologic injectable medications.

   e. Monitors for medication side effects and efficacy.

   f. Assists healthcare consumers with financial or insurance concerns.

   g. Provides psychosocial support to the healthcare consumer and family.

   h. Acts as consultant to acute care nurses,or other healthcare providers such as physical therapists, rehabilitation facilities, primary care practices.

   i. Communicates with healthcare consumer, family, and other providers of care.

   j. Coordinates care with other providers.

2. In academic or private practice research facilities, the rheumatology registered nurse:

   a. Manages complex clinical research trials as a coordinator or project manager.

   b. Advanced practice registered nurses (APRNs) can be the co-principal investigator in clinical trials or principal investigator in nursing research.

3. In infusion suites in private practices, free standing infusion centers, and hospital infusion suites, the rheumatology registered nurse:

   a. Is competent in infusion technique, intravenous access.

   b. Infuses BRMs, bisphosphonates, steroids.

   c. Is knowledgeable regarding adverse drug reactions, infusion reactions.

   d. Manages other infusion personnel.

   e. Maintains privacy for multiple patients in open suite.

C. Educational background of rheumatology registered nurses:

1. Diploma, associate degree, baccalaureate, master's or doctorally prepared registered nurses:

   a. May come from medical-surgical, pediatric, orthopaedic, rehabilitation, home health care, or other gerontology backgrounds before pursuing rheumatology nursing.

   b. Training and education are received on the job from other rheumatology professionals; continuing education may be obtained through journals, seminars, professional association conferences; publications.

   c. Currently no defined academic route available to nurses pursuing education in rheumatology.

   d. APRNs gain their master's and/or doctorate in nursing in such specialties as medical-surgical, gerontology, pediatrics, and then concentrate on rheumatology through the same learning process as the registered nurse, although the APRN may have physician mentoring.

   e. All registered nurses will be licensed by their respective state board of nursing and will adhere to state laws governing nursing practice.

D. Use of the scope and standards of practice.

1. Basis for quality improvement systems.

2. Development and evaluation of rheumatology nursing service delivery systems and organizational structures.

3. Position descriptions and performance appraisals.

4. Agency policies, procedures, and protocols.

5. Educational offerings.

6. Certification activities.

II. Standards of Professional Practice.

A. Standard 1. Assessment.

1. The rheumatology registered nurse:

   a. Collects comprehensive data pertinent to the healthcare consumer's (HCC) health or situation.

      (1) Includes comprehensive personal and family history, social history, expressed needs, knowledge of situation, economic situation relevant to health.

      (2) Uses evidence-based assessment tools (such as Health Assessment Questionnaire, Disease Activity Score 28, Ankylosing Spondylitis Activity Score).

      (3) Prioritizes data collection based on the HCC's immediate need.

      (4) Documents relevant data.

   b. Additionally, the APRN:

      (1) Initiates and interprets diagnostic data.

      (2) Assesses the individual's social systems regarding health and illness.

B. Standard 2. Diagnosis.

1. The rheumatology registered nurse:

   a. Derives and validates diagnosis, identifies barriers or risks to health and safety.

   b. Documents diagnoses and issues.

2. Additionally, the APRN:

   a. Develops the differential diagnosis.

   b. May collaborate with staff in the development of the diagnosis.

C. Standard 3. Outcomes identification.

1. The rheumatology registered nurse:

   a. Identifies expected outcomes in consideration with the healthcare consumer.

   b. Develops timelines for expected outcomes, with modifications as needed.

   c. Documents outcomes as measurable goals.

2. Additionally, the APRN:

   a. Identifies expected outcomes incorporating scientific evidence and cost/clinical efficacy/ healthcare consumer satisfaction.

   b. Differentiates between care process interventions and system-level interventions.

D. Standard 4. Planning.

1. The rheumatology registered nurse:

   a. Develops plans that describe strategies, set priorities, provide continuity, and consider the economic impact on the healthcare consumer and family. The plan is evidence-based and provides for modification if new evidence emerges.

   b. Defines plan under current rules and regulations.

   c. Documents the plan.

2. Additionally, the APRN:

   a. Identifies strategies and therapeutic interventions that meet the multifaceted needs of healthcare consumers with complex conditions.

   b. Participates in the development and continuous improvement of systems that support the planning process.

E. Standard 5. Implementation.

1. The rheumatology registered nurse:

   a. Implements the plan with inclusion of the healthcare consumer, the family, and others using evidence-based interventions.

   b. Provides for the safety of the healthcare consumer.

   c. Advocates for health care that is sensitive to diverse populations.

   d. Uses community and other resources to achieve goals.

1
1.1
1.2
1.3
1.4
1.5
1.6
1.7
1.8
1.9

1
1.1
1.2
1.3
1.4
1.5
1.6
1.7
1.8
1.9

e. Documents plans.

2. Additionally, the APRN:

a. Facilitates the plan.

b. Supports collaboration for implementation.

c. Assumes responsibility for implementation of the plan.

d. Participates in the development and improvement of systems that support the implementation of the plan.

F. Standard 5A. Coordination of care.

1. The rheumatology registered nurse:

a. Organizes the plan and manages the care to maximize independence and quality of life.

b. Assists in identifying options of alternative care.

c. Documents the coordination of care.

2. Additionally, the APRN:

a. Provides leadership for coordinated care.

b. Prescribes necessary system and community support measures.

G. Standard 5B. Health teaching and health promotion.

1. The rheumatology registered nurse:

a. Provides health teaching addressing healthy lifestyle activities, risk-reducing behaviors, and preventive self-care.

b. Provides information regarding intended effects, adverse effects, disease states, treatments, and comorbidities in a manner appropriate to the healthcare consumer's learning style.

2. Additionally, the APRN:

a. Uses research to design health information/ education programs.

b. Evaluates health information resources for accuracy and appropriateness.

c. Provides guidance for health promotion and prevention and risk reduction.

H. Standard 5C. Consultation.

1. The APRN provides consultation to influence the plan, enhance the abilities of others, and effect change.

I. Standard 5D. Prescriptive authority and treatment.

1. The APRN:

a. Prescribes evidence-based treatment and procedures; pharmacologic agents based on knowledge and clinical indicators.

b. Evaluates risk/benefits of pharmacologic and therapeutic treatments.

c. Provides healthcare consumer with information regarding treatments.

J. Standard 6. Evaluation.

1. The rheumatology registered nurse:

a. Evaluates outcomes in collaboration with the healthcare consumer and others.

b. Documents the results of the evaluation.

2. Additionally, the APRN:

a. Evaluates the effectiveness of the interventions, adapts the plan as needed.

b. Uses evaluation to make process or structural changes including policy, procedure, or protocol revision.

K. Standard 7. Ethics.

1. The rheumatology registered nurse:

a. Practices guided by the Code of Ethics for Nurses and Interpretive Statements (American Nurses Association, 2001).

b. Recognizes, preserves, and protects the centrality of the healthcare consumer.

c. Maintains appropriate professional interpersonal boundaries.

d. Protects confidentiality within legal and regulatory parameters.

e. Takes appropriate action against unethical, illegal, or inappropriate behavior that jeopardizes the healthcare consumer or the situation.

f. Advocates for equitable health care.

2. Additionally, the APRN:

a. Participates in inter-professional teams that address ethical risks, benefits, and outcomes.

b. Obtains informed consent or informed refusal.

L. Standard 8. Education.

1. The rheumatology registered nurse:

   a. Participates and shares ongoing educational activities.

   b. Is a lifelong learner.

   c. Maintains professional records providing evidence of competency and learning.

   d. Seeks learning opportunities, including clinical experience.

   e. Contributes to the education of others in the work environment.

2. Additionally, the APRN:

   a. Uses current healthcare research findings to expand clinical knowledge and skills to enhance role performance.

M. Standard 9. Evidence-based practice and research.

1. The rheumatology registered nurse:

   a. Uses current evidence-based nursing knowledge to guide practice.

   b. Shares research findings with peers.

2. Additionally, the APRN:

   a. Contributes to nursing knowledge by conducting or synthesizing nursing research.

   b. Promotes a climate of clinical inquiry.

   c. Disseminates research findings.

N. Standard 10. Quality of practice.

1. The rheumatology registered nurse:

   a. Demonstrates quality through documentation of the nursing process.

   b. Participates in quality improvement.

2. Additionally, the APRN:

   a. Provides leadership in the design and implementation of quality improvements.

   b. Evaluates the quality of nursing practice in relation to existing evidence.

   c. Uses results of quality improvement to initiate change in nursing practice and the healthcare delivery system.

O. Standard 11. Communication.

1. The rheumatology registered nurse and the APRN:

   a. Communicate effectively in a variety of formats in all areas of practice.

   b. Communicates health data, inter-professional continuity/transitional care plans, concerns regarding hazards or errors in care.

P. Standard 12. Leadership.

1. The rheumatology registered nurse:

   a. Retains accountability and responsibility for care given by others.

   b. Mentors colleagues, treats them with dignity and respect.

   c. Participates in professional organizations.

   d. Seeks ways to advance nursing autonomy and accountability.

   e. Participates in efforts to influence healthcare policy.

   f. Develops communication and conflict resolution skills.

2. Additionally, the APRN:

   a. Mentors colleagues.

   b. Influences decision-making bodies to improve healthcare environments and healthcare consumer outcomes.

   c. Is a role model for expert practice.

   d. Provides directions to enhance effectiveness of the healthcare team.

Q. Standard 13. Collaboration.

1. The rheumatology registered nurse:

   a. Engages in team work and team building to effect positive outcomes.

   b. Participates in building consensus and resolving conflict in the context of care.

   c. Promotes cooperation, respect, and trust by adhering to standards and codes of conduct.

2. Additionally, the APRN:

   a. Partners with other disciplines while including the healthcare consumer to enhance optimal outcomes.

   b. Leads in developing and sustaining collaborative relationships.

   c. Documents plan of care communications to improve outcomes.

1
1.1
1.2
1.3
1.4
1.5
1.6
1.7
1.8
1.9

R. Standard 14. Professional practice evaluation.

1. The rheumatology registered nurse:

   a. Provides appropriate care in a sensitive manner.

   b. Participates in peer review, self evaluation, formally and informally, and takes action to achieve goals identified during these processes.

   c. Provides evidence for practice decisions as part of the evaluation process.

   d. Provides constructive feedback to peers.

2. Additionally, the APRN:

   a. Engages in a formal process to gain feedback regarding his/her nursing practice.

S. Standard 15. Resource utilization.

1. The rheumatology registered nurse:

   a. Identifies healthcare consumer needs and assists with available resources as appropriate.

   b. Delegates care to other healthcare workers as appropriate.

   c. Advocates for resources that enhance nursing practice.

   d. Assists healthcare consumers and their families to identify appropriate services, factoring in expenses, risks, and benefits.

2. Additionally, the APRN:

   a. Uses available resources to formulate plans of care.

   b. Formulates innovative solutions that use resources effectively and maintain quality.

   c. Evaluates strategies for cost effectiveness, benefits, and efficacy.

T. Standard 16. Environmental health.

1. The rheumatology registered nurse:

   a. Is knowledgeable in environmental health concepts and promotes a healthy work environment that reduces risk to workers and healthcare consumers.

   b. Participates in strategies that promote healthy communities and workplaces.

2. Additionally, the APRN:

   a. Creates partnerships that promote sustainable environmental policies and conditions.

   b. Advocates for and supports other nurses in advocating for environmental principles in nursing practice.

Summary

The acknowledgment of rheumatology as a nursing specialty and the publication of the *Scope and Standards of Rheumatology Nursing Practice* by the American Nurses Association and the Rheumatology Nurses Society in 2013, delineates the basic competencies for all rheumatology registered nurses and APRNs. Stakeholders and others will look to this document when reviewing practice skills and standards for the care of rheumatology healthcare consumers. It is incumbent upon registered nurses and APRNs in rheumatology to be familiar with this document so they may understand and practice according to these professional expectations.

References

American Nurses Association. (2001). *Code of ethics for nurses with interpretive statements.* Silver Spring, MD: Author.

Klippel, J.H., Stone, J.H., Crofford, L.J., & White, P.H. (Eds.). (2008) *Primer on the rheumatic diseases.* New York: Springer.

American Nurses Association and Rheumatology Nurses Society. (2013). *Rheumatology nursing: Scope and standards of practice.* Silver Spring, MD: Nursesbooks.org

Institute of Medicine. (2010). *The future of nursing; Leading change, advancing health.* Washington, DC: National Academies Press. Retrieved from http://www.iom.edu/Reports/2010/The-Future-of-Nursing-Leading-Change-Advancing-Health.aspx

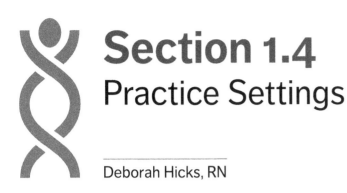

Section 1.4
Practice Settings

Deborah Hicks, RN

1
1.1
1.2
1.3
1.4
1.5
1.6
1.7
1.8
1.9

Introduction

The more than 100 types of rheumatologic diseases that may be primary, secondary, overlapping, or mimicking conditions create a unique complexity to the care and treatment of rheumatology healthcare consumers. Rheumatologic conditions are often chronic, painful, and complicated by co-morbidities. The disease states and treatment options require the rheumatology registered nurse to be knowledgeable about pathophysiology; the immune system; medication profiles/mechanisms of action and drug-drug interactions; financial assistance and insurance complexities; and collaborative treatment options provided by others such as physical and occupational therapists, nutrition counselors, joint replacement surgeons, and orthotic and prosthetics professionals. Therefore, in response to disease complexities and interdisciplinary care, the rheumatology registered nurse must be prepared to provide physical assessments and treatment monitoring, healthcare consumer education, psychosocial support, assistance with accessing financial assistance, and coordination of care with other healthcare providers as well as community resources.

Basic nursing education only provides a glimpse of immune-mediated disorders, and nursing school clinical experiences generally do not actively seek out patients with rheumatic conditions as a priority. Additionally, many registered nurses choose an acute care setting to begin their nursing careers. Therefore, most registered nurses choose rheumatology after gaining experience in other nursing areas such as medical surgical nursing, emergency room nursing, or critical care nursing. These registered nurses find rheumatology challenging on multiple levels. Rheumatology registered nurses can choose from a variety of practice settings. This chapter outlines the practice settings available to rheumatology registered nurses and highlights many of the responsibilities in each setting. The practice settings include, but are not limited to, outpatient clinics and private practice facilities, research facilities, and infusion suites. Additionally, rheumatology registered nurses may serve as consultants to pharmaceutical companies, acute care (hospital inpatient) facilities, rehabilitation facilities, home health agencies, and community based organizations, including faith-based nursing practice.

Learning Objectives

Upon completion of this chapter, the nurse will be able to:

1. Describe the practice settings available in the field of rheumatology nursing.

2. Identify the basic practice responsibilities within each practice setting.

I. Rheumatology registered nurses in outpatient clinics and private practice facilities: Pediatric, adult, or geriatric.

A. Responsibilities within the setting include the following:

1. Taking health histories and performing physical assessments, including the use of evidence-based measurement tools and joint counts.

2. Educating healthcare consumers and significant others about the healthcare consumer's conditions and treatment options.

   a. Disease/condition information including complications, chronicity, and potential outcomes with and without treatment.

   b. Medication risks/benefits, side-effect profiles, pre-screening, precautions.

   c. Vaccination schedules, recommendations including vaccines to avoid because of the medical condition or treatment regimen.

   d. Financial implications which may determine treatment options.

3. Educating, teaching proper technique, and demonstration of self-injectable medications including disease modifying anti-rheumatic drugs (DMARDs), biologic response modifiers (BRMs), and osteoporosis self-administered drugs.

4. Infusing biologic and other therapeutic agents under safe and recommended protocols.

5. Monitoring for side effects of medications as well as therapeutic outcomes.

6. Assisting the rheumatology healthcare consumer and significant others with insurance options and financial assistance as appropriate.

7. Providing psychosocial support and assistance to the rheumatology healthcare consumer and significant others:

   a. Discuss pain management options such as non-narcotic medications, exercise, massage therapy, meditation techniques.

   b. Open a discussion about sexual functioning.

   c. Talk about role adjustment in face of chronic disease.

   d. Discuss concerns of parents/guardians of children and adolescents.

   e. Be familiar with short- and long-term disability forms, Family and Medical Leave Act (FMLA) forms, long-term care insurance.

8. Creating an open dialogue in the coordination of care with other providers and community services.

9. Knowing and implementing the process of obtaining prior authorization for medications, procedures, and diagnostic testing.

10. Consulting with other health professionals about the care of rheumatology healthcare consumers in areas that do not have onsite rheumatology registered nurses.

    a. Rehabilitation facilities, postoperative or post-acute hospitalization for any reason.

    b. Acute care facilities where the healthcare consumer's hospitalization is not associated with the rheumatologic condition or the healthcare consumer is not under the care of a rheumatologist or advanced practice registered nurse (APRN) in rheumatology.

    c. Home health agencies caring for a healthcare consumer with an underlying rheumatologic condition that may affect general health status or the condition and treatment for which the agency is providing care.

    d. Community-based organizations such as mental health facilities, faith-based nursing, school nursing, and hospice that may be providing care for a condition or disease other than the healthcare consumer's rheumatologic condition.

II. Rheumatology registered nurses in research facilities.

A. Responsibilities as assigned by the principal investigator may include providing protocol management and good clinical practice. Regulatory adherence for rheumatology healthcare consumers involved in treatment, prevention, diagnostic, screening, quality of life, or behavioral clinical trials within this setting may include the following:

1
1.1
1.2
1.3
1.4
1.5
1.6
1.7
1.8
1.9

1. Identifying and screening rheumatology healthcare consumers according to the inclusion/exclusion criteria appropriate for each study.

2. Informing the rheumatology healthcare consumer of the risks and benefits of a particular study as well as alternatives to the research study. The informed consent process includes, but is not limited to, confidentiality measures, responsibilities of the rheumatology healthcare consumer and clinical trial healthcare team, reporting of adverse reactions, and the ability to refuse to participate or withdraw from the clinical trial at any time without penalty or loss of benefits.

B. The advanced practice registered nurses (APRNs) in rheumatology may serve as co-investigators, depending on the respective state's nurse practice act and the sponsors' operational guidelines for the clinical trial.

C. The rheumatology registered nurse in practice in other settings taking care of the rheumatology healthcare consumer participating in a clinical trial has the following responsibilities:

1. Be aware of the research protocol criteria so that standard of care will not conflict with the research protocol.

2. Keep the safety of the participant in a rheumatology clinical trial foremost.

3. Report any real and potential adverse effects to the appropriate research team.

4. Collaborate and cooperate with the clinical research team by assisting with data collection as required, scheduling office and procedure visits, and serving as a liaison between the study staff and the rheumatology healthcare consumer.

III. Rheumatology registered nurses in rheumatology infusion suites.

A. Responsibilities for providing care in infusion suites include the following:

1. Competency in regard to intravenous infusion techniques, guidelines, and regulations.

a. Vascular access, which may be challenging because of anatomical deformities caused by the rheumatic condition.

b. Use, safety, and maintenance of multiple types of access devices and administration equipment.

c. Use of aseptic technique for vascular access, and for the preparation of infusible agents.

d. Calculations for weight-based medication dosing.

2. Management of infusion suites including, but not limited to, staffing, scheduling of healthcare consumer's infusions, ordering medications and equipment, updating medication information as it becomes available, familiarizing staff with new medications and/or protocols, developing infusion protocols, obtaining prior authorization for infusions.

3. Being familiar with each infusible drug's expected outcome and the unique side-effect/adverse reaction profile.

4. Screening healthcare consumers for conditions that would interfere with timely infusions, such as concurrent infections, recent illnesses; scheduled surgeries or diagnostic tests that might complicate or be complicated by the infusion; any change in medication history including, but not limited to, vaccines, medication allergies, over-the-counter medicines and herbal supplements, and alternative therapies.

5. Being able to prepare for, identify, and react appropriately to infusion reactions.

6. Teaching healthcare consumers about medications, side effects, risks/benefits of drugs and conditions.

7. Providing ongoing assessment of healthcare consumer's status while monitoring for adverse reactions as well as expected outcomes.

8. Maintaining infusion technique competency by updating professional knowledge through evidence-based practice, as well as maintaining current references for the infusion suite.

1
1.1
1.2
1.3
1.4
1.5
1.6
1.7
1.8
1.9

9. Taking the opportunity to discuss additional information regarding healthy lifestyles; co-morbid conditions; new medications the healthcare consumer may have started; nutrition; financial information and financial assistance programs; and updated information regarding rheumatology medications while healthcare consumer is receiving infusions.

10. Communicating with the healthcare provider regarding the health status of the healthcare consumer.

Summary

Rheumatology nurses have an obligation to remain committed and involved in developing consumer-centric healthcare policy. Being involved in specialty nursing organizations, facility committees charged with developing procedures and protocols affecting the rheumatology healthcare consumer, and participating in nursing research when available and applicable will further the specialty of rheumatology nursing and continue to expand the excellence of care rheumatology registered nurses provide individuals with rheumatic conditions, regardless of the practice setting in which that care is provided.

Suggested Reading

American Nurses Association and Rheumatology Nurses Society. (2013). *Rheumatology nursing: scope and standards of practice.* Silver Spring, MD: http://nursesbooks.org

1
1.1
1.2
1.3
1.4
1.5
1.6
1.7
1.8
1.9

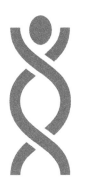

Section 1.5
Policies and Procedures

Vivian A. Gaits, RN, MSN, ACNS-BC, AOCN, CRNI

Introduction

Although each nurse practices under an individual license, it is the nurse's responsibility to know, understand, and abide by policies developed and espoused by the organization in which the nurse works. This ensures that the nurse practices in a manner that conforms to the goals and standards of the organization, and in a safe and effective way. Well-written policies and procedures protect employers, practitioners, and patients, and ensure standardized care. Frequently, nurses assist in the development of both policies and procedures. The process must be thoughtful and organized, and should be based on available scientific evidence, national standards, and practice guidelines. Policies and procedures should be simple and easy to read, understand, and use. They should be readily available for use by all stakeholders. They are often compiled into a policy and procedure manual. Licensing, accrediting, and regulatory bodies frequently require that policy and procedures be established, maintained, and reviewed.

Learning Objectives

Upon completion of this chapter, the nurse will be able to:

1. Describe the importance of policies and procedures in promoting safe and effective nursing practice.

2. Differentiate policies from procedures.

3. Describe the importance of developing policies and procedures using best available research findings, national guidelines, and standards of care.

4. List the steps to take when developing evidence-based policies and procedures.

5. Acknowledge that evidence–based practice evolves continuously, and thus, policies and procedures must be updated on a regular basis.

Content Outline

I. Definitions.

(Peabody, 2012; Rao, 2013).

A. Policy: Statement defining the "rule" or standard which should be met (but not how to meet it) - "WHAT SHOULD BE DONE AND WHO SHOULD DO IT."

1. Provides a consistent guide to how to behave in a particular setting or under a particular set of circumstances.

2. Defines the minimum standard to be met.

3. May be site-specific (i.e., outlines a rule for this practice site alone, or a general statement based on a national standard).

4. Should be specific enough to provide guidance but general enough to avoid locking practitioners into untenable practice requirements.

5. Should provide guidance for all "stakeholders" whose practice is reflected in the policy (i.e., licensed nurses and medical assistants who practice in the same area).

6. Change less frequently than procedures, as they are non-negotiable rules for behavior.

B. Procedure: A written guide for how a policy is to be met - "HOW TO PERFORM THE TASK/ MEET THE STANDARD."

1. Generally involves psychomotor skill(s).

2. Provides a sequence of steps, in chronological order, to follow in order to meet the associated standard.

3. Should provide a list of equipment to be used.

4. Should be clear and understandable for all users.

5. Should specify what documentation, if any, is required to substantiate achievement of the standard and where that should be made.

6. Should not be unnecessarily restrictive, so as to make the procedure unusable.

7. Procedures may change frequently, based on available tools, new technology, and staffing.

II. Developing policy statements.

A. Policies should reflect at least local standards of care and are often based on state, regional, or national standards set by licensing, accrediting, or regulatory bodies.

B. Policies specific to nursing define a minimum standard to be achieved in patient care.

1. Are relied on by practitioners to guide care.

2. Provide a basis for legal or disciplinary action.

3. Should be consistent with the scope of practice defined in the nurse practice act of each state.

C. Policies can be developed using published nursing research, guidelines, position statements, and standards of care.

1. Using published guidelines helps ensure that internal policies are consistent with best practices and current state of knowledge.

2. Published guidelines represent an accumulation and analysis of scientific evidence and thus, are evidence-based, providing a strong legal and clinical basis for practice.

3. Incorporating nursing research enhances the application of nursing science in practice (Hagle & Senk, 2010; Squires, Moralejo, & LeFort, 2007).

4. Position statements are developed and put forth by a variety of professional organizations, using an expert consensus-based approach that results in recommendations for action. The American Nurses Association, Oncology Nursing Society, and Infusion Nurses Society, for example, all have position statements that pertain to rheumatology nursing.

5. Policies may be wholly adapted from another healthcare institution, accrediting bodies, or from professional organizations (Brennan & Abrutyn, 1995).

D. Review of policies should occur at pre-determined intervals (e.g., biennially).

1. Minimum review interval should be specified in a policy.

1
1.1
1.2
1.3
1.4
1.5
1.6
1.7
1.8
1.9

1
1.1
1.2
1.3
1.4
1.5
1.6
1.7
1.8
1.9

2. Include a list of those responsible for the review.

3. Require an update of supporting literature.

4. Documentation of the review process should be noted on the policy or in another central location.

5. When new policies are established or old ones altered, this should be communicated to all stakeholders, as a means to ensure consistency of care.

III. Developing procedures.

A. Language should be clear and easily understandable.

B. Procedure must be clearly tied to the policy (i.e., procedure supports the achievement of the standard specified in the policy statement).

C. Procedures should be consistent with standards of care and best practices.

D. Procedures may also be adapted from published nursing procedure books, affiliating or national organizations.

E. Deviation from established procedures may be used in a legal or disciplinary proceeding; care should be used to ensure that procedures are complete and accurate as possible.

F. Procedures should be reviewed and revised on a predetermined basis or as needed when circumstances dictate (e.g., upon introduction of new equipment or staff).

1. Minimum review interval should be specified in a policy.

2. Should also include a list of those responsible for the review.

3. Should include updating supporting literature.

4. Documentation of the review process should be noted on the procedure.

5. When new procedures are developed or old ones altered, this is communicated to all stakeholders (MDHSS, 2006).

IV. Steps to developing a policy and procedure.

A. Identify organization goal, ideal, or standard that needs to be met.

B. Convene representative group of stakeholders to assist in the development of the policy.

C. Perform comprehensive literature review, gathering evidence that will support both the policy and procedure.

D. Write draft of the policy statement; review and revise with group.

E. Establish equipment needs (if any) and steps to be taken to achieve standard.

F. Identify persons responsible for performing the procedure.

G. Write a step-by-step procedure, including an equipment list; review and revise with group.

H. Include a list of references from literature review.

I. Use a consistent format when developing multiple policies and procedures as this enhances understandability. Examples are readily available in multiple print or online sources.

J. Accept the completed policy and procedure; incorporate into policy and procedure manual; and communicate to all stakeholders.

K. Review and revise policy and procedure according to pre-determined interval.

Summary

Policy and procedure manuals may be purchased whole or in part from a variety of organizations and booksellers, and may be adapted for use. Policies should reflect the goals and standards of an organization and be based on a variety of materials from professional sources and published literature. Because policies and procedures provide the underpinnings of professional nursing practice, it is critical that they are developed thoughtfully and critically, and are updated as often as practice changes require.

1
1.1
1.2
1.3
1.4
1.5
1.6
1.7
1.8
1.9

References

Brennan, P.J., & Abrutyn, E. (1995). Developing policies and guidelines. *Infection Control and Hospital Epidemiology, 16*(9), 512-517.

Hagle, M.E., & Senk, P.S. (2010). Evidence-based practice. In M. Alexander, A. Corrigan, L. Gorski, J. Hankins, & R. Perucca (Eds.), *Infusion nursing: An evidence-based approach* (3rd ed., pp. 10-21). St. Louis: Saunders Elsevier.

Missouri Department of Health & Senior Services (MDHSS). (2006). Public health nursing manual, Guidelines for Developing Policies and Procedures. Presented at the Public health nursing manual,. Retrieved 1 October 2014, from http://health.mo.gov/living/lpha/phnursing/procedures.php

Peabody, L. (2012). *How to write policies, procedures and task outlines* (3rd ed.). Lacey, WA: Writing Services.

Rao, P. (2013). *The policy and procedure manual: Managing "by the book."* Retrieved from http://www.asha.org/slp/healthcare/policy_procedures.htm.

Squires, J.E., Moralejo, D., & LeFort, S.M. (2007). Exploring the role of organizational policies and procedures in promoting research utilization in registered nurses. *Implementation Science,* 2(17). Retrieved from http://www.implementationscience.com/content/2/1/17 doi:10.1186/1748-5908-2-17

1
1.1
1.2
1.3
1.4
1.5
1.6
1.7
1.8
1.9

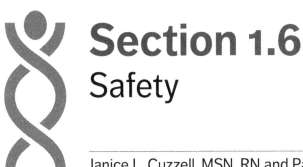

Section 1.6
Safety

Janice L. Cuzzell, MSN, RN and Pamela M. Vath, MS, FNP-BC

Introduction

The concept of safety encompasses a broad range of issues that directly affect the rheumatology nurse and nursing practice. Rheumatology nurses strive to maintain a safe work environment and ensure that patients achieve the best possible clinical outcomes. As part of the healthcare team, rheumatology nurses play a vital risk-assessment role when performing physical assessments, infusing biologics and other therapeutic agents, communicating key patient information to the physican and/or advanced practice clinician, educating healthcare consumers about self-care and adverse events, and monitoring for side effects of medications.

Patient safety has been described as instrumental to measuring the quality of care. However, most studies of patient safety and quality measures have been conducted in acute care settings, a factor that limits application of evidence-based findings in physicians' offices or outpatient infusion clinics. In *Patient Safety and Quality: An Evidence-Based Handbook for Nurses* (Hughes, 2008), the authors concluded that quality outcomes are heavily influenced by both the complex nature of the disease state and by the involvement of multiple healthcare providers and specialists. Given the complexity of caring for patients with rheumatic and immune-mediated disorders, the rheumatology nurse has an obligation to 1) maintain competency in his or her area of clinical practice or focus; 2) proactively participate in early assessment and mitigation of potential risk factors; 3) implement measures to prevent occurrence of adverse events; and 4) advocate for treatment decisions that are in the patient's best interest.

Learning Objectives

Upon completion of this chapter, the nurse will be able to:

1. Identify professional competencies required to provide safe care to patients with rheumatic diseases.

2. Identify the patient safety considerations unique to rheumatology nursing.

3. Recall the side effects of medications currently prescribed for patients with rheumatic disorders.

4. Discuss the challenges of providing a safe environment for infusion of complex biologics and other therapeutic drugs.

5. Describe the multifaceted patient education needs that affect patient safety.

1
1.1
1.2
1.3
1.4
1.5
1.6
1.7
1.8
1.9

Content Outline

I. Foundation for safe care - scope and standards of practice.

A. Healthcare provider competency.

1. Pursue and maintain a basic level of knowledge and skills necessary to provide safe patient care in the outpatient setting.

2. Maintain active professional licensure in state of practice and practice to the full extent of education and training (Institute of Medicine [IOM], 2010).

3. Maintain active basic life support (BLS) certification (minimum requirement for direct patient care).

4. Regularly demonstrate competencies specific to rheumatology practice setting and job responsibilities (IOM, 2010).

   a. Infection prevention and surveillance.

   b. Physical assessment and/or diagnosis of the rheumatology patient.

   c. High-risk medication management and expected outcomes.

   d. Management of infusion suites.

   e. Intravenous infusion techniques.

   f. Management of infusion-related adverse events.

   g. Clinical research.

   h. Long-term disability and fall prevention.

   i. Coverage and reimbursement issues.

   j. Care of children and adolescents.

   k. Healthcare consumer advocacy.

   l. Partnering with physicians and other healthcare professionals.

II. Patient safety considerations in rheumatology.

A. Increased infection risk.

1. Patients diagnosed with rheumatic and autoimmune diseases are immune compromised, have multiple comorbid complications, and are more susceptible to infections.

2. Immunosupressants are commonly used to treat patients in rheumatology and increase the risk for acquired infections.

   a. Corticosteroids.

   b. Non-biologic disease-modifying antirheumatic drugs (DMARDs).

   c. Biologic DMARDs.

B. Increased fall risk.

1. Patients diagnosed with rheumatic conditions are at increased risk for falls.

2. By 2025 the annual incidence of osteoporosis-related fractures and costs is projected to rise by almost 50% in the United States.

   a. The most rapid growth is estimated for people 65–74 years of age, with an increase >87%.

   b. An increase of nearly 175% is projected for Hispanic and other populations (Burge et al., 2006).

3. Rheumatic diseases are associated with a higher incidence of physical disability, falls, and related fractures compared to the age-specific general population (Davis, 2009).

   a. Impaired mobility due to joint pain and stiffness.

   b. Increased fatigue.

   c. Diminished bone strength.

   d. Impaired balance.

   e. Muscle weakness and atrophy.

   f. Pain medications with associated cognitive impairment.

C. Drug therapies used in rheumatology are complex and often prescribed in combination or for an extended period of time, increasing the potential for adverse events, drug-drug interactions, and development of therapeutic resistance.

1. Biologic therapies administered by intravenous infusion are associated with a high risk of adverse events requiring astute nursing assessment and intervention skills. The infusion nurse must:

   a. Prepare for safe and timely management of mild to severe infusion-related reactions (immediate and delayed).

1
1.1
1.2
1.3
1.4
1.5
1.6
1.7
1.8
1.9

b. Maintain current knowledge of the hypersensitivity reactions associated with each biologic.

c. Keep emergency supplies stocked and readily available (see Table 1).

d. Partner with the physician to develop emergency protocols to facilitate team response in emergent situations (see Table 2).

e. Provide post-infusion instructions for the patient to ensure timely reporting of delayed hypersensitivity reactions.

2. Exacerbation of concomitant medical conditions may occur during or after an infusion.

a. Assess for changes in the patient's medical condition or medication profile prior to each infusion.

b. Teach patients who require rescue intervention for chronic conditions (such as a bronchodilator for asthma or nitroglycerin for angina) to bring medications with them when scheduled for infusion.

3. Dosage calculation, mixing, and administration time varies with each biologic.

a. Weight-based or body surface area dosage calculations increase the potential for medication error.

b. Rate of administration requires accurate titration to manage the frequency and severity of infusion reactions.

4. A comprehensive nursing assessment mitigates the risk of therapy-related adverse events.

a. Record drug, food, and environmental allergies, any of which may potentiate adverse events and/or play a role in disease flare.

b. Assess for signs and symptoms of active and/or latent infection at each visit.

(1) Most DMARDs, corticosteroids, and biologic agents are not recommended for use in the presence of active infections, including but not limited to: Active or untreated latent TB, active herpes zoster infection, and life-threatening fungal infections.

Table 1: Infusion Equipment and Supplies

Equipment	Supplies	Emergency Medications
Safe, comfortable chair with cleanable surfaces that can tilt into Trendelenburg position (Brown, 2005)	Disposable gloves	Epinephrine IM
IV pole (or equivalent)	Disposable tourniquets (one per patient)	Acetaminophen PO
IV infusion pump (optional)	Angiocaths (variety of sizes)	Antihistamine PO and/or IV
Nurse call system	Antiseptic skin wipes	Corticosteroid IV
Table with cleanable surface for IV start equipment	Tape (paper, adhesive, plastic)	Sterile saline vials
Thermometer	Cotton gauze pads (sterile and/or unsterile)	Sterile water vials
Stethoscope	Normal saline IV bags (100 cc, 250 cc, 500 cc)	Sterile syringes and needles (variety of sizes)
Sphygmomanometer	D5W IV bags (100 cc, 250 cc, 500 cc)	Oxygen tank with stand and tubing/cannula/mask
	IV tubing (primary sets, secondary sets, extension tubing)	Albuterol inhaler (optional)
	Band-Aid® or equivalent	Amylnitrate (optional)
	Occlusive dressings for IV site	

Source: Author (Vath).

1
1.1
1.2
1.3
1.4
1.5
1.6
1.7
1.8
1.9

Table 2: Classification and Treatment of Infusion Reactions

Classification of Symptoms	Nursing Interventions (Treatments per standing orders or discretion of the provider)	Subsequent Infusions (Treatments per standing orders or discretion of the provider)
Mild (Grade 1) Localized cutaneous reactions such as mild pruritus, flushing, rash, dizziness, headache, < 20 point change in systolic BP.	» Stop or slow infusion and wait for symptoms to subside. After symptoms subside, resume infusion at ½ the rate. » Continue to evaluate patient, including close monitoring of vital signs. » Complete documentation of the infusion-related event.	» Some physicians may prefer to premedicate patient 0.5-1.5 hours prior to drug administration with: • Diphenhydramine 50 mg intravenous (IV). • Acetaminophen 650 mg. » Initiate subsequent infusions at ½ the usual rate, increasing titration slowly based on patient response.
Moderate (Grade 2) Above plus generalized rash or urticaria, palpitations, chest discomfort, shortness of breath, hypo- or hypertension with >20 point change in systolic BP.	» Stop drug infusion immediately and **NOTIFY** healthcare provider. » At physician's discretion treat with: • 0.9% Normal Saline Solution (aka NSS, NS, N/S, or NaCL) (~500-1000 mL hour IV). • Diphenhydramine 50 mg IV. • Acetaminophen 650 mg. • Methylprednisolone 20-40 mg IV (or equivalent). » After symptoms subside, resume infusion at ½ the rate and continue to monitor closely. Complete documentation of the infusion-related event.	» Pretreat patient 0.5-1.5 hours prior to study drug administration with any or all: • Diphenhydramine 50 mg IV. • Acetaminophen 650 mg. • Methylprednisolone 20-40 mg IV (or equivalent). » Initiate subsequent infusions at ½ the usual rate, increasing titration slowly based on patient response. Note: If a moderate infusion reaction recurs in same patient even with pretreatment, consider discontinuing any further infusions of drug.
Severe (Grade 3) Above plus fever with rigors, hypo- or hypertension with > 40 point change in systolic BP, wheezing, angioedema, or stridor.	» Stop drug infusion immediately; **NOTIFY physician.** » Evaluate patient, including close monitoring of vital signs. » Maintain airway, oxygen if available. » Treat patient immediately with: • 0.9% NSS (~500-1000 mL/hour IV). • Epinephrine for bronchospasm, hypotension, unresponsiveness to IV fluids, or angioedema. Dose and route as per standard of care for infusion center. • IV corticosteroids, solumedrol 100 mg or equivalent. • Diphenhydramine 50 mg IV. • Acetaminophen 500-650 mg. » **Transport to Emergency Dept:** Grade 3 wheezing, hypotension, or if angioedema is unresponsive to single dose of epinephrine. » Complete documentation of infusion-related event..	» Do not resume infusion. » Discontinue drug and do not rechallenge. » If an infusion reaction occurs during or after drug administration, the patient will remain at the center/office for a minimum of 1 hour for observation after resolution of symptoms and undergo the following procedures unless transferred to the emergency department. » Clinical evaluation, treatment, and stabilization of patient according to standard medical practice and/or with suggested approaches outlined above; » Close monitoring of vital signs. Every 5 to 10 minutes for Grade 1 or Grade 2 infusion reactions and every 2 to 5 minutes for Grade 3 or Grade 4 infusion reactions until stable
Life threatening (Grade 4) Defined as a reaction that is life threatening (potentially) requires pressor and/or ventilator support or shock associated with acidemia and impairing vital organ function due to tissue hypoperfusion. Drug infusion is stopped.	» Activate the Emergency Response System » Continue to monitor vital signs and standard medical practice in an emergent life-threatening situation » Maintain IV line of 0.9% NSS (~500-1000 mL/hour). » **Transport to Emergency Dept:** Grade 4 at the discretion of the healthcare provider.	» Document treatment and care appropriately. » Further care at order of physician.

Source: Adapted from Vogel, W. (2010). Infusion reactions: Diagnosis, assessment, and management. *Clinical Journal of Oncology Nursing, 14*(2), E10-26.

1
1.1
1.2
1.3
1.4
1.5
1.6
1.7
1.8
1.9

(2) Concomitant use of steroids and other immunosuppressive agents may mask common signs and symptoms of infection.

(3) Reactivation of latent tuberculosis infection (LTBI) can occur with biologic therapy.

    i)   Screen all patients for LTBI as recommended on the product label both prior to biologic therapy and annually thereafter if therapy is initiated.

    ii)   Assess patient's medical history to identify potential risk factors for tuberculosis (TB) infection including being homeless, previously residing in countries with a high prevalence of TB, intravenous drug use, and time spent in institutional settings.

    iii)   A tuberculin skin test (TST) or interferon-release assay (IGRA) should be performed for the initial screening (Singh et al., 2012).

    iv)   Patients with a positive initial or repeat TST or IGRA should have a chest radiograph and/or sputum examination to rule out active disease.

    v)   Patients diagnosed with rheumatoid arthritis have a higher incidence of false-negative skin tests and may require additional screening.

(4) Predisposition to or reactivation of viral infections can occur with biologic therapy.

    i)   Screen for hepatitis according to product label prior to intiating biologic therapy.

    ii)   Treatment with MTX, leflunomide, sulfasalazine (SSZ), minocycline, and biologic agents should be avoided in the presence of acute hepatitis B or C.

    iii)   In the presence of chronic hepatitis B or C (treated or untreated), the severity of compromised liver function is considered a key factor in making therapeutic decisions.

(5) Live vaccines are contraindicated during treatment with biologic agents (see Table 3).

c. Maintain a current, comprehensive patient medication list.

(1) Patients with rheumatic conditions often are followed by multiple healthcare providers who prescribe medications.

(2) Document all prescription and over-the-counter drugs, vitamins, minerals, herbal supplements, alternative medicine treatments, topicals, and home remedies.

Table 3: Commonly Prescribed Live and Inactivated Vaccines

Live Vaccines	Inactivated Vaccines
» Mumps Measles Rubella (MMR)	» Tetanus diphtheria/acellular pertussis (Td/Tdap)
» Varicella Zoster (VZV)	» Hepatitis A (HAV)
» Live attenuated influenza (LAIV)	» Hepatitis B (HBV)
» Herpes Zoster (HZV)	» Human Papiloma Virus (HPV)
» Yellow Fever	» Influenza A/B/H1N1 (TIV)
» Oral typhoid	» Menigococcal (MCV)
» Bacille Calmette-Guerin (BCG)	» Pneumococcal (PCV)
» Rotovirus (RV)	» Inactivated polio (IPV)
» Polio oral	» Rabies
» Adenovirus type 4, 7, oral	» Typhoid polysaccharide
» Smallpox (Vaccinia)	

Source: U.S. Food and Drug Administration. http://www.fda.gov/BiologicsBloodVaccines/Vaccines/ApprovedProducts/UCM093833.

1
1.1
1.2
1.3
1.4
1.5
1.6
1.7
1.8
1.9

d. Monitor results of recent lab work or diagnostic tests for contraindications to therapy.

   (1) A baseline complete blood count, liver transaminase level, and serum creatinine are recommended by the American College of Rheumatology (ACR) when starting or resuming therapy with a nonbiologic or biologic DMARD. Repeat lab work routinely per office protocol and report abnormal lab values to the prescriber prior to administering medications.

e. Inquire about recent or planned surgeries or dental work.

   (1) Therapy may need to be interrupted to prevent infection and promote healing.

   (2) The ACR recommends that, in general, biologic agents should not be used during the perioperative period, for at least 1 week prior to, and 1 week after surgery. Always refer to the label for product-specific recommendations.

   (3) The pharmacokinetic properties of a given biologic agent (e.g., half life) and type of surgery are additional factors that need to be considered when interrupting therapy.

   (4) Minor surgeries with a low risk of infection (e.g., cataract operations) may not require therapy interruption (Saag et al., 2008).

f. Document history of previous infusion reactions which:

   (1) Provides information about a patient's tolerance to immunomodulation with biologics and other intravenous medications.

   (2) Includes details of reaction including the type of therapy, how long into the infusion the reaction occurred, the symptoms the patient experienced, interventions performed, and outcome.

g. Have patient demonstrate an understanding of the risks of current therapy and educate regarding appropriate prevention strategies.

   (1) Review medication guide with patient and/or significant other.

   (2) Teach signs and symptoms requiring medical intervention.

      i) Adverse events associated with the prescribed treatment protocol.
      ii) Delayed hypersensitivity reactions to infusables or injection site reactions.
      iii) Symptoms of recurrent or active infection including fever, chills, productive cough.
      iv) Exacerbation of concomitant medical conditions such as congestive heart failure or diabetes.
      v) Disease flare.

   (3) Emphasize importance of patient's role in promptly communicating adverse events to the healthcare provider.

   (4) Assess for pregnancy risk and counsel as indicated.

   (5) Many therapies used in rheumatology are contraindicated during pregnancy and while breast feeding.

Summary

Although still in its infancy, rheumatology nursing is rapidly becoming recognized as an emerging specialty practice. Delivering optimal patient outcomes in this high-risk patient population requires an emphasis on safety. Rheumatology nurses must develop astute assessment and intervention skills in order to safely administer many of the therapies used to treat rheumatic diseases. In addition, rheumatology nurses play a vital role in maintaining a clean and safe practice environment.

References

Burge, R., Dawson-Hughes, B., Solomon, D.H., Wong, J.B., King, A., & Tosteson, A. (2006). Incidence and economic burden of osteoporosis-related fractures in the United States, 2005-2025. *Journal of Bone and Mineral Research, 22*(3), 465-475.

Brown SG (August, 2005). Cardiovascular aspects of anaphylaxis: implications for treatment and diagnosis. *Current Opinion in Allergy and Clinical Immunology* 2005; 5:359–364.

Davis, G.C. (January, 2009). Reduce the danger of falls: Common factors in arthritis patients increase falls risk. *The Rheumatologist*. Retrieved from http://www.the-rheumatologist.org/details/article/873455/Reduce_the_Danger_of_Falls.html

Hughes, R.G. (Ed.). (2008). *Patient safety and quality: An evidence-based handbook for nurses* (AHRQ Publication No. 08-0043). Rockville, MD: Agency for Healthcare Research and Quality.

Institute of Medicine. (2010). *The future of nursing: Leading change, advancing health.* Washington, DC: National Academies Press. Retrieved from http://www.iom.edu/Reports/2010/The-Future-of-Nursing-Leading-Change-Advancing-Health.aspx

Saag, K.G., Teng, G.G., Patkar, N.P., Anuntiyo, J., Finney, C., Curtis, J.R., ... Furst, D.E. (2008). American College of Rheumatology 2008 recommendations for the use of nonbiologic and biologic disease-modifying antirheumatic drugs in rheumatoid arthritis. *Arthritis & Rheumatism, 59*(6), 762-784.

Singh, J.A., Furst, D.E., Bharat, A., Curtis, J.R., Kavanaugh, A.F., Kremer, J.M., ... Saag, K.G. (2012). 2012 update of the 2008 American College of Rheumatology recommendations for the use of disease-modifying antirheumatic drugs and biologic agents in the treatment of rheumatoid arthritis. *Arthritis Care & Research, 64*(5), 625-639.

Suggested Readings

American Nurses Association and Rheumatology Nurses Society. (2013). *Rheumatology nursing: Scope and standards of practice.* Silver Spring, MD: http://nursesbooks.org.

Centers for Disease Control and Prevention. (2011). *Guide to infection prevention for outpatient settings: Minimum expectations for safe care.* Retrieved from http://www.cdc.gov/hicpac/pubs.html

Dao. K. & Cush, J. J. (Eds.) (2012). A vaccination primer for rheumatologists. *American College of Rheumatology: Drug Safety Quarterly, 4*(1). Retrieved from http://www.rheumatology.org/publications/dsq/index.asp.

Dexter, T.R. (2008). Role of the rheumatology infusion nurse. *John Hopkins Studies in Nursing, 6*(2), 39-44.

Kippel, J.H., Stone, J.H., Crofford, L.J., & White, P.H. (Eds.). (2008). *Primer on the rheumatic diseases* (13th ed.). New York: Springer.

Resources

Check for Safety: A Home Prevention Checklist for Older Adults. (2006). Atlanta, GA: Centers for Disease Control and Prevention (CDC). www.cdc.gov/ncipc/pub-res/toolkit/CheckListForSafety.htm

Quality and Safety Education for Nurses (QSEN). http://www.qsen.org/

1
1.1
1.2
1.3
1.4
1.5
1.6
1.7
1.8
1.9

1
1.1
1.2
1.3
1.4
1.5
1.6
1.7
1.8
1.9

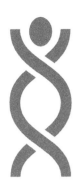

Section 1.7
Ethical and Legal Issues

Patricia Weinstein, PhD, ARNP, NP-C, CNE

Introduction

Rheumatology registered nurses commonly encounter clinical situations that present ethical dilemmas given that rheumatic disorders are often characterized by inequitable access to health care, challenges to self-management, and chronicity of illness. In addition, research trials and new therapies may pose risks without guarantee of benefit.

Nurses are in the best position to advocate for the rights of patients. An understanding of ethical principles and decision making as well as an awareness of factors that can increase the risk of ethical conflicts may assist nurses in analyzing and resolving ethical problems and alleviating moral uncertainty or distress.

Learning Objectives

Upon completion of this chapter, the nurse will be able to:

1. Identify ethical principles used in analyzing moral dilemmas.

2. Discuss common ethical/legal issues that arise in the care of patients with rheumatic disorders.

3. Describe the process of ethical decision making and moral resolution.

1
1.1
1.2
1.3
1.4
1.5
1.6
1.7
1.8
1.9

Content Outline

I. Bioethical principles
(Beauchamp & Childress, 2012).

A. Beneficence - duty to do good and prevent harm.

B. Nonmaleficence - obligation not to inflict harm intentionally; prima facie principle.

C. Autonomy - right to self-determination, respect for patient's right to make decision about and for self.

D. Justice - equitable distribution of risks and benefits.

E. Virtue - persistent, praiseworthy traits of human character that increase the chance of moral conduct.

F. Caring (feminist) ethics - characterized by nurturing with an emphasis on responsibilities to others.

II. Special issues.

A. Chronic illness (Jennings, Callahan, & Caplan, 1988).

1. Challenges normal moral boundaries of caring and family caregiver expectations.

2. Challenges understanding of social justice and community in view of community's health care and social services.

B. Threats to autonomy (Townsend, Adam, Cox, & Li, 2010).

1. Dependency upon healthcare providers to assume some decision making because of vulnerability in setting of chronic and often serious illness.

2. Complexity of newer technologies challenges informed decision making.

3. Low health literacy among some patients with rheumatic disorders (Swearingen et al., 2010).

C. Inequitable access to health care (Rom, Fins, & Mackenzie, 2007).

1. Racial/ethnic disparities in treatment (e.g., lower rates of total knee, hip replacements among African Americans and Hispanics compared to whites) (Bang et al., 2010).

2. Disease-related impaired mobility.

3. Loss of employment and employment-based private insurance secondary to pain and chronic illness.

4. High cost of pharmacologic agents (e.g., biologics).

D. Clinical trials.

1. Informed consent – participant's autonomous authorization (Beauchamp & Childress, 2012).

a. Pre-conditions.

(1) Mental competence.

(2) Voluntariness.

b. Information elements.

(1) Full disclosure of risks, benefits, and treatment alternatives to research protocols.

(2) Understanding of protocol, risks, benefits.

(3) Right to withdraw from study.

c. Consent elements.

(1) Decision to participate.

(2) Authorization.

2. Types of research (Sugarman & Bingham, 2008).

a. Early phase therapeutic trials.

(1) Potential toxicity may not be revealed in animal studies.

(2) Biological agents require targeted molecule expressed in disease; thus, patients rather than healthy volunteers may be needed as study participants.

(3) Study design may require patients who have not received other treatments with proven efficacy; thus, enrollment may delay effective treatment.

(4) Preliminary efficacy outcomes for early dose-ranging experiments may exclude patients with severe and/or refractory disease; thus, analysis of drug's risks and benefits limited or misleading.

(5) Participants should not be denied effective, standard-of-care treatment when enrolled.

b. Prevention studies.

(1) Asymptomatic/early-in-disease participants who may not develop specific disease or complication may be exposed to intervention-related risks.

(2) Study participants' misunderstanding that experimental intervention will prevent disease may alter decisions regarding other treatment options (Simon, Wu, Lavori, & Sugarman, 2007).

c. Post-marketing studies.

(1) Often long-term exposure to agent for treatment of rheumatic disorder.

(2) Participants must be informed of both expected and unexpected toxicities that may evolve over time.

3. Seeding or Sampling Case Studies

a. Marketing merit only; not considered medical research.

b. Participants may be given medication free for short period; clinicians may be reimbursed for "enrolling" participants.

c. Manufacturer-sponsored trials of approved drugs without evidence of scientific purpose may entice prescribers to prescribe new drug.

d. No scientific value.

III. Nursing implications.

A. Promotion of patient self-management (Redman, 2005).

1. Restoration/maintenance of patient autonomy.

a. Investment of educational resources to increase health literacy.

b. Negotiation for adherence to treatment regimen.

c. Use of adaptive equipment to increase independence.

2. Improvement in patient self-care competency in order to limit harm.

3. Advocacy of available community and social services for equitable distribution of resources.

B. Resolution of ethical dilemmas (Santa Clara University, 2012).

1. Ethical decision making and moral resolution.

a. Recognize the ethical issue.

b. Gather facts and identify stakeholders.

c. Evaluate alternative actions.

d. Make a decision and test it.

e. Implement and evaluate effects of action.

2. Reduction of moral distress (Zuzelo, 2007).

a. Open communication among nurses and healthcare professionals on ethical issues.

b. Involvement in and access to ethics committees/consultations.

c. Discussion of ethical issues in neutral setting.

d. Self-care.

(1) Reduction of workload.

(2) Acceptance of limitations.

(3) Self-examination of ethical values.

IV. Legal considerations (Guido, 2010).

A. Maintenance of nursing knowledge and competencies.

B. Adherence to professional standards of care and licensure.

C. Adherence to professional codes of ethics.

D. Compliance with Health Insurance Portability and Accountability Act (HIPAA).

E. Protection of research participants' rights.

1. Informed consent.

2. Confidentiality.

3. Protection from harm.

F. Reporting of unethical/illegal conduct.

1. Objective documentation of facts.

2. Report via proper chain of command.

3. Report to outside agencies if no response.

1
1.1
1.2
1.3
1.4
1.5
1.6
1.7
1.8
1.9

1
1.1
1.2
1.3
1.4
1.5
1.6
1.7
1.8
1.9

Summary

Nursing care of patients with rheumatologic disorders may be ethically complex. Thus, nurses should be able to recognize ethical issues relevant to the care of patients and engage in ethical decision making. This requires familiarity with principles of bioethics, knowledge of professional codes of ethics, identification of interdisciplinary resources, and effective communication with patients, their families, and other health professionals.

References

Bang, H., Chiu, Y. L., Memtsoudis, S. G., Mandl, L. A., Della Valle, A. G., Mushlin, A. I., . . . Mazumdar, M.(2010). Total hip and total knee arthroplasties: Trends and disparities revisited. *American Journal of Orthopedics,39*(9), E95-102.

Beauchamp, T. L., & Childress, J. F. (2012). *Principles of biomedical ethics* (7th ed.). New York: Oxford University Press.

Guido, G. W. (2010). *Legal & ethical issues in nursing* (5th ed.). Boston: Pearson.

Jennings, B., Callahan, D., & Caplan, A. L. (1988). Ethical challenges of chronic illness. *The Hastings Center Report, 18*(1), S1-S16.

Redman, B. K. (2005). The ethics of self-management preparation for chronic illness. *Nursing Ethics, 12*(4), 360-369.

Rom, M., Fins, J. J., & Mackenzie, C. R. (2007). Articulating a justice ethic for rheumatology: A critical analysis of disparities in rheumatic diseases. *Arthritis and Rheumatism, 57*(8), 1343-1345.

Santa Clara University. (2012). *Markkula Center for Applied Ethics: Ethical decision making*. Retrieved from http://www.scu.edu/ethics/practicing/decision/

Simon, A. E., Wu, A. W., Lavori, P. W., & Sugarman, J. (2007). Preventive misconception: Its nature, presence, and ethical implications for research. *American Journal of Preventive Medicine, 32*(5), 370-374.

Sugarman, J., & Bingham, C. O., III (2008). Ethical issues in rheumatology clinical trials. *Nature Clinical Practice: Rheumatology, 4*(7), 356-363.

Swearingen, C. J., McCollum, L., Daltroy, L. H., Pincus, T., Dewalt, D. A., & Davis, T. C. (2010). Screening for low literacy in a rheumatology setting: More than 10% of patients cannot read "cartilage," "diagnosis," "rheumatologist," or "symptom." *Journal of Clinical Rheumatology, 16*(8), 359-364.

Townsend, A., Adam, P., Cox, S. M., & Li, L. C. (2010). Everyday ethics and help-seeking in early rheumatoid arthritis. *Chronic Illness, 6*(3), 171-182.

Zuzelo, P. R. (2007). Exploring the moral distress of registered nurses. *Nursing Ethics, 14*(3), 344-359.

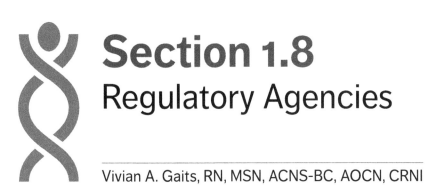

Section 1.8
Regulatory Agencies

Vivian A. Gaits, RN, MSN, ACNS-BC, AOCN, CRNI

1
1.1
1.2
1.3
1.4
1.5
1.6
1.7
1.8
1.9

Introduction

The American Nurses Association defines nursing as the "protection, promotion and optimization of health and abilities, prevention of illness and injury, alleviation of suffering through the diagnosis of human response and advocacy in the care of individuals, families, communities and populations" (American Nursing Association, 2014). Rheumatology nursing encompasses all these characteristics in the care of persons diagnosed with any of the rheumatic diseases. Whereas nursing practice was formerly measured against local practice standards, nationally developed and recognized standards and guidelines increasingly provide benchmarks for practice. The ever-expanding role of nursing requires an understanding of the organizations, regulatory agencies, and legal parameters that govern the practice of nursing.

Learning Objectives

Upon completion of this chapter, the nurse will be able to:

1. Characterize the role of the state, federal, and local agencies and organizations that promulgate laws, statutes, standards, and guidelines that influence rheumatology nursing practice.

2. Acknowledge that laws, statutes, and standards are relevant to one's own practice and practice environment.

3. Describe the most common areas where nursing practice may violate the law.

4. Describe the role of the state board of nursing.

5. Define scope of practice as it relates to nursing practice.

6. Differentiate voluntary and mandatory oversight of rheumatology nursing practice.

7. Identify various professional organizations that offer credentialing, standards of practice, and practice guidelines pertinent to rheumatology nursing practice.

1
1.1
1.2
1.3
1.4
1.5
1.6
1.7
1.8
1.9

Content Outline

I. Nurses are required to provide nursing care that is safe, reasonable, and, increasingly, evidence-based.

A. Failure to do so places the nurse at risk of violating laws, statutes, and standards.

B. Minimizing that risk requires an understanding of:

1. Law as it pertains to nursing.

2. Regulations that govern the practice of nursing.

3. Applicable standards of care and practice.

II. The legal regulation of nursing is the responsibility of the individual state's board of nursing enacted through the nurse practice act.

A. The nurse practice act, intended to ensure the health, safety, and welfare of state residents, generally includes educational requirements for licensure and defines scope of practice.

B. The nurse practice act creates the board of nursing (BON) and authorizes the board to enforce rules and regulations concerning the practice of nursing.

C. Scope of practice refers to the procedures and actions that are allowed under the practice act.

1. Scope of practice differs according to license granted.

2. Scope of practice differs specifically among registered nurses (RNs), licensed practical nurses (LPNs)/licensed vocational nurses (LVNs) and advanced practice registered nurses (APRNs)/nurse practitioners (NPs).

3. Nurse practice acts differ from state to state, with considerable variety in what is included and allowed.

4. Some nurse practice acts provide specific guidelines for individual acts that are allowed or disallowed; others are more general in nature.

5. LPNs often work under the supervision of RNs.

a. Their scope of practice is more restricted than an RNs (e.g., assessment functions are often limited by state practice acts).

6. Individual facility guidelines and job descriptions may be more restrictive than the state nurse practice act and supersede the nurse practice act.

D. States may have special provisions for mandatory continuing education for license renewal included in the nurse practice act.

E. The Nurse Licensure Compact allows for synchronous multistate licensure, without additional fees or applications but is limited to certain states.

F. Each nurse must be familiar with the nurse practice act for the state(s) in which the nurse practices, and under which license the nurse practices (Alexander & Webster, 2010; Westrick, 2009).

III. Sources of law that govern the practice of rheumatology nursing.

A. Four primary sources of law.

1. Constitutional law: Formal set of rules and principles that describes the rights of the people of the United States, including those in the Bill of Rights guaranteeing respect for all persons.

2. Statutory or legislative law: Includes laws written and enforced at federal, state, and local levels.

a. Examples include drug safety regulations from the Food and Drug Administration (FDA) and protection of healthcare workers from the Occupational Safety and Health Administration (OSHA).

b. Federal law supersedes any state or local regulation.

3. Administrative law: A form of law that is developed by an administrative agency, such as a state board of nursing.

4. Common law or case law: Results from interpretation at the court or judicial level.

a. Example is malpractice law.

1
1.1
1.2
1.3
1.4
1.5
1.6
1.7
1.8
1.9

b. When a wrong is committed against a person, it is referred to as a *tort* (Alexander & Webster, 2010).

B. Common areas in which nurses may violate the law in the practice of rheumatology nursing include:

1. Intentional tort: Intentional actions that result in harm, even if the harm is not intended.

   a. The most common are *assault* and *battery*.

   b. *Assault* is the <u>threat</u> of bodily harm without consent (e.g., the patient has refused a procedure, but the nurse applies exam gloves anyway).

   c. *Battery* is intentional physical touch to which the patient has not consented (e.g., the nurse examines the patient despite refusal, or administers medication despite a patient's refusal).

2. Unintentional tort: An unintended act, or failure to act, that results in harm.

   a. The most common is *negligence*, the failure to perform act(s) that any reasonable person would in the same circumstance.

   b. *Malpractice* is an act of negligence performed by a member of a profession, and is defined as deviance from a standard of practice that another, equally qualified professional would have followed in the same circumstance. Four conditions must be met:

      (1) A duty was owed (i.e., the nurse had responsibility for care of the patient).

      (2) The duty was breached (i.e., the nurse did not perform care relative to a standard of care).

      (3) The breach of care caused injury.

      (4) There must be a causal relationship between the breach of duty and injury.

   c. Malpractice may also be considered acting beyond the scope of practice as defined in the nurse practice act.

   d. Common areas of nursing negligence and thus malpractice include:

      (1) Failure *to follow standards of care and practice* (e.g., adhering to policies and procedures, standards of practice defined by professional organizations or practice acts).

      (2) Failure *to use equipment in a responsible manner* (e.g., infusion pumps, sphygmomanometers).

      (3) Failure *to communicate (*e.g., failure to notify a physician of a change in patient condition).

      (4) Failure *to document* (e.g., failure to document care rendered or a patient's response to treatment).

      (5) Failure *to assess and monitor (*e.g., failing to observe patient progress).

      (6) Failure *to act as a patient advocate* (Croke, 2003; Reising & Allen, 2007).

IV. **Many agencies contribute to monitoring healthcare facilities and practitioners, promoting safety and quality care, providing information about healthcare practices in general, and enforcing legal compliance.**

A. Federal, state, and local agencies establish rules and regulations for healthcare practitioners and facilities.

   1. Oversight is mandatory.

   2. Examples include the Centers for Medicare and Medicaid Services (CMS) and state boards of nursing.

B. Accrediting agencies help ensure quality in a variety of settings, through the provision and measurement of practice against standards of care.

   1. Oversight is generally voluntary, but failure to conform to standards may adversely affect reimbursement by federal agencies such as the Centers for Medicaid and Medicare Services (CMS).

   2. There are many accrediting agencies, including the Healthcare Facilities Accreditation Program among others. A widely known example is The Joint Commission (TJC):

      a. Accredits and certifies a variety of healthcare organizations, including hospitals, certain physician practices, and ambulatory care facilities.

      b. Accreditation is mandatory in certain states, as a condition for licensure, and required for state-administered Medicaid reimbursement.

C. Professional organizations provide ongoing education, standardized educational curricula, standards of practice and standards of care, and clinical practice guidelines.

1. Provide minimum criteria for practice, as well as promote excellence in specific areas of practice.

2. Although not legally binding, adherence to guidelines and standards and expectations for continuing education is regarded highly, and often used as a legal benchmark for professional practice.

3. Examples include the Rheumatology Nurses Society (RNS), American College of Rheumatology (ACR), and Association of Rheumatology Health Professionals (ARHP).

D. Local institutions and agencies also provide standards, policies, procedures, and guidelines for care.

1. Adherence to such guidelines is usually a condition for continued employment.

2. Employees may participate in the development of standards, policies and procedures, and guidelines, using the resources of and adhering to mandates from any regulatory, credentialing, or professional organizations to do so.

E. Various non-governmental credentialing bodies also offer certification in a specific area of nursing, demonstrating recognition of the nurse's increased knowledge and expertise.

1. Offered by a variety of organizations including the American Nurses Credentialing Center (ANCC), Infusion Nurses Certification Corporation (INCC), and the Oncology Nursing Certification Corporation (ONCC).

2. Voluntary, although more frequently being used as a condition for employment or advancement.

3. Goal is to promote both higher standards of practice as well as consumer confidence.

4. Provides additional expectations for performance that exceed those of the nurse prepared at the basic level, and may be used to benchmark practice.

5. Enables the practitioner to use an additional credential after professional designation (e.g., Certified Registered Nurse Infusion® [CRNI], Registered Nurse-Board Certified [RN-BC], Certified Pediatric Nurse® [CPN] (Fights, 2012).

6. Rheumatology Nurses Society (RNS) has partnered with the American Nurses Credentialing Center (ANCC) for the development of a rheumatology nursing board certification through portfolio. Other certifications may also be pertinent to rheumatology practice.

V. Federal or national agencies.

A. Food and Drug Administration (FDA):

1. Responsible for regulating the production and distribution of drugs and medical devices in the United States.

2. Ensures that prescription and over-the-counter-medications are safe and health benefits outweigh risks of use.

3. Provides ongoing information for nurses and other healthcare providers (HCPs) regarding medication safety and product withdrawals via public health advisories, drug safety podcasts.

4. Administers a voluntary adverse event reporting system (FAERS), a database on adverse events and medication errors.

5. Administers Risk Evaluation and Mitigation Strategy (REMS) plans, risk management plans for certain medications. REMS-specified elements to assure safe use (ETASU) often contain procedures that require the oversight or understanding of nurses (Merenda, 2011).

   a. Drugs used routinely in rheumatology practice have associated REMS.

   b. Examples include tocilizumab, teriparatide injection and pegloticase, among others.

B. Occupational Safety and Health Administration (OSHA):

1. Charged with helping both employers and employees avoid or reduce work-related injuries and deaths through development and subsequent enforcement of regulations.

2. Hazard Communication Standard (right-to-know law) mandates that employers disclose the presence of hazardous chemicals in the workplace, including cleaning products and medications that nurses use and administer.

3. Publishes standards regarding the handling of blood and blood products, as well as handling medications that pose risks to HCPs.

C. Centers for Disease Control (CDC):

1. Mission is to protect health and promote quality of life through prevention and control of disease, injury, and disability.

2. Provides guidance to healthcare providers (HCPs) through dissemination of practice guidelines, including those on preventing catheter-related infections, controlling and detecting tuberculosis, and immunization.

3. National Institute of Occupational Safety and Health (NIOSH), a division of the CDC, maintains a comprehensive list of hazardous drugs in the workplace and guidelines for their use.

D. Centers for Medicare and Medicaid Services (CMS) – a division of the U.S. Department of Health and Human Services:

1. Federal agency that administers Medicare program and parts of the Medicaid program.

2. Establishes standards for HCPs and healthcare organizations to ensure quality of care for Medicare and Medicaid recipients.

3. Nurses employed by any agency that cares for those recipients must abide by the standards and guidelines set by CMS. Failure to comply may result in financial and other penalties.

4. CMS also oversees regulation of laboratory services on humans offered in a variety of settings through the Clinical Laboratory Improvement Amendments (CLIA).

   a. Any facility performing diagnostic or monitoring tests on human tissue or fluids must adhere to federal requirements (e.g., urine analysis, fingersticks for blood glucose monitoring).

   b. Requirements are based on the complexity of the tests performed and vary accordingly.

5. CMS oversees the Physician Quality Reporting System (PQRS).

   a. Federally mandated program.

   b. Uses a variety of payment incentives and adjustments to promote the delivery and documentation of quality care.

   c. Measures assessed are different each year, and vary according to the type and setting of care.

   d. Clinical nurse specialists, nurse practitioners, and physician assistants are all eligible under this program, and nurses may participate in performing or documenting eligible quality services.

6. CMS regulations are complex and changing as a result of the Affordable Care Act.

E. U.S. Department of Health and Human Services (HHS):

1. Office for Civil Rights enforces the Health Insurance Portability and Accountability Act (HIPAA), which protects the privacy of health information and establishes standards for the security of electronic health information.

   a. Standards provide patients with access to health records and control over how health information is used.

   b. Most HCPs, including nurses, and agencies are required to abide by these regulations; significant financial penalties may be incurred for violations.

2. Agency for Healthcare Research and Quality (AHRQ).

   a. Mission is to improve the quality, safety, effectiveness, and efficiency of health care by sponsoring, conducting, and disseminating research.

   b. Funds research by and about nurses.

   c. Includes resources for evidence-based practice, patient safety, and nurse staffing research.

   d. Consumer Assessment of Healthcare Providers and Systems provides a national benchmarking database (currently under revision) for evaluating care.

F. National Committee for Quality Assurance (NCQA).

1. Offers a variety of voluntary certification and accreditation recognition programs for HCP practices that meet certain standards.

   a. Based on best practice criteria and standards in the areas of communication, care management, and patient self-management, among others.

1
1.1
1.2
1.3
1.4
1.5
1.6
1.7
1.8
1.9

1
1.1
1.2
1.3
1.4
1.5
1.6
1.7
1.8
1.9

b. Provides additional benchmark criteria against which practice is measured and demonstrated.

2. Maintains the Healthcare Effectiveness Data and Information Set (HEDIS).

   a. Includes a wide variety of performance measures intended to evaluate healthcare plan performance.

   b. Certain healthcare organizations must submit HEDIS data in order to provide services to Medicare Health Maintenance Organization (HMO) subscribers.

VI. State agencies.

A. May enact legislation that complements or enhances federal law but may not contradict federal statutes.

B. State departments of health.

   1. License a variety of healthcare facilities in each state, including hospitals, ambulatory care facilities, and nursing homes.

   2. Collect and publish data on quality indicator measures, staffing reports, patient safety, infections, discharges, and others that may be used as benchmarks as required by each state.

C. State board of nursing (BON):

   1. Outlines standards for safe nursing in each state via state-specific nurse practice act.

      a. Nurse practice act includes scope of practice, outlining what the licensee is able to do.

      b. Usually specifies the who-what-where-when-why of nursing practice.

      c. Scope of practice varies with each type of license.

   2. Administers National Council Licensure Exams for RNs and PNs (NCLEX-RN and NCLEX-PN).

   3. Issues licenses to practice nursing.

   4. Monitors licensees' compliance with state laws.

   5. Processes complaints against nurse licensees.

   6. Takes action against nurses who have demonstrated unsafe practice, ranging from fines and remediation to suspension or revocation of license.

7. Some BONs also mandate acquisition of continuing education as a condition for licensure (Westrick, 2009).

8. The National Council of State Boards of Nursing provides an arena for BONs to act together in matters of common interest.

   a. Provides a venue for consumers to lodge complaints about nursing care.

   b. Maintains nurse disciplinary statistics and nurse licensure verification for participating BONs.

D. State departments of health (DOH) and/or departments of environmental protection (DEP) also regulate the use of x-ray equipment and the disposal of hazardous wastes; regulations vary from state to state.

VII. Standards and guidelines.

A. Provide benchmark criteria against which to measure practice.

B. May be promulgated by professional or legislative organizations.

   1. Standards developed by professional organizations are generally voluntary.

   2. Standards developed by legislative bodies are mandatory (e.g., educational requirements for licensure; federal administration codes that specify nurse-patient ratios in federally-funded institutions).

   3. In a judicial setting, voluntary standards may be used to evaluate care performed by an individual.

C. Standards may apply to healthcare providers or facilities in general or to a specific subset of practitioners.

D. Standards may be published in professional journals or other sources of nursing literature.

E. Standard of care vs. standard of practice: Terms sometimes used interchangeably.

   1. Standard of care.

      a. Focus is on the patient.

      b. Represents practice that results in the best possible outcome for the patient.

1
1.1
1.2
1.3
1.4
1.5
1.6
1.7
1.8
1.9

c. Identifies the care a patient should expect to receive from any competent provider.

d. Based on professional literature, protocols, and expert opinion.

2. Standard of practice.

a. Focus is on the provider of care.

b. Defines minimum, acceptable level of practice.

c. Derived from policies and procedures, standards and scopes of practice, and nurse practice acts (Alexander & Webster, 2011; Dempski, 2009; Phillips, 2010).

F. Practice guidelines.

1. Generally developed by professional organizations or special committees convened specifically for this purpose.

2. Evidence-based.

3. Intended to provide general guidelines for care but not specific guidance for individual patients.

4. Although not legally binding, are used to benchmark individual and organizational practice.

G. Professional organizations that provide standards and guidelines pertinent to rheumatology nursing practice.

1. American Nurses Association (ANA).

a. Broadly specifies the scope and standards of practice of nursing in the United States, including advanced practice nursing.

b. Uses the nursing process – assessment, diagnosis, identification of outcomes, planning, implementation, and evaluation – as framework for practice.

2. Infusion Nurses Society (INS).

a. Identifies the scope of infusion nursing practice.

b. Establishes standards of practice related to infusion nursing.

c. Provides policies and procedures related to infusion nursing.

d. Develops nursing position papers (e.g., *The Use of Nursing Assistive Personnel in the Provision of Infusion Therapy*).

3. Oncology Nursing Society (ONS).

a. Specifies the scope of oncology nursing practice, including nurses who administer chemotherapy agents such as methotrexate (MTX) and cyclophosphamide.

b. Develops nursing position papers (e.g., *Education of the RN Who Administers and Cares for the Individual Receiving Chemotherapy and Biotherapy*).

c. Offers a course for non-oncology nurses: *Treatment Basics: Antineoplastic Therapy in the Non-Oncology* Setting.

4. American College of Rheumatology (ACR)/ Association for Rheumatology Health Professionals (ARHP).

a. ARHP is a division of the ACR open to non-physician health professionals.

b. Provides practice guidelines for a variety of rheumatologic conditions, including rheumatoid arthritis, gout, and osteoporosis, among others.

c. Provides an online, in-depth advanced rheumatology course for both physician and non-physician HCPs.

(1) Voluntary; does not confer a credential.

(2) Demonstrates achievement of advanced rheumatology knowledge.

5. Cochrane Collaboration.

a. International organization that provides systematic reviews of healthcare research.

b. Recognized for high standards in evidence-based health care.

c. Has conducted a variety of reviews specific to rheumatic disease.

6. European League Against Rheumatism (EULAR).

a. European equivalent of the American College of Rheumatology (ACR).

b. Offers a variety of educational programs, as well as Recommendations for Management (i.e., standards of care/practice guidelines) and Classification and Diagnosis Criteria for a variety of rheumatologic conditions.

c. EULAR Congress held annually in June.

1
1.1
1.2
1.3
1.4
1.5
1.6
1.7
1.8
1.9

Summary

It is critical for nurses to understand the legal and regulatory environment for nursing care in their specific venue of practice. In complex healthcare organizations such as hospitals, these considerations may be more apparent but may be less obvious in more isolated settings such as physician offices. Published practice guidelines and standards of care provide helpful information for the rheumatology nurse, and ongoing education and certification affirm the nurse's commitment to quality care, but these also provide benchmarks against which individual practice may be measured in legal or disciplinary settings.

References

Alexander, M.C., & Webster, H.K. (2010). Legal issues of infusion nursing. In M. Alexander, A. Corrigan, L. Gorski, J. Hankins, & R. Perucca (Eds.), *Infusion nursing: An evidence-based approach* (3rd ed., pp. 49-59), St. Louis: Saunders Elsevier.

American Nurses Association. (2014). What is Nursing? Retrieved from http://www.nursingworld.org/especiallyforyou/what-is-nursing

Croke, E.M. (2003). Nurses, negligence, and malpractice. *American Journal of Nursing, 103*(9), 54-63.

Dempski, K. (2009). Standards of care. In S.J. Westrick & K. Dempski (Eds.), *Nursing law and ethics* (pp. 15-18). Sudbury, MA: Jones and Bartlett Publishers.

Fights, S.D. (2012). Reap the benefits of certification. *American Journal of Nursing, 112*(1), 10-11.

Merenda, C. (2011). Understanding FDA's risk evaluation and mitigation strategy. *American Nurse Today, 6*(8). Retrieved from http://www.americannursetoday.com/article.aspx?id=8120&fid=8078

Phillips, L.D. (2010). *Manual of IV therapeutics* (5th ed.). Philadelphia: F.A. Davis

Reising, D.L., & Allen, P.N. (2007). Protecting yourself from malpractice claims. *American Nurse Today, 2*(2). Retrieved from http://www.americannursetoday.com/article.aspx?id=4186&fid=4172

Westrick, S.J. (2009). Regulation of nursing practice. In S.J. Westrick & K. Dempski (Eds.), *Nursing law and ethics* (pp. 6-9). Sudbury, MA: Jones and Bartlett Publishers.

Resources

Alexander, M. (Ed). (2011). Infusion nursing standards of practice. *Journal of Infusion Nursing, 34*(1S), S1-110.

Agency for Healthcare Research and Quality–Nursing http://www.ahrq.gov/about/nursing/

Agency for Healthcare Research and Quality–Benchmarking https://cahps.ahrq.gov/surveysguidance.htm

American Board of Nursing Specialties – Approved certification programs http://www.nursingcertification.org/accreditation-exams.html

American College of Rheumatology–Advanced rheumatology course http://www.rheumatology.org/education/ProfMeetingCourses/nppa.asp

American College of Rheumatology–Clinical practice guidelines http://www.rheumatology.org/practice/clinical/guidelines/

American Nurses Association–Standards http://www.nursingworld.org/MainMenuCategories/ThePracticeofProfessionalNursing/NursingStandards

American Nurses Credentialing Center http://www.nursecredentialing.org/

Centers for Disease Control–Guidelines http://stacks.cdc.gov/cbrowse/?parentId=cdc%3a100&pid=cdc%3a100&type=1&facetRange=960

Centers for Medicare and Medicaid Services–Affordable Care Act http://www.cms.gov/affordable-care-act-in-action-at-cms.html

Centers for Medicare and Medicaid Services–CLIA http://www.cms.gov/Regulations-and-Guidance/Legislation/CLIA/index.html?redirect=/clia

Centers for Medicare and Medicaid Services–Regulations http://www.cms.gov/Regulations-and-Guidance/Regulations-and-Guidance.html

Centers for Medicare and Medicaid Services–PQRS http://www.cms.gov/Medicare/Quality-Initiatives-Patient-Assessment-Instruments/PQRS/index.html

The Cochrane Collaboration http://www.cochrane.org/cochrane-reviews

European League Against Rheumatism http://www.eular.org/

Food and Drug Administration–Adverse event reporting (FAERS) http://www.fda.gov/Drugs/GuidanceComplianceRegulatoryInformation/Surveillance/AdverseDrugEffects/default.htm

Resources (continued)

1
1.1
1.2
1.3
1.4
1.5
1.6
1.7
1.8
1.9

Food and Drug Administration - Risk Evaluation and Management Strategy (REMS)
http://www.fda.gov/Drugs/DrugSafety/PostmarketDrugSafetyInformationfor PatientsandProviders/ucm111350.htm

Health Insurance Portability and Accountability Act
http://www.hhs.gov/ocr/privacy/hipaa/understanding/coveredentities/index.html

Infusion Nurses Certification Corporation
http://www.incc1.org/i4a/pages/index.cfm?pageid=1

Institute of Pediatric Nursing
http://www.ipedsnursing.org/ptisite/control/mission

The Joint Commission
http://www.jointcommission.org/

National Committee for Quality Assurance
http://www.ncqa.org/Clinicians.aspx

National Council of State Boards of Nursing
https://www.ncsbn.org/about.htm

National Institute for Occupational Safety and Health–Hazardous drugs http://www.cdc.gov/niosh/topics/hazdrug/

Nurse Licensure Compact
https://www.ncsbn.org/nlc.htm

Occupational Safety and Health Administration–Guidelines for hazardous drugs http://www.osha.gov/dts/osta/otm/otm_vi/otm_vi_2.html

Oncology Nursing Certification Corporation
http://www.oncc.org/

Oncology Nursing Society–Position statements
http://www.ons.org/Publications/Positions

Oncology Nursing Society – Treatment Basics course
http://www.ons.org/CNECentral/Chemo/TreatmentBasics

Pediatric Nursing Certification Board
http://www.pncb.org/ptistore/control/index

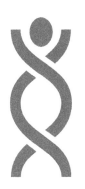

Section 1.9
Research in Rheumatology Nursing

Sheree C. Carter, PhD, RN

1
1.1
1.2
1.3
1.4
1.5
1.6
1.7
1.8
1.9

Introduction

The specialty practice of rheumatology nursing stands at the forefront of universal recognition and respect in the worldwide healthcare community. Research not only advances the practice of rheumatology nursing and documents outcomes for evidence-based practice, but also where human clinical trials are concerned, provides tremendous advances in practice as well as treatment options for the patient with a rheumatic condition. Many who call themselves rheumatology nurses in the U.S. today gravitated to the practice of rheumatology nursing through the management and conduct of clinical research trials of the biologic agents. International rheumatology nurses document the outcomes of specialized practice with patient satisfaction and education objectives. It is imperative for rheumatology nurses to understand and engage in rigorous research for clinical practice as well as to advance new treatment modalities and innovations.

Learning Objectives

Upon completion of this chapter, the nurse will be able to:

1. Define human subject protection.

2. Identify the regulating entities for the conduct of clinical trials.

3. Describe the research phases used in bringing a new clinical compound to the public.

4. Identify areas where research is needed in rheumatology nursing

Content Outline

I. Nursing Research.

A. Nursing research, specifically in the field of rheumatology nursing, is rather sparse in the U.S. nursing literature. It is, however, fairly prominent in the European literature but needs more, richly formulated studies. Nursing research is vital to rheumatology nurse specialists. At the 2012 Rheumatology Nurses Society (RNS) Conference a motion was made and subsequently passed to adopt the European League Against Rheumatism (EULAR) recommendations for the role of the nurse in the management of chronic inflammatory arthritis, which included the research agenda and educational agenda that appeared in the *Annals of Rheumatic Diseases* (van Eijk-Hustings et al., 2012). The research agenda is as follows with slight modification to add U.S. applicability:

1. Study the contribution of the nurse in improving access to care and in facilitating the effectiveness of care provided by members of the multidisciplinary team.

2. Study the role of nurses in optimizing "treat to target" in early disease.

3. Study the contribution of the nurse in improving patient-preferred outcomes.

4. Compare the different components of nursing care in each European country, in each U.S. state, and/or region in relation to knowledge and competencies.

5. Perform cost-effectiveness studies across different European countries and across the U.S. involving the role of the nurse in basic and advanced practice.

6. Study the long-term effects of interventions by a nurse on quality of life and the patient's psychosocial and general well-being.

7. Study the contribution of the nurse in improving patients' self-management and self-efficacy.

8. Study the effect of interventions by a nurse on the patient's employment status and social participation.

9. Define the contribution of the nurse in the prevention of co-morbidities.

10. Study the recommendations in different patient populations including ankylosing spondylitis and psoriatic arthritis.

B. Nursing research is defined as the application of scientific inquiry as it relates to nursing. The systematic investigation of patients and their health experience is the primary concern of nursing (Schlotfeldt, 1977).

C. Nursing research refers to the use of systematic, controlled, empirical, and critical investigation in attempting to discover or confirm facts that relate to a specific problem or question about the practice of nursing (Schlotfeldt, 1977).

D. Research is needed to evaluate the effectiveness of nursing treatment modalities, to determine the effect of nursing care on the health of patients, or to test theory. Nursing practice is undergoing tremendous changes and challenges. In order to meet social challenges and needs, nursing practice must be research based (Lanuza, 1999).

E. The overarching reasons for specific nursing research are to:

1. Contribute and build upon the body of nursing knowledge.

2. Describe, analyze, and validate improvements and specific outcomes of nursing care and practice that promote evidence-based practice.

3. Explore and evaluate the efficiency and cost-effective outcomes of specific nursing care and interventions.

4. Ensure credibility of the nursing profession.

5. Provide accountability.

F. There are a few methodological approaches to research a nurse may take to properly, ethically, and scientifically conduct nursing research:

1. Quantitative research methodology:

   a. Is vigorous, systematic, objective, measurable.

1
1.1
1.2
1.3
1.4
1.5
1.6
1.7
1.8
1.9

b. Generally has experimental and control groups with random selection.

2. Qualitative research methodology:

   a. Explores phenomena, perceptions; is subjective.

   b. May use surveys, interviews, or case reports.

3. Mixed methods research methodology:

   a. Uses a combination of both quantitative and qualitative methods to evaluate/explore a phenomenon that draws from the strengths and minimizes the weaknesses of either qualitative or quantitative research designs alone.

G. The nursing research process begins with an identified question or problem that is significant to nursing and the findings of the study will add to the knowledge of nursing either directly or indirectly. Other steps in this conceptualization process include but are not limited to:

1. Reviewing the literature.

2. Developing/identifying a theoretical framework.

3. Identifying the research variables.

4. Defining the objectives, purpose, and terms to be used in the study.

5. Formulating plans of action/evidence.

H. Any of the research methodologies identified are vital to the documentation of rheumatology nursing practice. Research by rheumatology nurses is encouraged, not only to provide evidence for practice but to preserve and further define the specialty so as to provide consistent, competent, and standardized care for patients with rheumatic conditions.

I. An equally important area for rheumatology nurses to understand and manage is the human clinical trials associated with rheumatology.

II. Human Clinical Trial Regulations.

A. There are federal laws located in the Code of Federal Regulations (CFR) Title 21 to serve as a basis for conducting all human clinical trials research (www.accessdata.fda.gov/scripts/cdrh/cfdocs/cfcfr/cfrsearch.cfm). Federal law is the minimum standard for research. However, institutional review boards (IRBs), another regulating oversight body, may have more stringent guidelines to conduct research; their standards may be stricter but cannot be lower than the federal standards found in 21 CFR.

B. There are also international guidelines for good clinical practice known as the International Conference on Harmonization of Technical Requirements for Registration of Pharmaceuticals for Human Use (ICH) as well as Good Clinical Practice (GCP) Guidelines known in the United States.

C. Many states have specific laws regarding insurance coverage. This is primarily seen with cancer studies and standards of care and some phase I studies, especially with life-threatening diseases. Generally, there are no specific state issues with clinical trials in rheumatology. However, it is always good to know the state's restrictions.

D. The Food and Drug Administration (FDA) requires an IRB to review and be given authority to approve, require modifications in, or disapprove all research activities covered by the IRB regulations [21 CFR 56.109(a)]. The IRB should also review the methods and materials that investigators propose to use to recruit subjects. The Department of Health and Human Services – Office of the Inspector General has special guidelines about conflict of interest and compliance.

E. The pharmaceutical industry also has special PhRMA guidelines and directives.

F. All human subjects are protected and must understand and sign an informed consent form (ICF) which explains their rights and duties during the trial as well as potential risks and harms of participation.

1
1.1
1.2
1.3
1.4
1.5
1.6
1.7
1.8
1.9

III. The Informed Consent.

A. What It Is:

1. A process.

2. A protection of rights.

3. Gives as much information as currently is known so an independent decision can be made about participating.

4. Gives information about what to expect by participating and resource information if there are questions.

B. What It Is Not:

1. A legally binding contract.

2. Participant giving up personal rights.

3. Not signing an informed consent will not upset the physician or the staff.

4. Stating that everything included in the informed consent will happen.

5. Be used to identify the patient to the public, on the news, or in a scientific paper.

C. What Is In The Title of the Study? – It will tell you the DESIGN.

D. Blind - Subject and investigator do not know which treatment the patient is receiving.

E. Single-Blind - Subjects do not know which treatment they are receiving but the investigator does know.

F. Double-Blind - Subject, investigator, and the monitor and data analyst do not know which treatment the subject is receiving.

G. Double-Dummy - Used in a tablet formulation study. Subjects receive a combination of tablets for both drugs being tested so that they will either receive active test drug and placebo comparator drug or placebo test drug and active comparator drug.

H. Double-Blind, Double-Dummy - Neither the physician nor the subject can tell which treatment the subject is receiving. To do this, both treatments must look identical. Sometimes this is not possible; perhaps one drug is a pill, and one is a liquid. A dummy liquid is made up to look like the active liquid, and a dummy pill is made up to look like the active pill. Subjects are given either the active pill and the dummy liquid or the active liquid and the dummy pill.

I. Randomized - The "gold standard" of clinical trials. Each subject is assigned to either the treatment or control (non-treatment) by a non-biased random generated program or mechanism.

J. Parallel Group - Each subject only receives one trial drug or placebo, or in another method the patient receives one active treatment or the standard of care treatment.

K. Crossover - Each subject receives all trial medications (i.e., each subject receives active and placebo treatments). There is a period between each treatment called the "wash-out period" where no medication is taken. The order of drug treatments is carefully determined through randomization.

L. Rescue - Generally the term for a generic drug to take while in a clinical trial when experiencing a crisis – such as acetaminophen for pain in an osteoarthritis drug trial or a specific rescue steroid protocol to follow when having a systemic lupus erythematosus flare.

M. Prospective - A trial conducted in a series of steps with each step depending on the results of the one before it.

N. Safety and Efficacy - Is the treatment safe and can it produce the desired benefit?

O. Open-label - Everyone knows what the subject is receiving.

P. Active Comparator - Also known as active control - when a treatment exists that is clearly better than doing nothing for the subject (i.e., giving the subject the placebo). The alternate treatment would be a standard-of-care therapy. The study would compare the test treatment to standard-of-care therapy. Methotrexate (MTX) is commonly seen as the active comparator in rheumatoid arthritis trials.

1
1.1
1.2
1.3
1.4
1.5
1.6
1.7
1.8
1.9

Q. Placebo - An inactive substance.

R. Cohort- A group of patients sharing a particular characteristic to be studied in a prospective or follow-up fashion.

IV. Phases of a Clinical Trial (see Table 1).

A. Concept and Discovery.

1. An idea is born – hypothesis.

B. Pre-clinical phase.

1. Refine/synthesize/ purify/ and acquire evidence.

2. 2 to 6 years on average for this phase, can take up to 20 years.

3. More or less 10,000 compounds are involved during this phase.

4. Looking for a desired effect/response.

C. Phase 0.

1. Phase 0 is presented here primarily because of the kindred relationship some of the biologic and the disease modifying drugs in rheumatology share with other medical specialty therapies. Not as likely to see this phase in rheumatology trials but it is useful information. The nurse may see some information in the investigators brochure with results from phase 0 studies particularly with the biologics used in cancer chemotherapy first. In 2006, the FDA updated its guidance on exploratory investigational new drug (IND) studies. The purpose was to expedite the discovery and development of new molecular entities to allow clinical evaluation before dose escalation, safety, and tolerance studies.

a. Phase 0 is an exploratory IND. This phase involves first-in-human testing of investigational agents at sub-therapeutic doses. (Not likely to produce treatment).

Table 1: Time and Money Trail for a New Drug

	Concept and Discovery	Pre Clinical	Phase 0	Phase 1	Phase 2	Phase 3	Phase 4
Number of Volunteers				20-100	100-500	Several 100(s) to several 1000(s)	1000(s)
Time Duration	2-20 Years	2-6 Years		6-12 Months	Several months up to 3 Years	2-3 Years	1-5 Years
Estimated Cost	$100 Million+	$100 Million+ per Year		$100 Million+	$150 Million+	$150 Million+	$100 Million+
Estimated number of drugs to pass Phase	5-10,000	5-10,000	250	4-5	2-3	1-2	1
Locations			Limited to Specialized Centers	Limited to Specialized Phase 1 Centers	Academic and Qualified Centers	Academic, Private Offices, and Qualified Centers	All Settings and International Centers

Sources: Adapted from Clinicaltrials.gov, U.S. Department of Health and Human Services (hhs.gov), Food & Drug Administration (fda.gov), and the Center for Drug Evaluation and Research (fda.gov/cder).

1
1.1
1.2
1.3
1.4
1.5
1.6
1.7
1.8
1.9

b. Phase 0 establishes an early opportunity before larger numbers of human subjects are tested to see if the agent is modulating its target.

c. Phase 0 establishes earlier in the pipeline whether further clinical development is warranted.

D. Phase I.

1. Safety phase - first-in-human studies.

2. This phase is the end of discovery and the beginning of development.

3. Prior to beginning this phase the IND study has been filed first with the FDA.

4. Phase I is closely monitored with healthy volunteers or low risk patients.

5. Approximately 20 to 80 patients over several weeks to several months are involved. It is a short-term design.

6. Phase 1 is designed to determine metabolism and pharmacologic actions of the drug in humans, side effects, associated pharmacokinetics and pharmacodynamics, and to gain early evidence on effectiveness.

E. Phase II.

1. Efficacy phase: Evaluates drug for effectiveness for a specific indication in subjects with a particular disease.

2. Determines common and short-term side effects such as nausea, vomiting, diarrhea, rash.

3. Evaluates and identifies associated risks.

4. Phase II trials are well controlled, closely monitored, and conducted with a relatively small number of subjects.

5. This is a pivotal phase in the drug development process; expect to see a drop of 66 to 75% of new formulations of drugs in trials at this phase.

6. Deeper Study.

a. Types of studies within this phase:

(1) Phase I/IIa, phase IIa, phase IIb, phase IIb/III.

(2) There is no official definition for each of these classifications, generally speaking:

(3) II, IIa will evaluate for absorption, metabolism, and pharmacodynamics of the drug.

(4) IIb, IIb/III generally evaluates more heavily for safety and efficacy and the clinical benefit.

F. Phase III.

1. Feasibility studies.

a. Success rate for a new drug during phase III is 25 to 30%. This is a pivotal phase in the life of the new drug.

b. Establishes safety and efficacy of primary endpoints with the selected dose in the intended population. Phase III sets the basic data for labeling and packaging.

c. Phase III is an expanded randomized controlled trial, generally blinded when comparing to a standard control, comparator, or placebo.

d. Phase III occurs only after success of phase II trials where the effectiveness has been established. Generally, this phase is more open to multicenter, international, private practices, and contract research organization centers.

e. Phase III further establishes safety and efficacy profile for an overall risk-benefit.

2. Deeper study.

a. Can also see a breakout of this phase, such as phase IIIa, and phase IIIb.

b. Phase IIIa is an FDA identifier that a new drug application is in process. It generates additional safety and efficacy data in very large numbers of subjects of the intended population as well as special populations with co-morbid conditions such as renal disease or post MI for two years. Phase IIIa includes a large amount of package insert information that is generated from the phase III and phase IIIa trials.

c. In phase IIIb trials the New Drug Application (NDA) has already been filed with the FDA. The drug is close to market but has not yet been approved. Phase IIIb studies may supplement earlier trials; may complete earlier trials such as extensions; and may examine quality-of-life issues and marketing issues.

1
1.1
1.2
1.3
1.4
1.5
1.6
1.7
1.8
1.9

G. Phase IV.

1. Phase IV trials are still controlled clinical trials on FDA-approved-for-market drugs.

2. They can be either post marketing surveillance studies which are observational and non-experimental, or they are marketing studies that support publications and gather evidence on how the drug is doing in the market.

3. Phase IV gathers data about medication interactions and information for different age groups and diverse populations. These trials:

a. Gather further safety and efficacy data.

b. Focus on an adverse event.

c. Study how the drug is doing in the market.

4. If there is a new label or a new indication desirable for this FDA-approved drug, the drug is returned to either a phase II or a phase III study for additional testing under an NDA. Phase IV is also used for detection of inadequately quantified adverse reactions and related risk factors.

Summary

Research in rheumatology nursing is designed to document, enhance, and validate the impact, both medically and economically, what rheumatology nurses have made and continue to make in practice, outcomes, and clinical research management. Rheumatology nurses everywhere are encouraged to embrace research procedures and methodologies to validate and document the profession. Educate yourself on the principals and guidelines of good clinical practice so that you may speak to those in your care with confidence regarding clinical trials.

References

Lanuza, D. M. (1999). Research and practice. In M.A. Mateo & K.T. Kirchoff (Eds.), *Using and conducting nursing research in the clinical setting (2nd ed., pp. 2-12). Philadelphia: W.B. Saunders.*

Schlotfeldt, R.M. (1977). Nursing research: Reflection of values. *Nursing Research, 26*(1), 4-8.

Stone, J. (2006). *Conducting clinical research.* Cumberland, MD: Mountainside MD Press.

U.S. Department of Health and Human Services, Food and Drug Administration Center for Drug Evaluation and Research (CDER). (2006). *Guidance for industry, investigators, and reviewers: Exploratory IND studies.* Washington, DC: Author.

1
1.1
1.2
1.3
1.4
1.5
1.6
1.7
1.8
1.9

SECTION 2

RHEUMATOLOGY NURSING ACROSS THE LIFESPAN:
PEDIATRICS

2
2.1
2.2
2.3
2.4
2.5
2.6
2.7
2.8
2.9
2.10
2.11

Contents of Section 2

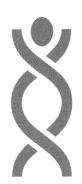

Section 2.1
Juvenile Idiopathic Arthritis

Maria Cusano-Sanzo, MSN, RN, CPN

Introduction

Mention the word arthritis and most people conjure up images of octogenarians with gnarly fingers walking with canes. But arthritis affects children as well. Close to 300,000 children in the United States suffer from some type of arthritis (www.rheumatology.org). This chapter will focus on addressing the specifics of juvenile idiopathic arthritis (JIA) (formerly referred to as juvenile rheumatoid arthritis.)

Learning Objectives

Upon completion of this chapter, the nurse will be able to:

1. Describe the significance of knowing the anti-nuclear antibody (ANA) value in children.

2. Identify the differences between types of JIA.

3. Identify three side effects of methotrexate (MTX).

4. Describe three biologics and their side effects.

Content Outline

I. Etiology/Epidemiology.

A. Unknown.

 1. Immune system goes into "overdrive" in response to a virus/illness and attacks body's healthy tissues in response.

 2. Synovial tissue swelling with increased production of synovial fluid.

 3. Cartilage is present, not worn away as in osteoarthritis.

 4. Because immobility increases pain and stiffness, symptoms are worse in the morning, after sleeping all night, naps, or long car rides.

 5. Blood work alone not a deciding factor in diagnosis.

B. Girls twice as likely to be affected as boys.

C. Most common age of onset is between 1 and 3 years of age.

D. Fifty percent of patients have oligoarthritis.

E. 16-43 per 100,000 children in U.S (Petty & Cassidy, 2011a).

II. Diagnosis.

A. Onset at < 16 years of age.

B. History of 6 weeks of arthritis (pain, swelling, limited range of motion).

 1. Joint pain, swelling, or limited range of motion of less than six weeks may be transient, reactive, or from trauma. It could also result from a septic joint or Lyme arthritis.

C. Onset type determined in first six months.

 1. Polyarthritis- 5 or more joints involved (Petty & Cassidy, 2011a).

   a. Usually of a more symmetrical presentation.

   b. Usually affects small joints of hands in teens, but in younger children, usually affects large joints (knees, ankles, wrists).

   c. Can be subcategorized into rheumatoid factor positive or negative.

 2. Oligoarthritis (pauciarticular disease) - 4 or fewer joints involved (Petty & Cassidy, 2011a).

   a. Arthritis is usually asymmetrical.

   b. Usually affects larger joints such as knees but not hips.

   c. Associated with highest rate of uveitis at 20% (Smith et al., 2005).

   d. Fifty to sixty percent of patients fall into this category.

   e. Can be subcategorized into persistent (stays as an oligo throughout disease) or extended (more than four joints after 6 months).

   f. "Severe pain out of proportion to the swelling is characteristic of leukemia and is a key feature that differentiates arthritis secondary to malignancy from JIA" (Punaro, 2011, p.166).

 3. Systemic-onset: Arthritis accompanied by rash and fever (Petty & Cassidy, 2011a).

   a. Rash is non-itchy, and evanescent salmon-colored.

   b. Fever is daily and spikes in the afternoon.

   c. Elevated white blood count (WBC) and decreased hemoglobin and hematocrit. Decreased WBC could also signify leukemia or macrophage activation syndrome (MAS).

   d. Fifteen percent will have an isolated episode with complete resolution of symptoms.

   e. May have associated pericarditis and or pleuritis.

   f. Ten percent of patients with JIA demonstrate systemic-onset.

 4. Psoriatic arthritis (Petty & Cassidy, 2011a).

   a. Arthritis associated with psoriasis; psoriasis may precede or follow symptoms of arthritis. Child must have arthritis of a finger or toe (called dactylitis) with associated tenosynovitis and a first degree relative with psoriasis.

 5. Enthesitis-related arthritis.

   a. Usually affects lower extremities and axial skeleton and is rheumatoid factor (RF) and ANA negative, but some may be HLA-B27 positive (Petty & Cassidy, 2011b).

   b. Lower back pain and stiffness.

c. Most common in males who may have a first-degree relative with the same diagnosis. Also often associated with inflammatory bowel disease and eye inflammation.

6. Undifferentiated arthritis (Petty & Cassidy, 2011a).

   a. A child who does not fit into the previous six categories or overlaps two or more categories.

III. Treatment.

A. Non-steroidal anti-inflammatory drugs (NSAIDs).

1. Used as a first-line medication.

2. Advise patient not to take with other NSAIDs.

3. Teach patient to take with food.

4. Lab work every six months to monitor liver and kidney function or as directed by the provider.

5. Most common side effects are gastrointestinal complaints (stomach upset).

B. Prednisone (orally or intravenously).

1. Ideally for short-term use as a "bridging medicine."

2. Warn about emotional lability, increased appetite, hyperactivity, and weight gain ("chipmunk cheeks").

3. Need to wean off and not stop abruptly.

C. Disease modifying anti-rheumatic drugs (DMARDs) are considered second-line medications. However, standard of care is to use early on to achieve better disease control with better short- and long-term prognosis for children with polyarticular and systemic disease:

1. Methotrexate (MTX):

   a. Works as an immunosuppressant.

   b. Used in pediatric oncology since the 1960s (COG, 2012) and childhood arthritis since the 1990s (Ruth & Passo, 2012).

   c. Instruct patient to hold MTX if febrile (> 101 degrees F) or for 24-48 hours if on antibiotics for an infection. Some recommendations are to hold MTX until off antibiotics completely.

d. Labs every two to three months to monitor white count (may drop) and liver function (may rise).

e. Most common side effects include nausea, mouth sores, and, rarely, hair loss.

f. Discuss birth control with sexually active patients as MTX can cause birth defects.

g. Can be given orally or subcutaneously once a week.

2. Sulfasalazine (SSZ) (Azulfidine®).

   a. Used as an anti-inflammatory/anti-bacterial (Ilowite & Laxer, 2011).

   b. Side effects include rash on sun-exposed skin, GI complaints, and, rarely, oral ulcers (Ilowite & Laxer, 2011).

   c. Given orally.

3. Hydroxychloroquine (Plaquenil®).

   a. Given orally daily.

   b. Need annual eye exam because of risk of retinal damage.

   c. Much more commonly used for adults with RA and children and adults with lupus. Less common today to treat children with JIA.

D. Biologics are the newer immune modulating therapies. Among the most common biologics used in rheumatology are:

1. Enbrel® (Etanercept).

   a. Tumor necrosis factor (TNF) alpha inhibitor.

   b. Given subcutaneously once or twice a week.

   c. Needs tuberculin skin test placed and read as negative before starting treatment.

   d. Warn patients about increased risk of infection and common injection site reactions.

   e. Teach patients to hold Enbrel® if febrile (temperature > 101 degrees F) or for the first 24-48 hours if on an antibiotic (or as directed by the physician).

   f. Common side effect is injection site reaction.

2. Humira® (Adalimumab).

   a. Tumor necrosis factor inhibitor.

   b. Given subcutaneously once every two weeks.

2
2.1
2.2
2.3
2.4
2.5
2.6
2.7
2.8
2.9
2.10
2.11

c. Needs tuberculin skin test placed and read as negative before starting treatment.

d. Warn patients about increased risk of infection and common injection site reactions. Teach patients to hold Humira® if febrile (temperature > 101 degrees F) or for first 24-48 hours if on an antibiotic (or as directed by the physician).

e. Common side effect is injection site reaction.

3. Remicade® (Infliximab).

a. Tumor necrosis factor inhibitor. Approved for GI (pediatric Crohn's disease and adult arthritis) but off label for JIA. Can be used when physician ordered and approved for off label use by insurance company.

b. Given intravenously at week 0, 2, and 4 and every 4 to 8 weeks thereafter, depending on how patient is doing.

c. Need tuberculin skin test placed and read as negative before initiating treatment.

d. Treatment must be held if febrile or ill.

e. Concern is for infusion reaction, especially after third infusion.

f. Pre-medicate with Tylenol® and Benadryl® per attending physician.

4. Kineret® (Anakinra).

a. Interleukin-1 medication given daily subcutaneously.

b. Used for systemic-onset JIA.

c. Redness and pain at injection site are common.

5. Orencia® (Abatacept).

a. T-cell inhibitor.

b. Given intravenously monthly at home or in clinic.

c. Also available in weekly subcutaneous form.

d. Common side effects include headache, dizziness, or itchiness with infusion.

6. Actemra® (Tocilizumab).

a. Interleukin-6 medication.

b. Given intravenously every two weeks for systemic JIA and every four weeks for polyarticular JIA.

c. Dizziness and headaches are common side effects.

d. Obtain CBC, sed rate, AST, ALT, GGT before every infusion and obtain cholesterol every three months.

7. Rituxan® (Rituximab).

a. B-cell inhibitor.

b. Given intravenously twice, two weeks apart.

c. Side effects include infection and infusion reaction.

d. Pre-medicate with hydrocortisone, acetaminophen, diphenhydramine, and ranitidine.

e. Monitor vital signs every 15 minutes during the first hour and every 30 minutes until infusion is complete.

f. First infusion is given at half the rate of second infusion.

8. Arcalyst® (Rilonacept).

a. Given subcutaneously once a week.

b. Injection site reactions a common side effect.

c. Serum lipid monitoring necessary (Ilowite & Laxer, 2011).

d. Swelling, pain, and redness at injection site are common.

9. Ilaris® (Canakinumab).

a. Interleukin-1 medication.

b. Given subcutaneously monthly.

c. Pain, redness, and swelling at injection site are common side effects. Cold and flu symptoms also are common side effects.

E. Physical Therapy.

1. Physical therapy for increasing strength and mobility is recommended with a regular exercise program.

F. Intra-articular joint injections.

1. If a child presents with one or two swollen joints, one option is to aspirate the joint of synovial fluid and inject a steroid directly into the joint. If successful (9-12 months of no symptoms), this alleviates the need for systemic, daily medications. Commonly used for children with oligoarthritis.

2
2.1
2.2
2.3
2.4
2.5
2.6
2.7
2.8
2.9
2.10
2.11

G. Nutrition.

1. It is helpful to refer to a nutritionist for education on healthy food choices and prevention of weight gain while on prednisone.

IV. Laboratory findings.

A. Complete blood count (CBC).

1. Normal white count in oligoarthritis and elevated or normal in other types unless low due to macrophage activation syndrome.

2. Decreased hemoglobin and hematocrit.

B. Erythrocyte sedimentation rate (ESR).

1. Non-specific marker of inflammation; may be elevated in arthritis.

2. May be elevated for other reasons, such as infection, recent illness, or even obesity.

C. Anti-nuclear antibody (ANA).

1. May be positive or negative in JIA. Ten percent or less of the population can have a positive ANA for no reason.

2. Important in determining frequency of eye exams and risk category for eye disease.

3. Often referred to as the "lupus test."

D. Rheumatoid factor (RF).

1. An antibody found in blood, more commonly in adults than in children (positive in children with rheumatoid factor positive JIA, usually teenage girls with small joint arthritis of hands and feet).

2. Often indicative of more erosive, chronic disease.

E. Cyclic citrullinated peptide (CCP).

1. A sensitive and specific antibody found in patients with rheumatoid arthritis, more common in adults than in children but also frequently positive in those children with rheumatoid factor positive JIA.

2. A newer lab test.

V. Co-morbid conditions.

A. Delay in sexual maturation.

B. Osteopenia/osteoporosis.

1. Due to prolonged steroid use.

C. Micrognathia.

D. Decreased fitness.

1. Multi-factorial: Weight gain with steroid intake, decreased activity with flare of disease, decreased lung capacity, parental overprotectiveness.

E. Dietary changes, weight gain/loss (helpful to see pediatric nutritionist).

F. Uveitis.

1. Most common among young girls with oligoarticular JIA who are ANA positive (Petty & Rosenbaum, 2011).

2. Follow-up with a pediatric ophthalmologist.

VI. Nursing implications.

A. Education.

1. Patient (and parent) education is of paramount importance, especially in the newly-diagnosed patient. Patients should be given handouts on the disease. Also helpful is a staff contact name and number if patients or families have questions once they get home. Families of newly diagnosed children can be asked if they would like to talk to a family with a child similar in age and diagnosis. If they agree and give permission, staff contacts an appropriate family and gives them the family's contact information. Support groups also are available through the local arthritis foundation chapter.

B. Psychosocial.

1. A child's sense of belonging may be affected when after-school activities and sports participation are interrupted by flares, physicians' appointments, or physical therapy appointments.

2. Play dates or trips to the shopping mall with peers may be cancelled or postponed because of fatigue or an exacerbation of symptoms, making children feel different.

3. If available, have the families speak with a pediatric social worker or someone from the family support program at the hospital.

2
2.1
2.2
2.3
2.4
2.5
2.6
2.7
2.8
2.9
2.10
2.11

C. Medications (see Treatment).

D. Resources (see Suggested Readings and Internet Resources).

E. Educational impact.

1. Children with arthritis may have disrupted sleep because of pain. Pain and lack of sleep lead to decreased ability to concentrate and thus interfere with learning.

2. Some children wake up an hour earlier to take NSAIDs, go back to bed to give the medications time to work, and then wake up to start the day and activities of daily living when their pain is better controlled.

3. Simple activities, such as holding a pencil or sitting cross-legged on the floor, may cause the child with arthritis to experience increased pain and stiffness.

4. Students with arthritis may benefit from an individualized education plan to include accommodations such as use of the elevator, having an extra set of books at home, having extra time to get from one class to another, and rest periods in the nurse's office, to name a few.

5. Because immobility increases pain and stiffness, physical education is encouraged on a self-limiting basis. Instead of running the mile, the child can run the quarter mile until he/she is not able to run without pain. At that point, instead of sitting out, the child continues by walking the remainder of the way, if possible. If wrist pain prevents the child from doing push-ups, perhaps sit-ups might be more tolerable.

F. Financial impact.

1. Parents of children with a chronic disease, not just those with arthritis, are faced with increased financial burdens (e.g., gas and parking expenses to get to physicians' appointments, co-pays for medications and physicians' appointments, and days missed from work).

2. Unscheduled visits and time off for flare of symptoms may increase financial stress. Parents should be encouraged to complete Family Medical Leave Act (FMLA) paperwork for their employers.

Summary

Unlike patients from two or three decades ago, those afflicted with JIA have a plethora of medication options to help them control their arthritis. The advent of biologics has improved the outcome of functionality, school attendance, and self-esteem and has decreased joint erosion and joint damage. The rheumatology nurse's role is critical to the education of patients and families dealing with this autoimmune disorder.

Acknowledgment

The author thanks Barbara Edelheit, MD, and Karen Damon Callahan, MLS, RN, for their help with proofreading this chapter.

References

COG, Childrens Oncology Group (2012). http://www.childrensoncologygroup.org/downloads/COG_Update_on_the_Methotrexate_Shortage.pdf

Ilowite, N. T., & Laxer, R. M. (2011). Pharmacology and drug therapy. In J. T. Cassidy, R. E. Petty, R. M. Laxer, & C. B. Lindsley (Eds.), *Textbook of pediatric rheumatology* (6th ed., pp. 71-126). Philadelphia, PA: Saunders Elsevier.

Petty, R. E., & Cassidy, J. T. (2011a). Chronic arthritis in childhood. In J. T. Cassidy, R. E. Petty, R. M. Laxer, & C. B. Lindsley (Eds.), *Textbook of pediatric rheumatology* (6th ed., pp. 211-235). Philadelphia, PA: Saunders Elsevier.

Petty, R. E., & Cassidy, J. T. (2011b). Enthesitis-related arthritis (juvenile ankylosing spondylitis). In J. T. Cassidy, R. E. Petty, R. M. Laxer, & C. B. Lindsley (Eds.), *Textbook of pediatric rheumatology* (6th ed., pp. 272-286). Philadelphia, PA: Saunders Elsevier.

Petty, R. E., & Rosenbaum, J. T. (2011). Uveitis in juvenile idiopathic arthritis. In J. T. Cassidy, R. E. Petty, R. M. Laxer, & C. B. Lindsley (Eds.), *Textbook of pediatric rheumatology* (6th ed., pp. 305-314). Philadelphia, PA: Saunders Elsevier.

Punaro, M. (2011). Rhuematologic conditions in children who may present to the orthopaedic surgeon. *Journal of the American Academy of Orthopedic Surgeons, 19*(3), 163-169.

Ruth NM, Passo MH. Juvenile idiopathic arthritis: management and therapeutic options. *Ther Adv Musculoskelet Dis.* 2012;4(2):99-110.

Smith, J. A., Thompson, D. J., Whitcup, S. M., Suhler, E., Clarke, G., & Smith, Barron, K.S. (2005). A randomized, placebo-controlled, double-masked clinical trial of etanercept for the treatment of uveitis associated with juvenile idiopathic arthritis. *Arthritis and Rheumatism, 53*(1), 18-23.

Suggested Readings

Living with Juvenile Rheumatoid Arthritis by S. H. Gray (2003).

The Child with Arthritis in the School Setting by Maria Sanzo (2008).

Kids Get Arthritis Too: A Wellness Letter for Families of Children with Arthritis. A bimonthly publication of the Arthritis Foundation. http://www.arthritis.org/media/kgat

It's Not Just Growing Pains: A Guide to Childhood Muscle, Bone and Joint Pain, Rheumatic Diseases, and the Latest Treatments by T.J. Lahman.

Questions & Answers About...Juvenile Arthritis. National Institutes of Health.

Keeping a Secret: A Story About Juvenile Rheumatoid Arthritis by E.M. Melas (2001).

Raising a Child with Arthritis: A Parent's Guide. The Arthritis Foundation (1998).

Your Child with Arthritis: A Family Guide for Caregiving by L.B. Tucker, B.A. DeNardo, J.A. Stebulis, & J.G. Schaller (1996).

Yoga for Arthritis by Loren Fishman and Ellen Saltonstall (2008).

Internet Resources

» www.arthritis.org
» www.rheumatology.org
» www.nih.gov

2
2.1
2.2
2.3
2.4
2.5
2.6
2.7
2.8
2.9
2.10
2.11

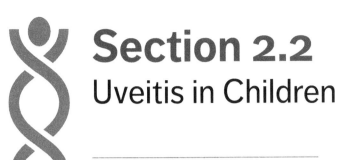

Section 2.2
Uveitis in Children

Cathy Patty-Resk, MSN, RN, CPNP

Introduction

Uveitis is an inflammatory eye condition. It can be diagnosed and treated by an opthalmologist. Uveitis precedes juvenile idiopathic arthritis (JIA) in approximately six percent of the cases. Uveitis can also be a co-morbidity of juvenile idiopathic arthritis. Studies have identified cytokines such as Interleukin 1Beta, IL-2, IL-6, interferon-y and TNF-alpha in the aqueous solution of patients with uveitis (Horai & Caspi 2011). These studies have also noted successful treatment of inflammatory uveitis with biologics. However, in many ophthalmology practices the ophthalmologist prefers to have a pediatric rheumatologist co-manage the patient when systemic immunmodulators are necessary to control the ocular inflammation.

Learning Objectives

Upon completion of this chapter, the nurse will be able to:

1. Understand the basic anatomy of the eye and which structures are involved in uveitis.

2. Identify the most common first-line ophthalmology treatment.

3. Identify at least two high risk groups.

4. Understand and explain to patients and families what uveitis is, their risk and the need for and importance of an eye examination.

5. Anticipate what type of medications and treatment their patients with uveitis may be taking or advancing toward.

Content Outline

I. Basic Eye Anatomy
(See Figure 1 and Figure 2).

II. Parts of the Ophthalmology Exam.

A. Visual Acuity.

B. Ocular Pressures.

C. Slit Lamp Exam.

   1. View anterior eye structures.

     a. Conjunctiva.

       (1) Anterior Chamber.

     b. Cornea.

     c. Iris - synechiae.

D. Dilated Exam.

   1. View posterior eye structures.

     a. Retina - looking for inflammatory cells in the vitreous, a jelly-like substance filling the back of the eye.

     b. Macula - looking for macular edema which indicates elevated pressure on the macula. If there are wrinkles in the macula, maculopathy is present due to low pressures. The macula is responsible for central vision.

III. Definition of Uveitis.

A. Uveitis is inflammation of the uvea, the middle layer of the eye that consists of the iris, ciliary body and choroid.

IV. Four Main Causes of Uveitis:

A. Eye injury.

B. Inflammatory diseases.

C. Infections.

D. Exposure to toxic chemicals (ie. pesticides, acids).

V. Basic statistics of JIA-associated inflammatory uveitis
(Cassidy, Petty, Laxer, & Lindlesly, 2011; Muthappan, 2010; and Foster, n.d.).

A. 64-80% of patients have eyes affected bilaterally.

B. 12% (approximately) with pauci JIA will go blind, usually due to chronic low grade inflammation of eye/eyes.

C. Highest risk of anterior uveitis is within 2 years after onset of JIA and declines >8 years and after onset of JIA.

Figure 1: Drawing of the Eye

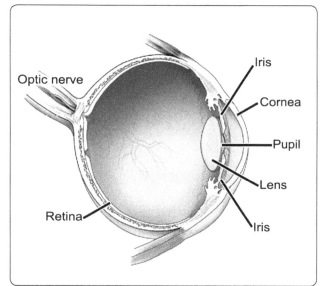

Source: National Eye Institute, National Institutes of Health.

Figure 2: Drawing of the Eye: Detail

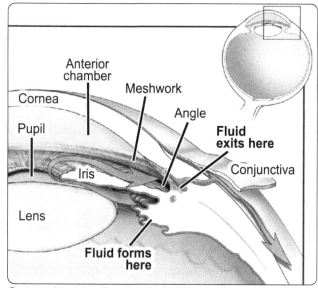

Source: National Eye Institute, National Institutes of Health.

D. Antinuclear antibody (ANA) negative children have more ocular complications, possibly due to less frequent screening.

VI. Risk stratification for children being diagnosed with JIA-associated inflammatory uveitis:
(Campanilho-Marques R, et al, 2014; Muthappan, 2014.)

A. Type of JIA.

1. Pauciarticular JIA > risk.

2. Systemic onset JIA (SOJIA) < risk.

B. Biomarkers.

1. High risk.
   a. +ANA.
   b. DR5(HLA-DR5).
   c. DR1(HLA-DR1).

2. Low risk.
   a. +RF less likely to develop uveitis.

C. Age.

1. Mean age 4 years ; younger age > risk.

D. Sex.

1. Female/male ratio 4.4 : 1.

2. Males have worse prognosis.

E. Years of disease.

1. Higher risk at onset of disease.

VII. Four Types of Inflammatory Uveitis.

A. Anterior uveitis is inflammation seen in the iris (iritis) or the iris and ciliary body.

1. Diagnosed by Slit Lamp Exam.

B. Intermediate uveitis is inflammation of the ciliary body or vitreous (peripheral retina) (Janigian, 2014).

1. Dilated Exam: Snowbanks, which is the presence of white exudates(blood vessels and other histologic debris) which are aggregates of snowballs which consist of inflammatory cells in the vitreous.

C. Posterior uveitis is inflammation of the retina or choroid.

1. Dilated Exam: Macular edema.

D. Diffuse uveitis (also called panuveitis) is inflammation of all areas of the uvea.

1. Slit Lamp and Dilated Exam: All above findings possible.

VIII. Signs & Symptoms.

A. Redness.

B. Pain.

C. Photophobia.

D. Tearing.

E. Lid puffiness or drooping.

F. Blurry vision.

G. Floaters.

H. Photopsia (seeing flashing lights).

I. Decreased visual acuity (mild usually 20/40).

IX. High Risk Groups
(Campanilho-Marques, 2014).

A. Pauci JIA.

B. +ANA (usually >1:360).

C. +HLA-B27 (Spondyloarthropathies).

D. +HLA-B51 (Behçet's).

E. Inflammatory Bowel Disorders.

F. Ankylosing Spondylitis.

G. Psoriatic Arthritis.

X. Less Common Risk Groups.

A. Sarcoidosis.

B. Interstitial nephritis.

C. Relapsing polychondritis.

D. Vasculitis.

2
2.1
2.2
2.3
2.4
2.5
2.6
2.7
2.8
2.9
2.10
2.11

XI. Treatment

(Cassidy, 2011; Janigian, 2014;
Semeraro, 2014; Muthappan, 2014).

A. Pharmaceutical Interventions.

1. Predforte 1% ophthalmic drops (if only anterior segment inflammation).

2. Periocular corticosteroid injections.

3. Atropine or homatropine (cycloplegics).

4. Intravitreal triamcinalone acetonide.

5. Methotrexate (MTX).

6. Infliximab.

B. Surgical Interventions:

1. Cataract removal.

2. Band keratopathy treatment.

XII. Prognosis

(Petty, 2011; Taylor et al, 2012).

A. More severe condition with macular edema; has guarded prognosis.

B. Anterior segment late findings:

1. Synechiae.

2. Band keratopathy.

3. Cataracts.

4. Glaucoma.

C. Later in disease course.

1. 28-50% more severe visual loss secondary to chronic macular edema.

2. 15% uveitic glaucoma.

3. 3-22% retinal detachment.

4. 6-28% vitreous hemorrhage.

5. 15-20% cataracts (not dependent on steroid use).

XIII. Ophthalmology Exam Schedule for Children with Uveitis.

A. Regular/Routine check-ups:

1. Every 3 months, 6 months or yearly depending on age and history of uveitis flares.

B. During uveitis flares:

1. Can be more than once a week, weekly or monthly; dependent upon severity and medications being used to treat.

Summary

Recent studies have shown that TNF alpha inhibitors are more effective than methotrexate (MTX) in treating uveitis that persists beyond initial treatment of predforte 1%. However, many providers continue to use MTX and then progress to infliximab or other TNF inhibitor. However, MTX is recommended as adjunct therapy to infliximab for the prevention of anti-chimeric antibody formation against the infliximab's mouse protein. It should be noted, at this time infliximab is still considered by the FDA as off label use in uveitis. To be successful with these appeals to document the medical necessity of such use, the rheumatology nurse must be knowledgeable of risk factors associated with uveitis, understand the condition of uveitis, its treatment and prognosis. Rheumatology nurses are in a prime position to make a very positive impact on the percentage of patients with chronic uveitis who are at risk for potential loss of sight.

References

Acta Reumatol Port. 2014 Apr-Jun;39(2):116-122. Prognostic value of antinuclear antibodies in juvenile idiopathic arthritis and anterior uveitis. Results from a systematic literature review. Campanilho-Marques R, Bogas M, Ramos F, Santos MJ, Fonseca JE.

Cassidy, J.T., Petty, R.E., Laxer, R.M. & Lindsley, C.B. (2011). Textbook of Pediatric Rheumatology (6th ed.). Philadelphi: Saunders.

Drug Des Devel Ther. 2014 Mar 24;8:341-8. Anti-TNF therapy for juvenile idiopathic arthritis-related uveitis. Semeraro F1, Arcidiacono B2, Nascimbeni G1, Angi M1, Parolini B2, Costagliola C3.

Foster, C. S. (n.d.), Juvenile idiopathic arthritis and uveitis: What is it and what is its effect on the eye? http://www.uveitis.org/docs/dm/juvenile_idiopathic_arthritis_and_uveitis.pdf

Horai R, Caspi RR (2011). Cytokines in autoimmune uveitis. *Journal of Interferon & Cytokine Research.* October 2011, 31(10): 733-744. doi:10.1089/jir.2011.0042.

Janigian Jr., Robert H., Filippopoulos, Theodoros, Welcome, Brian A. Medscape Intermediate uveitis (2014). http://emedicine.medscape.com/article/1208794-overview

Muthappan. Eyewiki 2014. http://eyewiki.aao.org/Juvenile_Idiopathic_Arthritis

Taylor SR, Lightman SL, Sugar EA, Jaffe GJ, Freeman WR, Altaweel MM, Kozak I, Holbrook JT, Jabs DA, Kempen JH. The impact of macular edema on visual function in intermediate, posterior, and panuveitis. Ocul Immunol Inflamm. 2012;20:171-81.

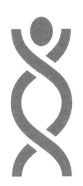

Section 2.3
Systemic Juvenile Idiopathic Arthritis

Samantha R. Judd, MSN, RN, CPNP

Introduction

Systemic juvenile idiopathic arthritis (JIA) accounts for 5–15% of patients diagnosed with some form of JIA in North American and European populations (Dewitt et al., 2013). Systemic onset juvenile idiopathic arthritis (SOJIA) is a subset of JIA that involves multiple organ systems and can result in life threatening complications. This chapter will focus on educating on the specifics of SOJIA and dangers during flares.

Learning Objectives

Upon completion of this chapter, the nurse will be able to:

1. Identify the three most common manifestations of SOJIA.

2. Describe the basic dysregulation of the immune system with SOJIA that can lead to life threatening events and death.

3. Describe three nursing interventions that should be done to help reduce the risk of severe complications of a patient on a biologic.

4. Identify three resources that families should be aware of when child is diagnosed with a lifelong disease.

Content Outline

I. Etiology/Epidemiology.

A. Unknown.

B. Deregulated innate immune response that results in an increase in the production of inflammatory cell markers.

C. Recent studies with untreated patients during the early phase of the disease showed over-representation of genes of the IL-6 and TLR/IL-1R pathways (Inflammatory pathway markers) (Dewitt et al., 2012).

D. Children of both sexes are affected equally (De Benedetti & Schneider, 2010).

E. Onset has a broad range of ages with most occurring between 1-5 years old, however it may occur <1 year or >5years (De Benedetti & Schneider, 2010).

II. Diagnosis.

A. According to the International League of Associations for Rheumatology (ILAR) (Dewitt et al., 2012) the diagnostic criteria for SOJIA includes:

1. Fever ≥2 weeks, quotidian in pattern (≥39°C at least once a day and returns to ≤37°C), documented daily for ≥3 days.

2. Arthritis in ≥1 joint (for ≥6 weeks).

3. At least one of the following: Evanescent erythematous rash, generalized lymph node enlargement, hepatomegaly and/or splenomegaly or serositis.

4. Salmon colored rash that may appear in linear streaks, or as macules surrounded by a zone of pallor and larger lesions with central clearing (DeBenedetti & Schneider, 2010) .

III. Complications.

A. Events that precipitate flares are not always identifiable. Life threatening complications of SOJIA can occur at any time with flares. These children are often moved to the Pediatric Intensive Care Unit (PICU) when the following occur:

1. Cardiac.
   a. Endocarditis.
   b. Pericardial effusion.
   c. Myocarditis.

2. Pulmonary.
   a. Pleural effusion.
   b. Pulmonary disease.

3. Hepatic.
   a. Hepatomegaly.
   b. Hepatitis.

4. Splenic.
   a. Splenomegaly.

5. Macrophage Activation Syndrome (MAS) (See Section on MAS). Most devastating (DeBenedetti and Schneider, 2010).

IV. Treatment.

A. According to Dewitt et al. (2012) there are several options of treatment plans:

1. Glucocorticoids: Either prednisone 1 mg/kg orally daily (max 60 mg/day) continue until improvement then taper the dose. Or methylprednisone (MP) 30 mg/kg IV daily (max 1 gm/day) for three days (equals one pulse treatment), may be repeated multiple times, MP pulses only once weekly.

   a. This therapy may be used by itself or in conjunction with methotrexate (MTX) or biologic DMARDs (disease modifying antirheumatic drug).

   b. Used mostly as a "bridging" medication for short term use as the DMARDs and biologics are initiated. As they eliminate cytokines to the point of the child reaching a state of improvement, the steroids are tapered.

   c. Always make sure the child is tapering doses over an appropriate amount of time that is reflective of the history of their steroid use. Make sure they never stop their steroids abruptly. This can lead to adrenal insufficiency and death in some cases.

   d. On high dose or long term steroid regimens, the child may develop cushingoid facies, hyperactivity, increased appetite with potential for weight gain, emotional lability and eventually may become immunocompromised. Make sure your families are well educated about these side effects. Many of these side effects can create a negative self-image for the child or adolescent.

2. MTX 0.5 mg/kg-1 mg/kg weekly (max of 25 mg) or 30 mg/m2 weekly.

   a. May be given PO, SQ, IV or IM. May be used in conjunction with glucocorticoids and/or NSAIDs.

   b. MTX is a DMARD. Believed to work by blocking enzymes (dihydrofolic acid reductase, purine & thymidylic acid to interfere with DNA synthesis, repair and cellular replication) that are involved in the immune system. However the direct effect that it has on arthritis is not determined (Cannon, 2012).

   c. Adverse effects could include: Stomatitis, mouth sores, stomach ache (PO), nausea and vomiting (PO), decrease in the immune response, possible liver and bone damage.

   d. Must be administered in conjunction with 1 mg of folic acid daily to replenish folic acid which will help prevent MTX toxicity. Folic acid deficiency may lead to oral sores/stomatitis.

   e. Live vaccines should be avoided.

   f. Discuss proper birth control with teens during therapy and up to 3 months after discontinuation due to the teratogenic effects of MTX.

3. Anakinra (ANK) (Kineret®) 2 mg/kg (max 100 mg) SubQ Daily.

   a. If the child is non-responsive to the ANK or is worsening, the dosage may be increased to 4 mg/kg to a max of 200 mg.

   b. ANK may be given in conjunction with glucocorticoids, MTX and NSAIDs.

   c. ANK is an anti-IL-1 treatment. It blocks receptors within the inflammatory pathway to help reduce the number of inflammatory cells being produced.

   d. Side effects include becoming significantly immunocompromised, putting patient at risk for infections as well as headaches, and local site reaction (Patel, 2012).

   e. Make sure child does not receive live vaccines.

   f. Make sure the child has a negative QuantiFERON® - TB Gold test done or a negative purified protein derivative (PPD) test for tuberculosis.

   g. It must be given each day at the same time, best if it is warmed to room temperature before given. Ice may be applied to the injection site prior to administration. Educate parents to not rub site after giving and sites must be rotated.

   h. Occasional local site injection reaction may occur. Re-educate family on the recommended injection guidelines (letting medication reach room temp. before administering and icing area immediately after injection).

   i. Discuss proper birth control with teens during therapy due to teratogenic effects.

4. Tocilizumab (TCZ) (Actemra®) 8 mg/kg (if >30 kg) or 12 mg/kg (if <30 kg) IV every 2 weeks.

   a. May be given by itself or in conjunction with Glucocorticoids, MTX or NSAIDs.

   b. TCZ is a recombinant humanized anti-IL6 receptor monoclonal antibody of the immunoglobulin IgG1K (American College of Rheumatology, 2013).

   c. QuantiFERON® - TB Gold blood test or PPD must be negative and a complete blood count and liver function tests must be done prior to beginning TCZ infusions.

   d. No live vaccine administration while child is on this medication!

   e. Do not administer if the child is displaying signs of an infection.

   f. Mild infusion reactions include: Chills and flushing. If this occurs slow down the infusion rate and monitor (American College of Rheumatology, 2013).

   g. Severe infusion reactions include: Hives, shortness of breath, anaphylaxis, swelling of face or hands, fever, chills, high or low blood pressure and chest pain (American College of Rheumatology, 2013). In the event that this occurs, stop the infusion and activate rapid response/ call 911. Make sure you have emergency equipment available such as IV access, oxygen supplementation and epinephrine. Do not hesitate to give epinephrine if the above signs of severe reaction occur.

   h. Discuss proper birth control with teens during therapy due to teratogenic effects.

2
2.1
2.2
2.3
2.4
2.5
2.6
2.7
2.8
2.9
2.10
2.11

V. Laboratory markers and Diagnostic Tests.

A. According to Burns et al. (2013) the initial work up for SOJIA should include:

1. Complete blood count: This would demonstrate signs of chronic inflammation such as a possible decrease in hemoglobin, an increase in platelet count or an elevated white count.

2. Acute phase reactants, such as: Erythrocyte sedimentation rate (ESR) and C-reactive protein(CRP). Both would be elevated. CRP would be significantly elevated.

3. Albumin levels would be low as a result of the inflammation.

4. Liver enzymes, such as alanine transaminase (ALT) and aspartate transaminase (AST), may be high. Gamma-glutamyl transferase (GGT) may be elevated with hepatic involvement.

5. Immunology tests, such as: ANA, C3/C4 levels, IgG, IgA, IgM, Rheumatoid Factor (RF) and cyclic citrullinated peptide (CCP).

6. When severe inflammation is present with overproduction of cytokines, evaluate for macrophage activation syndrome (MAS): One characteristic finding is extremely elevated ferritin levels (see section on MAS).

7. Other: Lactate dehydrogenase (LDH) was elevated in 90% of patients (Tsai, Lee, Yu, Wang, Yang...& Chiang, 2012).

B. Radiographs (X-rays) will typically reveal arthritis: Soft tissue and bone abnormalities. Joints that are most symptomatic and affected should have radiographs done to evaluate for joint damage. Radiographs generally show bony growth (inflammation) and joint space narrowing.

C. Magnetic resonance imaging (MRI) will show bone marrow edema and early erosions undectable by X-rays.

VI. Outpatient treatments:

A. Physical therapy and occupational therapy depending on joint involvement and disease state.

1. Best to wait until joint inflammation is under better control to allow for low pain or pain free PT/OT sessions for best results.

2. Take into consideration the fact that health insurance will only pay for a certain amount of sessions per calendar year.

3. Plan to maximize therapy to make sure child is getting most out of PT/OT.

B. Adjunctive treatments may include physical therapy, ice, heat and/ or splinting of affected joints, but the treatment for SOJIA, much like JIA, is largely pharmacologic. Complementary, alternative, and traditional medication(s) often are used by patients to manage symptoms, but the scientific data supporting their effectiveness are limited or nonexistent (Stanley & Ward-Smith, 2011).

C. Support groups for children with arthritis or SOJIA. The child will need support from peers that are experiencing similar stressors and alterations of childhood.

D. Encourage child to participate in low impact activities such as swimming, yoga or elliptical to help keep joints in motion without causing pain or damage to them.

VII. Nursing Implications:

A. Follow the infusion and injection guidelines strictly when administering immunosuppressive medications to the child.

B. Make sure **NO LIVE VACCINES** while undergoing immunosuppressive treatment.

C. Be aware of common strategies that would be helpful when the child is developing common injection site reactions such as rotating the site, applying ice before administration, allowing the medication to sit at room temperature for longer and not "rubbing" the site post administration.

D. Educate families on the importance of regular follow up with providers and taking medications as prescribed.

E. Encourage parents to have Individualized Educational Plans (IEPs) and 504 plans developed for their child to ensure school success and facilitate normalization in the school setting.

F. Educate on insurance that may be available to help supplement the cost of all of the encompassing treatments. This may be state programs besides Medicaid, pharmaceutical assistance programs or even hospital-based one-time assistance.

G. Encourage parents to have Family Medical Leave Act (FMLA) forms filled out so that their employment and health insurance will not be in jeopardy due to missing work while caring for their ill child or accompanying child to the many medical appointments.

Summary

The child with SOJIA presents many challenges to the provider, nurse and family. It is important that the parents are able to recognize early signs of disease flares to avoid the serious complications that can occur with rapid onset flares or flares with delayed treatment. The nurse plays a key role in educating parents on the many facets of this complicated systemic disease and how to grow up with as much normalcy as possible.

References

American College of Rheumatology, (2013). *Actemra® (tocilizumab)*. ARHP practice committee. Retrieved from: www.rheumatology.org

Burns, C.E., Dunn, A.M., Starr, N.B., and Blosser, C. (2013). *Pediatric primer care (5th edition)*. Philadelphia. Saunders.

Cannon, M. (2012). *Methotrexate (rheumatrex, trexall)*. American College of Rheumatology. Retrieved from: www.rheumatology.org.

Dewitt, E., Kimura, Y., Beukelman, T., Nigrovic P, P., Onel, K., Prahalad, S., & Wallace, C. (2012). Consensus treatment plans for new-onset systemic juvenile idiopathic arthritis. *Arthritis Care & Research, 64*(7), 1001-1010. doi:10.1002/acr.21625

De Benedetti, F. and Schneider, R.(2010). Systemic Juvenile Idiopathic Arthritis. In J.T. Cassidy, R.E. Petty, R.M. Laxer & C.B. Lindsley (Eds.), *Textbook of Pediatric Rheumatology* (6th ed., pp.236-247). Philadelphia, PA: Saunders Elsevier.

Patel, D. (2012). *Anakinra (Kineret®)*. American College of Rheumatology. Retrieved from: www.rheumatology.org.

Stanley, L. C., & Ward-Smith, P. (2011). The Diagnosis and Management of Juvenile Idiopathic Arthritis. *Journal Of Pediatric Healthcare*, 25(3), 191-194. doi:10.1016/j.pedhc.2010.12.003

Tsai, H., Lee, J., Yu, H., Wang, L., Yang, Y., & Chiang, B. (2012). Initial manifestations and clinical course of systemic onset juvenile idiopathic arthritis: A ten-year retrospective study. *Journal Of The Formosan Medical Association*, 111(10), 542-549. doi:10.1016/j.jfma.2011.06.013

2
2.1
2.2
2.3
2.4
2.5
2.6
2.7
2.8
2.9
2.10
2.11

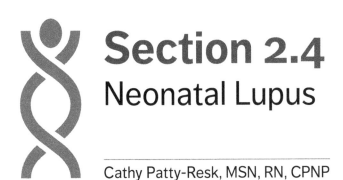

Section 2.4
Neonatal Lupus

Cathy Patty-Resk, MSN, RN, CPNP

Introduction

Neonatal lupus (NL) is a passively acquired autoimmune disease that occurs in a very small percentage of all fetuses and neonates. It occurs when a mother who has elevated SSA/Ro serum levels, and/or, SSB/La serum levels (both also referred to as extractable nuclear antigens [ENA]) transmits RoRNP autoantibodies through the placenta. Fetuses and neonates may present with congenital heart block (CHB) or skin features and less commonly both issues (Buyon, 2010). It is imperative that the nurse and nurse practitioner can identify fetus' and infants at risk for NL or those who present with signs of congenital heart block to decrease mortality in these infants.

Learning Objectives

Upon completion of this chapter, the nurse will be able to:

1. Identify mothers at high risk of delivering infant with NL.

2. Recommend safe pharmacologic therapy during pregnancy which may prevent development of NL.

3. Identify the two types of NL and list four signs of each.

4. Implement appropriate monitoring and testing of the neonate suspected of having NL or at high risk of NL.

5. Order appropriate testing of the mother who does not have a known history of rheumatologic disorder when her infant is suspected as having or has been born with NL

I. Risk factors for NL
(Buyon, Lindsley, & Silverman, 2011).

A. Mother with autoimmune disease.

   1. Systemic Lupus Erythematosus (highest risk).

   2. Sjögren's Syndrome (highest risk).

B. Mother with high SSA/Ro and/or SSB/La antibody titers.

C. Mother had previous child with NL skin or cardiac manifestations.

D. Mother had previous child with sinoatrial or atrioventricular (SA/AV) node firing or conduction abnormality.

E. Infant with high SSA/Ro and/or SSB/La antibody titers.

F. Note: A mother with an autoimmune disease or elevated SSA/Ro and/or SSB/La antibodies can safely breastfeed their infant without worry of transmitting NL. NL is not caused or worsened by breastfeeding (Buyon, Lindsley, and Silverman, 2011).

II. NL during the gestational period Best practice: Cardiac monitoring and passive treatment via mother (Buyon, 2014; Buyon, Lindsley, & Silverman, 2011).

A. Usually first identified when fetal bradycardia is identified.

   1. Bradycardia detected on Doppler examination during routine obstetrician (OB) visit.

   2. Very high fetal morbidity and mortality at this point.
      a. AV node fibrosis.
      b. Other congenital heart abnormalities also possible.

B. Doppler ultrasound frequency schedule determined by OB.

C. Pulsed Doppler fetal echocardiography 18th-26th week gestation; then every other week until 32 weeks (general recommendation but no formal guidelines) (Buyon, Lindsley, & Silverman, 2011).

   1. Doppler technique- mechanical PR interval (Buyon, 2014).

D. Maternal medications can help prevent CHB in fetus and neonate (Buyon, 2014).

   1. Hydroxychloroquine 400 mg orally daily from week six through entire pregnancy.
      a. Effects on fetuses well studied in mothers with SLE.
      b. Very low risk to baby.
      c. Has been used in pregnant women for many years.

   2. Intravenous Immunoglobulin (IVIG): Not proven to be effective.

   3. Dexamethasone.
      a. Poorly documented cases of untreated fetus'
      b. Reported very effective in some studies; but not proven to be effective vs. untreated fetus'
      c. Carry serious risks to mother and fetus.

III. Signs of NL in the neonate.

A. May first appear at birth or up to six months of age.

B. Bradycardia.

C. Doppler ultrasound.

   1. Heart block on electrocardiogram (ECG) (1st, 2nd and 3rd degree).

   2. Echocardiogram (ECHO).
      a. Detection of fibrosis.
      b. Other cardiac anomalies.

D. Skin rash (see Cutaneous NL below).

E. Elevated liver function tests (see Liver disease below).

IV. Two types of NL (Buyon, 2014; Buyon, Lindsley, & Silverman, 2011).

A. Cutaneous NL.

   1. Timing of rash.

2
2.1
2.2
2.3
2.4
2.5
2.6
2.7
2.8
2.9
2.10
2.11

a. Sometimes present at birth.

b. Most commonly develops within first few weeks of life.

c. Absent at birth or usually develops between 6-12weeks.

d. Can occurs any time after birth (0-6mos).

e. Polycyclic.

f. Rarely develops after 6mos. of age.

g. Resolves when maternal antibodies are no longer present.

h. Mean duration 17 weeks.

i. Cutaneous telangiectasis can occur at 6-12mos.

(1) Affects 10% infants with C-NL.

(2) Usually bilateral.

(3) Fade over time, sometimes takes years.

2. Distribution of rash.

a. Face and scalp most common distribution (not malar area).

b. Generalized rash to include palmar and plantar surfaces.

c. Around eyes in raccoon-like pattern.

3. Characteristics of rash.

a. Pink.

b. Discrete, round or elliptical plaques with fine scale that has central clearing.

c. Papulosquamous.

d. Similar to annular erythema.

e. Bullous lesions may be seen on plantar surfaces.

f. Sun exposure worsens rash.

g. Non-scarring.

4. Treatment of rash.

a. No steroids; increases risk of telangiectasis and could worsen them.

b. No treatment recommended.

B. Cardiac-NL (Buyon, 2014; Buyon, Lindsley, & Silverman, 2011).

1. 1st, 2nd degree heart block.

a. Can progress to complete heart block.

b. Continuous ECG monitoring.

c. Pediatric cardiology consultation and care.

2. Complete heart block (CHB).

a. Associated with endocardial fibroelastosis (EFE).

(1) Can require cardiac transplant in severe cases.

b. Continuous cardiac monitoring.

c. Pediatric cardiology consultation and care.

3. Structural cardiac defects may be present.

V. Other disease associated with NL
(Buyon, 2014; Buyon, Lindsley, & Silverman, 2011).

A. Liver disease.

1. May affect 15-25% of infants with NL.

2. Hepatomegaly with or without splenomegaly.

3. Elevated liver function tests [Gamma-Glutamyl Transferase (GGT), Aspartate Aminotransferase (AST), Alanine Aminotransferase (ALT), Lactate Dehydrogenase (LDH)].

4. Biopsy not usually needed unless severe liver dysfunction or persistent.

5. Usually spontaneous resolution without treatment.

6. Usually resolves spontaneously without any sequelae.

B. Hematologic disease.

1. Thrombocytopenia.

2. Less often but possible; anemia, neutropenia and thrombocytopenia (pancytopenia).

3. Spontaneous resolution.

VI. Overall Survival Rates
(Buyon, Lindsley, & Silverman, 2011).

A. Fetal death may occur before the end of 2nd trimester (1 in 7000-8000 pregnancies).

B. Earlier spontaneous abortions may occur.

C. Significant predictors of mortality (Buyon, 2014).

1. In-utero death (one or more of the following yields 10-fold increase in death).

2
2.1
2.2
2.3
2.4
2.5
2.6
2.7
2.8
2.9
2.10
2.11

a. Hydrops fetalis; the earlier the diagnosis the higher risk of death.

b. Endocardial fibroelastosis (EFE).

c. Gestational age <20 weeks.

d. Heart rate <50 bpm.

e. Impaired left ventricular function.

2. Neonatal period mortality (one or more of the following yields 6-fold increase in death) (Buyon, 2014).

a. Hydrops fetalis; the earlier the diagnosis the higher risk of death.

b. EFE.

c. Gestational age <20 weeks.

d. Heart rate <50 bpm.

e. Impaired left ventricular function.

Summary

Neonatal Lupus is a pediatric rheumatologic condition that is relatively uncommon. Consequently NL is infrequently seen in most newborn nurseries. However, it is very important for the fetal and neonatal survival to identify those at risk very early in pregnancy. Otherwise, the fetal/neonatal mortality and morbidity is increased significantly and the survival rate may be reduced significantly especially if 2nd or 3rd degree heart block is present during fetal growth or at birth.

References

Buyon, J.P. (2014) Neonatal Lupus. Retrieved from: www.uptodate.com

Buyon, J.P., Lindsley, C.B. & Silverman, E.D. (2011). Neonatal Lupus Erythematosus. In Cassidy, J.T., Petty, R.E., Laxer, R.M., & Lindsley, C.B., (Eds.), *Textbook of Pediatric Rheumatology, (6th Ed.)* (Chapter 23, pp.361-373). Philadelphia, PA: Saunders Elsevier.

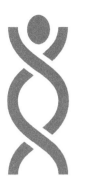

Section 2.5
Nursing Management of Pediatric Systemic Lupus Erythematosus

Dawn E. Isherwood, MSIR, BSN, RN

Introduction

Because of the heterogenic nature of lupus, as well as its ability to mimic other autoimmune diseases in physical presentation and laboratory findings, the diagnosis of lupus can be a prolonged and frustrating experience for both the patient and healthcare provider. To care effectively for a patient with lupus, the healthcare professional needs an up-to-dated understanding of the disease, its many manifestations, and its changing and often unpredictable course (Lupus Foundation of America (LFA), 2011).

Information about the pathogenesis and treatment of lupus has experienced an explosion in this century,

especially over the past 50 years (Lawrence et al., 1998). And while the knowledge about lupus has increased dramatically, there is still much to be learned, and research is ongoing to better diagnose and treat this disease process.

The purpose of this chapter is to review the pathophysiology, diagnostic criteria, physical/socio-economic impact, and standards of care in patients with systemic lupus erythematosus (SLE).

Learning Objectives

Upon completion of this chapter, the nurse will be able to:

1. Define and classify the various forms of lupus.

2. Describe the epidemiology and pathogenesis of lupus.

3. Identify the American College of Rheumatology symptoms and laboratory criteria for the diagnosis of lupus.

4. Identify the potential impact of lupus to the various parts of the body.

5. Describe current drug therapy and disease management of the patient with lupus.

6. Describe potential co-morbid conditions that may develop from lupus and the medications used to control the disease and its symptoms.

7. Identify short- and long-term considerations for lifestyle changes to develop a management plan to meet the individual patient's needs.

Content Outline

I. Pathophysiology of systemic lupus erythematosus.

A. The classification criteria for diagnosis established for SLE in adults has been applied successfully to children (Lahita, 2004).

B. The overall clinical manifestations of SLE occurring in children resemble those in adults (Lahita, 2004).

C. Lupus in children is more severe than in adults.

D. SLE is an autoimmune inflammatory disease that can progressively damage multiple organs. The pathophysiology of SLE involves antibody formation against self-molecules, including those directed against ribonucleic acid (RNA) and deoxyribonucleic acid (DNA).

E. The pathogenesis of lupus is thought to be a combination of predisposing genetic factors and environmental factors such as medication or infectious agents that trigger an abnormal immune response (see Figure 1).

F. This occurs when:

1. Suppressor T cells fail to suppress; in other words, there are defects in cell signaling (Wallace, 2008).

2. There are defects in immune tolerance.

3. Apoptotic cells (cells going through the normal dying process) promote the creation of auto-antibodies (Wallace, 2008).

4. There is loss of T regulatory cells that control auto-reactivity. This leads to the formation of autoantibodies and immune complexes, which promote inflammation and tissue damage (Wallace, 2008).

II. Etiology/epidemiology of systemic lupus erythematosus.

A. There are an estimated 1.5 to 2 million individuals diagnosed with SLE in the United States.

1. Approximately 25% of all cases of SLE begin in the first two decades of life (Lahita, 2004).

2. Extraordinarily rare in children under the age of 5 (Lahita, 2004).

3. A concordance of 57 – 67 percent is reported for identical twins (Lahita, 2004).

4. SLE is more prevalent in women than men.

   a. The increased frequency of SLE among women has been attributed in part to an estrogen hormonal effect (see hormonal factors) (Cooper et al., 1998; Costenbader, Feskanich, Stampfer, & Karlson, 2007).

   b. An estrogen effect is suggested by a number of observations including the female-to-male ratio of SLE in different age groups:

      (1) The ratio approaches 1:1 in very young children under 2 (Ilowite, 2011).

      (2) In children in whom sex hormonal effects are presumably minimal, the female-to-male ratio is 3:1 (Lahita, 1999).

      (3) In adults, especially in women of child-bearing years, the ratio ranges from 7:1 to 15:1 (Chakravarty, Bush, Manzi, Clarke, & Ward, 2007; Lahita, 1999).

      (4) In "older" individuals, especially post-menopausal women, the ratio is approximately 8:1(Chakravarty, Bush, Manzi, Clarke, & Ward, 2007; Lahita, 1999).

B. Investigators have found evidence to support several likely possibilities in the etiology of SLE.

1. Some believe there may be more than one type of SLE and that its etiology may vary from one person to the next.

C. Current studies are focusing on the following elements:

1. Immune system dysfunction – (see pathophysiology).

2. Genetics.

   a. Studies to date suggest that many different genes contribute to lupus susceptibility and that no single genetic abnormality causes the disease.

   b. It also appears that genes may be influential in determining the type or severity of lupus.

   c. Genes that have been associated with lupus in humans include.

(1) The immune system genes human leukocyte antigen (HLA)-DR3 (and B8 in older data), HLA-DR2, and complement C4 genes; other HLA-DR alleles; and alleles at HLA-DQ (National Institute of Arthritis and Musculoskeletal and Skin Diseases [NIAMS], 2006).

(2) Genes that ensure cells die at an appropriate time (apoptosis genes).

   i) Defective *fas* gene which contributes to apoptosis.

(3) Genes that regulate key inflammatory molecules, the cytokines.

3. Environmental influences (LFA, 2011).

  a. Ultraviolet rays from the sun.

  b. Ultraviolet rays from fluorescent light bulbs.

  c. Sulfa drugs, which make a person more sensitive to the sun, such as Bactrim®

and trimethoprim-sulfamethoxazole (Septra®) ; sulfisoxazole (Gantrisin®); tolbutamide (Orinase®); sulfasalazine (SSZ) (Azulfidine®); diuretics.

  d. Sun-sensitizing tetracycline drugs such as minocycline (Minocin®).

  e. Penicillin or other antibiotic drugs such as amoxicillin (Amoxil®); ampicillin (Ampicillin Sodium ADD-Vantage®); cloxacillin (Cloxapen®).

  f. An infection.

  g. A cold or a viral illness.

  h. Exhaustion.

  i. An injury.

  j. Emotional stress, such as a divorce, illness, death in the family, or other life complications.

Figure 1: A Model of the Pathogenesis of Systemic Lupus Erythematosus (SLE) That Implicates the Products of Disease-Associated Polymorphic Genes

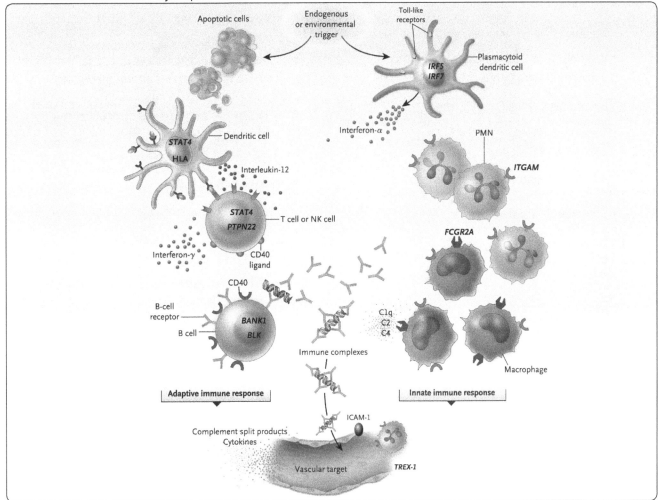

Source: Crow, Mary K. (2008). Collaboration, Genetic Associations, and Lupus Erythematosus. *New England Journal of Medicine*, 358, 956-961. doi: 10.1056/NEJMe0800096. Reprinted with permission.

k. Anything that causes stress to the body, such as surgery, physical harm, pregnancy, or giving birth.

l. Silica exposure.

4. Hormones.

a. Hormones are the body's messengers, and they regulate many of the body's functions.

b. In particular, the hormone estrogen appears to play a role in lupus.

(1) Female sex hormones have the ability to stimulate the helper T lymphocytes, so called because they help B lymphocytes to produce antibodies (Isenberg & Manzi, 2008).

(2) Male hormones encourage suppressor T lymphocytes, which tend to block the production of antibodies (Isenberg & Manzi, 2008).

III. Nursing assessment.

A. Asses flares.

1. Number of flares since last visit.

2. Severity of flare (impact on activities of daily living).

3. Symptoms associated with flare.

4. Triggers that bring on or are associated with flare.

B. Psychosocial history to include stress, school, work, social activities, and ability to accomplish activities of daily living.

1. Discuss with patient/family the possible need for evaluation and intervention of a social worker, mental health counselor, or psychologist.

2. Discuss the possible need for an individualized education plan (IEP) and a 504 plan. An IEP is a written plan for a child with a disability that is developed and implemented according to federal and state regulations. A 504 plan is a legal document created by the school for students with disabilities to assist with instructional services.

C. Current medication and supplements.

1. Adherence to treatment plan.

IV. Diagnosis.

A. The diagnosis of lupus is based on a combination of physical symptoms and laboratory results.

B. It is usually a diagnosis that evolves over time either toward more certainty or to the conclusion that the person does not have lupus.

C. The diagnosis of SLE is made by a careful review of:

1. Current symptoms.

2. Laboratory test results.

3. Medical history.

4. Medical history of close family members.

D. The American College of Rheumatology (ACR) established criteria for SLE in 1982, which were most recently revised in 1997 (Tan et al., 1997).

1. These criteria establish guidelines for diagnosis and consist of four cutaneous, four systemic, and three laboratory criteria.

V. American College of Rheumatology Criteria for Classifying SLE for Research Purposes.

A. Malar rash (LFA, 2011).

1. Lesions occur when systemic lupus is active.

2. Flattened areas of red skin on the face that resemble a sunburn.

3. When the rash appears on both cheeks and across the bridge of the nose in the shape of a butterfly, it is known as the "butterfly rash." However, the rash can also appear on arms, legs, and body.

B. Discoid rash (LFA, 2011).

1. Appears as disk-shaped, round lesions. The sores usually appear on scalp and face, but sometimes they will occur on other parts of the body as well.

2. Discoid lupus lesions are often red, scaly, and thick.

3. Usually they do not hurt or itch.

2
2.1
2.2
2.3
2.4
2.5
2.6
2.7
2.8
2.9
2.10
2.11

C. Photosensitivity.

D. Oral ulcers.

E. Arthritis (Arthritis, 2013).

   1. Polyarthralgia and polyarthritis, defined as arthralgias or arthritis affecting 5 or more joints, are the most common joint problems seen in people with SLE.

   2. Over 50% of lupus patients manifest arthralgias upon their initial diagnosis.

   3. Both large joints, such as the knees, shoulders, and elbows, and small joints, such as the toe and finger joints, can be affected by lupus arthritis.

F. Serositis (pleuritis or pericarditis).

   1. Pleuritis and pericarditis are the most frequent pulmonary and cardiac manifestations of SLE. A prevalence of serositis at disease onset of 17% with a cumulative incidence of 36% (Kean & Lynch, 2000).

   2. Pleuritic chest pain may occur during the course of lupus in up to 60% (Kean & Lynch, 2000).

   3. Manifestations of serositis (Kean & Lynch, 2000; Tincani, Rebaioli, Taglietti, & Shoenfeld, 2006).

      a. Chest pain may be unilateral or bilateral and usually is located at the costophrenic margins, either anterior or posterior.

      b. Cough and dyspnea.

      c. Pericarditis usually manifests as precordial pain aggravated by deep breathing and decubitus, typically improving with sitting up.

      d. Friction rubs may be heard.

G. Renal disorder (persistent proteinuria or cellular casts).

   1. Manifestations of lupus nephritis (John Hopkins, 2013).

      a. High blood pressure.

      b. Dark urine.

      c. Flu-like symptoms.

      d. Joint pains and aches.

      e. Swelling (edema) of the legs, ankles, eyes, and hands.

      f. Weight gain, caused by water retention when the kidneys do not filter properly.

   2. Some patients may have few and subtle symptoms or none at all in the early stages of the disease.

H. Neurological disorder (seizures or psychosis).

   1. Neuropsychiatric systemic lupus erythematosus (NPSLE) is arguably the least understood manifestation of SLE, as it is associated with a complicated and often baffling range of clinical presentations (Hermosillo-Romo & Brey, 2002).

   2. NP-SLE can involve the central nervous system (CNS), peripheral nervous system, and/or the autonomic nervous system.

   3. Manifestations can include (ACR Ad Hoc Committee, 1999; Bertsias, et al., 2010):

      a. Central nervous system.

         (1) Acute confusional state.

         (2) Cognitive dysfunction.

             i) Mild to moderate.

             ii) Severe (dementia).

         (3) Headache.

         (4) Aseptic meningitis.

         (5) Myelopathy.

         (6) Movement disorders.

         (7) Demyelinating syndromes.

         (8) Seizures.

      b. Psychiatric disturbances.

         (1) Psychosis.

         (2) Mood and anxiety disorders.

             i) Severe depression.

             ii) Anxiety.

      c. Peripheral nervous system.

         (1) Cranial neuropathy.

         (2) Guillain-Barrè syndrome.

         (3) Plexopathy.

         (4) Autonomic neuropathy.

         (5) Myasthenia gravis.

   4. Cognitive impairment from NPSLE can affect any or all of the following cognitive functions (Brunner & Klein-Gitelman, 2009):

2
2.1
2.2
2.3
2.4
2.5
2.6
2.7
2.8
2.9
2.10
2.11

a. Simple or complex attention.

b. Reasoning.

c. Executive skills (e.g., planning, organizing, sequencing).

d. Memory (e.g., learning, recall).

e. Visual-spatial processing.

f. Language (e.g., verbal fluency).

g. Psychomotor speed.

I. Hematologic disorder (anemia, leukopenia, or lymphopenia on two or more occasions, thrombocytopenia).

1. Immunologic disorder (abnormal anti-dsDNA or anti-Sm, positive antiphospholipid antibodies).

2. Abnormal anti-nuclear antibody (ANA) titer.

a. Auto-Antibody Testing.

(1) Anti-nuclear antibody test (ANA).

i) Antinuclear antibodies (ANA) are antibodies that connect, or bind, to the nucleus -- the "command center" -- of the cell.

ii) This process damages and can destroy the cells.

iii) The ANA blood test is a sensitive test for lupus since these antibodies are found in 97 percent of people with the disease.

iv) When three or more typical features of lupus are present -- such as involvement of the skin, joints, kidneys, lungs, heart, blood, or nervous system -- a positive ANA test can help confirm a diagnosis of lupus.

v) A positive ANA test result does not always mean an individual has lupus.

1) The ANA can be positive in people with other illnesses or positive in people with no illness.

2) The ANA can also change from positive to negative or negative to positive in the same person.

3) The ANA may show a negative reading in some patients who have received immunosuppressant therapy only to later return to a positive reading.

4) Immune fluorescence pattern can help distinguish different auto-immune disease:

(a) Homogeneous or rimmed patterns are suggestive of SLE.

(b) Speckled pattern is the most common but least specific. Suggestive of:

(i) SLE.

(ii) *Sjögren's* syndrome.

(iii) Mixed connective tissue disease.

(iv) Scleroderma.

(c) Nucleolar pattern is suggestive of scleroderma or CREST syndrome.

(2) Antibodies to double-stranded DNA.

i) Anti-dsDNA antibodies are found in 50 percent of the people with SLE.

1) The antibodies form in response to DNA exposed during apoptosis and can bind to proteins and deposit in tissues (such as in the kidney) and damage the organ.

ii) The disease can still be present even if these antibodies are not detected.

(3) Anti-Sm antibodies.

i) Target Sm proteins in the cell nucleus.

ii) Found in 30-40 percent of people with SLE.

iii) The presence of this antibody almost always confirms the diagnosis of SLE.

(4) Antibodies to phospholipids (aPLs).

i) Nearly 30 percent of people with lupus will test positive for antiphospholipid antibodies.

ii) The most commonly measured aPLs are lupus anticoagulant, anticardiolipin antibody, and anti-beta2 glycoprotein I.

iii) Can cause narrowing of blood vessels, leading to blood clots in the legs or lungs, stroke, heart attack, or miscarriage.

(5) Antibodies to Ro/SS-A and La/SS-B.

i) Ro and La are the names of proteins in the cell nucleus.

2
2.1
2.2
2.3
2.4
2.5
2.6
2.7
2.8
2.9
2.10
2.11

1) Often found in people with Sjögren's syndrome.

(6) Antibodies to RNP target ribonucleoproteins.

    i) Help to control chemical activities of the cells.

    ii) Anti-RNPs are found in many autoimmune conditions and will be at very high levels in patients whose symptoms combine features of several diseases, including lupus.

(7) Antibodies to histone.

    i) A protein that surrounds the DNA molecule.

    ii) Sometimes found in people with systemic lupus but more often seen in people with drug-induced lupus.

(8) Complements.

    i) A group of proteins that protect the body against infections.

    ii) Complement proteins are used up by the inflammation caused by lupus.

       1) People with inflammation due to active lupus often have decreased complement levels.

    iii) There are nine protein groups of complement, so complement is identified by the letter C and the numbers 1 through 9.

       1) The most common complement tests are CH50, C3, and C4.

       2) CH50 measures the overall function of complement in the blood. Low levels of C3 or C4 may indicate active lupus.

b. Other laboratory testing.

(1) CRP (C-reactive protein) binding.

    i) A protein produced by the liver.

    ii) High levels may indicate inflammation due to lupus.

(2) Erythrocyte sedimentation rate (ESR or "sed" rate).

    i) Indicator of inflammation in the body.

    ii) Measures the amount of a protein that makes the red blood cells clump together.

    iii) May be elevated in people with active lupus, but it can also be high due to other reasons, such as an infection.

(3) Complete Blood Count.

    i) Anemia.

       1) About 40 percent of individuals with lupus experience anemia.

       2) May be caused by iron deficiency, gastrointestinal (GI) bleeding, medications, and autoantibody formation to RBCs, or "chronic disease" (NIAMS, 2006).

    ii) Leukopenia and thrombocytopenia.

       1) Abnormalities in the white blood cell (WBC) and platelet counts are an important indicator of SLE.

       2) Around 40 percent of lupus patients have a low level of total white cells (Isenberg & Manzi, 2008).

       3) Approximately 80 percent of lupus patients have low levels of lymphocytes (Isenberg & Manzi, 2008).

       4) Occurs in 25 to 35 percent of patients with SLE (NIAMS, 2006).

VI. Treatment.

A. Treatment varies depending on the organ systems involved in the individual's disease.

  1. The treatment plan for children with SLE must be based on a careful assessment of the extent and severity of the disease versus the risk of treatment (Lahita, 2004).

  2. Consideration of the need for growth and normal function at home and in school (Lahita, 2004).

B. Goal of treatment:

  1. Reduce inflammation caused by lupus.

  2. Suppress an overactive immune system.

  3. Prevent flares and treat them when they occur.

  4. Control symptoms like joint pain and fatigue.

  5. Minimize damage to organs.

C. Medications used to treat SLE.

  1. Anti-inflammatories.

    a. Aspirin has pain-reducing, anti-inflammatory, and anticoagulant

2
2.1
2.2
2.3
2.4
2.5
2.6
2.7
2.8
2.9
2.10
2.11

properties that can control some of the symptoms of lupus.

b. Non-steroidal anti-inflammatory drugs (NSAIDs).

   (1) Suppress inflammation.

   (2) Decrease joint pain and stiffness.

   (3) Commonly used NSAIDs:

      i) Ibuprofen (Motrin®)

      ii) Naproxen (Naprosyn®)

      iii) Indomethacin (Indocin®)

      iv) Nabumetone (Relafen®)

      v) Celecoxib (Celebrex®)

c. Side effects (NIAMS, 2006).

   (1) Gastrointestinal (GI): Dyspepsia, heartburn, epigastric distress, and nausea; less frequently, vomiting, anorexia, abdominal pain, GI bleeding, and mucosal lesions. Misoprostol (Cytotec®), a synthetic prostaglandin that inhibits gastric acid secretion, may be given to prevent GI intolerance. It prevents gastric ulcers and their associated GI bleeding in patients receiving NSAIDs. Another product, Arthrotec®, combines misoprostol with the NSAID diclofenac sodium in a single pill.

   (2) Genitourinary: Fluid retention, reduction in creatinine clearance, and acute tubular necrosis with renal failure.

   (3) Hepatic: Acute reversible hepatotoxicity.

   (4) Cardiovascular: Hypertension and moderate to severe noncardiogenic pulmonary edema. All NSAIDS now carry a warning that they may increase the risk of myocardial infarction.

   (5) Hematologic: Altered hemostasis through effects on platelet function.

   (6) Other: Skin eruption, sensitivity reactions, tinnitus, and hearing loss.

2. Antimalarial (NIAMS, 2006).

a. Anti-inflammatory action of these drugs is not well understood.

b. Anti-coagulant properties to reduce the risk of blood clots.

c. Decrease in plasma levels.

d. Types of antimalarial medications:

   (1) Hydroxychloroquine sulfate (Plaquenil®)

   (2) Chloroquine (Aralen®)

e. Side effects.

   (1) Central nervous system: Headache, nervousness, irritability, dizziness, muscle weakness, and tinnitus.

   (2) Gastrointestinal: Nausea, vomiting, diarrhea, abdominal cramps, and loss of appetite.

   (3) Ophthalmologic: Visual disturbances and retinal changes are manifested by blurring of vision and difficulty in focusing. A very serious potential side effect of antimalarial drugs is damage to the retina. Because of the relatively low doses used to treat SLE, the risk of retinal damage is quite small: About 1 in 5,000. However, patients should have a thorough eye examination before starting this treatment and yearly thereafter.

   (4) Dermatologic: Dryness, pruritus, alopecia, skin and mucosal pigmentation, skin eruptions, and exfoliative dermatitis.

   (5) Hematologic: Blood dyscrasia and hemolysis in patients with glucose 6-phosphate dehydrogenase (G6PD) deficiency.

3. Corticosteroids (NIAMS, 2006).

a. Hormones secreted by the cortex of the adrenal gland.

b. Highly effective in reducing inflammation and suppressing the immune response.

c. These drugs may be used to control exacerbation of symptoms and are used to control severe forms of the disease.

d. Types of corticosteroids:

   (1) Prednisone (Orasone®, Meticorten®, Deltasone®, Cortan®, Sterapred®)

   (2) Hydrocortisone (Cortef®, Hydrocortone®)

   (3) Methylprednisolone (Medrol®)

   (4) Dexamethasone (Decadron®)

e. Side effects (*long-term effects).

   (1) Central nervous system: Depression, mood swings, and psychosis.

   (2) Cardiovascular: Congestive heart failure (CHF) and hypertension* .

2
2.1
2.2
2.3
2.4
2.5
2.6
2.7
2.8
2.9
2.10
2.11

(3) Endocrine: Cushing's syndrome, menstrual irregularities, and hyperglycemia.

(4) Gastrointestinal: GI irritation, peptic ulcer, and weight gain.

(5) Dermatologic: Thin skin, petechiae, ecchymoses, facial erythema, poor wound healing, hirsutism, urticaria, and acne.

(6) Musculoskeletal: Muscle weakness, loss of muscle mass, and osteoporosis.

(7) Ophthalmologic: Increased intraocular pressure, glaucoma, exophthalmos, and cataracts.

(8) Other: Immunosuppression and increased susceptibility to infection.

4. Immunosuppressive (NIAMS, 2006).

    a. Although they have different mechanisms of action, each type functions to decrease or prevent an immune response.

    b. Types of immunosuppressive medications:

       (1) Azathioprine (Imuran®). Azathioprine, one of the most widely used immunosuppressives for lupus, is an antimetabolite. Antimetabolites work by blocking metabolic steps within immune cells, thus interfering with immune function. Used to control the underlying disease process, azathioprine has fewer serious side-effect risks than some other drugs used to control lupus.

       (2) Cyclophosphamide (Cytoxan®). An alkylating agent and strong immunosuppressive, cyclophosphamide is reserved for treating lupus with kidney disease or other internal organ involvement. It works by targeting and damaging autoantibody-producing cells, thereby suppressing the hyperactive immune response and reducing disease activity. It has the potential for severe side effects, including risk of serious infection.

       (3) Methotrexate (MTX) (Rheumatrex®). Originally developed as a cancer treatment and later approved for rheumatoid arthritis, MTX, like azathioprine, is an antimetabolite. It is predominantly used for lupus arthritis. It requires monitoring of the CBC and liver function tests. To reduce toxicity, daily folic acid is prescribed.

       (4) Cyclosporine (Neoral®). Originally developed to prevent the body from rejecting transplanted organs, cyclosporine is now commonly used to treat rheumatic diseases, including lupus. Cyclosporine is an antimetabolite.

       (5) Mycophenolate mofetil (CellCept®). A strong immunosuppressive drug developed to prevent the rejection of transplanted organs, mycophenolate is sometimes used as an alternative to cyclophosphamide for lupus with kidney involvement. Mycophenolate works by keeping T and B lymphocytes from replicating.

    c. Side effects.

       (1) Immunosuppressives can have serious side effects.

       (2) Patients/family need to understand that side effects are dose-dependent and are generally reversible by reducing the dose or stopping the medication.

       (3) Immunosuppression (resulting in increased susceptibility to infection).

       (4) Bone marrow suppression (resulting in decreased numbers of RBCs, WBCs, and platelets).

       (5) Development of malignancies.

       (6) Dermatologic: Alopecia (cyclophosphamide and MTX).

       (7) Gastrointestinal: Nausea, vomiting, stomatitis, esophagitis, and hepatotoxicity.

       (8) Genitourinary: Hemorrhagic cystitis, hematuria, amenorrhea, impotence, and gonadal suppression (cyclophosphamide only).

       (9) Hematologic: Thrombocytopenia, leukopenia, pancytopenia, anemia, and myelosuppression.

       (10) Respiratory: Pulmonary fibrosis.

       (11) Other: Increased risk of serious infections.

5. Monoclonal Antibody (mAbs).

    a. The monoclonal antibody approach has been used to target both B and T lymphocytes, the white blood cells responsible for autoantibody production in lupus (LFA, 2011).

2
2.1
2.2
2.3
2.4
2.5
2.6
2.7
2.8
2.9
2.10
2.11

b. While several monoclonal antibody therapies are used in the treatment of SLE, only BENLYSTA® has been approved by the FDA for use in adults with moderate to severe lupus. It has not been approved for use in children and there are no clinical trials at this time.

c. Types of monoclonal antibody medications:

(1) Rituximab (Rituxan®, anti-CD20). Targets a specific protein known as CD20 that appears on the surface of B cells. Rituxan® binds to CD20 and is believed to work with the body's own immune system to attack and kill the marked B cells (LFA, 2013). This is not FDA approved for the treatment of lupus.

6. Intravenous immunoglobulin (*IVIG*).

a. A preparation of pooled human plasma containing primarily IgG.

b. IVIG has been used in studies for children with lupus nephritis with mixed results.

VII. Co-morbid Conditions.

A. Osteoporosis.

1. A high prevalence of osteoporosis and osteopenia is present in SLE (Pineau, Lee, Ramsey-Goldman, Clarke, & Bernatsky, 2007).

2. Although part of this increase in risk is because of recognized risk factors (corticosteroid use, decreased physical activity, decreased sun exposure, etc.), lupus activity may also play a role (Pineau, Lee, Ramsey-Goldman, Clarke, & Bernatsky, 2007).

B. Cardiovascular disease.

1. Patients with lupus have a significant increased risk of cardiovascular events (Pineau, Lee, Ramsey-Goldman, Clarke, & Bernatsky, 2007).

2. This increase in risk is related to an increased number of traditional risk factors (e.g., hypertension, hyperlipidemia), but lupus-related factors (e.g., steroid exposure, SLE activity) may also be important (Pineau, Lee, Ramsey-Goldman, Clarke, & Bernatsky, 2007).

3. Because patients with lupus are at high risk of cardiovascular disease (CVD), they should have regular screening for the presence of traditional risk factors and aggressive risk reduction (Pineau, Lee, Ramsey-Goldman, Clarke, & Bernatsky, 2007).

C. Malignancy and SLE.

1. SLE is associated with an increased risk of malignancies, particularly lymphoma and lung cancer (Pineau, Lee, Ramsey-Goldman, Clarke, & Bernatsky, 2007).

2. Though immunosuppressive therapy may not be the principal driving factor for overall cancer risk in autoimmune diseases such as SLE, it may contribute to an increased risk of some hematological malignancies (Pineau, Lee, Ramsey-Goldman, Clarke, & Bernatsky, 2007).

3. Lymphoma risk in SLE may in part be driven by disease activity, but work in progress aims to differentiate the effects of lupus treatment from lupus activity (Pineau, Lee, Ramsey-Goldman, Clarke, & Bernatsky, 2007).

VIII. Nursing implications.

A. Special considerations in children and adolescents with SLE in collaboration with other interdisciplinary team members).

1. Emotional support.

a. Encourage patient and family to:

(1) Talk openly about the condition in order to build trust.

(2) Listen to questions and concerns, even if repetitive.

(3) Talk openly to other people in the child's life.

(4) Educate everybody in the family about the disease; make sure they do not have unnecessary fears or misconceptions.

(5) Continue regular activities; keep things as normal as possible, including doing chores.

(6) Allow the patient to have some "say" and control over illness where age appropriate.

2. Body image.

a. Need for acceptance by peers is at its peak in adolescence.

(1) Hair loss.

(2) Dermatitis.

(3) Vasculitic lesions.

2
2.1
2.2
2.3
2.4
2.5
2.6
2.7
2.8
2.9
2.10
2.11

b. Physical growth.

   (1) Girls who acquired lupus before age 12 had significant reductions in growth, especially after having lupus for at least a year (Rygg et al., 2011).

   i) Delayed pubertal onset.

   ii) Delayed or absent menarche.

   iii) Irregular menses or suspension of periods after initiation of menses.

   (2) In males, there were no significant associations among disease characteristics, treatments, growth failure, or pubertal delay (Rygg et al., 2011).

3. Social interaction.

   a. Important to ensure that the patient does not become estranged from his or her peer group.

   (1) Patients who isolate themselves from their peers tend to have exacerbations of disease twice as frequently as those who remain socially active (although cause and effect here are difficult to determine) (Lahita, 2004).

4. School issues for children with lupus.

   a. Challenges related to absenteeism, physical education class, cognitive functioning, teasing.

   b. Meet with the school.

   c. Obtain a letter from the physician.

   d. Request an IEP.

   e. Request a 504.

5. Contraception and pregnancy.

   a. Estrogen-containing oral contraceptives have been associated with exacerbation of SLE (Lahita, 2004).

   b. Progesterone does not induce flares (Lahita, 2004).

   c. The inability to bear children often concerns young women with SLE (Lahita, 2004).

6. Vaccinations.

   a. Except for live virus vaccines routine childhood vaccines are recommended.

   b. Vaccines not recommended:

   (1) MMR.

   (2) varicella (chicken pox).

   (3) influenza nasal spray.

B. Osteoporosis.

   1. Screening for osteoporosis with bone mineral densitometry should be considered in all patients with SLE, especially in the presence of osteoporosis risk factors (Pineau, Lee, Ramsey-Goldman, Clarke, & Bernatsky, 2007).

   2. Early and aggressive measures for bone preservation should be considered in all patients treated with corticosteroids (Pineau, Lee, Ramsey-Goldman, Clarke, & Bernatsky, 2007).

C. Cardiovascular disease.

   1. Because patients with lupus are at high risk of CVD, they should have regular screening for the presence of traditional risk factors, and aggressive risk reduction (Pineau, Lee, Ramsey-Goldman, Clarke, & Bernatsky, 2007).

D. Medication adherence (LFA, 2011; NIAMS, 2006).

   1. Non-compliance is 59% in adolescents required to take steroids (Lahita, 2004). Explain consequenses of non-adherence.

   2. Create rapport with patients.

   3. Fully explain all medications to include possible side effects and potential problems that may result from non-adherence.

   4. Provide the patient with strategies on how to integrate medication treatment plan into daily activities of living.

   5. Prepare medications in advance by using a pill box to help organize one or even two weeks' worth of medications.

   6. Use alarm clock or cell phone alarm to alert patient when it is time to take medication.

   7. Encourage family and friends to form a support system with the patient (particularly for teens and young adults) to help reinforce medication adherence.

   8. Verify adherence with medication treatment plan during follow-up appointments.

   9. Remain vigilant for signs of non-adherence, as the patient may be embarrassed and not admit to being non-adherent.

2
2.1
2.2
2.3
2.4
2.5
2.6
2.7
2.8
2.9
2.10
2.11

10. Consider intravenous medications when concerns about non-adherence affect disease management.

E. Photosensitivity (LFA, 2011; NIAMS, 2006).

1. Teach the patient to minimize direct exposure to UV from sun and/or fluorescent and halogen light bulbs, including tanning beds. Glass does not provide complete protection from UV rays (NIAMS).

2. Instruct the patient to use sunscreen of SPF 30 or greater and encourage the use of broad-brimmed hats and tightly-woven, loose-fitting clothing with long sleeves and long pants.

3. Teach patients about the benefits of shields that cover fluorescent bulbs to minimize indoor exposure. Recommend shields with nanometer readings of 380 to 400.

4. Assess the need for window films on the patient's car (if a teen or young adult).

5. Instruct the patient that certain drugs can increase sensitivity to the sun, including antihistamines, diuretics, non-steroidal antiinflammatory drugs (NSAIDs) and antibiotics, including tetracycline or "sulfa" antibiotics. Extra precautions should be taken if patient is on these medications.

6. Special emphasis on the effects of photosensitivity should be given to people of color (e.g., African American, Hispanic, Asian, and Native American).

F. Extreme fatigue (LFA, 2011; NIAMS, 2006).

1. Assess the patient's general fatigue level.

2. Assess for the presence of depression, anxiety, and other stressors.

3. Conduct an assessment to determine the patient's daily activities that contribute to fatigue.

4. Help the patient develop an energy-conserving plan for completing daily and other activities and school. Many people with lupus need to take a daily nap. Encourage a nap earlier in the day to prevent any issues with insomnia.

5. Encourage the patient to get 8 to 10 hours of sleep at night.

6. Encourage exercise as tolerated.

G. Diet and nutrition (LFA, 2011; NIAMS, 2006).

1. Assess the patient's prescription and nonprescription drug regimen and dosages for medications that may affect patient's nutritional status.

2. Assess the patient's usual daily dietary intake by recommending that the patient keep a food diary.

3. Educate patient about which medications to take with food.

4. Develop a dietary plan with the patient that encourages healthful eating. If the patient has nutrition-related lupus complications, refer to a dietician for counseling.

5. Encourage exercise as tolerated.

6. Record the patient's weight at each visit.

7. Instruct the patient to weigh at home once a week, record it, and bring to all patient visits.

H. Smoking (LFA, 2011; NIAMS, 2006).

1. Assess smoking habits of the patient/family. Encourage prevention of smoking for non-smoking adolescents.

2. Provide support, guidance, and instruction on the safest techniques of smoking cessation.

3. Provide contacts for local smoking cessation classes.

I. Infection (LFA, 2011; NIAMS, 2006).

1. Assess the patient's current medications, particularly those that promote susceptibility to infection such as corticosteroids and immunosuppressive medications.

2. Teach the patient/family to use good hand-washing and personal-hygiene techniques.

3. Teach the patient/family the signs and symptoms of infection and reinforce the importance of reporting them to the healthcare provider.

4. Encourage the patient/family to eat a balanced diet with adequate calories to help preserve the immune system.

5. Teach the patient/family to minimize exposure to crowds and people with infections or contagious illnesses.

2
2.1
2.2
2.3
2.4
2.5
2.6
2.7
2.8
2.9
2.10
2.11

6. Check the patient's current immunization status.

7. Teach the patient/family that infections can be minimized with immunizations.

8. Encourage the patient/family to consult the healthcare provider about vaccines and/or allergy shots that are being considered.

J. Stress (LFA, 2011; NIAMS, 2006).

1. Assess for presence and degree of anxiety or life stressor.

2. Encourage patient to find positive coping mechanisms for stressor.

3. Encourage the patient to accept help from others, such as counseling or a support group.

4. Discuss complementary coping activities such as biofeedback, yoga, and/or acupuncture.

5. Encourage development of a consistent exercise regimen.

K. Depression (LFA, 2011; NIAMS, 2006).

1. Assess the patient for the signs and symptoms of depression.

2. Assess the patient's interpersonal and social support systems.

3. Encourage the patient to express feelings.

4. Proper emotional support in the form of group or individual discussion with professionals trained to care for children with SLE.

5. Initiate a referral to a mental health professional.

L. Neuropsychiatric issues (LFA, 2011; NIAMS, 2006).

1. Assess the patient for any changes in cognition, memory, and/or mental status.

2. Provide patient/family tips that may help ease the frustrations of cognitive impairment caused by lupus.

a. Patient should focus attention when receiving new information. Repeat information back to the provider, ask for clarification, ask for memory tools, and/or write the information down. Verify any details.

b. Focus on one task at a time.

c. Encourage exercise, heart healthy diet, and adequate sleep.

d. Learn and use memory techniques, such as associating a person's name with an image, or repeating the name several times in conversation.

e. Try to stay organized. One helpful hint is to use a year-long calendar notebook so that all appointments, plans, contact information, and reminders can be kept in one place.

3. Initiate a referral for neuropsychiatric evaluation if ordered by healthcare provider.

Summary

Pediatric SLE is a chronic condition that requires understanding of the disease state and its multiple presentations, treatment options, and potential side effects. Additionally the nurse must develop a trusted relationship with the patient and family to help them navigate the complexity of the disease, the treatment options, the potential side effects of treatment as well as the complications of non-adherence, through the developmental stages of childhood.

References

ACR Ad Hoc Committee on Neuropsychiatric Lupus Nomenclature. (1999). The American College of Rheumatology nomenclature and case definitions for neuropsychiatric lupus syndromes. *Arthritis and Rheumatism, 42*, 599-608.

Arthritis. (2013). Retrieved from http://www.hopkinslupus.org/lupus-info/lupus-affects-body/lupus-arthritis/

Bertsias G.K., Ioannidis, J.P.A., Aringer, M., Bollen, E., Bombardieri, S., Bruce, I.N., ... Boumpas, D.T. (2010). EULAR recommendations for the management of systemic lupus erythematosus and neuropsychiatric manifestations: Report of a task force of the EULAR standing committee for clinical affairs. *Annals of Rheumatic Disease, 69*, 2074-2082.

Brunner, H., & Klein-Gitelman M. (2009, March). *Lupus in the child's mind: Unique neuropsychiatric problems require a unique approach. The Rheumatologist.* Retrieved from Unique neuropsychiatric problems require a unique approach

Chakravarty, E.F., Bush, T.M., Manzi, S., Clarke, A.E., & Ward, M.M. (2007). Prevalence of adult systemic lupus erythematosus in California and Pennsylvania in 2000: Estimates obtained using hospitalization data. *Arthritis and Rheumatism, 56*(6), 2092-2094.

Cooper, G.S., Dooley, M.A., Treadwell, E.L., St. Clair, E.W., Parks, C.G., & Gilkeson, G.S. (1998). Hormonal, environmental, and infectious risk factors for developing systemic lupus erythematosus. *Arthritis and Rheumatism, 41*(10), 1714-1724.

Costenbader, K.H., Feskanich, D., Stampfer, M.J., & Karlson, E.W. (2007). Reproductive and menopausal factors and risk of systemic lupus erythematosus in women. *Arthritis and Rheumatism, 56*(4), 1251-1262.

Hermosillo-Romo, D., & Brey, R.L. (2002). Neuropsychiatric involvement in systemic lupus erythematosus. *Current Rheumatology Reports, 4,* 337-344.

Isenberg, D., & Manzi, S. (2008). *Lupus the facts* (2nd ed.). New York: Oxford University Press.

Ilowite, N. T. (2011). *15 questions with Dr. Norman Ilowite – pediatric lupus.* Retrieved from http://www.lupus.org/webmodules/webarticlesnet/templates/new_learnclinical.aspx?articleid=4139&zoneid=531

John Hopkins Children's Hospital. (2013), *Lupus nephritis.* Retrieved from https://www.hopkinschildrens.org/Lupus-Nephritis.aspx

Kean, M.P., & Lynch, J.P. (2000). Pleuropulmonary manifestations of systemic lupus erythematosus. *Thorax, 55,* 159-166.

Lahita, R.G. (1999). The role of sex hormones in systemic lupus erythematosus. *Current Opinion in Rheumatology, 11*(5), 352-356.

Lahita, R.G. (2004). *Systemic lupus erythematosus* (4th ed.). New York: NY: Academic Press.

Lawrence, R.C., Helmick, C.G., Arnett, F.C., Deyo, R.A., Felson, D.T., Giannini, E.H., ...Wolfe, E. (1998). Estimates of the prevalence of arthritis and selected musculoskeletal disorders in the United States. *Arthritis and Rheumatism , 41*(5), 778-799.

Lupus Foundation of America, Inc. (2011). *Learn about lupus.* Retrieved from www.lupus.org

National Institute of Arthritis and Musculoskeletal and Skin Diseases (NIAMS). (2006). *Lupus: A patient care guide for nurses and other health professionals* (3rd ed.). Bethesda, MD: Author.

Pineau, C. A., Lee, C., Ramsey-Goldman, R., Clarke, A.E., & Bernatsky, S. (2007). The second hit: Co-morbidities in systemic lupus erythematosus. *Future Rheumatology, 2*(5), 497-506.

Rygg, M., Pistorio, A., Ravelli, A., Maghnie, M., Di Iorgi, N., Bader-Meunier, B., Ruperto, N. (2011, October 13). A longitudinal PRINTO study on growth and puberty in juvenile systemic lupus erythematosus. *Annals of the Rheumatic Diseases* (Epublication).

Tan, E., Cohen, A.S., Fries, J.S., Masi, A.T., McShane, D.J., Rothfield, N.F., & Winchester, R.J. (1982). The 1982 criteria for the classification of systemic lupus erythematosus. *Arthritis and Rheumatism, 25*:1271-77.

Tincani, A., Rebaioli, C.B., Taglietti, M., & Shoenfeld, Y. (2006). Heart involvement in systemic lupus erythematosus, anti-phospholipid syndrome and neonatal lupus. *Rheumatology* (Oxford), *45*(Suppl 4), 8-13.

Wallace, D. J. (2008). Lupus: The essential clinician's guide. New York: Oxford American Rheumatology Library.

Suggested Readings

Hochberg, M.C. (1985). The incidence of systemic lupus erythematosus in Baltimore, Maryland, 1970-1977. *Arthritis and Rheumatism, 28*(1), 80-86.

Krajewski, D. (2011, May 7). *Endocrine manifestationsin systemic lupus erythematosus.* Department of Endocrinology Georgetown University Hospital.

Pons-Estel, G.J., Alarcón, G.S., Scofield, L., Reinlib, L., & Cooper, G.S. (2010). Understanding the epidemiology and progression of systemic lupus erythematosus. *Seminars in Arthritis and Rheumatism, 39*(4), 257-268.

Serdula, M.K., & Rhoads, G.G. (1979). Frequency of systemic lupus erythematosus in different ethnic groups in Hawaii. *Arthritis and Rheumatism, 22*(4), 328-333.

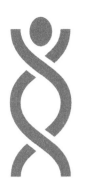

Section 2.6
Juvenile Dermatomyositis

Maria Cusano-Sanzo, MSN, RN, CPN

Introduction

Juvenile dermatomyositis (JDMS) is a rare childhood disease that affects muscle and skin. It is characterized by muscle inflammation, weakness and rash accompanied by elevated muscle enzymes. Children with JDMS will often ask to be carried and may be thought of as "clumsy." This chapter will focus on the diagnosis, treatment and nursing implications of children with JDMS.

Learning Objectives

Upon completion of this chapter, the nurse will be able to:

1. List three classic symptoms of JDMS.
2. List three treatment options and modes of action.
3. Identify three abnormal lab findings in JDMS.
4. List two co-morbid conditions of JDMS

Content Outline

I. Pathophysiology/Etiology.

   A. Autoimmune disorder.

   B. Cause is unknown but may be triggered by viral illness. Immune system attacks healthy muscles, damaging muscles which causes a "leak" of muscle enzymes. Infection and environmental triggers may also play a role (Li & Imundo, 2006).

II. Epidemiology.

   A. Incidence is a little over 3 cases per 1 million (Rider, Lindsley, & Cassidy, 2011).

   B. Slightly higher incidence in girls than boys.

   C. Average age of onset is 6-7 years of age (Rider & Miller, 2007).

   D. Most common inflammatory myopathy of childhood (Cooper et al., 2007).

   E. Caucasian prevalence is ~ 65 %; Hispanic is ~14 %; and African-American is ~11 % (Mendez, et al., 2003).

III. Diagnosis.

   A. Onset is usually gradual as opposed to sudden and usually affects proximal muscles bilaterally.

   B. Reddish purple rash on eyelids, referred to as a heliotrope rash, is sometimes accompanied by eyelid swelling (see Figure 1).

   C. Red, scaly rash on knuckles, elbows, knees referred to as Gottron's papules (see Figure 2).

   D. Elevated muscle enzymes (AST, ALT, Aldolase, LDH, CK.) AST and ALT will be elevated and gamma glutamyl transferase (GGT) will remain normal, differentiating between muscle enzyme elevation versus liver. Muscle enzymes will improve before muscle strength does.

   E. Patients may require an electromyography (EMG); however, diagnosis can be confirmed without this; it is a somewhat uncomfortable procedure to undergo. EMGs are rarely done.

Figure 2: Gottron's papules

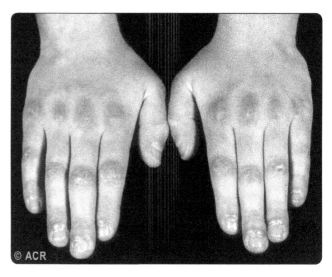

© ACR

» Gottron's papules over the extensor surface of the interphalangeal and metacarpophalangeal joints. Some areas are hypo pigmented with depressions suggestive of atrophic scars. These lesions are typical of dermatomyositis and are distinct from similar lesions found in systemic lupus erythematosus in which the erythema is located between rather than on the joints.

Source: © 2014 American College of Rheumatology. Used with permission.

Figure 1: Heliotrope rash

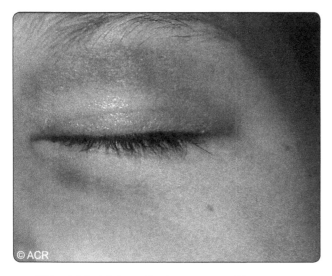

© ACR

» This child with juvenile dermatomyositis demonstrates heliotrope (lilac colored) discoloration and edema of the upper eyelid.

Source: © 2014 American College of Rheumatology. Used with permission.

F. Muscle biopsy and/or magnetic resonance imaging (MRI) may be necessary to confirm diagnosis but not mandatory.

G. Diagnosis requires presence of skin findings and three other of the above signs.

IV. Clinical features.

A. Child will complain of fatigue, crankiness, not being able to keep up with friends on the playground, difficulty climbing the steps of the school bus or trouble lifting arms up over his or her head to pull off a shirt or top.

B. Weakness in neck muscles may cause difficulty swallowing and may need barium swallow to assess.

C. Change in voice quality may be indicative of weak chest muscle and/or weakness of the soft palate (Pachman & Lindsley, 2007).

D. Low grade fevers may be present at onset of symptoms.

V. Treatment.

A. Steroids, either orally or intravenously, are first line medications.

1. 50-75 % achieve complete remission with steroids alone (Olsen & Wortmann, 1997) but the majority of patients now receive a combination of steroids and methotrexate (MTX).

B. MTX (may be given orally or subcutaneously).

C. Intravenous immunoglobulin (IVIG).

1. Considered very safe (Manlhiot et al., 2008).

2. Side effects may include headache, nausea, fever abdominal cramps, malaise, lethargy and myalgia (Manlhiot et al., 2008).

D. Other immunosuppressive agents are used for those patients who are steroid resistant.

1. Cyclosporine is used for patients who are not responding to conventional treatments. Its response is quick, typically within 2 to 4 weeks (Yocum, 1997).

2. Cyclophosphamide (Cytoxan®).
   a. Given intravenously.

3. Mycophenolate Mofetil (CellCept®).
   a. Only one study of 50 patients studied use of Mycophenolate Mofetil (Rouster-Stevens, Morgan, Wang, & Pachman, 2010).

E. Hydroxycholorquine (Plaquenil®).

1. Used for the cutaneous manifestations of JDMS but not recognized as a beneficial treatment for muscle inflammation (Olsen & Wortmann, 1997).

F. Physical therapy helps with muscle strengthening and prevention of contractures and possible muscle atrophy.

G. Rituximab (Rituxan®).

1. B-cell inhibitor given intravenously weekly x 4 infusions.

2. Small case report of four pediatric patients (Cooper et al., 2007).

H. Tacrolimus (Prograf®).

1. Inhibits T-cell activation.

2. Little is known about its efficacy (Hassan, van der Net, & van Royen-Kerkhof, 2008).

I. Thalidomide (Thalomid®).

1. Immunomodulatory drug.

2. One case report documented (Miyamae et al., 2010).

VI. Co-morbid conditions.

A. Eye issues.

1. Cataracts and glaucoma from prolonged steroid use.

B. Associated vasculitis.

1. Child may have gastrointestinal symptoms; (e.g. blood in stool, severe abdominal pain, or cutaneous ulcerations). Changes may be seen in nail fold capillaries using oil and an ophthalmoscope.

C. Calcinosis (see Figure 3).

1. Calcium deposits form as small, superficial bumps that may pop and ooze. Additionally, joint mobility can be affected by sheets of calcium that form an exoskeleton (Li & Imundo, 2006).

2
2.1
2.2
2.3
2.4
2.5
2.6
2.7
2.8
2.9
2.10
2.11

2. May occur one to three years after illness and may cause more disability than the muscle inflammation (Miyamae et al., 2010).

3. Considered to be a sign of active disease in pediatrics (Riley et al., 2008).

4. Some success reported with use of sodium thiosulfate.

D. Lipodystrophy.

1. Children with chronic or very active disease may develop lipodystrophy. These patients often have associated insulin resistance, hyperinsulinemia, diabetes, hypertriglyceridemia, hypertension, liver disease and short stature (Li & Imundo, 2006).

VII. Nursing implications.

A. Education.

Figure 3: Calcinosis

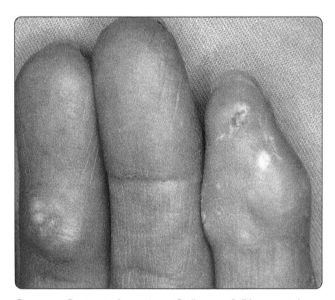

Source: © 2014 American College of Rheumatology. Used with permission.

1. Explain to patients short-term side effects of steroids may include emotional lability, increased appetite, weight gain and "chipmunk cheeks." Encourage healthy snacks to avoid additional weight gain. Remind them that this is the first medication the physician will try to wean off.

2. Explain that potential side effects of MTX may include a rise in liver function tests and/or a drop in white count, necessitating blood work every two to three months (or more frequent if changes in values.) Other side effects may include nausea and/or mouth sores. Instruct patients that while on MTX, they should not take the medication if febrile (>101) or for the first 48 hours of antibiotic therapy.

3. Stress need for annual eye exam with visual field testing while on Plaquenil® because of rare risk of retinal damage.

4. Encourage parents and patients to comply with physical therapy regime as its benefits will help with progress and improvement of symptoms.

5. If undergoing muscle biopsy, explain pre- and post-op procedures to patient and involve help of a child-life specialist to accompany patient to the operating room.

6. Develop a rapport with the school nurses. They are often yours and the parents' eyes and ears while children are in school.

7. If your clinic is large enough and fortunate enough to have social workers, nutritionists, physical therapists and psychologists on the team, collaboratively use a team approach to benefit the child with JDMS.

8. Warn parents of potential exacerbation of dermatological symptoms with increased/extended sun exposure and encourage use of sunscreen.

Summary

Children with JDMS require a multidisciplinary approach to diagnosis and treatment. The nurse may be the best member of the healthcare team to coordinate this effort. Recognizing the medical and social implications of JDMS will better prepare the nurse for this task.

2
2.1
2.2
2.3
2.4
2.5
2.6
2.7
2.8
2.9
2.10
2.11

Acknowledgments

The author wishes to thank Lawrence Zemel, MD and Tegan Willard, BSN, RN for their help with this chapter.

References

Cooper, M. A., Willingham, D. L., Brown, D. E., French, A. R., Shih, F. F., & White, A. J. (2007). Rituximab for the treatment of juvenile dermatomyositis. *Arthritis and Rheumatism, 50*(9), 3107-3111.

Hassan, J., van der Net, J. J., & van Royen-Kerkhof, A. (2008). Treatment of refractory juvenile dermatomyositis with tacrolimus. *Clinical Rheumatology, 27 (11)*, 1469-1471.

Li, S. C., & Imundo, L. F. (2006). Major rheumatic diseases. In I. S. Szer, Y. Kimura, P. N. Malleson, & T. R. Southwood (Eds.), *Arthritis in children and adolescents. Juvenile idiopathic arthritis* (pp. 86-115). Oxford: Oxford University Press.

Manlhiot, C., Tyrrell, P. N., Liang, L., Atkinson, A. R., Lau, W., & Feldman, B. M. (2008). Safety of intravenous immunoglobulin in the treatment of juvenile dermatomyositis: Adverse reactions are associated with immunoglobulin A content. *Pediatrics, 121*, e626-e630. Retrieved from http://pediatrics. aappublications.org/content/early/2008/02/25/ peds.2007-1218/T3.expansion

Mendez, E.P., Lipton, R., Ramsey-Goldman, R., Roettcher, P., Bower, S., Dyer, A., and Pachman, L. (2003). US incidence of juvenile dermatomyositis, 1995-1998: results from the National Institute of Arthritis and Musculoskeletal and Skin Diseases Registry. *Arthritis Rheum.* 2003 Jun 15;49(3):300-5.

Miyamae, T., Sano, F., Ozawa, R., Imagawa, T., Inayama, Y., & Yokota, S. (2010). Efficacy of thalidomide in a girl with inflammatory calcinosis, a severe complication of juvenile dermatomyositis. *Pediatric Rheumatology, 8*, 6. Retrieved from http://www.ped.rheum.com/ content/8/1/6

Olsen, N. J., & Wortmann, R. L. (1997). Inflammatory and metabolic diseases of muscle. In J. H. Klippel, C. M. Weyand, & R. L. Wortmann (Eds.), *Primer on the rheumatic diseases* (11th ed., pp. 276-282). Atlanta, GA: The Arthritis Foundation.

Pachman, L. M., & Lindsley, C. B. (2007). First signs of illness. In L. G. Rider, L. M. Pachman, F. W. Miller, & H. Bollar (Eds.), *Myositis and you. A guide to juvenile dermatomyositis for patients, families and healthcare providers* (pp. 43-51). Washington, DC: The Myositis Association.

Rider, L. G., & Miller, F. W. (2007). What is juvenile myositis?. In L. G. Rider, L. M. Pachman, F. W. Miller, & H. Bollar (Eds.), *Myositis and you. A guide to juvenile dermatomyositis for patients, families and healtcare providers* (pp. 9-22). Washington, DC: The Myositis Association.

Rider, L. G., Lindsley, C. B., & Cassidy, J. T. (2011). Juvenile dermatomyositis. In J. T. Cassidy, R. E. Petty, R. M. Laxer, & C. B. Lindsley (Eds.), *Textbook of pediatric rheumatology* (Sixth ed., pp. 375-413). Philadelphia, PA: Saunders Elsevier.

Riley, P., McCann, L. J., Maillard, S. M., Woo, P., Murray, K. J., & Pilkington, C. A. (2008). Effectiveness of infliximab in the treatment of refractory juvenile dermatomyositis with calcinosis. *Rheumatology, 47*, 877-880. Retrieved from htttp://creativecommons. org/licenses/by-nc/2.0/uk

Rouster-Stevens, K. A., Morgan, G. A., Wang, D., & Pachman, L. M. (2010). Mycophenolate Mofetil: A possible therapeutic agent for children with juvenile dermatomyositis. *Arthritis Care & Research, 62*(10), 1446-1451.

Yocum, D. E. (1997). Cyclosporine and other experimental immunomodulatory agents. In W. J. Koopman (Ed.), *Arthritis and allied conditions. A textbook of rheumatology* (13th ed., pp.761-775). Baltimore, MD: Williams and Wilkins.

Suggested Readings

Myositis and You: A Guide to Juvenile Dermatomyositis for Patients, Families, and Healthcare Providers edited by Lisa G. Rider, MD, Lauren Pachman, MD, Frederick W. Miller, MD, PhD, Harriet Bollar (2007.)

Polymyositis/Dermatomyositis: NIAMS Information Package provided free of charge by the National Institute of Arthritis and Musculoskeletal and Skin Diseases (NIAMS) and National Institute of Health (NIH.) 1-877-22-NIAMS

Juvenile Dermatomyositis, an information sheet provided by the Arthritis Foundation (AF), can be obtained by calling 1-800-283-7800 or by visiting the AF website: www.arthritis.org

Internet Resources:

» www.arthritis.org
» www.rheumatology.org
» www.nih.gov
» www.myositis.org
» www.curejm.com

2
2.1
2.2
2.3
2.4
2.5
2.6
2.7
2.8
2.9
2.10
2.11

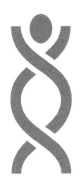

Section 2.7
Behçet's Disease in Children

Cathy Patty-Resk, MSN, RN, CPNP

Introduction

Behçet's Disease (BD) was first described in 1927 by the Turkish dermatologist, Hulusi Behçet. He identified this vasculitic disease with the triad of aphthous stomatitis, genital ulcerations and uveitis. About twenty years later, superficial thrombophlebitis was identified as a fourth criteria. The history of this disease has been traced back to the route of the Silk Road and follows the patterns of emigration in the twentieth century (Dilsen, 1996; Ozen, 2011). Nonetheless, it affects many races and nationalities today. It is a rare disease but is seen in most larger pediatric and adult academic rheumatology practices in the U.S. Since the original triad of signs, arthritis has also been added to the list. Current research is focusing on genetics, molecular biology and immunology in hopes of finding better diagnostic and treatment options (VanDaele, 2009). So far, researchers know the innate immune system plays a significant role in BD because of the hyperactive neutrophils and the inflammation mediated by the innate immune system. There also seems to be an antibody-mediated process since transient neonatal BD has been observed in infants of mothers with BD (Ozen, 2011). Specific etiology and pathogenesis is unknown which has made treatment of this disease very difficult in severe cases.

Learning Objectives

Upon completion of this chapter, the nurse will be able to:

1. Identify three characteristics of Behçet's Disease and characteristics that differentiate it from other look-alike diseases like common aphthous ulcers (AU) and herpes simplex virus (HSV) infections.

2. Understand the basic autoimmune response that precipitates the condition.

3. Understand the importance of pathology and microbiology in diagnosis.

4. Provide rationale for three common pharmacologic treatments.

5. Develop a comprehensive plan of care for the Behçet's Disease patient.

Content Outline

I. Who is affected?

A. 5-13% have childhood onset.

B. Mean age of onset around 12 years of age.

C. May or may not know of family member with BD.

II. Criteria of the International Study Group (ISG) diagnosis of BD (96% specificity, sensitivity 91%) (Ozen, 2011).

A. Recurrent oral ulcers.

   1. Negative HSV and microbial cultures.

   2. Ulcers <0.5cm diameter.

   3. Biopsy pathology negative for granulomatous disease or oncologic process.

B. Plus two of the following:

   1. Recurrent genital ulcers (negative for HSV and other pathogens).

   2. Pathergy (state of both immune and non-immune reactions).

   3. Eye inflammation.
     a. Uveitis: Anterior or posterior.
     b. Retinal vasculitis.

   4. Skin lesions.
     a. Erythema nodosum.
     b. Pseudo folliculitis.
     c. Papulopustular lesions.
     d. Cystic acne (while not on steroids).

III. Other criteria.

A. Arthritis accompanying above criteria.

B. HLA B51 positive (in 50-80% pts. with BD).

IV. What if it doesn't meet enough criteria required by ISG?

A. Can have diagnosis of incomplete or partial BD.

B. ISG criteria has not been validated.

V. Course of the disease.

A. Oral and genital ulcers.

   1. Oral ulcers present in 87% of BD patients.

   2. Occur in crops.

   3. Painful.

   4. Periods of exacerbations may vary significantly without known influences.

   5. Can occur throughout the entire GI tract.

   6. Oral ulcers do not scar when healed.

   7. Genital ulcers may scar when healed.

   8. Genital ulcers usually occur after puberty (present in approximately 6% of BD patients).

   9. Classified as minor aphthae <1cm diameter.

   10. Classified as major aphthae >1cm diameter.

B. Ocular disease.

C. Vascular disease.

   1. BD is the only vasculitis that involves arterial and venous systems and vessels of all sizes.

   2. Thrombus more common in adults (5-15% of children).
     a. Can occur in any size artery or vein.
     b. Significantly increases morbidity and mortality.

   3. Aneurysms.

   4. Periungual dilatation with dropouts present (75% of adults).

D. Musculoskeletal disease.

   1. Arthritis (50-75% of children).
     a. Non-erosive.

   2. Sacro-iliac arthritis (adults).

   3. Myositis not common.
     a. May mimic thrombus.

E. Central nervous system disease.

   1. Meningoencephalitis - fever, headache, stiff neck, and difficulty with coordination.

F. Gastrointestinal disease.

2
2.1
2.2
2.3
2.4
2.5
2.6
2.7
2.8
2.9
2.10
2.11

1. Uncommon manifestation.

2. Mimics Crohn's disease.

   a. Diarrhea.

   b. Abdominal pain.

   c. Exacerbations and remissions.

   d. Ulcerations present.

3. Hepatic vein occlusion may lead to Budd-Chiari syndrome.

G. Renal disease.

   1. Amyloidosis.

   2. Glomerulonephritis.

   3. Renal artery stenosis or aneurysm.

   4. Renal vein thrombosis.

   5. Microvasculature interstitial disease.

VI. Pathology.

A. BD is an occlusive vasculitis in arterioles and veins.

B. Synovial fluid - predominately neutrophils.

C. Muscle biopsies - fibrosis, perivascular infiltrates, necrosis.

VII. Treatment.

A. No pediatric controlled studies; research is based on adult population with BD.

B. Very difficult to treat; treatment is site/symptom/co-morbid disease specific and depends on severity.

C. Arthritis - Colchicine and nonsteroidal anti-inflammatory drugs (NSAIDs) typically used in juvenile idiopathic arthritis (JIA). (if not controlled with colchicine alone).

D. Oral & Genital Ulcers.

   1. Mild disease.

      a. Topical therapies.

         (1) Topical sucralfate, viscous lidocaine preparations, oral hydrocortisone (generally not very effective as treatment; comfort measures).

      b. Systemic therapies.

         (1) Colchicine and glucocorticoids (mixed results).

   2. Severe disease (Vandaele, 2009; Petty, 2011).

      a. High dose methylprednisone pulses; sometimes followed by oral prednisone.

      b. Thalidomide (risk of peripheral neuropathy).

      c. Methotrexate (MTX).

      d. Infliximab (Remicade®).

      e. Abatacept (Orencia®).

      f. Anakinra (Kineret®) (currently being studied for BD).

      g. Interferon (higher doses more effective and longer remissions).

      h. Etanercept (Enbrel®) (for nodular skin lesions and oral ulcers).

E. Uveitis.

   1. Cyclosporine and azothioprine have protective effects.

   2. Infliximab (Remicade®) (to help control uveitis flares).

F. Pyoderma gangrenosum.

   1. Complicated by pathergy phenomenon.

      a. Sterile needle pricks lead to cutaneous lesions and any debridement of such results in local expansion of wound.

      b. Extensive debridement is not recommended.

G. Erythema nodosum.

   1. Unlike erythema nodosum in other diseases, in BD there is medium vessel vasculitis directly underneath.

      a. Treat with systemic glucocorticoids.

H. Neurologic disease.

   1. Aseptic meningitis.

   2. Encephalitis, focal parenchymal lesions and medium vessel vasculitis.

I. Large artery vasculitis.

VIII. Nursing considerations.

A. Pain management.

B. Hydration.

2
2.1
2.2
2.3
2.4
2.5
2.6
2.7
2.8
2.9
2.10
2.11

C. Other specialty referrals (ie. Opthalmology, GI, Nephrology, Neurology).

D. Parent/child missed days of work/school - initiate FMLA for work and IEP for school.

E. Anticipate patient's needs during family or individual vacations and summer camps (ie. bring prednisone and other needed meds for outbreak management, physician contact information, preferred medical facility and location near vacation/camp).

F. Education - regular ophthalmology check-ups, disease, cause, rarity, limited research based treatment for pediatric patients, BD home management.

G. Emotional support - child and parent; the more severe condition the more support required.

Summary

Rheumatology nurses can be most effective in providing care to these patients with a solid knowledge base of BD and monitoring of the evidence-base in research.

Nurses will continue to play a very important role from diagnosis to treatment in the lives of BD patients and their families. They will continue to fill the knowledge gap and help patients/families better understand their disease, how unpredictable it can be, how to manage the early signs more effectively at home and provide the extensive emotional support that is needed.

References

Dilsen, N. (1996). History and development of Behçet's disease. *Revue du Rhumatisme (English Edition),* 63(7-8), 512-519. Retrieved from http://www.ncbi.nlm.nih.gov/pubmed/8896069

Ozen, S., and Petty, R.E. (2011). Behçet disease. In Cassidy, J.T., Petty, R.E., Laxer R.M., & Lindsley, C.B., (Eds.), *Textbook of Pediatric Rheumatology* (6th ed.), pp. 552-558. Philadelphia, PA: Saunders Elsevier.

van Daele, P. L., Kappen, J. H., van Hagen, P. M., & van Laar, J. A. (2009). Managing Behçet's disease: An update on current and emerging treatment options. *Therapeutics and Clinical Risk Management,* 5(2), 385-390. Retrieved from http://www.ncbi.nlm.nih.gov/pmc/articles/PMC2697543/

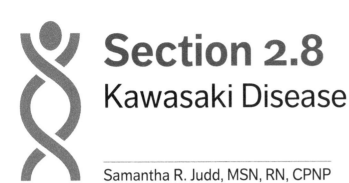

Section 2.8
Kawasaki Disease

Samantha R. Judd, MSN, RN, CPNP

Introduction

Kawasaki disease (KD) is also known as mucocutaneous lymph node syndrome or infantile polyarteritis and is characterized by an acute generalized systemic vasculitis occurring throughout the body (Burns et al., 2013). The disease is self-limiting and approximately 15-25% of the children affected develop coronary aneurysms or ectasia (Newburger et al., 2004). Therefore KD is the most common cause of acquired heart disease in children in Japan and the US (Wood & Tulloh, 2009).

Learning Objectives

Upon completion of this chapter, the nurse will be able to:

1. Identify the diagnostic criteria that is most common with KD.

2. Identify the importance of identification and initiation of therapy.

3. Be able to provide parents with information regarding treatment and special considerations.

Content Outline

I. Etiology and Epidemiology.

A. The etiology of Kawasaki disease is unknown. It is believed ubiquitous infection(s) trigger an abnormal host inflammatory response, leading to KD in genetically predisposed children (Golshevsky, Cheung & Burgner, 2013).

B. More than 85% of cases occur in children younger than 5 years of age (Wood & Tulloh, 2009).

C. Genetic susceptibility is probably an important contributor as evidenced by the racial incidence with Asian-American children being highest, followed by African American and Hispanic children. Lowest incidence is Caucasian children, and higher rates of occurrence being among siblings (Burns et al., 2013).

D. It exhibits seasonal outbreaks with increases in late winter and early spring (Burns et al., 2013).

E. Between 9.1 and 32.5 per 100,000 children (depending on race) contract KD each year in the U.S (Wood & Tulloh, 2009).

F. TNF-alpha appears to be an important facilitator in the inflammatory cascade for KD (Newburger et al., 2004).

II. Diagnosis.

A. KD is characterized by prolonged fever of > 102° F / 39° C plus four of the five cardinal clinical diagnostic criteria; a polymorphous rash, non-exudative conjunctivitis, mucosal changes, erythema or desquamation of extremities and cervical lymphadenopathy (Yim, Curtis, Cheung & Burgner, 2013).

B. The first day of fever is considered the onset of illness. Important to keep a timeline of the illness because of the progression of potential serious complications without the initiation of treatment.

C. According to Burns et al. (2013) there are 4 stages of illness:

1. Stage 1: Acute Phase (days 0-14). High fever, significant irritability, rash, conjunctival injection, strawberry tongue, fissuring of lips, tachycardia, erythema of hands and feet.

2. Stage 2: Subacute phase (2-4 weeks after illness onset). Resolution of fever. This phase lasts until all other symptoms subside. Desquamation of the fingers, then the toes, transient jaundice, abnormal liver enzymes, arthralgia or arthritis, transient diarrhea, orchitis, facial palsy and sensorineural hearing loss may occur. Coronary artery aneurysms appear during this time.

3. Stage 3: Convalescent phase (6-8 weeks). All clinical signs of KD have resolved, however lab values have not returned to normal. This phase is complete when all blood values have returned to normal.

4. Stage 4: Chronic Phase (40 days on into adult hood). Coronary complications may persist on to adulthood.

D. According to Newburger et al (2004):

1. Patients with fever for >5 days and <4 principal features can be diagnosed as having KD when coronary artery disease is detected by 2D echocardiography (2DE) or coronary angiography.

2. In the presence of >4 principal criteria, the diagnosis of KD can be made on day 4 of illness.

3. KD should be considered in the young child with unexplained fever for >5 days that is associated with any of the principal clinical features of this disease.

E. Mood alterations, behavioral changes, gastrointestinal upset and diarrhea (20%), pain or arthritis affecting large joints (30%), hydrops of the gall bladder (10%) and deranged liver function are other reported sequelae of the disease (Wood & Tulloh, 2009).

F. Arthritis associated with KD is possibly non-erosive synovitis with excellent outcome but initially indistinguishable from an early stage of JIA (Izumi et al., 2011).

G. Mild, diffuse dilatation of coronary arteries usually begins on day 10 from fever onset. If left untreated, 25% of these patients progress to true aneurysms, with 1% becoming 'giant aneurysms' (>8 mm internal diameter) (Golshevsky, Cheung and Burgner, 2013).

III. Treatment

Treatment is time sensitive in KD. The goal is to prevent any irreversible damage.

A. Intravenous Immunoglobulin (IVIG).

1. According to Yim et al. (2013):

   a. Effective treatment that has been shown to decrease the amount of coronary lesions.

   b. Most effective if given within the first 10 days of illness however, if inflammation is still present after the 10th day, then IVIG is appropriate .

   c. One time dose IVIG of 2 g/kg over a period of 12 hours.

   d. Follow strict infusion instructions (see product insert instructions) when administering.

B. High dose aspirin (ASA).

1. According to Yim et al. (2013):

   a. In the US the standard dosing is 80-100 mg/kg/day and in Japan and the UK it is 30-50 mg/kg/day divided into 4 doses.

   b. Institutions vary in the protocols for ASA dosing that they use.

2. According to Wood and Tulloh (2009):

   a. High-dose aspirin is initially used for its anti-inflammatory effect, but after the acute phase the dose of aspirin is reduced to 5 mg/kg/day, and acts as an inhibitor of platelet function.

   b. ASA can then be continued up to 6 weeks if no evidence of coronary involvement. However if there was coronary involvement, low dose ASA therapy would be continued.

C. Corticosteroids.

1. According to Newburger et al. (2013):

   a. Corticosteroids are not standard first line treatment for KD; it is mainly used for children who fail IVIG therapy.

   b. Studies of steroids in the initial therapy for KD, as well as in therapy for patients with persistent or recrudescent fever despite treatment with IVIG and aspirin, have shown that corticosteroids reduce fever and inflammatory acute phase reactants C-reactive protein (CRP) and erythrocyte sedimentation rate (ESR).

   c. The effects of steroids on coronary artery abnormalities are still uncertain.

   d. The dosing is IV Methylprednisolone 30 mg/kg (1 gm max) for 2-3 hours once daily for 1-3 days.

D. Alternative treatments in the event of IVIG failure to treatment; according to Newburger et al. (2013) & Cassidy et al. (2011):

1. Failure to respond usually is defined as persistent or recrudescent fever >36 hours after completion of the initial IVIG infusion. Most experts recommend re-treatment with another dose of IVIG at 1-2 g/kg over 12 hours.

2. Introduce pulse corticosteroids with methylprednisolone 30 mg/kg (1 gm max) for 2-3 hours once daily for 1-3 days.

3. Infliximab (Remicade®):

   a. According to a research study recently done by Tremoulet, et al (2014): The addition of infliximab (Remicade®) to primary treatment in acute KD did not reduce treatment resistance. Infliximab (Remicade®) was safe, well tolerated, and reduced fever duration. Markers of inflammation such as the left anterior descending coronary artery Z score, and intravenous immunoglobulin reaction rates were reduced.

   b. Immunocompromising to the child. **No live vaccines to be given for at least four weeks after LAST infusion.**

   c. Need to have outpatient infusions done every couple of weeks.

   d. Need to follow proper infusion protocols, follow product information preparation and disposal and have emergency equipment (i.e. oxygen, epinephrine, suction) at bedside in case of anaphylaxis.

IV. Laboratory and Diagnostic Findings.

A. According to Burns et al. (2013), in Stage 1 findings are generally: Elevated ESR and

2
2.1
2.2
2.3
2.4
2.5
2.6
2.7
2.8
2.9
2.10
2.11

platelet count (as high as 700,000/mm3), elevated CRP, leukocytosis with left shift, slight decreases in red blood cells and hemoglobin, hypoalbuminemia, increased Alpha-2 globulin and sterile pyuria.

B. Rule out other sources of infection is necessary. Possible blood culture, rapid strep and throat culture, cerebrospinal fluid and urine culture needed.

C. Raised C-reactive protein (CRP) (>35 mg/L) is seen in approximately 80% of cases and a raised erythrocyte sedimentation rate (ESR) (>60 mm/h) in 60% (Yim et al., 2013).

D. 2D echo may show cardiac artery changes.

   1. According to Burns et al. (2013), repeat 2D echocardiograms need to be done 2 weeks and 6-8 weeks after onset of fever.

V. Nursing Implications.

A. Recent studies suggest that children with KD may have long-term sequelae, even when there is no overt coronary artery involvement in the acute stage of the disease. Affected children should therefore be kept on long-term follow-up, and instructed to avoid known cardiovascular risk factors, such as sedentary lifestyle, being overweight, high-lipid and caloric meals, alcohol or tobacco use (Pinto, Laranjo, Paramés, Freitas & Mota-Carmo, 2013).

B. Educate families on the importance of following up due to the nature of the disease and possible long term consequences.

C. According to Furukawa et al. (1994) (as cited in Newburger et al., 2004):

   1. Measles and varicella immunizations should be deferred for 11 months after a child receives high-dose IVIG. A child in whom the risk of exposure to measles is high may be vaccinated earlier and then be re-immunized >11 months after IVIG administration if the child has an inadequate serological response.

D. In the event the child was to receive infliximab (Remicade®), high dose steroids or a cytotoxic agent, make sure that no live vaccines are given.

   1. Follow the strict guidelines and product information for each infusion and continuously monitor the patient for adverse reactions.

Summary

Kawasaki disease is a vasculitis that has an unknown etiology with some possibly devastating complications if not treated. Only a small percentage of children will go on to develop coronary artery aneurysms with complications, however this small, yet significant, number could also be contributed to the recognition and current treatments of the disease. It is imperative that the rheumatology nurse continues to address the frequent follow-ups and medication compliance as well as other needs the family or child may need.

References

Burns, C. E., Dunn, A. M., Brady, M. A., Starr, N. B., & Blosser, C. (2013). *Pediatric primary care (5th ed.).* Philadelphia: Saunders.

Cassidy, J.T., Petty, R.E., Laxer, R.M. & Lindsley, C.B. (2011). Textbook of Pediatric Rheumatology (6th ed.). Philadelphi: Saunders.

Golshevsky, D., Cheung, M., & Burgner, D. (2013). Kawasaki disease - The importance of prompt recognition and early referral. *Australian Family Physician, 42*(7), 473-476.

Izumi, G., Narugami, M., Saita, Y., Matsuzawa, T., Sugawara, O., Kawamura, N., & Kobayashi, I. (2011). Arthritis associated with Kawasaki disease: MRI findings and serum matrix metalloproteinase-3 profiles. *Pediatrics International, 53*(6), 1087-1089. doi:10.1111/j.1442-200X.2011.03393.x

Newburger, J., Takahashi, M., Gerber, M., Gewitz, M., Tani, L., Burns, J...& Taubert, K. (2004). Diagnosis, treatment, and long-term management of Kawasaki disease: a statement for health professionals from the Committee on Rheumatic Fever, Endocarditis, and Kawasaki Disease, Council on Cardiovascular Disease in the Young, American Heart Association. *Circulation, 110*, 2747-2771.

Pinto, F., Laranjo, S., Paramés, F., Freitas, I., & Mota-Carmo, M. (2013). Long-term evaluation of endothelial function in Kawasaki disease patients. *Cardiology In The Young*, *23*(4), 517-522. doi:10.1017/S1047951112001357

Tremoulet, A., Jain, S., Jaggi, P., Jimenez-Fernandez, S., Pancheri, J., Sun, X., & ... Burns, J. (2014). Infliximab for intensification of primary therapy for Kawasaki disease: a phase 3 randomised, double-blind, placebo-controlled trial. *Lancet*, *383*(9930), 1731-1738. doi:10.1016/S0140-6736(13)62298-9

Wood, L., & Tulloh, R. (2009). Kawasaki disease in children. *Heart*, *95*(10), 787-792. doi:10.1136/hrt.2008.143669

Yim, D., Curtis, N., Cheung, M., & Burgner, D. (2013). An update on Kawasaki disease II: Clinical features, diagnosis, treatment and outcomes. *Journal Of Paediatrics & Child Health*, *49*(8), 614-623. doi:10.1111/jpc.12221

2
2.1
2.2
2.3
2.4
2.5
2.6
2.7
2.8
2.9
2.10
2.11

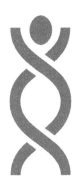

Section 2.9
Henoch-Schönlein Purpura

Samantha R. Judd, MSN, RN, CPNP

Introduction

Henoch-Schönlein purpura (HSP) is the most common form of vasculitis in childhood (Penny, Fleming, Kazmierczak and Thomas, 2010). HSP is self-limiting and is most commonly mild in its course, however, it may have serious life threatening involvement. Most commonly, the serious life threatening complications include renal involvement. This chapter will focus on HSP.

Learning Objectives

Upon completion of this chapter, the nurse will be able to:

1. List three common manifestations of HSP.

2. Understand the various forms of HSP involvement.

3. List three common nursing implications about the treatments of HSP.

Content Outline

I. Etiology and epidemiology:

A. Unknown etiology, however there is evidence that IgA is involved in the pathogenesis of HSP (Burns et al., 2013).

B. Several antigens such as infective agents, vaccinations, drugs, insect bites and different foods have been found to trigger the disease (Penny et al., 2010).

C. The incidence of HSP seems to increase in the autumn and winter following an upper respiratory infection (Penny et al., 2010).

D. Incidence is higher in 4-6 year old children and in boys more so than girls (Penny et al., 2010).

II. Diagnosis.

A. The diagnosis is based on the presence of two or more of the following four findings: Palpable purpura, bowel angina/abdominal pain, diagnostic biopsy (granulocytes found in the walls of arterioles or venules on histologic exam) and pediatric age group (less than 20 years old at onset of symptoms) (Burns et al., 2013).

B. Frequently associated with skin, joint and gastrointestinal manifestations, as well as renal involvement in approximately 50% of the patients (Ninchoji et al., 2011).

C. Arthritis occurs in approximately 80% of the patients and is very painful with an acute onset. Joints that are most often affected include ankles and knees (Burns et al., 2013).

D. Henoch-Schönlein purpura nephritis (HSPN) ranges from relatively common transient isolated microscopic hematuria to nephrotic syndrome, rapidly progressive glomerulonephritis and renal failure (Ninchoji et al., 2010).

III. Treatment:

A. Supportive treatment unless there is significant involvement of systems.

B. Careful attention is given to maintaining hydration and electrolyte balances (Burns et al., 2013).

C. In mild to severe HSPN without nephrotic syndrome, Ninchoji et al. (2011) state that ACE-1 (Angiotensin-converting enzyme) and ARB (Angiotensin II Receptor Blocker) therapy can be used. Ninchoji et al. (2011) recommend the following:

1. ACE-1 (Lisinopril 0.1- 0.4 mg/kg with max dose of 20 mg/day).
   a. 1st line therapy.
   b. Tetratogenic - proper birth control measures for the sexually active adolescent.
   c. If patient develops dry cough or has allergic reaction, then it needs to be immediately stopped and changed to ARB.
   d. If little or no benefit after several months, then ARB should be added.

2. ARB (candesartan 0.05 mg/kg and increased to 0.2 mg/kg. Max dose 20 mg).
   a. Can be given by itself or in conjunction with the ACE-1. Special attention needs to be made to renal function and blood pressure when given in conjunction with ACE-1.
   b. Tetratogenic- proper birth control measures should be in place for sexually active adolescents.
   c. Monitor renal function and liver function during therapy.
   d. Monitor blood pressures.

3. If the ARB added to ACE-I offered little benefit after several months and massive proteinuria with hypoalbuminemia is detected, the patient should be given the combination therapy described under severe HSPN.

4. These findings indicate that ACE-I and/ or ARB can be used successfully in HSPN patients without nephrotic syndrome, and it is not necessary for moderate–severe cases to be treated aggressively with steroids, immunosuppressive agents, tonsillectomy, or plasma exchange even if heavy proteinuria persists (Ninchoji et al., 2011).

D. In severe HSPN with nephrotic syndrome one research study done by Ninchoji et al.

(2011) found that the use of combination therapy helped to restore renal function. Ninchoji et al (2011) recommended:

1. Corticosteroids:

    a. 2 mg/kg/day prednisolone, given in three divided doses (maximum dose, 80 mg/day) for the first 4 weeks, followed by prednisolone at 2 mg/kg given as a single dose every other morning for 8 weeks. The dose was then decreased by 0.5 mg/kg every 2 weeks.

    b. There is little evidence suggesting that corticosteroids prevent any gastrointestinal (GI) or renal involvement (Gibson, Amamoo and Primack, 2008). However it will help to suppress the inflammatory process, and therefore allow already damaged tissue to heal.

    c. The child may develop obesity or cushingoid facies due to the steroid use.

    d. The child may also become immunocompromised from long term steroid use.

2. Azathioprine (2 mg/kg/day as a single dose; maximum dose 100 mg) or mizoribine (5 mg/kg/day as a single dose; maximum dose 300 mg), and were maintained for 6 months.

    a. Comes in pill form or IV infusion.

    b. Follow strict administration protocols when giving IV infusion.

    c. Monitor for life threatening reactions during IV infusion such as anaphylaxis and have emergency equipment at the bedside (i.e. Epinephrine, IV fluids, Oxygen and suction).

    d. Immunosuppressant drugs, do not give live vaccines while patient is on this medication.

    e. Make sure that the child has a QuantiFERON® - TB Gold test done before initiation of therapy and that it is negative.

    f. Make sure that adequate birth control measures are being taken for the sexually active adolescent as this medication is a teratogen.

3. Warfarin 1 mg/day in the morning.

    a. Anticoagulant therapy.

    b. Monitor International Normalized Ratio (INR) and for bleeding (while on anticoagulation therapy should be 1.5-2 times normal value).

    c. Teratogenic- Make sure adequate birth control is in place.

4. Dipyridamole 3 mg/kg/day divided into 3 doses and increased to 6 mg/kg/day (max 300 mg/day) and maintained for 8 weeks then stopped.

    a. Antiplatelet therapy.

    b. The child is at risk for bleeding, monitor INR weekly (1.5-2 times normal value).

    c. Teratogenic- make sure adequate birth control is in place.

    d. Severe contraindication when given with warfarin.

    e. Educate families on adverse effects of medication such as chest pain, angina exacerbation, abnormal ECG, headache, and dizziness and when to seek medical attention and stop medication.

IV. Laboratory and Diagnostic findings:

A. Erythrocyte sedimentation rate (ESR), C-reactive protein (CRP), and white blood cell (WBC) count are elevated. Platelet count is normal or even high (Burns et al., 2013).

B. Other tests are ordered based on system involvement (i.e. GI involvement with abdominal x-ray).

C. Urinalysis is done to rule out renal involvement. If it is suspected a renal biopsy may be done to assist with grading of involvement.

V. Management:

A. Monitor for GI blood loss, hematuria and proteinuria. Refer to GI and nephrology if any blood or protein are present.

B. Monitor for hypertension by primary care provider (PCP) weekly. If hypertension present refer to nephrology immediately.

C. Monitor pain and the use of over-the-counter (OTC) analgesics.

D. Refer to nephrology if there is renal involvement suspected.

E. Monitor INR, blood urea nitrogen (BUN), creatinine (Cr), glomerular filtration

2
2.1
2.2
2.3
2.4
2.5
2.6
2.7
2.8
2.9
2.10
2.11

rate (GFR), hemoglobin (Hgb), and liver function test (LFT) while patient is undergoing treatment with ACE-1, ARB, or immunosuppressive drugs.

VI. Nursing special considerations:

A. Be aware that there is an increased risk of intussusception with HSP and GI involvement (Penny et al., 2009).

B. Families may feel as if they have no control and become anxious when they learn that there is no treatment for HSP.

C. Reassure families that the child may pass blood in the stool and that this is temporary. However, advise them on what is normal and what requires immediate attention by a provider.

D. If the child is on immunosuppressive therapy such as high dose steroids or immunosuppressive drugs, the child may not receive any live vaccines.

E. Depending on the extent of disease involvement/untoward sequelae, educate the parents on Family and Medical Leave Act (FMLA) papers and the importance of making sure their child has support from his/her teachers at school.

Summary

HSP for the most part has more "look than bite". Most families become very concerned about their child's skin manifestations or symptoms, as they should, however most cases are simple and straight forward and require minimal intervention. Although, when there is significant involvement action must be taken to help preserve organ function. More research is being done to help find the best treatment with the least adverse effects. The role of the rheumatology nurse with these patients is to help educate and comfort the families as they go through the treatment process and to continually assess the child and family's needs.

References

Burns, C. E., Dunn, A. M., Brady, M. A., Starr, N. B., & Blosser, C. (2013). *Pediatric primary care (5th ed.).* Philadelphia: Saunders.

Gibson, K., Amamoo, M., & Primack, W. (2008). Corticosteroid therapy for Henoch Schönlein purpura... Pediatrics. 2007 Nov;120(5):1079-87. *Pediatrics, 121*(4), 870-872.

Ninchoji, T., Kaito, H., Nozu, K., Hashimura, Y., Kanda, K., Kamioka, I., & ... Matsuo, M. (2011). Treatment strategies for Henoch-Schönlein purpura nephritis by histological and clinical severity. *Pediatric Nephrology, 26*(4), 563-569. doi:10.1007/s00467-010-1741-5

Penny, K., Fleming, M., Kazmierczak, D., & Thomas, A. (2010). An epidemiological study of Henoch-Schönlein purpura. *Paediatric Nursing, 22*(10), 30-35.

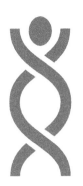

Section 2.10
Benign Joint Hypermobility Syndrome

Cathy Patty-Resk, MSN, RN, CPNP

Introduction

Musculoskeletal pain of non-inflammatory origin affecting widespread joints is common in childhood. Benign Joint Hypermobility Syndrome (BJHS) applies to children that do not have hypermobility of joints due to an underlying cause or hereditary hypermobility syndrome. Many dancers and athletes are hypermobile, which contributes to their athletic skill. These patients often refer to themselves as being double jointed and take pride in being able to contort their joints in ways most people cannot. However, many times the patient, parent or primary care physician does not link the extreme flexibility to the joint pain. BJHS can cause chronic pain of joints that mimics other rheumatologic conditions such as juvenile idiopathic arthropathies (JIA) or connective tissue disease (CTD).

Learning Objectives

Upon completion of this chapter, the nurse will be able to:

1. List populations at risk for experiencing BJHS.

2. Identify at least three ways to check a patient for hypermobility.

3. Explain satisfactorily to patients and parents how their hypermobility causes pain.

4. Develop an effective treatment plan of care for the benign hypermobile patient

Content Outline

I. Populations at risk for BJHS and frequency (Leblanc & Houghton, 2011).

A. Whites 8-20%

B. Chinese.

C. Arabic.

D. Blacks.

E. Inuits.

F. Children ages 3-10 years of age most strongly effected.

G. Girls twice as often as boys.

II. Usual presentation (Leblanc & Houghton, 2011).

A. Intermittent pain to thighs, calf area or joints.

B. Pain worse with activity or after.

C. No morning stiffness to joints.

D. Repeated joint sprains.

E. No joint swelling or minimal swelling.

F. Patellofemoral pain common.

G. Back pain in adults.

H. Can affect temporomandibular joint (TMJ).

I. Pain worse at night.

III. Criteria for hypermobility (Leblanc & Houghton, 2011).

A. Three of five are required to establish diagnosis.

  1. Touch thumb to velar forearm.

  2. Hyperextend metacarpalphalangeal (MCP) joints so fingers parallel forearm.

  3. >10 degree hyperextension of elbows.

  4. >10 degree hyperextension of knees.

  5. Bend at waist and touch palms to floor with knees straight.

IV. Other common features of children with hypermobility (not diagnostic criteria) (Cleveland Clinic, 2009; Leblanc & Houghton, 2011).

A. Put heel behind head.

B. Excessive internal rotation of hip.

C. Excessive ankle dorsiflexion.

D. Excessive eversion of foot.

E. Passively touch elbows behind back.

F. Frequently "crack knuckles" (not harmful).

V. Treatment of BJHS (Cleveland Clinic, 2009; Leblanc& Houghton, 2011).

A. Physical therapy (PT) and occupational therapy (OT) for strengthening of muscles surrounding joints.

B. Orthopedic taping.

C. Bracing in severe cases.

D. Orthotics.

E. Supportive and well-cushioned footwear.

F. Post activity nonsteroidal anti-inflammatory drugs (NSAIDs).

G. Night time splints may help joints recover from active day.

H. Apply ice/cold.

I. Proprioceptive (balancing) exercises may be helpful.

VI. Helpful suggestions for patients with BJHS.

A. Be mindful of body positions.

  1. Don't show off hypermobility with "tricks".

  2. Don't hyperextend elbows when lifting or carrying objects.

  3. Don't sit on chairs with knees flexed and heels to buttocks.

  4. Don't sit "crisscross applesauce".

2
2.1
2.2
2.3
2.4
2.5
2.6
2.7
2.8
2.9
2.10
2.11

5. Stand with knees slightly bent.

B. Avoid overuse especially during athletics that cause pain afterward.

VII. Growing up and out of hypermobility.

A. Teens girls have an increased risk for anterior cruciate ligament (ACL) tears.

1. Increase in hormones affect tendons and ligaments to allow for rapid growth.

2. Risk tends to decrease as they approach end of teen years.

B. By late teen years most patients report an improvement in frequency of pain, severity of pain and fewer joint sprains.

C. Generalized joint laxity decreases with age.

D. Not common in older adults.

VIII. Hereditary syndromes of hypermobility: (these are NOT BJHS).

A. Marfan Syndrome.

B. Homocystinuria Syndrome.

C. Stickler Syndrome.

D. Ehlers-Danlos Syndrome.

E. Osteogenesis Imperfecta Syndrome.

F. Williams Syndrome.

G. Down Syndrome / Trisomy 21.

2
2.1
2.2
2.3
2.4
2.5
2.6
2.7
2.8
2.9
2.10
2.11

Summary

It can be very difficult for patients and parents/guardians to understand that something like benign hypermobility can cause so much discomfort or even swelling. They commonly believe there is something much more sinister and serious occurring. Treatment strategies focus on the patient experiencing pain-free and healthy joints. Optimal understanding, compliance with treatment strategies, and management of BJHS in everyday circumstances is crucial in order to afford patients the best possible outcome.

References

Cleveland Clinic (2009), *Benign hypermobility syndrome* in Diseases & Conditions, Cleveland Clinic Website. Retrieved from http://my.clevelandclinic.org/disorders/benign_hypermobility_joint_syndrome/hic_benign_hypermobility_syndrome.aspx

LeBlanc, C., and Houghton, K. (2011). Systemic Juvenile Idiopathic Arthritis. In J.T. Cassidy, R.E. Petty, R.M. Laxer & C.B. Lindsley (Eds.), *Textbook of Pediatric Rheumatology 6th Ed.*, (Chapter 14) pp. 697-717). Philadelphia, PA: Saunders Elsevier.

Section 2.11

Understanding the Benefits of Physical Therapy and Occupational Therapy

Cathy Patty-Resk, MSN, RN, CPNP

Introduction

As noted in previous sections, most rheumatologic conditions affect the joints, muscle and skin which often lead to pain, loss of function, mobility, work and school along with isolation of peers (Cakmak & Bolukbas, 2005; Kuchta & Davidson, 2011). Research has proven repeatedly that inactivity with arthritis is a key indicator of poor prognosis (Westby & Li, 2006). The Physical and Occupational Therapists (PT/OT) are key team members as their therapies provide a critical role in the preservation and restoration of joint function in rheumatic diseases. Patients and families should understand it is everything the team is doing together that will help manage the disease most and not just a single form of treatment.

Before understanding what the Physical and Occupational Therapists do to assist patients with maximizing their physical abilities, it is important to understand why joints are painful in arthritis. Pain due to arthritis is most always due to cytokines present in the synovial fluid that initiates a cascade of inflammatory events. Children with Juvenile Idiopathic Arthritis (JIA) and adults with Rheumatoid Arthritis (RA) tend to keep their joints in their most comfortable positions, usually flexion. During flexion, joints can accommodate the increased fluid from the synovial proliferation and effusion with less pressure on the already thickened synovium. This inflammatory cascade also causes the surrounding soft tissue to undergo fibrosis and contracture (Kuchta & Davidson, 2011; Rhodes, 1991). The synovium leaks through foramens in the bone and along the tendon sheaths, causing what is known as tenosynovitis. When a joint is kept in the flexed position for comfort, the extensor muscles become weak and contractures develop. Over time, as the patient tries to compensate for the weakness they begin to develop even more contractures with other muscle groups becoming weak (Cakmak & Bolukbas, 2005; Kuchta & Davidson, 2011). This phenomenon of decreased muscle mass surrounding arthritic joints has been documented since the 1800's when autopsies were performed to study diseases.

Learning Objectives

Upon completion of this chapter, the nurse will be able to:

1. Recognize when to refer the rheumatology patient for PT or OT services.

2. Initiate basic PT and/or OT exercises.

3. Know what specific services to order for work/school evaluations.

4. List the many benefits PT and OT services can offer the patient besides muscle strengthening.

5. Understand the use of splinting and its limitations

Content Outline

2
2.1
2.2
2.3
2.4
2.5
2.6
2.7
2.8
2.9
2.10
2.11

I. **Indications for referral** (Cakmak & Bolukbas, 2005; Kuchta & Davidson, 2011; Rhodes, 1991; Westby & Li, 2006).

A. Decreased mobility.

B. Difficulty performing activities of daily living (ADL).

C. Any restrictive range of motion (ROM).

D. Symptoms of active disease.

E. Pain.

F. Fatigue.

G. Morning stiffness or gelling.

H. Changes in activity participation or inactivity.

I. Mood or behavior changes.

J. Isolation from peers due to effects of disease.

K. Sleep disturbances related to disease.

II. **Information to Send to PT/OT Therapist** (Cakmak & Bolukbas, 2005; Kuchta & Davidson, 2011).

A. Last clinic letter: Diagnosis, extent of joint or systemic involvement, identified co-morbidities, medications and medical treatment plan.

III. **Physical Therapy Evaluation Includes** (Cakmak & Bolukbas, 2005; Kuchta & Davidson, 2011; Rhodes, 1991; Westby & Li, 2006).

A. Baseline examination; serial evaluations are to document progress.

B. Patient history.

1. Morning stiffness and duration, fatigue, perceived pain of patient/parent.

2. Independence of ADLs.

3. Functional mobility- at work or school and endurance.

4. Use of assistive devices, specialized equipment or splints.

5. Exercise program participation outside of PT/OT.

C. Examination.

1. Spine.

2. Joints; effusions, warmth, redness, swelling, synovial thickening.

3. Pain (occurs with movement; active, passive or weight bearing) and tenderness (occurs with touch or palpation).

4. Measurement of ROM to spine and extremities.

5. Muscle; manual strength, atrophy, asymmetry, developmental abilities (for pediatric patients).

6. Postural assessment.

7. Gait.

8. Functional mobility; proficiency to complete task from beginning to end, movement quality, speed of performance, endurance to perform multiple repetitions of an activity.

9. Assessment, design, manufacturing and proper fitting of splints.

IV. **Occupational Therapy Evaluation Includes** (Kuchta & Davidson, 2011; Rhodes, 1991).

A. Baseline examination; serial evaluations are to document progress.

1. Dressing.

2. Bathing.

3. Eating and drinking.

4. Toileting.

5. Meal preparation, cooking and clean up.

6. Laundry.

7. Writing, keyboarding.

8. Hobbies; gardening tools, painting, drawing, and similar activities.

9. Sports; gripping golf club, baseball, and similar activities.

10. Work/school related tasks; ergonomic desk environment.

11. Visual and physical safety at home, work and school.

12. Assessment, design, manufacturing and proper fitting of splints.

V. Goals of PT/OT Will Include
(Cakmak & Bolukbas, 2005; Kuchta & Davidson, 2011; Rhodes, 1991):

A. Restore ADL.

B. Decrease pain.

C. Increase muscle strength and length.

D. Improve quality of sleep.

E. Increased social participation by facilitating integration into school/work.

F. Increase ROM.

G. Increase energy and activity tolerance.

H. Proper use of splints.

I. Proper use of adaptive equipment.

J. Prevent loss of motion, disuse atrophy and long term goal of preventing osteoporosis (Rhodes, 1991).

K. Development of home PT/OT plan.

L. Coordinate medication timing with exercise and ADLs for optimal benefit.

M. Decrease and eliminate compensatory movements due to lack of muscle strength or stamina.

N. Improve quality of movement and balance.

O. School/work accommodation suggestions and adaptive measures for environment.

VI. Individualized Physical Therapy Techniques (Cakmak & Bolukbas, 2005; Kuchta & Davidson, 2011).

A. Measures to provide comfort; heat, cold, alternating heat/cold and transcutaneous electrical nerve stimulation (TENS) therapy.

B. Active, active-assistive, passive ROM.

C. No vigorous active or passive stretching.

D. Isometric exercises.

E. Contract/relax techniques.

F. Strengthening.

G. Deep heat (for adults only) using ultrasound and diathermy.

VII. Individualized Occupational Therapy Techniques (Kuchta & Davidson, 2011; Rhodes, 1991).

A. Paraffin and heat treatments.

B. Fine motor coordination, stamina and strength exercises.

C. Educate patient using proper ergonomics in school/work environments.

D. Teach energy conservation.

E. Evaluate home safety and modification recommendations; proper placement of assist bars.

F. Adaptive measures for ADLs; i.e. built ups, jar opener, non-skid rugs, toilet seat lift.

G. Assist with visually impaired services; i.e. finding large print book libraries, learning braille, schools for visually impaired.

VIII. Rationale for Splinting
(Cakmak & Bolukbas, 2005; Kuchta & Davidson, 2011; Rhodes, 1991).

A. Help relieve muscle contractures and stretch other soft tissues.

B. Resting splints; weakening and shortening of quadriceps muscle in knee arthritis is why flexion is a more comfortable position for patients, ankle splints to help prevent heel cord shortening in ankle arthritis since extension is the most comfortable position for them.

C. Finger splints, ring splints; help straighten fingers that have developed contractures

2
2.1
2.2
2.3
2.4
2.5
2.6
2.7
2.8
2.9
2.10
2.11

from arthritis damage in the phalanges or the inflammatory response leading to a fibrotic process as in sclerosing seen in scleroderma, can be used day or night.

D. In-shoe orthotic devices; to correct ankle, hind foot or forefoot deviations.

IX. Facilitating Compliance with Home OT/PT Maintenance Plan.

A. Adequate family support and supervision at home.

B. Continued daily emotional support.

C. Use creative motivational support.

D. Chart home progress on progress chart.

E. Use reward system particularly useful with children.

F. Have a therapy buddy to do exercises with patient (good for kids and seniors).

G. Take a warm bath before and encourage stretching on days that patient is having an unusually achy, sore day (don't skip personal plan frequently or completely).

X. Overcoming Social Isolation: Role of the OT/PT (Kuchta & Davidson, 2011).

A. Ability to drive car; step toward independence by enhancing community access.

   1. Driving assessment, instruction and handicap parking permit.

B. Power mobility; vehicle that can transport power wheelchair or scooter.

C. Therapy animal: Seeing eye dog, therapy dog.

D. "Field trips" into the patient's community with patient and OT/PT; allows real-time problem solving for patient, assesses their readiness and ability to successfully navigate and integrate into their community all while allowing the OT/PT to evaluate for safety and unexpected barriers.

E. Evaluation of stamina for social activity, work or school and assist with plan to escalate social endurance.

F. Assess psychological readiness for peers, strangers/community, schoolmates and co-workers; particularly when the following have occurred or are present:

   1. Disfigurement and/or skin changes from arthritis or sclerosis.

   2. Physically visible splints, casts or central lines.

   3. Use of ambulatory assistive devices.

   4. Newly adaptive school/work environment.

G. Encourage camps for children and adolescents with rheumatologic disorders.

   1. Learn from older peers and counselors with their diseases.

   2. Socialization with same age peers.
      a. Common diagnosis.
      b. Common medications and side effects.
      c. Frequent medical appointments.
      d. Common school challenges.
      e. Common social challenges.
      f. Social networking.

   3. Support system that will likely continue after camp.

   4. Friendships that reunite yearly.

H. Assist and encourage when ready, how to locate support groups for specific disease and age group (i.e. kids, teens, adults, seniors).

Summary

By maximizing the team approach to care the patient will be able to achieve the best possible outcome for health of body and mind. At the same time, recognize that not all patients will have access to timely PT/OT services and some may not have access at all due to access or living in rural areas where these services have limited availability. The following appendix pages are some of the common OT home therapies nurses and providers can utilize to get their pediatric and even adult patients heading in the right direction.

2
2.1
2.2
2.3
2.4
2.5
2.6
2.7
2.8
2.9
2.10
2.11

References

Cakmak, A., & Bolukbas, N. (2005). Juvenile rheumatoid arthritis: Physical therapy and rehabilitation. *Southern Medical Journal, 98*(2), 212-216.

Kuchta, G., & Davidson, I., (2011) Occupational and physical therapy for childhood rheumatic diseases. In Cassidy, J., Petty, R., Laxter, R., and Lindsley, C., (Ed[s]), *Textbook of Pediatric Rheumatology (6th Ed.)*, (Chapter 12, pp.198-210). Philadelphia, PA: Saunders Elsevier.

Rhodes, V., J., (1991). Physical therapy management of patients with juvenile rheumatoid arthritis. *Physical Therapy*, 71, 910-919.

Westby, M., and Li, L., (2006). Physical therapy and exercise for arthritis: Do they work? *Geriatrics and Aging.* 9, 624-630.

2
2.1
2.2
2.3
2.4
2.5
2.6
2.7
2.8
2.9
2.10
2.11

Visual motor integration is the ability to put together what we see with what we need to do. These include copying from a blackboard, catching a ball, or writing within the lines. Visual perception is how our brain interprets what we see, or what our brain "sees" when we are looking at something. Problems which can be seen are: The child can write letters and words from memory, but has difficulty copying them from the board, difficulty cutting on a line, inability to keep the pencil within the maze, poor placement of letters on a line, poorly spaced letters, or no spaces between words.

Compensatory strategies:

» Give the child more time to write.

» Give the child a copy of spelling words to put on their desk.

» Use tactile paper when writing or practicing letters (paper with ridges or textures).

» Mark outside of coloring or writing lines with red paper, puffy paint or glue to provide a border for the child to stay in-between.

Activities

» Trace letters and shapes with fingers before drawing them.

» Create a stand or salt box and have the child draw mazes for you or siblings and vice versa.

» Practice cutting on straight, curvy, or jagged lines.

» Play pick-up sticks.

» Play Frisbee® or catch.

» Mazes.

» Puzzles.

» Dot-to-Dots.

» Hidden pictures.

» Color by-numbers.

» Sorting objects (coins, marbles, socks, laundry).

» Cross words / word searches.

» Card games.

» Video games.

» Checkers.

» Dominoes.

» Pinball.

» Balloon volleyball.

» Baseball / tee-ball.

» Search books (Where's Waldo, I Spy).

» Connect Four®

» Walking or wheeling on lines.

» Drawing letters in the air with empty paper towel rolls, stick, finger, etc.

» Jumping on a trampoline while reading letter or pictures aloud off a chart, book or flash cards in their field of vision.

» Visual tracking- have the child follow your finger or a pen or other small object without moving their head in a horizontal line, vertical line, and diagonally. Have the child follow your finger, pen etc, as it moves closer to the tip of their nose. Have the child keep the object in focus as they turn their head to the side. Repeat tracking exercises with one eye covered, repeat with the other eye covered.

» Have the child on their back and track a tennis ball on a string.

» Have the child track a flashlight beam on the wall by pointing as you move it from wall to wall

Tactile activities are helpful in developing the hand's ability to manipulate objects and learn from touch. The sense of touch includes light touch, pressure, vibration, temperature, and pain. Here are some examples of ways to increase your child's tactile awareness and begin to learn from touch:

Activities

» Rub the child's body all over with towels. This is a fun activity after bathing or swimming.

» Give your child "fidget" toys; stress balls made of different textures, rubber, plastic, knobby rubber.

» Do massage and back rubs using a variety of lotion or powder on child while identifying body parts. Some children enjoy vibration from vibrating massage products, such as pillows or massagers.

» Pretend to paint the body with a clean paintbrush, then rub the "paint" off with a towel.

» Playing with water, or pouring water on the child.

» Playing with foam soap in the bathtub.

» Wrapping the whole body up in a blanket.

» Playing in a small wading pool filled with packing peanuts or sand or plastic balls.

» Log rolling on the floor.

» Soap paint on the body (available at toy stores).

» Face and body paints.

» Playing in the sandbox with only shorts on to get good tactile input all over the body. Encourage weight bearing positions such as hands and knees, prone on elbows, kneeling, and standing to give additional tactile stimulation.

» Find hidden shapes and objects (small game pieces, coins, buttons) in different textures such as dry beans, rive, sand, macaroni noodles, Styrofoam packing pieces. Playing hide-and-seek with different objects, finding puzzle pieces and putting a puzzle together.

» Feely-Meely game- fill a box or bag with different objects, have the child reach in and try to identify the objects by touch. You can use shapes, letters, coins, paperclips, textured cloth.

» Make collages using fabric pieces, yarn, paper, etc.

» Make texture books with rough, smooth, hard, soft, fuzzy, scratchy types of objects or fabrics for the child to experience. Some suggestions are burlap, feathers, suede, sandpaper, felt, cotton, corduroy, silk, terrycloth, etc.

» Have the child help you in the kitchen with kneading dough, mixing cookie batter.

» Edible finger painting with pudding or whipped cream or applesauce.

» Use piles of shaving cream on a garbage bag or vinyl tablecloth outside. Finger paint letters, pictures in shaving cream, make a beard or gloves or shoes with the shaving cream on the child's face, hands and feet.

» Play-doh®, Silly Putty®.

» Gak®, Gooze®, Silly String®.

» Blowing bubbles and popping them.

» Paper Mache.

» Play dress up with different textured clothes.

» Crawl or walk over different textured surfaces: Sand, carpet, tile, grass.

» Rub lotions and powders- be carful of skin allergies, if there is any open skin or the child develops a rash, try something else.

2
2.1
2.2
2.3
2.4
2.5
2.6
2.7
2.8
2.9
2.10
2.11

Some of the following activities may not be suitable for patients with arthritis because they require substantial weight bearing on joints. However, these activities would be beneficial for individuals without arthritis.

The following are examples of home exercises to continue to increase your child's arm strength, grip strength, and endurance in gross motor activities involving the upper extremities:

Activities:

» Write or draw overhead on a chalkboard, dry erase board, or paper taped on a wall.

» Stir, knead with hands and roll cookie dough with a rolling pin.

» Make pictures with stamps.

» Experiment with manipulative activities using resistant materials (for example-- clay, putty, Play-doh®, dough). Have your child roll out a "snake", flatten into a "pancake", make a "ball", etc.

» Hide small objects like beads or pennies in a round ball of putty or Play-doh® and have child manipulate the putty to find/ retrieve the hidden objects.

» Play with pop beads or interlocking toys that can be pulled apart or pushed together.

» Play tug of war with the child seated on the floor (for safety).

» Push cart (Fisher Price™ grocery cart) with heavy objects or weights inside.

Only do the following if you nurse, OT or medical provider say it is ok:

» Take wheelbarrow walks.

» Walk like a crab.

» Do push-ups (in a modified position on knees or doing "dips" supported by arms on a chair placed behind them).

» Climb on play equipment, with supervision.

Bilateral integration is the ability to use both sides of the body in symmetrical and asymmetrical motions. This includes the ability to cross midline or reach across the body with the opposite arm or leg. Examples of bilateral tasks are clapping, banging on a drum, rubbing stomach and patting the head at the same time, etc. Problems seen in children with bilateral integration difficulty are a hesitation or jerk at the midline when drawing a horizontal line, inability to use the non-writing hand to hold the paper, inability to hold an object in one hand while manipulating it with the other.

Activities to encourage bilateral integration:

- » Any toy that requires the use of both hands.
- » Fastening clothes, buttoning, zippers, snaps, buckling belts.
- » Opening and closing jars and other containers.
- » Pushing/ rolling large balls.
- » Flattening Play-doh® with a rolling pin.
- » Songs with motions that go with them (Itsy Bitsy Spider, Wheels on the Bus, Patty-cake).
- » Cutting large pieces of paper.
- » Using templates to draw around or inside.
- » Drawing with both hands at the blackboard.
- » Musical instruments and clapping.
- » Finger painting.
- » Pop beads and interlocking toys.
- » Donkey kicks alternating sides.
- » Theraband® activities with both hands.
- » Jumping jacks, galloping, skipping.
- » Stringing beads.
- » T-Ball, tether ball.
- » Rub stomach and pat head at the same time.
- » Deal cards and sort them.
- » Make shadow pictures with hand gestures.
- » Bounce and catch various size balls.
- » Touch thumb to each finger- now faster! Both hands at once!
- » Make snow angels- now lift hand and arm at the same side together, now try left leg and right arm and left arm and right leg.

Fine motor skills are dependent on the strength of the small muscles in the hands. They involve the small movements we make with our hands. These skills begin with swiping at objects and progress to grabbing them, and eventually moving them in very delicate ways. These skills are required to do many daily activities such as buttoning buttons, typing on a computer, or writing on paper with a pencil. On this page are some activity ideas to work on at home. You can think of other ideas, too! Just look at a toy or activity and think about what your child needs to play the game or complete the activity and determine how much work it will be for the hands and fingers.

Activities

» Apply hand lotion and have the child rub it into their hands and fingers.

» Finger painting.

» Letter/ line/ shape formation in shaving cream, pudding, whipped cream, or frosting.

» Finger puppets.

» Push-button toys and games.

» Drop coins into a slot (empty coffee can with slit in lid, coin bank, etc).

» Turning pages in a book.

» Pick small objects out of a bucket of dry ice, dry beans, or sand- using thumb and index finger.

» String necklace of cheerios, fruit loops, macaroni, beads, etc. onto a string or pipe cleaner.

» Games that require thumb and index finger grasps including Connect Four®, Barnyard Bing®, Memory®, etc.

» Lacing cards.

» Drawing on chalkboard.

» Lego's®, Duplos®, or Lincoln Logs®.

» Stamp pads or stamps.

» Helping at home with snapping beans, planting flowers, folding papers, stacking plastic cups and plates, sticking stamps, etc.

» Flick wads of paper across a table, alternating using all four fingers with the thumb- play soccer or hockey with the wad of paper .

» Make an "o" by touching the thumb to finger tips one at a time.

» Crumple a sheet of paper, towel or sheet by pulling the fingers into a fist.

» Turning handles.

» Shaking dice.

» Turning pennies over.

» Pulling pennies or dry beans out of Theraputty® or Play-doh®.

» Scissors- use index and middle fingers as "blades" cutting imaginary line.

» Finger flicks- alternate flicking each finger off thumb.

» Peg boards.

» Trace shapes, letters on carpet.

» Rapid finger touch- touch tip of each finger to thumb with increasing speed with each hand, then both hands, then with eyes closed!

» Squeezing water bottles with index and middle finger while holding the bottle neck with thumb, ring finger and small finger.

» Squirreling- pick up small objects (pennies, beads, cheerios) with thumb, index and middle fingers, move the object from the fingertips to store it in the palm under the ring finger and small finger. Then, do the opposite moving one object at a time to release each one into a small container or coin slot.

» Sealing Ziploc® bags.

» Use tongs or tweezers to move game pieces.

» Play jacks.

» Pop beads or Styrofoam beads from Toys R' Us™, which are cylindrical that pop up when you pinch them.

2
2.1
2.2
2.3
2.4
2.5
2.6
2.7
2.8
2.9
2.10
2.11

Flour dough, Play-doh® and Silly Putty® can be used as a substitution for Theraputty® if needed.

Theraputty® is a substance that comes in varying resistance from extra soft to heavy to increase hand strength and manipulate skills. Here are a few ideas to make hand exercises fun:

Activities:

» Roll theraputty into a hotdog or snake; use pennies to make polka-dots or stripes on the snake; try pinching the putty all the way between your index finger and thumb- Try pinching with the other fingers! You can also try to form letters by rolling pieces of theraputty and putting them together.

» Mash theraputty into a pancake; pinch the edges to make a "pie crust"; use both hands at midline or one hand on the table to ash the putty- try it standing up and sitting down- you can also try writing letters once the theraputty is flat.

» Squeeze the theraputty as hard as you can with one hand, then pass it to the other hand and repeat! Try to spin the theraputty in one hand and squeeze over and over.

» Roll the theraputty into a ball by making circles with both hands at midline, try it by placing putty on the table and rolling with one hand making circles to form a ball.

» Pull the putty apart and make shapes and objects out of it, circles, squares, cars etc.

» Pull the putty apart and then roll it into a ball to make "spaghetti and meatballs".

» Poke your index finger into the putty to work on finger isolation.

SECTION 3

RHEUMATOLOGY NURSING ACROSS THE LIFESPAN:
REPRODUCTIVE YEARS

3
3.1
3.2

Section 3.1

Fertility, Medicinal Teratogens, and Rheumatic Disease

Cathy Patty-Resk, MSN, RN, CPNP

Introduction

Fertility and childbearing in rheumatic disease can be quite complicated. There are considerations that must be researched and thought through by the provider, discussed with the patient and continually re-evaluated during treatment. Nurses have always played a key role in patient care and education. Frequently the patient turns to the nurse for counseling and information related to all aspects of their disease, including fertility and pregnancy risks.

Learning Objectives

Upon completion of this chapter, the nurse will be able to:

1. The rheumatology nurse will be able to explain what a teratogen is to a reproductive age women.

2. The rheumatology nurse will understand basic sequence of events after fertilization with regard to effects of teratogens on the fetus.

3. The rheumatology nurse will be knowledgeable of the FDA classes of medication based on teratogenicity.

4. The rheumatology nurse will discuss comfortably the importance of choosing the most efficacious form of contraception while taking medications in FDA Class D and X.

5. The rheumatology nurse will advocate for patients use of contraception with evidence-based data regardless of age.

6. The rheumatology nurse will understand that ages 11 years and older are considered of reproductive age with regard to teratogenic medications.

7. The rheumatology nurse will recognize developmental barriers to teen contraceptive use.

8. The rheumatology nurse will understand how motivational interviewing can be used to establish contracts with teens.

9. The rheumatology nurse will discuss the Teen Pregnancy Contract with the adolescent and parent in ways that strengthen the patient's commitment to pregnancy prevention.

Content Outline

I. Understanding Gonadal Function and Fertility in Rheumatic Disease.

A. Infertility is the impairment of reproductive capability. This can be due to:

1. Problems preventing successful gamete union leading to infertility;

2. Obstacles in effective implantation of the uterine wall;

3. Difficulties in maintaining pregnancy post-implantation, and;

4. Complications during labor (Hickman & Gordon, 2011).

B. In general, the pubertal and post-pubertal ovaries and testes are more likely to be effected by cytotoxic drugs than in pre-pubertal stages of development. In males the cytotoxic drugs may decrease the number of sperm produced (oligozoospermia), effect their motility (asthenozoospermia), or cause abnormal morphology of sperm (teratozoospermia) (Soares, 2007). In females the cytotoxic drugs may decrease the ovarian reserve, number of eggs that can successfully be fertilized.

C. Male and Female associated infertility in rheumatology patients may be disease related or related to medication. Male infertility due to disease (systemic lupus erythematosus [SLE]) has been thought to be due to anti-sperm antibodies. However, fertile patients have also been shown to have anti-sperm antibodies. Soares et al. (2007) showed a link between testis volume which correlated with the degree of sperm abnormalities. There are also inconsistencies in reports of infertility due to Primary Ovarian Failure (POF) caused by anti-corpus luteum antibodies with raised follicle-stimulating hormone (FSH) levels, an autoimmune related menstrual dysfunction. Hickman & Gordon (2011) found that juvenile SLE patients had normal or low FSH levels during menstrual abnormalities and adult SLE women who had fertility difficulties actually had elevated FSH levels. POF is associated with decreased ovarian reserves making fertility very difficult or impossible. POF can be disease related or associated with alkylating agents, such as cyclophosphamide (CTX) (Cytoxan®) during or after puberty (Hickman & Gordon, 2011) (Keane, Hobbie, & Ruccione, 2006).

D. In a study of 245 RA patients by Brouwer et. (2014), they found that total time to pregnancy (TTP) was longer in those patients who were older or nulliparous, had higher disease activity, used nonsteroidal anti-inflammatory drugs (NSAIDs) or prednisone >7.5 mg daily. The conclusion was for preconception treatment strategies to aim at maximum suppression of disease activity, taking account of possible negative effects of NSAIDs use and higher prednisone doses. They also found that smoking, disease duration, rheumatoid factor, anti-citrullinated protein antibodies, past methotrexate (MTX) use, and preconception sulfasalazine (SSZ) use did not prolong TTP.

Table 1: Federal Drug Agency Teratogenic Classes of Medications

FDA Category	Description
D	Adequate well-controlled or observational studies in pregnant women have demonstrated a risk to the fetus.
	However, the benefits of therapy may outweigh the potential risk. For example, the drug may be acceptable if needed in a life-threatening situation or serious disease for which safer drugs cannot be used or are ineffective.
X	Adequate well-controlled or observational studies in animals or pregnant women have demonstrated positive evidence of fetal abnormalities or risks.
	The use of the product is contraindicated in women who are or may become pregnant.

Source: Adapted from the U.S. Food and Drug Administration (FDA).

II. Understanding Medicinal Teratogens in Rheumatic Disease.

A. The mechanisms in which certain medications affect fetal development depends on the stage of fetal development as well as the strength and frequency of dosing of medication. Substances known to interfere with fetal development causing or relating to birth defects are teratogenic. Currently, medications used in rheumatology known to be teratogenic are azathioprine (AZA) (Imuran®), cyclophosphamide (CTX) (Cytoxin®), leflunomide (LEF) (Arava®), methotrexate (MTX) (several trade names), and mycophenolate mofetil (MMF) (CellCept®).

B. According to a study by Schwarz, et al., (2013), almost half of all women prescribed teratogenic medications did not receive counseling regarding the medication's teratogenic effects. The women were more likely to report counseling occurred if the provider was a female. The women who received counseling were more likely to use contraception after prescribed a teratogenic medication than women who did not receive any counseling (Schwarz, et al., 2013).

C. Women who filled Class A or B medications were no more likely to have received counseling than women who filled Class D or X medications; 48% vs 51% of prescriptions. In the U.S. 6% of all pregnancies have some exposure to Class D or X teratogenic medications. Prescriptions filled by women using contraceptive methods of the highest efficacy, such as intrauterine device (IUD), implant, or sterilization were least likely to become pregnant within the first three months of exposure to teratogens. (Schwarz, Postlethwaite, Hung, & Armstrong, 2007). Due to the nature of the rheumatic diseases and use of known teratogenic medications, specifically widley used methotrexate (MTX) as a gold standard of treatment, it is imperative the rheumatology nurse understand teratogens to educate the patients in potential child-bearing years.

III. Fetal Development: Teratogen medication exposure with regard to basic fetal development timeline (Sachdeva, Patel, & Patel, 2009).

A. Fertilization to implantation: Little known, if any, effects.

B. Blastogenesis.

1. 15-21 days after conception.

2. The development of an embryo during cleavage and germ layer formation.

3. Highly resistant to birth defects.

Table 2: Anti-rheumatic Drugs Known to be Teratogenic

Drug Class	FDA Category	Clinical recommendations
Alkylating Agent		
Cyclophosphamide (CTX)	D	Discontinue 3 months before conception, and pregnancy test before next infusion
DMARDs		
Azathioprine (AZA)	D	The risk for this drug must be weighed against the benefits of the drug because of increased risk of fetal abnormalities.
Mycophenolate mofetil (MMF)	D	Discontinue 6 weeks before conception.
Methotrexate (MTX)	X	Discontinue 3-6 months prior to conception; contraindicated during pregnancy. Patient should remain on folic acid supplements after discontinuation of MTX.
Leflunomide (LEF)	X	Discontinue 2 years before pregnancy; contraindicated during pregnancy. Can also do cholestyramine washout if absolutely necessary. (Østensen, 2008).

Source: Adapted from Organization of Teratology Information Specialists (OTIS) and various sources.

4. All or nothing effect from most drugs (range of no harm to killing of fetus).

C. Organogenesis.

   1. 3rd- 8th week after conception.

   2. Rapid organ development.

   3. Fetus at highest risk for deformities.

      a. Spontaneous abortion.

      b. Mild birth defects.

      c. Severe birth defects.

      d. Subtle but permanent defect that may not be detected or problematic until later in life.

   4. 9th week after conception onward.

      a. Fetus is growing in size and maturing organs.

IV. Federal Drug Agency teratogenic classes of medications (see Table 1).

A. Teratogenic Agents Used In Rheumatology (see Table 2):

   1. Alkylating agents (AA).

      a. Cyclophosphamide (CTX) (Cytoxan®).

   2. Disease modifying anti-rheumatic drugs (DMARDS):

      a. Azathioprine (AZA) (Imuran®)

      b. Mycophenolate mofetil (MMF) (CellCept®).

      c. Methotrexate (MTX).

      d. Leflunomide (LEF) (Arava®).

   3. Only known safe medication used in rheumatology for pregnancy.

      a. Hydroxychloroquine (HCQ) (Plaquenil®).

V. Reducing the risk of birth defects:

A. Birth control options:

   1. Short acting reversible contraception (SARC):

      a. Oral contraceptive pills:

         (1) Daily, ingested at same time; only recommended if patient meets the following criteria:

            i) Punctual.

            ii) Mature.

            iii) Proven reliability and detail oriented.

            iv) Long standing history of excellent compliance.

            v) Not at high risk for thrombosis.

   2. Long acting (LARC):

      a. Etonogestrel/ethinyl estradiol vaginal ring (NuvaRing®):

         (1) Self-insertion.

         (2) Once every 3 weeks.

         (3) Hormone infused.

      b. Medroxyprogesterone acetate (Depo-Provera®) hormone injection:

         (1) Every 3 months.

         (2) Documentation of each when administered.

      c. Intrauterine Devices (IUD).

         (1) One time insertion:

            i) Copper IUD (ParaGard®)

               1) No hormones.

            ii) Levonorgestrel-releasing intrauterine system (Mirena®) IUD.

               1) Hormone infused.

      d. Etonogestrel implant (Implanon®).

         (1) Implanted under skin by physician.

         (2) Lasts for 3 years without maintenance.

         (3) Pregnancy possible as soon as removed.

         (4) May cause irregular bleeding or spotting.

         (5) May not be effective in overweight or obese women.

      e. Permanent sterility / one surgery:

         (1) Highly efficacious.

         (2) Usually older females.

         (3) Multiparous females.

         (4) Patient's life would be in danger due to pregnancy.

   3. Preferred contraceptive methods for use with Class D & X medications:

      a. Long Acting Reversible Contraceptive (LARC) methods.

         (1) Intrauterine Device (IUD).

            i) May be recommended for some adolescents.

         (2) Injectable hormones.

            i) Recommended for adolescents.

(3) Vaginal ring.

    i) Not recommended for adolescents.

VI. The role of the nurse in contraceptive counseling and education:
(Gilger, 2004; Schwartz et al., 2007).

A. Supply patient with best known information on various methods.

B. Explain that only LARC methods can be used while on teratogenic medication.

C. Provide education on use, safety and effectiveness of various contraception methods.

D. Advocate for the adolescent and be a liaison between adolescent and parent.

E. Assist patient with adapting chosen method to real life for optimal success.

F. Require the patient provide written/ documented proof of LARC.

G. Document exactly what was taught and discussed at each visit.

H. Pregnancy Contract for Teens.

  1. Informed Contract Agreement:

    a. Agreement to medical care.

    b. Understands his/her condition.

    c. Understands treatment:

      (1) Risks.

      (2) Benefits.

      (3) Risk of foregoing treatment.

      (4) Teratogenic risks.

    d. Onus goes back to teen and caregiver.

  2. Contract has been used successfully for other conditions.

    a. Suicide (No-Suicide Contract, Kevin Caruso, Suicide.org Founder, Executive Director, Editor-in-Chief).

  3. Multi-purpose:

    a. Opens dialogue regarding sexual activity.

    b. Education regarding teratogenic effects.

    c. Discussion of birth control.

    d. Emphasizes seriousness of issues.

    e. Empowers teen.

  4. Motivational Interviewing (Miller & Rollnick, 2013):

    a. Promotes awareness and change of unhealthy behaviors.

    b. Conversation starter.

    c. Strengthen commitment to birth control.

    d. Assesses teen commitment/adherence.

  5. Elements of a Pregnancy Contract for Teens (see Appendix A):

    a. Description of diagnosis and medical treatment.

    b. Why is in necessary for patient's health and potentially survival.

    c. Nature of treatment.

    d. Risks and benefits of treatment.

    e. Available alternative treatments.

    f. Risks of foregoing treatment.

    g. Commitment to be seen by Gynecologist.

    h. Demonstrate proof of reliable birth control.

    i. Option to not take teratogenic medication.

    j. Option to take safer medication even if not as effective.

    k. Option to cancel contract at any time after discussing with provider.

    l. Shared responsibility with parent/guardian.

VII. Special considerations for adolescents ages 11-19 (Steyn & Goldstuck, 2014).

A. Research has shown some common reasons the sexually active adolescent is more likely to seek contraception is:

  1. If she perceives pregnancy as a negative outcome,

  2. Has long-term educational goals.

  3. Has family, friends, and/or a clinician who endorse the use of contraception.

B. Some parents suspect their teens are already sexually active but believe assisting with more effective contraceptive methods is endorsing sexual activity. Therefore, they defer.

C. Two common barriers can be removed for the adolescent to seek effective contraception by discussing this topic openly and having the parent, physician, and nurse's support for contraception.

D. The best contraceptive method for the adolescent must be simple to use, safe, and very effective (Steyn & Goldstuck, 2014).

VIII. Male/Female fertility preservation.

A. Infertility is very distressing (Keane, Hobbie, & Ruccione, 2006).

B. The American Society for Reproductive Medicine (2013) reported oocyte cryopreservation may be a viable alternative for those women with high potential for ovarian failure for whom embryo freezing is not an option.

C. Males have had remarkable success in gamete cryopreservation prior to gonadotoxic chemotherapy.

IX. Awareness and options.

A. Educate patients and parents of the untoward or potentially untoward effects certain rheumatology medications have on fertility and gonadotoxicity.

1. Fertility must be discussed between the provider, parents/guardians, spouse and patient prior to initiation of treatment.

2. Include pediatric/adolescent patients in these discussions.

3. For males:

    a. Absence of ever having nocturnal ejaculations or ejaculation with masturbation decrease likelihood of fertility being affected from treatment.

    b. Post-pubertal males ordinarily will be capable of ejaculation and can provide sperm for storage.

    c. Epididymal sperm aspiration and testicular sperm extraction can be a consideration for sperm banking.

X. Sperm banking.

A. To arrange for sperm banking the provider or nurse should contact their local American Society for Reproductive Medicine (ASRM) accredited sperm banking facility. The facility can be found by using the American Society for Reproductive Medicine's website, www.asrm.com.

B. The nurse/provider should contact the sperm bank to get forms that the provider may need to sign certifying the medical reason requiring sperm banking and the most up to date information for patients/parents.

C. Questions should be asked regarding privacy, number of specimens required, location of specimen collection(at facility or home), transporting specimens, cost of initial sperm collection and possible sources of financial assistance, including testing for baseline sperm counts and motility, yearly storage fees and disposition of stored specimens in case of patient death.

D. The patient's health insurer should also be contacted for information on possible coverage of these services that are required due to the toxic effects of chemotherapy.

E. One of the more controversial topics associated with fertility preservation methods relate to the directions for disposition of stored gametes, embryos and gonadal tissue in the case of patient death. Specific directions should be written into the fertility storage contract with the storage facility. This is a topic the nurse should encourage the family to discuss to prevent possible future emotional distress and legal battles.

XI. Future recommendations and research.

A. The American College of Rheumatology (ACR) at the Reproductive Health Summit on the Management of Pregnant and Lactating Women with Autoimmune Diseases is challenging the Federal Drug Association's (FDA's) classification of several rheumatology medications, including leflunomide (Arava®).

B. The ACR is concerned some patients may be terminating pregnancies unnecessarily due to poor communication regarding the teratogenicity of rheumatology medications between rheumatology providers, primary care physicians and OB/GYN providers (Dao, Cush, Kavanaugh, & Weiseman 2014).

C. The mechanisms of infertility in males and females with rheumatologic disease have many remaining unknowns. More research is needed to find ways to preserve or optimize patients' fertility so there is no need for medical intervention for conception and patients no longer feel they need to hurry to become pregnant before they are emotionally, financially, or physically ready due to fear of their "biological clock" running out of time.

Summary

There are multiple medications used in the treatment of rheumatic diseases that are known to be teratogenic agents. These are azathioprine (Imuran®), cyclophosphamide (Cytoxin®), leflunomide (Arava®), methotrexate (MTX) (several trade names), and mycophenolate mofetil (CellCept®). Special considerations for the rheumatology nurses role involves contraceptive education and counselling for the patients of potential child bearing age. The rheumatology nurse is also in a unique position to educate the patient on a health-promoting lifestyle prior to conception. Use of gonadotoxic therapies to treat rheumatic diseases should alert the nurse to be aware of fertility preservation options and make appropriate resources available to their patients (ASRM Position Statement Article). Counseling by a qualified mental health professional and genetic counselor, when appropriate, should also be offered. The most established strategy for preservation of female fertility is for a woman to undergo a cycle of In Vitro Fertilization (IVF) and create embryos for later use. This option is available only if there is time before treatment to undergo a cycle of stimulation to obtain eggs and a safe method of ovarian stimulation exists.

References

American College of Rheumatology(2014). Drug Safety Quarterly. Vol. 5(1) Spring Online publication of the ACR Drug Safety Committee.

Bayer Healthcare Pharmaceuticals Inc., (2014). Mirena®: Prescribing information. Whippany, NJ: Author.

Bristol-Myers Squibb Company (2005). Cytoxan®: Prescribing information. Deerfield, IL: Author.

Brouwer J, Hazes JM, Laven JS, Dolhain RJ. (2014). Fertility in women with rheumatoid arthritis: influence of disease activity and medication. *Ann Rheum Dis.* 2014 May 15. pii: annrheumdis-2014-205383. doi: 10.1136/annrheumdis-2014-205383.

Children's Oncology Group. (2014) http://www.childrensoncologygroup.org/index.php/hormonesandreproduction/malereproductivehealth.

Dao, K., Cush, J.J., Kavanaugh, A. and Weiseman, M. (2014) ACR reproductive health summit on the management of pregnant and lactating women with autoimmune diseases. American College of Rheumatology. Drug Safety Quarterly. Vol. 5(1) Spring. Online publication of the ACR Drug Safety Committee.

Ethics Committee American Society of Reproductive Medicine (ECASRM). Fertility Preservation and Reproduction in Patients Facing Gonadotoxic Therapies: A Committee Opinion. (2013). Elsevier Inc. Fertility and Sterility® Vol. 100, No. 5, November.

Genentech USA, Inc. (2013). CellCept®: Prescribing Information. South San Francisco, CA: Author.

Gilger, EA (2004). The Pediatric Chemotherapy and Biotherapy Curriculum. Section 12 Ethical and Legal Considerations. Association of Pediatric Oncology Nurses.

Hickman, R.A. and Gordon, C. (2011). Causes and management of infertility in systemic lupus erythmatosus. Rheumatology 2011; 50: 1551-1558. doi: 10.1093/rheumatology/ker105.

Keene N., Hobbie, W.L., & Ruccione, K., (2006) Cancer survivors: A practical guide to your future. 2nd ed. Sebastopol,CA: O'Reilly Press.

Merck & Co., Inc., (2014). Implanon®: Prescribing information. Whitehouse Station, NJ: Author.

Merck & Co., Inc., (2012). NuvaRing®: Prescribing information. Whitehouse Station, NJ: Author.

Miller, W.R. and Rollnick, S. (2013) Motivational interviewing: Helping people change. Third Edition. The Guilford Press.

No-Suicide Contract, Kevin Caruso Suicide.org. http://www.suicide.org/no-suicide-contract-form.html.

Østensen, M., Lockshin, M., Doria, A., Valesini, G., Meroni, P., Gordon, C., Brucato, A. and Tincani, A. (2008). Update on safety during pregnancy of biological agents and some immunosuppressive anit-rheumatic drugs. Rheumatology, 47; iii28-iii31. doi: 10.1093/rheumatology/ken 168.

Pfizer (2006). Depo-Provera®: Prescribing information. New York, NY: Author.

References (continued)

Sachdeva, P., Patel, B.D. and Patel, B.K., (2009). Drug use in pregnancy: A point to ponder! Indian Journal of Pharmacological Science, 71(1): 1-7.

Sanofi-Aventis (2014) Arava®: Prescribing information. Macquarie Park, NSW: Author.

Sanofi-Aventis Canada Inc. (2014). Plaquenil®: Prescribing information. Laval, Quebec: Author.

Schwarz, E.B., Parisi, S.M., Handler, S.M, Koren, G., Shevchik, G., Fischer, G.S., (2013). Counseling about medication-induced birth defects with clinical decision support in primary care. J Womens Health (Larchmont) Oct; 22(10): 817-24.

Schwarz, E.B., Postlethwaite, D., Hung, Y. and Armstrong, M., (2007). Documentation of contraception and pregnancy when prescribing potentially teratogenic medications for reproductive-age women. Annals of Internal Medicine. September 18; 147(6): 370-376.

Soares, P.M.F., Boarba, E.F., Bonfa, E., Hallak, J., Correa, A.L. and Silva, C.A.A. (2007). Gonad evaluation in male systemic lupus erythematosus. Arthritis & Rheumatism, 56: 2352-2361. doi: 10.1002/art.22660.

Steyn, P.S., Goldstuck, N.D., (2014). Contraceptive needs of the adolescent. Best Practice & Research Clinical Obstetrics and Gynaecology, doi.org/10.1016/j.bpobgyn.2014.04.012.

Teva Pharmaceuticals USA, Inc., (2013). Paragard®: Prescribing information. Sellersville, PA: Author.

3
3.1
3.2

I,_____, hereby agree that I will not become pregnant while taking

_____medication because it will likely cause an unborn baby to have severe birth

defects or cause miscarriage.

Furthermore, I agree that I will take the following actions to prevent pregnancy:

1. I will see a gynecologist to determine the most reliable and safest form of birth control for me.

2. I will bring documentation of my birth control to my Rheumatology appointments.

3. If I think I may want to become pregnant, I will discuss this with my Rheumatologist **BEFORE** I stop any medications or birth control.

4. It is MY choice to use birth control or not to use birth control.

5. I understand that if I do not use birth control my treatment options may include medications which have proven to be less effective than the treatment that is currently being recommended as above because they are not known to carry the same risk of severe birth defects or miscarriages.

6. If I become pregnant at any time I understand that I will not be able to see my current pediatric rheumatology provider and will have to immediately transfer my care to an adult rheumatologist.

_____   _____

PATIENT SIGNATURE   DATE

As the parent/guardian of _____, I agree to assist her in fulfilling

her contract obligations above. I will also share the responsibility of getting the proper birth control proof

documentation to her Rheumatologist.

_____   _____

PATIENT SIGNATURE   DATE

_____   _____

PROVIDER SIGNATURE   DATE

_____   _____

WITNESS SIGNATURE   DATE

3
3.1
3.2

Section 3.2

Maternal Health Considerations

in Rheumatoid Arthritis and Systemic Lupus Erythematosis Patients

Deanna L. Owens, MSN, RN

3
3.1
3.2

Introduction

The relationship between pregnancy and rheumatic disease remains a topic of interest that is in need of further clinical research to better determine treatment options ensuring optimal maternal and fetal health outcomes. The clinical management of pregnant patients with rheumatoid arthritis (RA) and systemic lupus erythematosus (SLE) involves various challenges. There are marked differences among disease activity within the pregnant population that are dependent on each particular diagnosis.

Learning Objectives

Upon completion of this chapter, the nurse will be able to:

1. Identify the effects of pregnancy on rheumatic disease.
2. Describe effective treatment strategies compatible with pregnancy.
3. Name medications incompatible with pregnancy.
4. Describe the mechanisms by which pregnancy affects the disease activity in patients with rheumatoid arthritis (RA).
5. Describe proper disease management in pregnant patients with RA.
6. List the possible pregnancy complications of patients with systemic lupus erythematosus (SLE).
7. Describe the mechanisms by which pregnancy affects the incidence of flares in patients with SLE.
8. Describe proper disease management in pregnant patients with SLE.

Content Outline

I. Effects of pregnancy on maternal disease: Rheumatoid arthritis (RA).

A. Observed changes in disease activity (Hazes et al., 2011).

1. Confirmed improvements of RA symptoms during pregnancy.

2. Increased risk of flare during postpartum period.

3. Symptomatic improvements usually begin in the first trimester and often peak in the second and third trimesters.

B. Mechanisms by which pregnancy affects disease activity:

1. Hormonal and immunologic changes during pregnancy result in noticeable improvement of symptoms.

2. Amelioration of RA during pregnancy is thought to be due to significant hormonal changes and immunologic factors (Man & Hazes, 2009).

   a. Immunological changes in cytokines and t-cell counts (Man & Hazes, 2009).

   b. Decreased pro-inflammatory cytokines (IL-12 & TNF alpha).

   c. Decreased production of T-helper1 (Th1) cytokines.

   d. Increased production of T-helper 2 (Th2) cytokines.

   e. Hormonal changes in cortisol levels, female sex hormones, and biochemical changes in alpha-2 pregnancy associated globulin (PAG).

   f. Studies demonstrate changes in serum levels of sex horomones, cortisol, and alpha-2 pregnancy-associated globulin, but did not yield any conclusive explanation for the improvement of RA symptoms during pregnancy (Hazes et al., 2011).

   g. An increase in estrogen and progesterone during pregnancy combined with elevated levels of cortisol and Vitamin D may have a direct effect on lowering specific pro-inflammatory cytokines, IL-12 and TNF-alpha (Hazes et al., 2011).

C. Treatment of RA during pregnancy.

1. Treatment of RA during pregnancy can be difficult because of medication contraindications during pregnancy and post partum if breast-feeding.

2. Limited number of therapeutic options because of lack of clinical trials concerning drug safety in patients who are pregnant.

3. U.S. Food and Drug Administration provides categories for drug safety (Hazes et al., 2011) (see Table 1).

4. Non-steroidal anti-inflammatory drugs (NSAIDs) can be used during the first part of pregnancy, but should be discontinued after 30 weeks because of increased risk of premature closure of the ductus arteriosus.

5. Disease modifying anti-rheumatic drugs (DMARDs) with teratogenic effects should be discontinued (See Table 2). The risk of maternal disease flare should be carefully weighed against risk of drug exposure to the fetus (Dhar & Sokol, 2006).

   a. Anti-malarial agents: Hydroxycholoroquine (HCQ) is compatible with pregnancy and can be continued to control symptoms of RA. Previous controversy surrounding the use of HCQ was due to increased risk of ototoxicity and retinal toxicity with the treatment of chloroquine during pregnancy (Hazes et al., 2011).

   b. Sulfasalazine (SSZ) is generally considered to be safe during pregnancy and should be combined with folic acid supplements. Risks and benefits should be discussed with treating provider (ACR, 2012).

6. Biologic agents should not be administered during pregnancy with the possible exception of TNF-inhibiting drugs during the conception period or during the first trimester (Hazes et al., 2011).

   a. TNF inhibiting drugs are considered Category B medications with animal studies resulting in no teratogenicity, embryotoxicity, or maternal toxicity (Roux, Brocq, Breuil, Albert, & Euller-Ziegler, 2007).

   (1) Note: Depending on the circumstance of each individual patient, the physician may choose to continue biologic therapy. Guidance and vigilant monitoring is necessary due to the

3
3.1
3.2

lack of research concerning effects of medication in women who are pregnant.

    (2) There are no well controlled human studies that link TNF-inhibiting drugs with teratogenic effects on a fetus or increased pregnancy loss (Roux et al., 2007). Anti-TNF medications are still likely to be discontinued based on the lack of research and ethical concerns about drug safety in patients who are pregnant.

    (3) Infliximab crosses the placenta in 2nd & 3rd trimesters of pregnancy (Østensen, 2008).

D. Table 2 depicts various anti-rheumatic drugs and associated risks during pregnancy (Hazes et al., 2011; Organization of Teratology Information Specialists, n.d.) (see Table 2).

E. Obstetric risks and complications (Man & Hazes, 2009).

  1. A small number of studies showing greater risk for the following.

    a. Pre-eclampsia.

    b. Cesarean section.

    c. Prematurity.

    d. Low birth weight.

  2. There is not an increased risk for fetal loss.

F. Patient education.

  1. Counseling prior to conception concerning possible fetal and maternal complications.

    a. Symptomatic improvements usually begin in the first trimester and often peak in the second and third trimesters.

    b. Increased risk of flare during postpartum period.

    c. Labor and delivery in patients with RA is often uneventful and there is no increased risk of fetal loss (Man & Hazes, 2009).

  2. Treatment options.

    a. Medication safety has not been well studied in patients who are pregnant; therefore the plan of treatment should be decided between the patient and the healthcare provider.

3
3.1
3.2

Table 1: Categories for Drug Safety

FDA Category	Description
A	Adequate, well-controlled studies in pregnant women have not shown an increased risk of abnormalities to the fetus in any trimester of pregnancy.
B	Animal studies have revealed no evidence of harm to the fetus; however, there are no adequate and well-controlled studies in pregnant women. OR Animal studies have shown an adverse effect, but adequate and well-controlled studies in pregnant women have failed to demonstrate a risk to the fetus in any trimester.
C	Animal studies have shown an adverse effect, and there are no adequate and well-controlled studies in pregnant women. OR No animal studies have been conducted, and there are no adequate and well-controlled studies in pregnant women.
D	Adequate well-controlled or observational studies in pregnant women have demonstrated a risk to the fetus. However, the benefits of therapy may outweigh the potential risk. For example, the drug may be acceptable if needed in a life-threatening situation or serious disease for which safer drugs cannot be used or are ineffective.
X	Adequate well-controlled or observational studies in animals or pregnant women have demonstrated positive evidence of fetal abnormalities or risks. The use of the product is contraindicated in women who are or may become pregnant.

Source: Adapted from the U.S. Food and Drug Administration.

3. Understanding the changes in disease state because of pregnancy-related biologic and hormonal changes.

   a. During pregnancy, the patient can expect an improvement in symptoms possibly because of increased levels of sex hormones and decreased levels of pro-inflammatory cytokines.

   b. 90% of patients experience a flare in symptoms within 6 months during postpartum period (Man & Hazes, 2009).

4. Drug effectiveness and safety.

   a. Methotrexate (MTX) should be discontinued 3-6 months prior to conception due to risk of fetal harm.

Table 2: Anti-rheumatic Drugs and Associated Risks

Drug Class	FDA Category	Clinical recommendations
Alkylating Agent		
Cyclophosphamide (CTX)	D	Discontinue 3 months before conception, and pregnancy test before next infusion.
SYMPTOM-MODIFYING DRUGS		
NSAIDs	B	First part of pregnancy up to 30 weeks gestation; After 30 weeks, consider class C drug because of increased risk of premature closure of the ductus arteriosus.
Corticosteroids (CSs)	C	Increased risk of adrenal insufficiency and oral cleft in the newborn; associated with increased incidence of premature delivery.
DMARDs		
Sulfasalazine (SSZ)	B	There is no increased risk for congenital malformations; should be combined with folic acid supplements.
Azathioprine (AZA)	D	The risk for this drug must be weighed against the benefits of the drug because of increased risk of fetal abnormalities.
Mycophenolate mofetil (MMF)	D	Discontinue 6 weeks before conception (Østensen, 2008).
Methotrexate (MTX)	X	Discontinue 3-6 months prior to conception; contraindicated during pregnancy. Patient should remain on folic acid supplements after discontinuation of MTX.
Leflunomide (LEF)	X	Discontinue 2 years before pregnancy or after cholestyramine washout (Østensen, 2008).
ANTI-MALARIALS		
Hydroxychloroquine (HCQ)	C	Compatible with pregnancy; no association with congenital malformations although risks are shown with Chloroquine.
BIOLOGICS		
Anti-TNF Therapies » Infliximab » Etanercept » Adalimumab » Certolizumab » Golimumab	B	Discontinue after positive pregnancy test or missed period; anti-TNF antibodies do not cross the placenta in the first trimester and have not been seen to cause teratogenic effects in animal reproduction studies.
Abatacept	C	Discontinue 10 weeks before conception; no human pregnancy data available. Crosses the placenta (Østensen, 2008).
Rituximab	C	B cell depletion in fetus. Known to resolve in first 6 months of life. Crosses placenta after week 16. Is not present in breast milk (Østensen, 2008).
Tocilizumab	C	Discontinue 10 weeks before conception; no human pregnancy data available.

Source: Adapted from Organization of Teratology Information Specialists (OTIS) and various sources.

   b. Leflunomide (LEF) should be discontinued 2 years prior to conception due to long half-life of medication in plasma, or after cholestyramine washout (Østensen, 2008).

   c. Prednisone (although considered a Category C medication) is inactivated in the placenta and can be continued at a low dose during pregnancy to control symptoms of RA.

   d. NSAIDs can be used in the first part of pregnancy, but should be discontinued after 30 weeks due to increased risk of premature closure of ductus arteriosis.

II. Effects of pregnancy on maternal disease: Systemic lupus erythematosus (SLE).

A. Observed changes in disease activity include:

1. Increased frequency of flares.

   a. Rash.

   b. Pleurisy.

   c. Pericarditis.

   d. Renal failure.

2. Severity of flares is unchanged in patients who are pregnant.

   a. Disease manifestations often result from necessary changes in medication during pregnancy.

3. Mechanisms by which pregnancy affects disease activity.

   a. SLE is more prevalent in females because of the strong association of female sex hormones and disease mechanism of action.

   b. Female sex hormones increase (specifically prolactin) during pregnancy causing increased risk for frequency of flares (Man & Hazes, 2009).

   c. Prolactin receptors are expressed through various cells in the body including T- and B-lymphocytes and are known to have possible links to worsening symptoms of SLE in patients who are pregnant (Man & Hazes, 2009).

4. Obstetric risks and complications.

   a. Risk of carrying antiphospholipid syndrome (APLS).

     (1) APLS causes hypercoagubility of blood resulting in umbilical venous and/or arterial clots that can lead to miscarriage.

     (2) The preferred treatment for APLS is a combination of low dose aspirin and heparin that can be given throughout the duration of the pregnancy (Man & Hazes, 2009).

       i) With appropriate management, greater than 70% of patients will deliver a viable live baby (Fosca, et al., 2011).

   b. Patients with SLE are at an increased risk to develop the following during pregnancy (Man & Hazes, 2009).

     (1) Hypertension.

     (2) Antiphospholipid syndrome (APLS).

     (3) Pre-eclampsia.

     (4) Diabetes mellitus.

     (5) Hyperglycemia.

     (6) Bladder infections.

     (7) Premature rupture of membranes.

     (8) Uterine rupture.

     (9) Retinal detachment during labor.

     (10) Severe retinopathy.

     (11) Deep vein thrombosis.

     (12) Liver necrosis.

     (13) Stroke.

5. Patient education.

   a. Counseling prior to conception concerning possible fetal and maternal complications.

     (1) Caesarean sections are common because of the high-risk nature of pregnancies in patients with SLE.

     (2) APLS increases the risk for clots in arteries and veins, miscarriage, hypertension during pregnancy, and prematurity (Man & Hazes, 2009).

     (3) The American College of Rheumatology (2012) suggests patients with SLE who also have poor kidney function and/or high blood pressure should be advised against getting pregnant.

   b. Understanding the changes in disease state due to pregnancy-related biologic and hormonal changes.

3
3.1
3.2

(1) A rise in female hormones (specifically prolactin) during pregnancy causes an increased risk for frequency of flares (Man & Hazes, 2009).

c. Drug effectiveness and safety.

(1) Prednisone (although considered a Category C medication) is inactivated in the placenta and can be continued at a low dose during pregnancy to control symptoms of SLE.

(2) Hydroxycholoroquine (HCQ) is compatible with pregnancy and can be continued to control lupus flares.

(3) Antihypertensive medications are often necessary because of the increased risk of high blood pressure during pregnancy and should be monitored by a physician.

(4) ACE inhibitors are not recommended because of their effects on kidney development in the fetus (Man & Hazes, 2009).

(5) Intravenous belimumab is a b-lymphocyte specific inhibitor used to treat adult patients with moderate to severe SLE who are also on a combination of additional disease maintenance medications (www.Benlysta.com).

i) Providers should discuss with patients, the potential risks versus benefits of continuing belimumab (Category C) therapy as there are no human studies or pregnancy data available.

Summary

The rheumatology nurse plays a critical role in educating the patient on adequate control of disease activity, medication management, and treatment strategies compatible with fetal development. Numerous immunologic and hormonal changes have been studied during pregnancy. Such research has fallen short of any definitive association between these biologic changes and pregnancy-associated improvements in rheumatoid arthritis (RA). In patients with systemic lupus erythematosus (SLE), disease flares are more prevalent both during pregnancy and throughout the postpartum period. Healthcare providers must pay close attention to patients who are pregnant or considering pregnancy to maintain a healthy, safe, and therapeutic treatment regimen.

References

American College of Rheumatology (2012). Patient Resources: Medications. Retrieved from www.rheumatology.org.

BENLYSTA® (belimumab): FDA-Approved Treatment for Lupus. (n.d.). Retrieved from http://www.benlysta.com/

Dhar, J., & Sokol, R., (2006). Lupus and Pregnancy: Complex Yet Manageable. Clinical Medicine & Research. Dec 2006; 4(4): 310-321.

Fosca, D., Valenti, O., Hyseni, E., Giorgio, E., Faraci, M., Renda, M., De Domenico, R., & Monte, S. (2011). Antiphospholipid syndrome during pregnancy: the state of the art. Journal of Prenatal Medicine, 5(2): 41-63.

Hazes, J., Coulie, P., Geenen, V., Vermeire, S., Carbonnel, F., Louis, E., ...& De Keyser, F. (2011). Rheumatoid arthritis and pregnancy: Evolution of disease activity and pathophysiological considerations for drug use. Rheumatology, 50, 1955-1968. doi: 10.1093/rheumatology/ker302.

Man, Y., & Hazes, J. (2009). Pregnancy in rheumatic diseases: An overview (3rd ed.). Oxford: University Press.

Organization of Teratology Information Specialists. (n.d.). Retrieved from http://www.mothertobaby.org/

Østensen, M., Lockshin, M., Doria, A., Valesini, G., Meroni, P., Gordon, C., Brucato, A. and Tincani, A. (2008). Update on safety during pregnancy of biological agents and some immunosuppressive anit-rheumatic drugs. Rheumatology, 47; iii28-iii31. doi: 10.1093/rheumatology/ken 168.

Roux, C., Brocq, O., Breuil, V., Albert, C., & Euller-Ziegler, L. (2007). Pregnancy in rheumatology patients exposed to anti-tumor necrosis factor (TNF)-α therapy. Rheumatology, 46, 695-698. doi: 10.1093/rheumatology/kel400

SECTION 4

RHEUMATOLOGY NURSING ACROSS THE LIFESPAN:
ADULT YEARS

Contents of Section 4

4
4.1
4.2
4.3
4.4
4.5
4.6
4.7
4.8
4.9
4.10

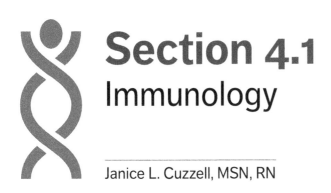

Section 4.1
Immunology

Janice L. Cuzzell, MSN, RN

Introduction

The immune system is composed of an elaborate network of organs, tissues, and cells designed to protect the body against attacks by foreign invaders such as bacteria, viruses, and fungi. Despite constant exposure to a potentially harmful environment, a normal immune system ensures prompt recognition and targeting of pathogens. However, serious disease states such as sepsis, cancer, and autoimmune disease can result if the immune response is suppressed or misses its target (Abbas & Lichtman, 2009; Janeway, Travers, Walport, & Shlomchik, 2005).

The secret to the immune system's success is a very complex and efficient communication system that is initiated as soon as an invader is detected. Millions of immune cells release chemical signals that not only regulate their own behavior but also recruit and direct other immune cells to help contain the invasion. The result is a precise and well-orchestrated response that serves to maintain a state of homeostasis (Sompayrac, 2008).

Malfunctions of the immune system such as autoimmune disease, infection, and hypersensitivity reactions are commonly encountered in rheumatology practice. For example, the immune system becomes hyperactive in autoimmune disease, thus requiring therapies that suppress the immune system. A review of the normal immune response not only builds a foundation for understanding the pathophysiology of autoimmune disease states, it also helps explain the mechanism of action and adverse events associated with the biologic therapies used to treat many rheumatic diseases.

Learning Objectives

Upon completion of this chapter, the nurse will be able to:

1. List the sub-populations of T-cells and how each contributes to chronic inflammation.

2. Discuss the role of B-cells and antibodies in protecting the body from pathogens.

3. Describe the role of cytokines in mounting an immune response.

4. Describe the role of the innate immune system and the protective function of inflammation.

5. Discuss the adaptive immune response and how it differs from innate immunity.

Content Outline

The Normal Immune Response

I. Organs of the immune system (lymphoid organs).

A. Bone marrow.

1. Bone marrow is comprised of soft, spongy, vascular tissue that fills bone cavities.

2. Hematopoietic stem cells in the marrow give rise to the cellular components of blood.

   a. Myeloid lineage: Includes monocytes, macrophages, neutrophils, basophils, eosinophils, erythrocytes, platelets, and dendritic cells.

   b. Lymphoid lineage: Includes T lymphocytes (T-cells), B lymphocytes (B-cells), and natural killer cells (NK cells).

3. Cells in the hematopoietic marrow have both long-term and short-term potential to regenerate.

B. The thymus.

1. The thymus is located in front of the heart and behind the sternum (anterior superior mediastinum).

2. T-cells, an important immune cell in the adaptive immune response, are "educated" in the thymus so that they can differentiate between "self" and "non-self" molecules.

C. Lymph nodes.

1. Lymph nodes are oval-shaped structures that are distributed widely throughout the body and connected by lymphatic vessels.

2. Clusters of lymph nodes are found in the neck, armpit, abdomen, and groin.

3. Specialized compartments in each lymph node serve as zones where the different types of lymphocytes congregate.

   a. T-cells from the thymus reside in the paracortex.

   b. B-cells develop in and around the germinal centers.

   c. Plasma cells reside in the medulla.

4. Lymphocytes leave the lymph node and periodically circulate throughout the body patrolling for foreign antigens.

5. Antigens in the blood or lymph fluid enter and leave the lymph nodes by way of incoming and outgoing lymphatic and blood vessels.

   a. A lymph node enlarges (lymphadenopathy) when lymphocytes in the node recognize a circulating protein as "foreign" and respond with rapid proliferation.

D. The spleen.

1. The spleen is located in the upper left quadrant of the abdomen and acts primarily as a blood filter.

2. This organ is similar in structure to a lymph node, with specialized compartments where T lymphocytes and B lymphocytes congregate and are activated to remove foreign antigens.

E. The tonsils, adenoids, and appendix.

1. These lymphoid tissues are anatomically positioned in the body to intercept foreign antigens that enter through the respiratory and digestive tracts.

II. Cells and other components of the immune system (see Table 1).

A. All immune cells begin as immature stem cells in the bone marrow.

1. Immature stem cells respond to chemical signals (cytokines and chemokines) that are initiated during an immune response.

2. These chemical signals regulate the differentiation of stem cells into specific cell types including neutrophils, monocytes, macrophages, dendritic cells, mast cells, T lymphocytes, and B lymphocytes.

3. The type and amount of cells produced during an immune response depend on the identity of the foreign protein and the severity of the threat to homeostasis.

B. B lymphocytes (B-cells).

1. The primary function of a B-cell is to recognize free-floating foreign proteins (antigens) and produce immunoglobulin (antibodies) against them.

2. B-cells differentiate into plasma cells when they are activated against a specific antigen.

3. The type of immunoglobulin produced by a plasma cell depends on the type of cytokine that was present during activation.

4. Some B-cells mature into memory cells that reside in the lymph node where they can react quickly to subsequent attacks by the specific antigen.

C. Immunoglobulin (Ig).

1. An immunoglobulin or antibody is a large protein molecule released by B-cells into the circulation and body secretions in response to an antigen.

2. Immunoglobulin provides protection against antigens through several mechanisms:

a. Neutralization or inactivation of foreign substance.

b. Opsonization or coating of the antigen with antibody and complement protein, promoting phagocytosis of the antigen.

c. Complement activation.

d. Agglutination or clumping of multiple antibody/antigen complexes.

e. Mobilization of natural killer cells.

f. Antibody dependent-cell mediated cytotoxicity (ADCC).

Table 1: Cells of the Immune System

Cell Type	Function
Basophil	» Plays a major role in immediate hypersensitivity reactions. » Produces some mediators of hypersensitivity reactions.
B-Cell	» Is responsible for humoral immunity. » Secretes antibodies that target highly-specific antigens. » Functions as an antigen-presenting cell to amplify the immune response.
Cytotoxic T-Cell	» Induces death of pathogen-infected cells, tumor cells, and allografts (via cell lysis).
Dendritic cell	» Presents antigen to T lymphocytes.
Eosinophil	» Kills parasites by phagocytosis or by directly releasing granules onto the surface of the large organism. » Directly involved in immediate type hypersensitivity reactions.
Macrophage	» Stimulates lymphocytes to mount a defense against pathogens. » Engulfs and destroys pathogens and cellular debris (via phagocytosis).
Mast cell	» Mediates local or systemic immediate hypersensitivity reactions and allergic reactions. » Contains vasoactive mediator histamine.
Monocyte	» Promotes migration, phagocytosis, chemotaxis, granule release, and killing (intracellular pathogens). » Processes and presents antigens to lymphocytes. » Kills tumor cells. » Participates in the inclusion of monocytes into thrombi.
Natural Killer (NK) cell	» Protects host by recognizing tumors and virus-infected cells (innate immune system). » Produces granules that kill the altered/infected cells via lysis
Neutrophil or Polymorphonuclear cell (PMN)	» Is recruited to the site of infection where they phagocytose invading organisms. » Contributes to collateral tissue damage that occurs during inflammation.
Th1 lymphocyte	» Produces IFN-gamma, IL-2, TNF. » Evokes cell-mediated immunity and phagocyte inflammation.
Th2 lymphocyte	» Produces IL-4, IL-5, IL-6, IL-9, IL-10 and IL-13. » Causes antibody responses, including IgE class. » Inhibits phagocytosis.
Plasma cell	» Produces high levels of antibodies. » Varies in cell life from days to months to years.

4
4.1
4.2
4.3
4.4
4.5
4.6
4.7
4.8
4.9
4.10

3. The classic Ig structure is Y-shaped protein.

    a. The two arms of the Y are fragment antigen binding sites ("Fab") that vary from one antibody to the next and are customized to a unique antigen.

    b. The base of the Y is referred to as the fragment crystallizable (Fc) portion of the antibody and remains similar from one antibody to the next.

    c. The Fc portion binds to complement protein or immune cells by way of antibody receptors.

4. Five classes of immunoglobulin.

    a. Immunoglobulin G (IgG).

        (1) Comprises 70% of the total immunoglobulin in human serum.

        (2) The longest-lived immunoglobulin with a half-life of about three weeks.

        (3) The predominant antibody produced in response to repeated attack by the same antigen.

        (4) A potent complement activator when bound to antigen.

        (5) Able to cross the placenta and provide initial immunity following birth.

    b. Immunoglobulin A (IgA).

        (1) Found in two forms in the human body: Serum IgA and secretory IgA.

        (2) Comprises 15-20% of the total immunoglobulin in human serum.

        (3) Produced by plasma cells in the bone marrow, lymph nodes, and spleen.

        (4) Capable of both anti-inflammatory and pro-inflammatory effects.

        (5) Provides the first line of defense against pathogens that can enter the body by way of the mucous membranes.

        (6) Provides immune protection to newborns since it is secreted in breast milk.

    c. Immunoglobulin M (IgM).

        (1) Found on the cell surface of B-cells and functions as an antigen receptor.

        (2) The first antibody to be produced by newly activated B-cells.

        (3) Primarily produced in the spleen.

        (4) An indicator of recent infection when levels are elevated.

        (5) Activates complement system proteins that are specific to the target antigen.

        (6) Neutralizes viruses by binding to them and preventing cellular infection.

    d. Immunoglobulin E (IgE).

        (1) Found in very small amounts in human serum.

        (2) Able to bind readily to Fc receptors on mast cells and basophils in the absence of antigen.

        (3) Able to guard against parasitic infections.

        (4) Thought to play a role in cancer surveillance.

    e. Immunoglobulin D (IgD).

        (1) Expressed by immature B-cells.

        (2) Plays an important role in B-cell differentiation and initiation of the adaptive immune response.

D. T lymphocytes (T-cells).

1. T-cells are programmed in the thymus to attack non-self antigen.

2. Unlike the B-cell, a T-cell does not recognize free-floating antigen but rather identifies a foreign invader with T-cell receptors (TCR) on the surface.

3. Randomly rearranged gene segments are used to generate TCRs, making it possible for each T-cell to attack a different or unique antigen.

4. Proper function of the immune system depends on the ability of T-cells to discriminate between self and non-self in order to prevent autoimmune disease.

5. T-cell subpopulations.

    a. Helper T-cells.

        (1) Designated as CD4+ because of a specific surface molecule marker.

        (2) Further designated as Th1 or Th2 based on type of cytokine the T-cell secretes (see Table 1).

        (3) Activate other immune cells to amplify the immune response, including B-cells, macrophages and other T-cells.

    b. Cytotoxic T Lymphocytes (CTLs).

        (1) Designated as CD8+ T-cells because of a specific surface molecule marker.

4
4.1
4.2
4.3
4.4
4.5
4.6
4.7
4.8
4.9
4.10

(2) Recognize antigen fragments bound to major histocompatibility complex (MHC) molecules, proteins on the surface of cells that help the immune system distinguish between self and non-self.

(3) Directly attack cells in the body recognized as infected or cancerous.

c. Regulatory T-cells (Treg).

(1) Down regulate the immune response through production of inhibitory cytokines that suppress inflammation.

(2) Actively inhibit activation of the immune system to prevent pathological self-reactivity (autoimmune disease).

(3) Are still being researched because the role of the suppressor T-cell is poorly understood.

6. T-cells only recognize an antigen if it is carried on the surface of a cell by the body's own major histocompatibility complex (MHC) molecules.

a. MHC molecules are proteins that allow T-cells to distinguish between self and non-self.

b. Normal cells in the human body are covered with MHC proteins that are unique to each person.

c. In humans, MHC antigens are called human leukocyte antigen (HLA).

(1) MHC class I molecules present foreign proteins that have been digested within the cell and attract Killer T-cells.

(2) MHC class II molecules present foreign proteins from outside of the cell to T-lymphocytes.

(3) Proliferation of T-helper cells stimulates B-cells to produce antibodies to the specific antigen.

(4) Self-antigens are suppressed by suppressor T-cells.

(5) The MHC of an organ recipient must be closely matched to the MHC of the donor to prevent T lymphocytes from attacking the new organ, leading to graft rejection.

E. Natural killer cells (NKCs).

1. Are programmed to recognize fatty substances (lipids and glycolipids) that are bound to MHC non-self-molecules.

2. Have the potential to attack many different types of foreign proteins.

3. Can contribute to the development of asthma and autoimmune diseases such as Type 1 diabetes and cancers if they fail to function properly.

F. Leukocytes.

1. Leukocytes are phagocytes, white blood cells that engulf and digest microbes and other foreign debris.

2. Phagocytes found in the blood stream are called monocytes.

a. Monocytes that migrate from the blood vessels into tissues develop into macrophages.

b. Macrophages act as scavengers to rid the body of old cells and foreign debris. Macrophages.

(1) Serve as antigen-presenting cells (APCs) in the tissue by presenting fragments of ingested antigen to other immune cells and activating them.

(2) Release specialized signaling proteins known as monokines, a type of pro-inflammatory cytokine. These monokines include tumor necrosis factor-alpha and interleukin 1, which help mobilize neutrophils.

(3) Have a specialized immune function in many organs including the liver, lungs, brain, and kidneys.

3. Granulocytes are white blood cells that play a key role in the innate immune response.

a. Granulocytes phagocytize microbes and destroy them using "prepackaged" antimicrobial granules contained in the cytoplasm.

b. Neutrophils or polymorphonuclear neutrophils (PMNs) are the most abundant type of granulocyte.

(1) PMNs play a key role in the innate immune response by being one of the first responders to microbial invasion.

(2) PMNs are subdivided into segmented neutrophils (segs) and banded neutrophils (bands).

(3) Neutrophil counts are increased (neutrophilia) in response to

4
4.1
4.2
4.3
4.4
4.5
4.6
4.7
4.8
4.9
4.10

pyrogenic infections and acute inflammatory conditions such as heart attacks and burns.

(4) Neutrophil counts are decreased (neutropenia) in disorders of the bone marrow, as a result of chemotherapy treatment, in autoimmune neutropenia, and with certain medications.

c. Eosinophils and basophils are types of granulocytes responsible for:

(1) Combating multicellular parasites and certain infections.

(2) Helping regulate mechanisms associated with asthma and allergy.

G. Mast cells.

1. Similar in appearance and function to basophils but not classified as a leukocyte.

2. Contain granules that are rich in histamine and heparin.

3. Are found in the skin, lungs, tongue, conjunctiva, and mucous membrane linings of the respiratory and intestinal tracts.

4. Express high-affinity receptors for the Fc region of IgE molecules, triggering allergic and anaphylactic reactions when activated by allergens (antigens).

5. Play an important role in wound healing and defense against pathogens.

H. Dendritic cells.

1. Antigen-presenting cells (APCs) found in tissues that come in direct contact with the external environment such as the skin and mucous membranes.

2. Become activated when they come in contact with and process antigen.

3. Migrate to lymphoid tissue where they present antigen to T-cells and B-cells, thus initiating the adaptive immune response.

4. Communicate with other immune cells via cell-to-cell contact and cytokine release.

5. Play a major role in autoimmune disease and allergy.

III. Cytokines.

A. Cytokines are small proteins that function as chemical signals during an immune response to initiate, sustain, or down-regulate inflammation.

1. Cytokines play an essential role in the intercellular communication that occurs during an immune response.

2. Each cytokine has a matching receptor present on cell surfaces that allows signals to be received and processed.

B. Cells can respond to a cytokine by:

1. Producing other cytokines.

2. Increasing the number of cell surface receptors that can attach to other molecules and modify cell function.

3. Suppressing cellular activity.

C. The cytokine family of proteins includes tumor necrosis factors as well as a variety of interleukins, interferons, and growth factors, many of which have overlapping or similar functions (see Table 2).

D. Inflammatory chemokines are cytokines that:

1. Are released by cells at the site of invasion or injury.

2. Chemically attract other cells such as neutrophils, monocytes, and lymphocytes to the site of inflammation (chemotaxis) in order to help defend or repair tissue.

3. Control the movement of immune cells during immune surveillance, such as directing lymphocytes to certain lymph nodes for antigen processing.

IV. Complement.

A. The complement system is comprised of more than 25 small proteins that work together to amplify an immune response by:

1. Initiating the classic inflammatory response to injury or infection:

a. Vasodilation and edema.

b. Increased redness.

c. Localized pain.

d. Loss of function.

4
4.1
4.2
4.3
4.4
4.5
4.6
4.7
4.8
4.9
4.10

Table 2: Cytokines

Cytokine	Source	Function
TNF-α	Macrophage T lymphocyte B lymphocyte	» Recruits neutrophils and macrophages to sites of infection. » Acts on hypothalamus to produce fever. » Promotes production of acute phase proteins by hepatocytes. » Interferes with catabolism in muscle and fat leading to cachexia.
IL-1	Macrophage Monocyte Fibroblast Dendritic cell	» Stimulates the proliferation and differentiation of T and B lymphocytes. » Activates macrophages, fibroblasts, osteoblasts, and epithelial cells. » Stimulates reabsorption of bone by osteoclasts. » Acts on hypothalamus resulting in prostaglandin-induced fever. » Acts on muscle cells resulting in prostaglandin-induced proteolysis.
IL-5	Eosinophil	» Stimulates growth of B-cells and antibody production. » Regulates eosinophil behavior and accumulation in tissues, particularly during allergic reactions.
IL-6	T lymphocyte Macrophage	» Stimulates growth and differentiation of T lymphocytes, B lymphocytes, and haemopoietic cells. » Stimulates hepatocytes to synthesize acute phase proteins.
IL-9	T lymphocyte	» Simulates cell proliferation. » Prevents programmed cell death (apoptosis).
IL-10	Monocyte Lymphocyte	» Inhibits human cytokine synthesis factor (also known as anti-inflammatory cytokine). » Down regulates secretion of Th1 cytokines, MHC class II antigens, and co-stimulatory molecules on macrophages. » Enhances B-cell survival, antibody production, and proliferation. » Is involved with JAK-STAT signaling pathway.
IL-12	Macrophage	» Stimulates T-cell differentiation (also known as T cell stimulating factor). » Stimulates production of interferon gamma, NK cells, and tumor necrosis factor-alpha.
IL-13	T lymphocyte	» Mediates allergic inflammation and disease.
INF-α INF-β	Lymphocyte Macrophage Fibroblast Endothelial cell Osteoblast	» Stimulates macrophages and NK cells for anti-viral responses. » Is active against tumor cells. » Is a pyrogenic factor. » Causes release of prostaglandins. » Contributes to reducing pain.
INF-Y	T lymphocyte Natural Killer (NK) cell	» Is a Type 2 interferon (also known as immune interferon). » Is the primary cytokine for definition of Th1 helper cells. » Is critical for innate and adaptive immunity against bacterial and viral infections. » Inhibits viral replication. » Promotes NK cell activity. » Promotes adhesion and binding of leukocytes for migration. » Activates inducible nitric oxide synthase. » Increases antigen presentation and phagocytosis by macrophages. » Is key cytokine in granuloma formation. » Suppresses osteoclast formation.
Chemokines	Cells	» Is a small cytokine that affects chemotaxis in other cells.

4
4.1
4.2
4.3
4.4
4.5
4.6
4.7
4.8
4.9
4.10

2. Enhancing phagocytosis of antigen (opsonization).

3. Activating the chemotaxis of neutrophils and macrophages.

4. Lysing foreign cells.

5. Ridding the body of antibody-coated antigen.

V. Mounting an immune response.

A. The innate immune response.

1. Primitive, non-specific response to infection or injury common to all vertebrates.

2. Employs two lines of defense:

a. Stops or neutralizes pathogens *before* they can invade the body through establishment of a physical barrier:

(1) Intact skin and acid mantle.

(2) Mucous membranes lining the respiratory, gastrointestinal, and reproductive tracts.

(3) Bodily secretions (e.g., tears, sweat).

b. Initiates an immediate vascular and cellular response to contain and/or destroy a foreign pathogen *after* it has breached a protective barrier.

(1) Tissue macrophages engulf and digest (phagocytize) invading pathogens, causing the release of cytokines and chemokines.

(2) Cytokines and chemokines mediate an acute inflammatory response.

(3) Nerve endings are stimulated and mast cells release histamine (clinical symptom: Increased pain).

(4) Blood vessels dilate resulting in increased blood flow to site of invasion (clinical symptom: Increased warmth and redness).

(5) Permeability of capillaries increases causing leakage of plasma proteins and fluid into tissue (clinical symptom: Localized edema).

3. Neutrophils and monocytes receive chemical signals that attract them to the site of inflammation (clinical symptom: Elevated white blood cell count).

a. Monocytes differentiate into macrophages and release cytokines that signal the recruitment of additional immune cells by chemotaxis.

b. Cytokine release causes the temperature to rise in order to inhibit further proliferation of the pathogen (clinical symptom: Fever).

c. Dead neutrophils and other cellular debris are eventually phagocytized by macrophages (clinical symptom: Pus formation).

4. Natural killer cells receive signals that mobilize them to recognize and kill virally infected cells and tumor cells.

5. Complement proteins in the blood and tissue are activated by the presence of bacteria resulting in immediate destruction of the invading pathogen.

6. Acute inflammation becomes chronic if the foreign pathogen persists without normal down-regulation of the inflammatory cascade by cytokines.

B. The adaptive immune response.

1. Works in conjunction with the innate immune system to protect the body from invasion by foreign proteins and pathogens.

2. Is a learned response to a specific antigen.

3. Requires prior exposure in order for the immune system to acquire a memory to the antigen.

4. Includes components common to the innate immune response including cytokines, complement proteins, phagocytic macrophages, and natural killer cells.

C. The two components of an adaptive immune response include cell-mediated immunity and humoral immunity.

1. Cell-mediated immunity is regulated by activation of T-cells.

a. Naïve T-cells require 2 signals to become activated (co-stimulation).

b. Experienced or memory T-cells do not require co-stimulation.

c. A single activated T-cell "clones" itself into multiple T-cells with specificity to the same antigen.

4
4.1
4.2
4.3
4.4
4.5
4.6
4.7
4.8
4.9
4.10

d. Antigen-specific T-cells migrate to site of inflammation.

e. Some activated T-cells remain behind as memory T-cells in order to facilitate antigen recognition during subsequent exposures.

f. The body naturally destroys T-cells that recognize self-antigen.

g. Failure of the body to destroy abnormal T-cells results in an autoimmune disorder.

2. Humoral or antibody-mediated immunity is regulated by B-cells.

a. Each B-cell is programmed to recognize and bind to one specific antigen.

b. There are two methods by which naïve B-cells become activated:

(1) T-cell dependent activation requires two separate signals.

(2) T-cell independent activation allows for a more rapid and effective response.

c. Activated B-cells mature into plasma cells that are dedicated to antibody secretion.

d. Some B-cells mature into memory cells that reside in the lymph node where they can react quickly to subsequent attacks by the same or a similar antigen.

Summary

A normally functioning immune system is a complex communication system with the unique ability to discriminate between self and non-self molecules, a mechanism known as immune tolerance. This natural mechanism is designed to prevent the immune system from attacking healthy body tissue. However, in some individuals who are genetically predisposed, a triggering event such as infection can result in an autoimmune disease. Rheumatoid arthritis, systemic lupus erythematosus, Sjögren's syndrome, systemic sclerosis, polymyositis, and dermatomyositis are just a few of the autoimmune diseases treated in rheumatology practice (Fauci & Langford, 2006).

A variety of injectable and infusible biologic therapies are available to treat autoimmune disease. These agents work by targeting one or more of the signaling pathways used by immune cells to produce, amplify, and sustain the abnormal inflammatory response. Maintaining a state of low disease activity remains the goal of therapy until more is understood about the causes and mechanisms of autoimmunity.

4
4.1
4.2
4.3
4.4
4.5
4.6
4.7
4.8
4.9
4.10

References

Abbas, A.K., & Lichtman, A.H. (2009). *Basic immunology: Functions and disorders of the immune system* (3rd ed.). Philadelphia: Saunders Elsevier.

Fauci, A.S., & Langford, C.A. (2006). *Harrison's rheumatology* (16th ed.). New York: McGraw-Hill.

Janeway, C.A., Travers, P., Walport, M., & Shlomchik, M.J. (Eds.). (2005). *Imunobiology: The immune system in health and disease.* New York: Garland Science.

Sompayrac, L. (2008). *How the immune system works* (3rd ed.). Malden, MA: Blackwell Publishing.

Section 4.2
Pain Management in Rheumatology

Deborah Hicks, RN

Introduction

4
4.1
4.2
4.3
4.4
4.5
4.6
4.7
4.8
4.9
4.10

Patients with rheumatic conditions often have co-morbid conditions that must be considered when assessing and treating pain. Age, polypharmacy, social history, cultural differences, and lifestyle are just some of the factors necessary to incorporate into the consideration of any management program, including that for pain. Pain alleviation can often be achieved by treatment of the rheumatic condition. But when pain is not relieved by treating the underlying cause, management of that pain must be undertaken. "Pain should be addressed as a disease entity not as a sensory entity." (Winfield, 2008, p. 620) "Self-report is always the most reliable indication of pain." (McGuire, 2010, p. 36.) This statement requires healthcare providers to examine their own biases about pain management. Pain management plans must be individualized to each patient's needs. Goals should be realistic and patients should have expectations that match therapeutic goals.

Healthcare providers in the practice of rheumatology treat many painful conditions. Being familiar with pain management guidelines will make choices of modalities and explanations to patients both evidence-based and rational. This chapter will describe basic pain mechanisms, evidence-based pain management guidelines, drug groups used in the treatment of pain, and other non-pharmacologic modalities for the treatment of common painful rheumatologic conditions.

Learning Objectives

Upon completion of this chapter, the nurse will be able to:

1. Name categories of pain.
2. Make a thorough pain assessment.
3. Describe the step-wise approach to pain management.
4. Identify pharmacologic as well as non-pharmacologic modalities to treat pain.
5. List patient barriers to adequate pain control

Content Outline

I. Implication of untreated or undertreated pain in patients with rheumatic conditions.

A. Quality-of-life impact.

1. Lost productivity/income.

2. Interference with activities of daily living.

3. Depression, anxiety, fear, sleeplessness, anger.

4. Impairment of family, work and social relationships.

B. Physiologic impact.

1. Prolongs stress response.

2. Increases heart rate, blood pressure, oxygen demands.

3. Decreases GI motility.

4. Causes immobility.

5. Decreases immune response.

6. Delays healing.

7. Increases the risk of chronic pain.

II. Mechanisms of pain.

A. Nociceptive.

1. Stimulation of peripheral pain receptors on thinly myelinated Aδ fibers (more rapid conduction, sharp pain) and/or demyelinated (C) afferents (slower conduction, burning pain) (So, Sprott, & Brune, 2012) during inflammation or injury of tissues.

2. Stimuli that threaten or provoke actual tissue damage (Bajwa & Smith, 2012).

3. Somatic pain.
   a. Skin and subcutaneous tissue; sharp, burning (skeletal muscle spasms).
   b. Visceral pain; poorly localized, diffuse, cramping (colitis).

4. Pain "matches" noxious stimulus.

5. Examples of nociceptive pain in rheumatologic conditions:
   a. Systemic inflammatory or degenerative conditions.
   b. Regional musculoskeletal pain (tenosynovitis).
   c. Compression neuropathies.
   d. Bursitis.
   e. Nerve entrapment syndromes.
   f. Localized forms of arthritis.

6. Pharmacologic approach includes non-narcotic and opioid analgesia.

B. Neuropathic.

1. May follow injuries or diseases that directly affect the nervous system (peripheral and central nervous systems).

2. Paroxysmal, perceived as electric shock-like discomfort or burning.

3. Contributions: Central sensitization and ectopic firing of peripheral neurons, developed during movement.

4. May be associated with hyperpathia (persistence after the stimulus has ended, spreading or worsening in crescendo fashion with repeated touching).

5. Conditions associated with neuropathic pain:
   a. Peripheral neuropathy.
      (1) Post-herpetic neuralgia.
      (2) Vasculitic neuropathy.
      (3) Radiculopathic pain due to injury to spinal nerve roots.
   b. Central neuropathic pain.
      (1) Central post-stroke pain.
      (2) Spinal cord injury pain.

6. Pharmacologic approach includes antidepressants, serotonin/norepinephrine reuptake inhibitors (SNRIs), tricyclic antidepressants (TCAs), and calcium channel alpha 2-delta ligands (pregabalin, gabapentin); opioids and tramadol are second line.

C. Chronic pain of complex etiology formerly called functional pain syndromes, now called central sensitivity syndromes.

1. Based on the absence of structural pathology.

2. Maladaptive (pain perception malfunction); hyperalgesia (increased response to a

4
4.1
4.2
4.3
4.4
4.5
4.6
4.7
4.8
4.9
4.10

normally noxious stimulus, sensitization of local nociceptors) and/or allodynia (painful response to normally non-noxious stimuli, central sensitization such as tender points in fibromyalgia).

3. Psychophysiologic/neurophysiologic dysregulation.

4. Stress response.

   a. Sympathetic nervous system activated.

   b. H-P-A response (hypothalamic-pituitary-adrenocortical axis), release of cortisol, becomes maladaptive (Winfield, 2008).

   c. Neuroplasticity: Dynamic processes that modify the circuits of neural transmission.

      (1) Modulation occurs at the spinal level but can occur at a higher level.

      (2) May explain the interactions between cognition, behavior, and pain perception often seen in clinical practice (So, Sprott, & Brune, 2012).

   d. Chronic painful conditions associated with rheumatology:

      (1) Fibromyalgia (FMS).

      (2) Irritable bowel syndrome (IBS).

      (3) Temporomandibular disorders (TMJ).

      (4) Migraine headaches.

D. Psychogenic.

   1. Somatoform and somatization disorders.

   2. Hysteria.

III. Pain assessment.

A. Specifically seek and evaluate pain.

   1. Treat pain as a disease entity, not as a sensory entity (Winfield, 2008).

B. Validate the patient's pain.

   1. Use pain intensity/pain relief scales (visual, descriptive, percentage).

   2. McGill-Melzack Pain Questionnaire (McGuire, 2010).

C. Describe location.

   1. Confined to site of origin (localized).

   2. Projected pain along specific nerve or nerves.

3. Radiating pain is diffuse around the site of origin, not well localized.

4. Referred pain is perceived in an area distant from site of painful stimuli.

D. Description of pain.

   1. Use visual analog scales, number rating scales, descriptive word scales (Pasero & McCaffrey, 2011).

   2. Wong-Baker FACES scale may be more useful in culturally-diverse patients with language barriers, developmentally disabled, children (McGuire, 2010).

   3. Common pain indicators that can be observed and documented (McGuire):

      a. Facial expression (grimacing, crying).

      b. Verbalizations or vocalizations (screaming).

      c. Body movements (restlessness).

      d. Changes in interpersonal interactions.

      e. Changes in activity patterns or routines.

      f. Mental status changes (confusion, increased confusion).

E. Determine course of the pain.

   1. Aggravating and relieving factors.

   2. Setting and associated features:

      a. Local (bony enlargements).

      b. Constitutional (fatigue, weight loss).

      c. Emotional (depression).

   3. Duration of pain (since time of origin).

F. Complete a full psychosocial and cultural assessment of the patient.

   1. Factors that may contribute to pain:

      a. History of poor parental health.

      b. Parental pain history.

      c. Childhood abuse, particularly sexual abuse.

      d. Poor family environment.

   2. Factors that may interfere with pain management:

      a. Fear of addiction.

      b. Patient wants to be a "good patient."

      c. Patient does not want to bother healthcare provider or caregiver.

4
4.1
4.2
4.3
4.4
4.5
4.6
4.7
4.8
4.9
4.10

d. Negatively biased attitude of healthcare provider may discourage patient complaint.

G. Determine etiology of pain.

    a. Pain associated with treatable/ underlying condition.

      (1) Treat condition appropriately.

    b. Pain as result of rheumatic condition under treatment.

      (1) May require pain management (acute or chronic).

      (2) Consider multiple modalities, starting with those with lowest risk.

IV. Pharmaceutical management.

A. World Health Organization analgesic ladder (see Table 1).

B. Non-opioid analgesics: First line therapy for mild to moderate pain.

    1. Aspirin.

      a. Analgesic effects are similar to acetaminophen.

4
4.1
4.2
4.3
4.4
4.5
4.6
4.7
4.8
4.9
4.10

Table 1: World Health Organization (WHO) analgesic ladder

Opioid
(morphine, fentanyl, etc.)
+/-non-opioid
+/-adjuvant
Moderate to severe pain
↑
Opioid
(codeine, tramadol, etc.)
+/-non-opioid
+/-adjuvant
Mild to moderate pain
↑
Non-opioid
(acetaminophen, aspirin, NSAID)
+/-adjuvant
Mild pain

Source: Adapted from World Health Organization (WHO)

b. Side effects:

    (1) GI disturbances (dyspepsia, gastritis, GI bleeding).

    (2) Prevents platelet aggregation (bleeding, bruising).

c. Drug names:

    (1) Aspirin (used less frequently because of GI side effects).

    (2) Non-acetylated salicylates (choline magnesium trisalicylate, salsalate).

      i) Lower risk of gastropathy.

      ii) No inhibition of platelet function.

d. Acetaminophen (Tylenol®)

    (1) Most commonly administered over-the-counter oral analgesic.

    (2) Not anti-inflammatory; not as effective as NSAIDs.

    (3) Useful for the management of hip or knee osteoarthritis.

    (4) Maximum dose is 3000 mg daily, toxic dose margins are lower than other medications (Bajwa & Smith, 2012).

    (5) Acetaminophen is the most common cause of acute liver failure in the U.S (Bajwa & Smith, 2012).

      i) Assess liver function.

      ii) Assess patient's other medications.

      iii) Assess social habits such as alcohol consumption, nutritional status.

      iv) Educate patient regarding over use, need for abstaining from excessive alcohol use, need for adequate hydration and nutritional intake.

      v) Make patient aware that some drugs may contain acetaminophen; adjust daily dose so as not to exceed daily maximum dose.

2. Non-steroidal anti-inflammatory drugs (NSAIDs/COX 2 inhibitors).

    a. Anti-inflammatory because they inhibit prostaglandin.

    b. Used for soft tissue injury, strains, sprains, headaches, arthritis, low back pain (LBP).

    c. When used in conjunction with opioids, they have a synergy, producing a dose-sparing effect.

d. Significantly more side effects than acetaminophen.

  (1) Inhibition of platelets (potential promotion of bleeding).

  (2) Gastrointestinal insult (dyspepsia/ gastric ulceration).

  (3) Renal insult:

    i) Nephrotoxicity/reversible renal insufficiency.

    ii) Fluid retention (use with caution in patients with hypertension, heart failure, and renal insufficiency).

  (4) Contraindicated in patients with a history of venous thrombosis due to possible prothrombotic effects.

  (5) Hepatotoxicity (elevations of liver enzymes are generally mild and reversible with discontinuation of the drug).

  (6) Allergic reactions.

  (7) Avoid when possible in older adults, those with history of GI disease, renal insufficiency, heart failure, hypertension, liver disease.

3. Drugs.

  a. Naproxen (Naprosyn®) (reversibly inhibits platelet function).

  b. Fluorbiprofen (ANSAID®).

  c. Diclofenac sodium (Voltaren®).

  d. Sulindac (Clinoril®) (hepatotoxicity).

  e. Oxaprozin (Daypro®).

  f. Etodolac (Lodine®).

  g. Indomethacin (Indocin®)(GI, central nervous system (CNS) adverse events may be more severe).

  h. Piroxicam (high incidence of gastropathy above 20 mg).

  i. Meloxicam (Mobic®).

  j. Ibuprofen (Motrin®).

  k. Nabumetone.

4. Topical NSAIDs may be a reasonable option.

  a. Capsaicin cream.

  b. Diclofenac gel (Voltaren® gel).

5. Cyclo-oxygenase 2 inhibitors (COX-2 inhibitors): (Celecoxib/Celebrex®)

  a. Selective NSAID, blocks COX 2.

  b. Equal efficacy to selective NSAIDs with fewer gastrointestinal side effects.

  c. Doses greater than 200 mg/ day have been associated with increased cardiovascular risk.

  d. Precautions similar to those for NSAIDs.

C. Opioids.

1. Bind to the mu, kappa, or delta opioid receptors (predominantly mu for analgesic effects) in the regions of the brain involved in integrating pain to pre- and postsynaptic terminals of peripheral nerves.

2. Current therapeutic opioids are derivatives of morphine. Derivatives of opium are called opiates (morphine, hydromorphone, codeine). Synthetic analogues are called opioids (all others).

3. Should be used only in patients with moderate to severe chronic pain who are experiencing an adverse impact on function or quality of life (Bajwa & Smith, 2012).

  a. Use in chronic non-cancer pain remains controversial.

  b. Dose with analgesic activity equivalent to 10 mg morphine (equianalgesia); equianalgesia useful when switching from one opioid and/or route of administration to another.

4. Risk/benefit assessment should include risk of substance abuse, misuse, or addiction.

5. Titration may take several weeks or months.

6. Frequent monitoring required for re-evaluation, efficacy, and side effects.

7. Tapering may take 2-3 weeks.

8. Side effects:

  a. Constipation (teach prevention: Push fluids, diet high in bulk and roughage, encourage activity, stool softeners/laxatives).

  b. Nausea and vomiting (may be initial and temporary, tolerance is achieved quickly, use anti-emetics prn; assess for other causes).

  c. Sedation (tolerance generally appears after 2-3 days, eliminate any other unnecessary sedating medications, consider opioid rotation; consider adjustment according to age).

4
4.1
4.2
4.3
4.4
4.5
4.6
4.7
4.8
4.9
4.10

d. Cognitive impairment (rule out other causes; assess, adjust dose and/or drug; assess for drug interactions).

e. Miosis (papillary constriction) (may be of concern with glaucoma and/or cataracts).

f. Myoclonus (muscle jerking).

g. Urinary retention (use with caution in patients with history of benign prostatic hypertrophy (BPH), urinary retention; teach patients to be aware of urinary output, symptoms of distention).

h. Respiratory depression (rare in patients with chronic pain; effects of all opioids may be greater in older patients, those who have reduced blood volume, or who receive other central nervous system depressants).

i. Older patients are more sensitive with respect to efficacy and side effects; starting doses should be reduced by 25-50%.

9. Risk of opioid overdose increases with increased dosing, at initiation of therapy, and with dose changes.

10. Evidence of efficacy for long term use in terms of pain relief or improved functional outcomes is limited; review of literature found that, compared to placebo and non-opioid analgesics, use of opioids did not result in significant improvement in pain scores (Bajwa & Smith, 2012).

a. Patients with neuropathic pain may require opioids but should only be initiated after anticonvulsants (1st line) and antidepressants (2nd line) are used first.

D. Drugs: Schedule for Controlled Substances (see Table 2).

Table 2: Schedule for Controlled Substances

Schedule I drugs: High abuse potential
» No accepted use in medical practice, cannot be prescribed » Heroin, lysergic acid diethylamide (LSD), mescaline
Schedule II drugs: High potential for abuse and dependence
» Accepted medical indications with severe restrictions » Require non-refillable written prescriptions » Morphine, codeine, methadone, oxycodone, hydromorphone, meperidine, fentanyl, cocaine, amphetamines, secobarbital, hydrocodone
Schedule III drugs: Abuse potential less than Schedule II
» Compounds with limited quantities of controlled substances » Accepted medical indications » Prescriptions refillable up to 5 times within 6 months » Acetaminophen combined with codeine, buprenorphine
Schedule IV drugs: Abuse potential less than Schedule III drugs
» Accepted medical indications » Prescriptions refillable up to 5 times within 6 months » Benzodiazepines, modafinil, propoxyphene, phentermine, pentazocine, phenobarbital, tramadol
Schedule V drugs: Abuse potential less than Schedule IV drugs
» Preparations containing limited quantities of certain opioids and stimulants » Accepted medical indications » Includes non-prescription antitussive and antidiarrheal medications » Diphenoxylate, propylhexedrine, pregabalin

Source: Adapted from Bajwa, Z., & Smith, H.(2012). Overview of the treatment of chronic pain. *Up To Date*®. Philadelphia: Wolters Kluwer Health.

4
4.1
4.2
4.3
4.4
4.5
4.6
4.7
4.8
4.9
4.10

1. Short-acting:

    a. Schedule II.

        (1) Morphine sulfate (Roxanol®)

        (2) Codeine.

        (3) Hydrocodone (Lortab®)

        (4) Hydromorphone (Dilaudid®)

        (5) Methadone (Dolophine®)

        (6) Oxycodone (Percocet®)

    b. Schedule IV.

        (1) Tramadol (Ultram®)

2. Long-acting:

    a. Schedule II.

        (1) SR-Morphine (MS Contin®)

        (2) SR-Oxycodone (Oxycontin®)

        (3) Transdermal fentanyl (Duragesic®)

E. Antiepileptic drugs.

    1. Inhibit neurotransmitter release (gabapentin) or lipophilic gamma aminobutyric acid (GABA) analog to facilitate diffusion across the blood-brain barrier (pregabalin).

    2. Calcium channel alpha 2-delta ligands.

        a. Particularly useful for post-herpetic neuropathy, diabetic neuropathy, vasculitic neuropathy, radiculopathy.

    3. Carbamazepine (Tegretol®), analgesic mechanism of action unknown.

        a. Especially useful in trigeminal neuralgia.

        b. Box warning per package insert.

        c. Precautions in patients with mixed seizure disorder; history of cardiac conduction disturbances, hepatic damage, renal damage, adverse hematologic disorders, hypersensitivity reactions.

        d. Review of package insert recommended.

    4. Side effects of gabapentin (Neurontin®)

        a. Dizziness (often resolves after the first few days).

        b. Peripheral edema.

        c. GI upset.

        d. Abnormal gait.

        e. Visual disturbances.

        f. Make patients aware of potential side effects, avoid driving initially, report peripheral edema, do not use with alcohol, may potentiate CNS depression with alcohol.

    5. Side effects of pregabalin (Lyrica®)

        a. Dizziness, somnolence.

        b. Edema.

        c. Dry mouth.

        d. Visual disturbances (blurring).

        e. Weight gain.

        f. Make patients aware of possible adverse events; dizziness usually resolves before the end of the first week, avoid driving; report adverse events; do not use alcohol; monitor suicidal tendencies.

        g. Schedule V controlled substance.

F. Tricyclic antidepressants (TCAs).

    1. Used to treat a number of chronic pain conditions with or without depression.

        a. Theorized that the analgesic properties are associated with drugs' action as serotonin and norepinephrine reuptake inhibitors.

        b. TCAs with the greatest effect on serotonin seem to have the greatest analgesic effect (Bajwa & Smith, 2012).

    2. Most frequently used TCAs.

        a. Amitriptyline (most potent anticholinergic adverse effects such as dry mouth, orthostatic hypotension, constipation, urinary retention; mostly seen at higher doses).

        b. Nortriptylline.

        c. Doxepin.

        d. Imipramine.

        e. Desipramine.

    3. Antecholinergic effects can be mitigated by starting at low dose several hours before bedtime (after the evening meal) and slowly titrating to higher doses as needed.

        a. Drowsiness may be seen with these agents and may work in favor of providing restful sleep (sleep disorders accompany many chronic pain syndromes such as fibromyalgia).

    4. Nursing implications.

        a. If patients awaken with a "hang over" the medication should be taken earlier in the evening.

4
4.1
4.2
4.3
4.4
4.5
4.6
4.7
4.8
4.9
4.10

b. Patients should understand that it may take weeks for analgesia to occur.

c. Many unpleasant side effects may diminish over time.

d. Insufficient therapeutic effect may be overcome with drug substitution.

e. It is important to be supportive, recognizing that these individuals may need additional psychosocial support to achieve pain relief and adhere to the pain management program.

G. Serotonin norepinephrine reuptake inhibitors (SNRIs).

1. Inhibition of serotonin and norepinephrine reuptake.

2. Similar efficacy as TCAs without the anticholinergic effects.

3. Have been shown in clinical trials to reduce pain, improve function, have positive effects on pain threshold and quality of life.

4. Well tolerated; most common side effects are headache and nausea.

5. Drugs:

a. Duloxetine (Cymbalta®); FDA approved for diabetic neuropathies, fibromyalgia, chronic musculoskeletal pain, LBP, osteoarthritis, FMS, major depression, anxiety, and stress urinary incontinence.

b. Venlafaxine (Effexor XR®); FDA approved for diabetic peripheral neuropathies, painful polyneuropathies of different origins.

c. Milnacipran (Savella®); FDA approved for FMS but not for depression.

H. Muscle relaxants.

1. Centrally acting skeletal muscle relaxants have modest benefit for nociceptive pain associated with muscle strain.

2. Used intermittently or as a single evening dose to relieve secondary muscle spasms in back pain and other chronic painful conditions (FMS).

3. Drugs include.

a. Cyclobenzaprine (Flexeril®).

b. Carisoprodol (Soma®).

c. Baclofen (Lioresal®).

d. Methocarbamol (Robaxin®).

4. Side effects.

a. Can cause CNS depression.

b. Somnolence.

c. Antecholinergic effects as listed for TCAs.

I. Topical agents.

1. Advantages over systemic agents.

2. Delivery at site of insult.

3. Lower initial rates of systemic absorption, although significant systemic concentrations can be achieved with topical agents.

4. Patient preference.

5. Patient perception of safety.

6. Agents.

a. 5% lidocaine (gel/patch).

(1) Used for peripheral neuropathic pain such as postherpetic neuralgia, and allodynia.

(2) Effective monotherapy but often used as an adjunct to systemic medication.

b. Capsaicin.

(1) An alkaloid derived from chili peppers.

(2) Repeated application is thought to deplete substance P from primary afferent neurons.

(3) May be most useful as adjunctive therapy.

(4) Must be applied 3-4 times daily with maximum efficacy achieved after 6-8 weeks.

(5) Major adverse events: Burning, stinging, erythema at site of application (leading to intolerance in up to one-third of patients).

c. Topical NSAIDs (gel, spray, cream).

(1) Modest relief for acute musculoskeletal pain; less effective for chronic low back pain, widespread musculoskeletal pain, peripheral neuropathic pain.

i) Diclofenac (Voltaren gel®) (for relief of knee osteoarthritis [OA] pain; well tolerated).

ii) Topical salicylates (response rates lower than for topical NSAIDs).

J. Injection therapies.

1. Local anesthetic injections.

2. Injection of trigger points such as myofascial pain.

3. Side effects are rare.

4. Epinephrine should not be used because of risk of ischemic necrosis.

    a. Botulinum toxin type A (BTX-A).

       (1) Potent neurotoxin.

       (2) May be effective in reducing opioid use in patients with severe postherpetic neuralgia.

    b. Glucocorticoid injections.

       (1) Use with lidocaine (for anesthetic properties).

       (2) Aspiration/injection can be used for diagnosis as well as treatment of localized pain.

       (3) Local corticosteroids may relieve inflammation.

       (4) Local injections are an efficient way to administer high concentrations of glucocorticoids directly into target tissue, maximizing desired effect, minimizing many side effects from systemic use.

       (5) Ultrasound guidance provides more accurate placement.

       (6) Reasonable expectation of clinical benefit when glucocorticoids are injected into joints, synovial cysts, peritendinous structures, bursal sacs, ligamentous attachments, tender points, periarticular tissues.

       (7) Single joint or soft tissue target should not be injected more than 3 times per year (Winfield, 2007).

       (8) Contraindicated in local or systemic infection, coagulopathy, tendon tear.

       (9) These injections can be painful; fully prepare the patient.

K. Epidural injections.

1. Usually performed by pain management specialists but referral may be appropriate for chronic back pain.

2. Interventional procedures.

    a. Intercostal nerve blockade, spinal injections, occipital nerve injections, other peripheral nerve injections.

    b. May provide short-term analgesia, evidence of long term outcome improvements is limited.

V. Non-pharmacologic Interventions.

A. Physical Interventions.

1. Physical/occupational therapy.

    a. Stretching key to normal range of motion (ROM).

    b. Muscle conditioning (improve stability, function, and pain).

    c. Aerobic exercise.

    d. Acupuncture.

    e. Chiropractic and/or osteopathic manipulation.

    f. Ultrasonic stimulation.

    g. Electrical neuromodulation.

       (1) Transcutaneous electrical nerve stimulation (TENS).

       (2) Safe, non-invasive, self-applied.

       (3) Can deliver variable frequency, pulse duration, intensity, and type of output.

       (4) Research is inconclusive regarding efficacy in chronic pain management.

2. Spinal cord stimulation (SCS).

    a. Spinal neuromodulation analgesic system.

    b. Option for chronic neuropathic pain.

    c. Minimally invasive, reversible.

    d. Found to be efficacious in failed back surgery syndrome and complex regional pain syndrome type 1.

3. Thermal applications (heat/cold).

4. Massage.

B. Behavioral medicine approaches.

1. Cognitive behavioral therapy (focuses on environment, behavior, and cognition).

    a. Structured.

    b. Goal directed/problem focused.

    c. Time limited.

    d. Behavioral skill training involves education related to behavioral principles

4
4.1
4.2
4.3
4.4
4.5
4.6
4.7
4.8
4.9
4.10

(conditioning, reinforcement, pain/illness behaviors) and how the principles interact with pain and disability.

   e. Relaxation and controlled breathing exercises.

   f. Patients learn to monitor situational factors that trigger pain/stress.

   g. Can be administered in a variety of formats including via computer or telephone.

2. Biofeedback.

   a. Very useful for migraine headaches and tension-type headaches; greatest impact on headache frequency.

   b. Significant effects on anxiety and medication consumption.

3. Relaxation therapy.

4. Psychotherapy and individual or group counseling.

   a. Patient education.

   b. Patient should understand that the goals of therapy are to reduce pain and improve function; goals and expectations should be realistic.

   c. Multidisciplinary approach leads to better outcomes.

   d. Medication should not be the focus of treatment.

Summary

Pain can be overwhelming and become the focus of a patient's life. Pain can be temporary or it can become chronic. Pain is complex and multifaceted; a management plan requires the integration of pharmacologic and non-pharmacologic strategies. The rheumatology nurse should be familiar with commonly used drugs and adjuvant modalities so the nurse can offer comprehensive care to patients with painful rheumatic conditions.

Acknowledgment

The author acknowledges the contributions of Nancy Crigger, PhD, FNP-BC, and Barbara Voshall, DNP, RN, to this chapter.

References

Bajwa, Z., & Smith, H.(2012). Overview of the treatment of chronic pain. *Up To Date®*. Philadelphia: Wolters Kluwer Health.

McGuire, L. (2010). Pain: The fifth vital sign. In D. Ignatavicius & L. Workman (Eds.), *Medical surgical nursing: Patient centered collaborative care* (pp. 35-61). St. Louis: Saunders Elsevier.

Pasero, C., & McCaffery, M. (2011). *Pain assessment and pharmacologic management*. St. Louis, MO: Mosby Elsevier

So, A., Sprott, H., & Brune, K. (2012). Pain: Mechanisms and management. In J. Bijlsma (Ed.), *EULAR textbook on rheumatic diseases* (pp. 1199-1217). London: BMJ Group.

Winfield, J. (2007). The patient with diffuse pain. In J. Imboden, D. Hellman, & J. Stone, (Eds), *Current diagnosis and treatment: Rheumatology* (pp. 138-145). New York: The McGraw Hill Companies.

Winfield, J. (2008). Pain management. In J. Klippel, J. Stone, L. Crofford, & P. White (Eds.), *Primer on the rheumatic diseases* (pp. 620-627). New York: Springer Science + Business Media.

Suggested Readings

Institute of Medicine. (2011). *Relieving pain in America: A blueprint for transforming prevention, care, education, and research*. Washington, DC: National Academies Press.

International Association for the Study of Pain. (1994). *Classification of chronic pain. Description of chronic pain syndromes and definitions of pain terms*. New York: Elsevier, Goldenberg, D.. (2012). Differential diagnosis of fibromyalgia. *Up to Date®*. Philadelphia: Wolters Kluwer Health.

Jarzyna, D., Janguquist, C.R., Pasero, C., Willens, J.S., Nisbet, A., Oakes, L., ... Polomano, R. C. (2011). American Society of Pain Management Nursing guidelines on monitoring for opioid-induced sedation and respiratory depression. *Pain Management Nursing, 12*(3), 118-145.

Resnick, B. & Pacala, J.T. (2012). American geriatrics society updated Beers criteria forpotentially inappropriate medication use in older adults. *Journal of the American Geriatrics Society, 60*(4), 612-613. DOI: 10.1111/j.1532-5415.2012.03923.x

St. Marie, B. (Ed). *Core curriculum for pain management nursing* (2nd ed.). Dubuque, IA: Kendall Hunt Publishing Company.

4
4.1
4.2
4.3
4.4
4.5
4.6
4.7
4.8
4.9
4.10

Section 4.3
Nursing Management of Patients with Rheumatoid Arthritis

Vanessa K. Hill, MSN, NP-C, Linda Cowden, RN, and Victoria Ruffing, RN, CCRP

Introduction

This chapter is designed to educate the rheumatology nurse about rheumatoid arthritis. The rheumatology nurse should have a thorough understanding of the disease including the pathophysiology, etiology, treatment, and nursing implications.

Learning Objectives

Upon completion of this chapter, the nurse will be able to:

1. Explain the pathophysiology of rheumatoid arthritis (RA).

2. Describe the role of autoimmunity in patients with RA.

3. Identify possible causes and contributing factors that may lead to the development of RA.

4. Identify patient populations at risk for the development of RA.

5. List supporting criteria used to confirm the diagnosis of RA.

6. Describe laboratory monitoring parameters.

7. Identify drug toxicities and extra-articular manifestations of RA.

8. Identify treatment options and list possible side effects and contraindications to therapy.

9. Explain the importance of maintaining physical abilities in patients with RA.

I. Pathophysiology.

A. Rheumatoid arthritis (RA) is a chronic, systemic, inflammatory autoimmune disease that primarily affects the musculoskeletal system (Gibofsky, 2012).

B. The inflammatory process that occurs in RA is caused by an incorrect immune response where the immune system attacks healthy connective tissues. (see Figure 1).

   1. Autoimmunity refers to the process that occurs when the immune system lacks the ability to distinguish normal tissue from foreign objects or damaged tissues. Healthy tissues are targeted and damaged by the immune system resulting in inflammation of the tissues.

   2. In a normal immune response, the immune system should target and destroy abnormal cells or foreign objects such as bacteria and viruses.

   3. The disregulated immune system in patients with rheumatoid arthritis is the culprit for connective tissue damage. Drug therapies designed to treat rheumatoid arthritis target specific cells of the immune system in order to stop the inflammatory process which is responsible for damaging connective tissues.

C. RA tends to target the synovial membrane of joints much more often than other organ systems.

   1. Musculoskeletal: Patients with RA will likely complain of morning stiffness lasting for at least one hour, joint pain, swelling, and erythema which may lead to joint destruction with deformity. Swan neck deformity occurs with abnormal extension of the proximal interphalangeal joint (PIP) and flexion of the distal interphalangeal joint (DIP). Ulnar deviation is noted with drifting of the fingers toward the ulna. Boutonniere deformities occur with abnormal flexion of the MCP and extension of the DIP.

   2. Typically, joint involvement is distributed in a symmetrical fashion, meaning if a joint on one side of the body is involved the same joint on the other side of the body will also be involved. Because of the autoimmune process, an abnormal inflammatory response occurs within diarthrodial joints. The inflamed synovium overproduces synovial fluid leading to synovitis of the joint which causes severe pain with range of motion, decreased range of motion, tenderness on palpation, obvious synovitis, and may lead to joint destruction and deformity (see Figure 2). Chronic effusions may lead to joint laxity because of stretched tendons and ligaments. Firm nodules, known as rheumatoid nodules, may form over bony prominences.

Figure 1: RA Joint Illustration

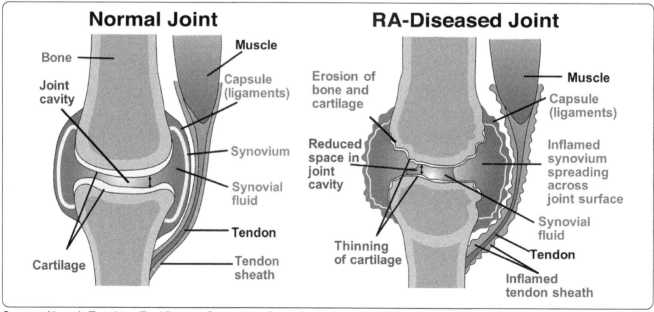

Source: *Nurse's Teaching Tool Patient Counseling Guide for Patients With Rheumatoid Arthritis.*
Rheumatology Nurses Society

D. The autoimmune process in patients who have RA may affect other organ systems causing many symptoms not related to the musculoskeletal system.

1. Constitutional symptoms: Patients may complain of chronic fatigue which may be accompanied by low grade fever not attributed to any other cause.

2. Immunologic: RA patients are at an increased risk for infection and malignancy most likely due to a disregulated immune system.

3. Cardiac: Pericarditis, inflammation of the lining of the heart, may cause chest pain and shortness of breath. Common causes of mortality in RA include cardiovascular disease, which accounts for approximately one third to one half of RA-related deaths, and infection, which is associated with approximately one quarter of such deaths (Mikuls, 2003).

4. Pulmonary: Pleurisy, inflammation of the lining of the lungs, may also cause chest pain, shortness of breath, and pain with breathing. Interstitial lung disease, the most common pulmonary manifestation in RA patients, affects the interstitium of the lungs and is more common in patients who have severe RA (Antin-Ozerkis, Evans, Rubinowitz, Jomer, & Matthay, 2010; Lake, 2011). Interstitial lung disease may be asymptomatic, but patients may complain of nonproductive cough and progressive shortness of breath with or without exertion. Pulmonary function tests will reveal restricted lung volume. Interstitial lung disease may be caused by rheumatoid arthritis or result from disease-modifying antirheumatic drugs (DMARDs) such as methotrexate (MTX).

5. Ocular: Scleritis, inflammation of the eye, may cause eye pain, redness, blurred vision, and photosensitivity. Many patients with RA also complain of dry eyes. This is known as keratoconjunctivitis sicca finding in Sjögren's Syndrome, which affects up to 25% of patients with RA (Dana, 2012).

Figure 2: Synovitis of the Left Knee

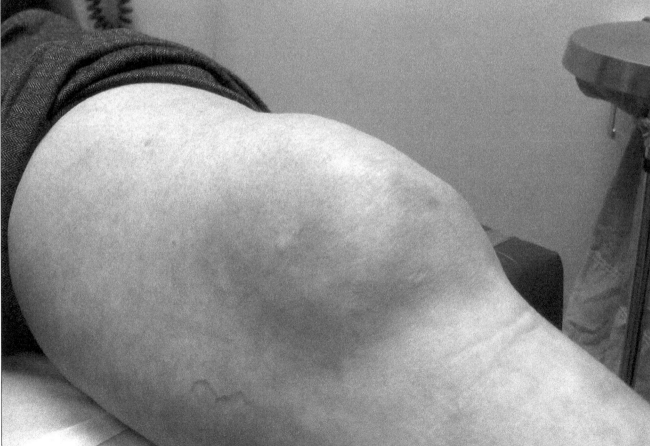

Source: Author, Victoria Ruffing

6. Integumentary: Patients who have a positive rheumatoid factor are at risk for developing nodules, known as rheumatoid nodules, over bony prominences such as on fingers and elbows.

7. Vascular: Vasculitis, the inflammation of blood vessels, may cause many symptoms depending upon which vessels are involved. As a result of vasculitis, tissue necrosis, blood vessel occlusion, and ischemia can occur damaging the skin, heart, eyes, nerves, lungs, and kidneys. Cutaneous vasculitis is the most common vascular manifestation affecting up to 90% of patients with rheumatoid vasculitis resulting in nail fold lesions or deep cutaneous ulcers on the lower extremities (Whelan & Stone, 2011).

8. Hematologic: Anemia and other cytopenias such as leukocytopenia are common in patients with rheumatoid arthritis. Anemia of chronic disease and iron deficiency anemia are most common and are thought to be present in up to 90% of patients with RA (Ehrenfeld & Shoenfeld, 2010).

9. Neurologic: Patients with RA are at risk for developing vasculitis which could cause complications such as ischemia, infarction, or bleeding resulting in transient ischemic attacks, stroke, and paralysis. Neuropathy may develop due to synovitis invading structures such as the spinal cord and peripheral nerves leading to myelopathy, radiculopathy, and entrapment neuropathies. Carpal tunnel syndrome is one of the most common neurologic manifestations of RA (Piecyk & Schur, 2012).

10. Renal: Renal disease may result from rheumatoid vasculitis, drug therapy used to treat RA, or from other co-morbid conditions (Rose, 2011).

II. Epidemiology / Etiology.

A. Rheumatoid arthritis affects approximately 1% of the population (Gibofsky, 2012).

B. Females are 2.5 times more likely to have RA than males.

C. Although rheumatoid arthritis may present at any age, onset is most common in the third to sixth decades (Symmons et al., 1994).

D. The incidence of RA increases after the sixth decade of life.

E. The etiology of RA is unclear but it is believed that many factors play an important role in the development of the disease.

1. People who have first degree relatives with RA are 1.5 times more likely to develop the disease than the general population.

2. Environmental factors such as pollution and cigarette smoke have been implicated as an initiating factor of disease development in genetically predisposed individuals (Klareskog, Stolt, & Lundberg, 2006).

3. Illnesses such as bacterial and viral infections are also believed to lead to the onset of RA.

F. RA may go into remission during pregnancy.

III. Diagnostic criteria.

A. The American College of Rheumatology (ACR) and the European League Against Rheumatism (EULAR) collaborated on establishing a new set of criteria for classifying RA (see Table 1).

1. The new diagnostic criteria are based on a point system.

a. A patient must present with at least one joint with synovitis, with no other diagnosis that would explain that synovitis. Then a score is garnered from 4 domains. A total of 6 or higher would confirm a diagnosis of RA. A patient presenting with a bony erosion, demonstrated on X-ray, bypasses the scoring system and is given the diagnosis of RA.

B. History: The health history is extremely important when assessing patients who may have rheumatoid arthritis in order to differentiate RA from other causes of inflammatory arthritis.

1. RA usually follows a pattern of insidious onset of joint pain and swelling, developing over weeks or months, multiple joint involvement which tends to be symmetrical, and is usually accompanied by constitutional symptoms such as fever, fatigue and weight loss (Haque & Bathon, 2005).

4
4.1
4.2
4.3
4.4
4.5
4.6
4.7
4.8
4.9
4.10

2. The most common joints affected include the wrists, metacarpophalangeal (MCP) joints, proximal interphalangeal (PIP) joints, and metatarsalphalangeal (MTP) joints.

3. Morning stiffness lasting longer than one hour is a symptom highly indicative and supportive of RA.

4. Systemic features of RA, such as pulmonary, cardiac, vascular, and ocular symptoms, typically occur after musculoskeletal complaints in patients who have or have had severe disease.

5. Constitutional symptoms related to RA include fever and fatigue. Increased fatigue may precede a rheumatoid arthritis flare.

6. History of, or presence of, hematologic abnormalities include leukocytopenia, anemia, thrombocytosis, or thrombocytopenia.

7. History of diseases or chronic illness may precede the diagnosis of RA as it is believed that illnesses may provoke the development of the disease.

8. Work and environmental exposures are also important as it is believed environmental exposure could also contribute to disease development.

9. Remember, not all patients will present with a typical pattern.

C. Physical exam: The physical exam is extremely important in diagnosing rheumatoid arthritis.

1. The clinician will perform a thorough physical exam to obtain data on not only musculoskeletal involvement, but other system involvement as well.

2. The musculoskeletal system exam includes inspecting for erythema, performing range of motion (ROM), and palpating for tenderness, and synovitis of each joint. Muscular strength is also assessed.

3. The integumentary exam includes observing for rash, evidence of vasculitis, and the presence of rheumatoid nodules.

4. The cardiopulmonary exam includes auscultation of heart and lung sounds.

5. The ophthalmology exam includes observing the eyes for redness, ulcers, and dry membranes.

6. Neurologic exam includes assessing sensory and motor function.

7. The vascular exam includes thorough skin assessment for ulcerations and nail fold lesions.

D. Laboratory: Multiple laboratory values may be obtained when a patient is evaluated for rheumatoid arthritis. It is important to remember negative values do not negate the diagnosis of RA and positive values alone do not support the diagnosis of RA. Laboratory and other diagnostic procedures are used to assist in the confirmation of the disease when combined with information gathered by obtaining a thorough health history and physical exam.

1. Rheumatoid factor (RF) is an autoantibody that can be detected using a blood sample. It is present in about 70% of patients who have rheumatoid arthritis. It may also be present in healthy individuals or those who have other autoimmune diseases, chronic infections, or

4
4.1
4.2
4.3
4.4
4.5
4.6
4.7
4.8
4.9
4.10

Table 1: ACR - EULAR Classification Criteria for RA

Stage	Points
Joint involvement	1-5 Points are given based on the size and number of joints.
Serology	2-3 Points are given based on low-positive or high positive RF or ACPA
Acute phase reactants	1 Point is given for abnormal ESR or CRP
Duration of symptoms	1 Point is given for duration greater than 6 weeks

» Patients should be considered as having RA if they have at least one joint with clinical synovitis which can not be explained by another disease and who score 6 of 10 points.

Source: Adapted from Aletaha, D., Neogi, T., Silman, A. J., Funovits, J., Felson, D. T., Bingham, C. O.,... Hawker, G. (2010). 2010 Rheumatoid Arthritis Classification Criteria. Arthritis & Rheumatism, 62(9), 2569-2581. http://www.rheumatol-ogy.org/ACR/practice/clinical/classification/ra/2010_revised_criteria_classification_ra.pdf

malignancies. Higher levels of RF correlate with more severe disease activity and extra-articular manifestations (Morehead, 2008).

2. Anti-cyclic citrullinated peptides antibodies (anti CCP or ACPA) are much more specific to RA. ACPA positivity combined with RF positivity correlates with a higher likelihood of joint erosions (Morehead, 2008).

3. Erythrocyte sedimentation rate (ESR) is an acute phase reactant, which is often elevated in the presence of inflammation or infection in the body. It is not specific to the cause of inflammation or infection.

4. C-reactive protein (CRP) is an acute phase reactant, which is often elevated with the presence of inflammation or infection in the body. It is not specific to the cause of inflammation or infection.

5. Complete blood count (CBC) is very important when assessing a patient with rheumatoid arthritis. It is important to establish base values prior to initiating disease-modifying antirheumatic drugs (DMARDs). Patients may present with anemia. Platelet counts could be elevated due to the presence of inflammation in the body. DMARD therapy may cause cytopenias.

6. Comprehensive metabolic profile should be obtained for baseline values. Kidney and liver function are important as these may also be affected by DMARD therapy. These values must also be considered when deciding on which medications are safe for the patient.

7. TB skin test or quantiferon gold and chest radiograph, if indicated, should be performed on patients prior to initiation of certain RA medications.

8. Hepatitis B and C should also be tested as this will affect the use of certain medications that could be liver toxic.

E. Radiographic: Conventional radiographs (X-rays) will reveal joint abnormalities such as bony erosions and joint space narrowing. Radiographic evidence of joint damage may occur within the first six to twelve months of the disease (Haque & Bathon, 2005); it may also appear prior to the diagnosis of RA.

F. Ultrasound: Musculoskeletal ultrasound may be used to detect synovitis in joints when it is not detectable using palpation. Ultrasound is also useful for detecting bony erosions. Ultrasound will also detect hyperemia, increased blood flow, in a joint which suggests the presence of intra-articular inflammation.

G. Magnetic Resonance Imaging (MRI): MRI is capable of detecting small defects which may occur with early arthritis not yet detectable by conventional radiographs.

H. Arthrocentesis: Performed by aspirating synovial fluid from an involved joint. The procedure may be done in the office setting with or without ultrasound guidance. Assessment of synovial fluid to determine cell counts and to assess for crystals is very important to rule out infection and crystal-induced disease, such as gout (Frye, 2008).

IV. Nursing Assessment.

A. Constitutional symptoms: Document patient complaints of fatigue and fever. Many patients with RA suffer from chronic fatigue which may worsen before or during an acute flare. Fever may also be present during disease flare.

B. Musculoskeletal: Assess individual joints for range of motion (ROM), pain with ROM, tenderness, redness, and swelling. The nurse should also note joint deformities and joint replacements or fusions. Swelling and erythema cannot be assessed in the hip joints, but the nurse should assess for limited or painful ROM. Unsteady gait may be present if the hips, knees, ankles, or toes are affected.

C. Immunological: Document infections and illness as patients with RA are immunocompromised and many medications used to treat RA may increase the risk of infection. The nurse should also understand that bacterial and viral illnesses may cause acute flares in RA patients.

D. Cardiopulmonary: Document complaints of chest pain and shortness of breath which could be indicative of cardiac or pulmonary inflammation. Auscultate

4
4.1
4.2
4.3
4.4
4.5
4.6
4.7
4.8
4.9
4.10

and document cardiac rate and rhythm, respiratory rate, and breath sounds.

E. Ocular: Document complaints of changes in vision, eye pain, photosensitivity, dryness, and redness. Visualize conjunctiva and sclera and document abnormalities.

F. Oral/Nasal: Document complaints of dry oral mucosa and incidence of oral or nasal ulcers. Mucosal ulceration could be a side effect of drug therapy and should not be ignored.

G. Integumentary/Vasculature: Document presence of nodules and skin lesions. Inspect fingers and toes for digital ulcers as well as lower extremities for skin ulceration.

H. Hematologic: Review and report laboratory values. Drug therapy may cause multiple cytopenias and affect kidney and liver function. RA may cause chronic anemia. Active inflammation can cause an increased sedimentation rate and C-reactive protein level. MTX and other DMARDs may also cause anemia due to bone marrow suppression.

I. Neurologic: Document complaints such as tingling and numbness in hands and fingers as this could be a sign of carpal tunnel syndrome. Patients may also complain of decreased sensation in digits, hands, and feet because of neuropathy.

J. Gastrointestinal: Long term use of steroids and nonsteroidal anti-inflammatory drugs (NSAIDs) may lead to the development of gastrointestinal ulceration and other complications. Document nausea, vomiting, diarrhea, and the presence of dark tarry or bright red blood in the stool. Assessment includes auscultation and palpation of the abdomen.

K. Renal: Monitor renal function including blood urea nitrogen (BUN), creatinine, glomerular filtration rate (GFR), and urinalysis. NSAID therapy and MTX may lead to renal impairment. Medication adjustment may be necessary with impaired renal function.

L. Hepatic: Monitor liver function tests closely. MTX and leflunomide as well as other DMARDs and chronic NSAID therapy may cause an elevation in liver enzymes.

M. Vaccinations: Patients with RA should receive regular vaccinations to prevent certain infections. Patients with RA who are on immunosuppressive medications should never receive any type of live virus (i.e., shingles vaccination), but the rheumatology nurse should encourage patients to receive routine influenza, pneumococcal, and hepatitis B vaccinations (Shur, Maini, & Gibofsky, 2012). Decision-making regarding live vaccines is complex and should be assessed on a case by case basis.

V. Treatment.

A. The goals of treatment are 1.) achieving the lowest possible level of arthritis disease activity and remission, if possible, 2.) minimizing joint damage and 3.) enhancing physical function and quality of life. In order to reach these goals, the following four steps must be taken:

1. Early disease recognition.

2. Early institution of disease modifying therapy.

3. Continuous reassessment of patient response to current regimen.

4. Recognition of potential medication toxicities.

B. Intensive management and clinical measurement of RA reduces disease activity (Grigor et al,. 2004).

C. A plethora of measurement tools are available.

1. The most common include: Disease Activity Score 28 (DAS28), Simplified Disease Activity Index (SDAI), Clinical Disease Activity Index (CDAI), Rheumatoid Arthritis Disease Activity Index (RADAI), Patient Activity Scale (PAS), and Routine Assessment Patient Index Data (RAPID).

2. Most disease activity measurements combine patient reported information with clinical information to reach a score; for example, physical function with C-reactive Protein.

4
4.1
4.2
4.3
4.4
4.5
4.6
4.7
4.8
4.9
4.10

Multi-biomarker disease activity scores are derived from labortory tests only.

3. These scores can be tracked over time to demonstrate effectiveness of treatment. Measurements of disease activity must be taken at each visit to the healthcare provider.

D. Non-pharmacologic.

1. Exercise: Joint contractures, muscle atrophy, and loss of function may occur due to avoiding use of affected joints (Shur, Maini, & Gibofsky, 2012). Range of motion exercises, weight bearing exercises, and aerobic exercise are recommended not only to maintain joint function but to also achieve and/or maintain healthy weight.

2. Rest: It is very important for patients to rest and protect inflamed joints. Rest will also improve fatigue which may be associated with rheumatoid arthritis.

3. Healthy diet and weight: Excess weight increases stress on joints. Proper nutrition should be used in order to maintain a healthy weight in individuals who tend to be overweight and in individuals who may become anorexic because of poor dietary intake.

4. Physical Therapy - may be used to improve or maintain joint function by using heat and cold application, massotherapy, passive and active range of motion, and fitting assistive devices for ambulation (Shur, Maini, & Gibofsky, 2012).

5. Occupational Therapy offers splinting and teaching use of assistive devices (Shur, Maini, & Gibofsky, 2012).

E. Pharmacologic.

1. NSAIDs.

a. Non-selective Cox inhibitors: Nonsteroidal anti-inflammatory drugs are useful in treating pain and inflammation associated with rheumatoid arthritis. Careful consideration should be used with elderly patients or those with renal impairment or a history of gastrointestinal ulceration. Renal function should be monitored as NSAIDs may cause renal impairment. Patients who have existing renal impairment should limit the use of or avoid NSAID therapy. Patients with impaired hepatic function should also avoid NSAID therapy.

NSAIDs increase bleeding tendency and should not be used in combination with anticoagulants or antiplatelet medications. There are many NSAIDs on the market, both prescription and over the counter. The following are examples of commonly used non-selective NSAIDs.

(1) Ibuprofen (Motrin®, McNeil, 2012): 200-800 mg usually given every 6-8 hours. The maximum dose for a 24 hour period is 2400 milligrams.

(2) Meloxicam (Mobic®, Boehringer Ingelheim Pharmaceuticals, 2010): 7.5-15 mg per day. The maximum dosage is 15 milligrams a day. Available by prescription only.

(3) Naproxen (Aleve®, Bayer HealthCare, 2011): Dosage is 220 mg every 8-12 hours with a maximum dosage of 3 tablets in a 24 hour period.

b. Selective Cox inhibitors: Selective Cox inhibitors are considered to be less harmful to the gastrointestinal (GI) tract as they do not target the prostaglandins responsible for the production of the protective mucosal lining along the GI tract. There is only one selective Cox inhibitor currently available.

(1) Celocoxib (Celebrex®, Pfizer, 2013a): 100-200 mg twice a day. Available by prescription only.

2. Steroid therapy is commonly used as short term therapy in acute situations or as adjunctive therapy. Long term use of high dose steroids may lead to osteoporosis, cardiovascular disease, cataracts, weight gain, gastrointestinal ulceration, and elevated blood glucose levels. Most patients respond quickly to steroids and have marked decrease in pain and swelling related to inflammation caused by rheumatoid arthritis within just days of beginning therapy. Some patients may require long term use of steroids in order to control the disease but typically patients are placed on other DMARDs in order to prevent steroid use. There are many types of steroids which may be given in different forms and routes. Oral steroids may be given daily or on an as needed basis in order to help control inflammation. Intra-muscular (IM) steroids may be given to patients in an acute situation needing immediate relief from severe joint pain involving multiple joints.

4
4.1
4.2
4.3
4.4
4.5
4.6
4.7
4.8
4.9
4.10

Intra-articular steroid injections may be given in a situation where a patient may have severe inflammation in one or two joints.

a. Oral.

(1) Prednisone: 5-60 mg per day in divided doses of 1-4 times per day (Drugs.com, 2013).

(2) Methylprednisolone: 4-48 mg orally per day for immunosuppression (Drugs.com, 2013).

(3) Betamethasone: 0.6-7.2 mg daily (Drugs.com, 2013).

b. IM.

(1) Depomedrol: 20-80 mg once as needed (Drugs.com, 2013).

c. IA.

(1) Triamcinolone: 5-40 mg once depending on the size of the joint. The average for the knee is 25 mg. The maximum weekly dosage is 75 mg (Drugs.com, 2013).

(2) Depomedrol: Dosage is 40-120 mg IA based on the size of the joint. For large joints, it is 20-80 mg IA. For medium joints, it is 10-40 mg IA and for small joints, it is 4-10 mg (Drugs.com, 2013).

3. Traditional Disease-Modifying Antirheumatic Drugs (DMARDs) actually alter the disease process of rheumatoid arthritis. Prior to the development of DMARD therapy, rheumatologists were limited in the selection of medications which could be used to treat RA. Unfortunately, as a result of limited therapy, patients with RA suffered serious consequences such as permanent disability. Now there are many DMARDs available to treat rheumatoid arthritis. The goal of DMARD therapy is to prevent inflammation and connective tissue damage.

a. Common DMARDs.

(1) MTX is commonly the first DMARD therapy used to treat RA. The usual dose is 7.5-25 mg given once weekly. The medication may be given orally as a 2.5 mg tablet or as injection. Injectable MTX is available as 25 mg/ml and may be given subcutaneously or intramuscularly. MTX should be used very carefully in patients with impaired hepatic function or liver disease. Liver function should be monitored frequently for toxicity. Dose modification may be necessary in those with renal impairment. MTX may also cause interstitial lung disease. Most common side effects reported by patients include nausea and fatigue (Drugs.com, 2013).

(2) Leflunomide (Arava®, Sanofi-Aventis, 2012) may be given in conjunction with MTX or as an alternative to MTX. It is given in oral form of 10-20 mg daily. It may be given to patients who have interstitial lung disease and may be used as an alternative to MTX if patients are unable to tolerate MTX. Most common side effect is diarrhea. Liver functions must be monitored as this drug may also be liver toxic. Must not be used in patients who are pregnant or planning to become pregnant.

(3) Sulfasalazine (SSZ): This medication may also be used in conjunction with other DMARDs. Patients should drink adequate amounts of water to prevent kidney stone formation. This is a delayed release tablet and should never be crushed. The initial dose is 500 mg daily for one week and then titrated 500 mg daily in 2 divided doses to reach a maximum of 3,000 mg daily. Patients may have orange-yellow discoloration of the urine or skin when taking this drug (Drugs.com, 2013). Annual eye exam are recommended.

(4) Hydroxychloroquine may be used initially in patients with low disease activity or in conjunction with other DMARD therapy. It is an oral medication available in 200 mg tablet. The usual dose is 400 mg daily which may be given as a single dose or divided doses. Most patients tolerate this medication well but may report nausea or rash. Laboratory monitoring includes CBC; the drug is not liver toxic. Dose modification may be necessary in the presence of renal impairment (Drugs.com, 2013). Annual eye exams are recommended.

b. Less commonly used agents.

(1) Minocycline. Initial dosage is 200 milligrams, then 100 milligrams every 12 hours or 50 milligrams four times a day (Drugs.com, 2013).

(2) Cyclosporine. Initial dose is 1.25 milligrams per kilogram twice a day. This may be increased by 0.5-0.75 milligrams per kilogram per day after

4
4.1
4.2
4.3
4.4
4.5
4.6
4.7
4.8
4.9
4.10

8 weeks. The dose may be increased again after 12 weeks with a maximum dosage of 4 mg/kg/day. Monitor renal function (Drugs.com, 2013).

4. Biologic DMARDs. These medications target specific entities of the immune cascade. Prior to initiation of any of these biologic medications, a TB test, hepatitis panel, and baseline blood work should be performed. Patients with any type of active infection should not be given biologic therapy.

a. Tofacitinib (Xeljanz®, Pfizer, 2013b) a Janus Kinase Inhibitor is approvedto treat RA. Dosage is 5 milligrams normally twice a day. It may cause an elevation in liver enzymes and cholesterol so these levels should be monitored during therapy. It is approved as monotherapy, or may be used in conjunction with other non-biologic DMARDs.

b. Anti Tumor Necrosis Factor Alpha therapy, known as anti-TNF therapy, targets tumor necrosis alpha factor therefore inhibiting the initiation of the immune cascade.

   (1) Infliximab (Remicade®, Janssen Biotech, 2013a): Recommended dose is 3 mg/kg given IV infusion at weeks 0, 2, and 6, followed by a maintenance regimen of 3 mg/kg every 8 weeks. The dosage may be adjusted up to 10 mg/kg or treating as often as every 4 weeks, but the risk of serious infections is increased at higher doses.

   (2) Etanercept (Enbrel®, Amgen, 2012): Given as a subcutaneous injection of 25-50 mg every week. This medication may be self-administered.

   (3) Adalimumab (Humira®, AbbVie, 2013): Dosage is 40 mg subcutaneous injection every other week but may be increased to weekly dose if full efficacy not achieved. This medication may be self-administered.

   (4) Golimumab (Simponi®, Janssen Biotech, 2013b): Subcutaneous dosage is 50 mg subcutaneous injection once a month. This medication may be self-administered. Golimumab IV (Simponi Aria®) is administered at 2 mg/kg every 8 weeks after 2 loading doses 4 weeks apart. Administration is over 30 minutes.

   (5) Certolizumab Pegol (Cimzia®, UCB, 2012): Initial dosage is 400 mg subcutaneously at weeks 0, 2, and 4, then 200 mg every 2 weeks. This medication may be self-administered.

c. IL-6 inhibitors bind to IL-6 in order to prevent activation of the inflammatory cascade.

   (1) Tocilizumab (Actemra®, Genentech, 2013): Dosage is 4-8 milligrams per kilogram of body weight with a maximum dose of 800 milligrams. This is given through an IV infusion every 4 weeks. Monitor the patient's cholesterol and liver enzymes. Tocilizumab subcutaneous is self administered via prefilled syringe of 162 mg per dose every 1-2 weeks.

d. T cell depletion.

   (1) Abatacept (Orencia®, Bristol-Myers Squibb, 2012): Can be given through an intravenous infusion or a subcutaneous injection. The dosage is based on weight for IV infusion. If the patient weighs less than 60 kilograms, give 500 mg. If the patient weighs 60-100 kilograms, give 750 mg. If the patient weighs more than 100 kilograms, give 1,000 mg every 4 weeks. Administer as a 30 minute IV infusion. The dose is repeated at 2 and 4 weeks after the initial dose, then every 4 weeks thereafter. For the subcutaneous injection, the patient may be given the IV infusion loading dose. Without the loading dose, patients may start with a 125 mg subcutaneous injection once weekly. Patients being changed from IV to subcutaneous administration should be given the subcutaneous injection when the next infusion is due and then weekly.

e. B cell depleting therapies destroy certain B cells in circulation in order to prevent the immune cascade.

   (1) Rituximab (Rituxan®, Genentech, 2012): Always pre-medicate the patient with acetaminophen and an antihistamine. Methylprednisolone 100 mg IV is recommended 30 minutes prior to the infusion. Rituximab is given as two 1,000 mg infusions separated by 2 weeks. Subsequent courses should be administered every 24 weeks or based on clinical evaluation, but not sooner than 16 weeks.

4
4.1
4.2
4.3
4.4
4.5
4.6
4.7
4.8
4.9
4.10

5. Treat to Target or tight control is a concept used in treating patients with rheumatoid arthritis (see Figure 3). The concept of treating to target revolves around early diagnosis along with early and aggressive treatment in order to adequately control the disease and prevent joint damage as well as other complications of rheumatoid arthritis. Patients should be monitored frequently and treatment changes should be made according to the patient's disease status. The goal of using treat to target is to achieve remission, but in patients with severe, refractory, or long history of rheumatoid arthritis, low disease activity is the best second option (Vermeer et al., 2011).

F. Surgical intervention.

1. Joint replacement may be necessary if severe destruction leads to decreased function and progressive pain in joints. Common joints which may be replaced include shoulders, hips, knees, and ankles. Small joints such as the metacarpal phalangeals (MCPs) may also be replaced.

2. Joint fusion may be necessary for immobilization and pain relief in a joint.

Ankles, wrists, and MTPs are commonly fused joints. Unfortunately, fusing a joint does not improve function.

VI. Co-morbid Conditions.

A. Secondary osteoarthritis may form in joints affected by RA.

B. Osteoporosis or osteopenia may be due to RA and/or the administration of glucocorticoid therapy.

C. Patients who have RA are at an increased risk for developing cardiovascular disease.

D. There is also an increased risk of infection and some cancers related to the RA disease process as well as the use of immunosuppressive medications used to treat the disease.

VII. Nursing Implications.

A. The rheumatology nurse plays a vital role in the rheumatology setting. As health care changes, the nurse is expected to

Figure 3: Treat to Target

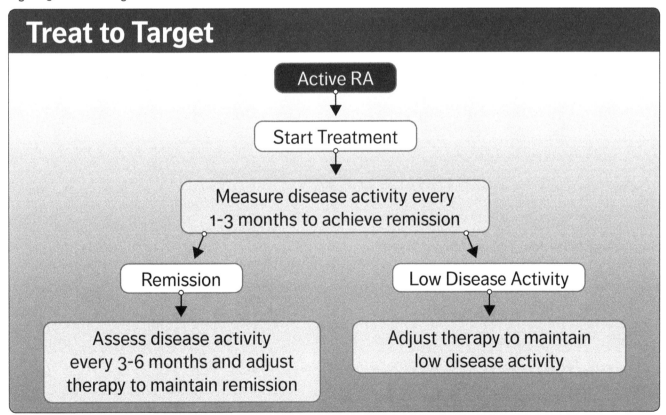

Treat to Target

Active RA
↓
Start Treatment
↓
Measure disease activity every 1-3 months to achieve remission

Remission
↓
Assess disease activity every 3-6 months and adjust therapy to maintain remission

Low Disease Activity
↓
Adjust therapy to maintain low disease activity

Adapted from: Smolen et al., 2010, Annals of the Rheumatic Diseases, 69(6), 964-975.

fill in many gaps, especially in patient education. It is extremely important to staff rheumatology clinics with trained rheumatology nurses in order to safely and effectively meet patients' needs.

B. Adherence to any treatment plan can be influenced by the rheumatology nurse (see Table 2). Factors contributing to poor adherence include poor knowledge regarding an illness, lack of motivation to manage the illness, lack of confidence (self-efficacy) in the ability to manage the illness, forgetfulness, stress, expectations regarding the outcome of treatment and consequences of poor adherence, low attendance at follow-up appointments, and not understanding treatment instruction, among others. Additionally, condition-related factors such as less severe symptoms, co-morbidities, and available treatments may also affect a patient's adherence to a treatment plan. Rheumatology nurses should also be aware of a patient's socio-economic status regarding ability to pay for medication, transportation, living conditions, family support system, and cultural beliefs when developing a treatment plan (Curkendall et al., 2008; Garcia-Gonzalez et al., 2008; Sabate, 2003).

C. Education of the patient:

1. Thoroughly explain rheumatoid arthritis using appropriate terms the patient can understand.

2. Teach what signs and symptoms to expect and what to report to the rheumatology nurse and/or other healthcare provider.

3. Effectively teach medication management including possible side effects and what to report to the healthcare provider.

4. Educate patients about non-pharmacologic therapeutic modalities such as proper nutrition, weight, exercise, rest, and counseling.

5. Provide a list of reputable websites patients may visit for credible and reliable information.

6. Provide reading level appropriate teaching material for the patient to take home.

D. Education of the rheumatology nurse:

1. Stay abreast of new treatment options to enable discussion about these with patients as the need arises.

2. Be knowledgeable about current treatments including the usual dose, frequency, route, possible side effects, and what patients should expect and report.

Table 2: Strategies for Successful Patient Education and Adherence to a Treatment Plan

» Assess the patient's level of understanding
» Discuss the patient's expectations
» Provide multiple forms of education (written, verbal, tactile)
» Include family or other support systems in discussion
» Pace education over time rather than all at once
» Use simple and understandable language
» Be honest and friendly
» Summarize essential points to increase retention
» Set mutual goals and outline responsibilities to be met within a specified timeframe
» Ask the patient to repeat important instructions

Source: Author, Victoria Ruffing

3. Read current articles.

4. Become a member of professional nursing societies and engage in ongoing learning experiences.

5. Ask questions. Always discuss any questions with knowledgeable healthcare providers. Network with other rheumatology nurses to share experiences and learn from others.

Summary

Rheumatoid arthritis is a systemic, inflammatory disease for which there is no cure. Joint pain and swelling are the hallmark characteristics of rheumatoid arthritis. Early diagnosis and treatment are imperative for favorable outcomes. Treatment goals are clinical remission, minimization of joint damage, and maintenance of physical function and quality of life. Treatment plans for the patient with RA will combine medical, social, and emotional support for the patient and family. Intensive management of RA should include clinical measurements in order to minimize disease activity. Medication regimens can be complicated. Patients must be educated on expected time of onset as well as side effects of medications. Patients receiving biologic DMARDs should be educated on reporting any signs and symptoms of infection to prevent serious complications.

Nurses play a vital role in the care and management of patients with rheumatoid arthritis.

References

AbbVie. (2013). *Humira®*: Prescribing information. North Chicago, IL: Author.

Amgen. (2012). *Enbrel®: Prescribing information*, Thousand Oaks, CA: Author.

Antin-Ozerkis, D., Evans, J., Rubinowitz, A., Homer, R.J., & Matthay, R.A., (2010), Pulmonary manifestation of rheumatoid arthritis. *Clinics in Chest Medicine,* 3(3), 451-478.

Bayer HealthCare. (2011). *Aleve®*: Prescribing information. Morristown, NJ: Author.

Bristol-Myers Squibb. (2012). *Orencia®*: Prescribing information. Princeton, NJ: Author.

Curkendall, S., Patel, V., Gleeson, M., Campbell, R.S., Zagari, M., & Dubois, R (2008). Compliance with biologic therapies for rheumatoid arthritis: Do patient out-of-pocket payments matter? *Arthritis & Rheumatism,59*, 1519-1526.

Dana, R. (2012, March 6). Ocular manifestations of rheumatoid arthritis. UpToDate®. Philadelphia: Wolters Kluwer Health. Retrieved from http://www. uptodate.com/contents/ocular-manifestations-of-rheumatoid-arthritis

Drugs.com (August, 2014) [Internet]. Prednisone Tablets, USP, (Available from: http://www.drugs.com/pro/prednisone-tablets.html

Ehrenfeld, M., & Shoenfeld, Y. (2010, February 11). Hematologic manifestations of rheumatoid arthritis. *UpToDate®*. Philadelphia: Wolters Kluwer Health. Retrieved from http://www.uptodate.com/contents/hematologic-manifestation-of-rheumatoid-arthritis

Frye, K.H., (2008). Arthrocentesis, synovial fluid analysis, and synovial biopsy. In J. H. Klippel, J. H. Stone, L. J. Crofford, & P. H. White (Eds.), *Primer on the rheumatic diseases* (13th ed., pp. 21-27). New York: Springer.

Garcia-Gonzalez, A., Richardson, M., Popa-Lisseanu, M.G., Cox, V., Kallen, M.A., Janssen, N.,,...Suarez-Almazor, M.E. (2008). Treatment adherence in patients with rheumatoid arthritis and systemic lupus erythematosus. *Clinical Rheumatology,27*(7), 883-889. Doi: 10.1007/s 10067-007-0816-6

Genentech. (2012). *Rituxan®* : Prescribing information. San Francisco, CA: Author.

Genentech. (2013). *Actemra®* : Prescribing information. San Francisco, CA: Author.

Gibofsky, A. (2012). Overview of epidemiology, pathophysiology, and diagnosis of rheumatoid arthritis. *The American Journal of Managed Care, 18* (13), S295-S302.

Grigor, C., Capell, H., Stirling, A., McMahon, A.D., Lock, P, Vallance, R.. . . Porter, D. (2004). Effect of a treatment strategy of tight control for rheumatoid arthritis (the TICORA study): A single-blind randomized controlled trial. *The Lancet*; *364*(9430), 263-269.

Haque, U. J. & Bathon, J.M. (2005). The role of biologicals in early rheumatoid arthritis. *Best Practice & Research Clinical Rheumatology*, 19(1), 179-189.

Janssen Biotech. (2013a). *Remicade®*: Prescribing information. Horsham, PA: Author.

Janssen Biotech. (2013b). *Simponi®*: Prescribing information. Horsham, PA: Author.

4
4.1
4.2
4.3
4.4
4.5
4.6
4.7
4.8
4.9
4.10

Klareskog, L., Stolt, P., Lundberg, K., Kallberg, H., Bengtsson, C, Grunewald, J., ... Alfredsson. (2006). A new model for an etiology of rheumatoid arthritis: Smoking may trigger HLA-DR (shared epitope)-restricted immune reactions to autoantigens modified by citrullination. *Arthritis & Rheumatism,54*(1), 38-46.

Lake, F. R. (2011, June 7). Interstitial lung disease in rheumatoid arthritis. *UpToDate®*. Philadelphia: Wolters Kluwer Health. Retrieved from http://www.uptodate.com/contents/interstitial-lung-disease-in-rheumatoid-arthritis

McNeil. (2012). *Motrin®: Prescribing information*. Fort Washington, PA: Author.

Mikuls, T.R. (2003). Co-morbidity in rheumatoid arthritis. *Best Practice & Research Clinical Rheumatology,17*(5), 729-752

Morehead, K. (2008). Laboratory assessment. In J. H. Klippel, J. H. Stone, L. J. Crofford, & P. H. White (Eds.), *Primer on the rheumatic diseases* (13th ed., pp. 15-20). New York: Springer.

Pfizer. (2013a). *Celebrex®*: Prescribing information. New York: Author.

Pfizer. (2013b). *Xeljanz®*: Prescribing information. New York: Author.

Piecyk, M., & Schur, P. (2012, March 22). Neurologic manifestations of rheumatoid arthritis. *UpToDate®*. Philadelphia: Wolters Kluwer Health. Retrieved from http://www.uptodate.com/contents/neurologic-manifestations-of-rheumatoid-arthritis

Rose, B. (2011, February 11). Renal disease in patients with rheumatoid arthritis. *UpToDate®*. Philadelphia: Wolters Kluwer Health. Retrieved from http://www.uptodate.com/contents/renal-disease-in-patients-with-rheumatoid-arthritis

Sabate, E. (2003). *Adherence to long-term therapies: Evidence for action*. Geneva: World Health Organization.

Sanofi-Aventis. (2012). *Arava ®: Prescribing information*. Bridgewater, NJ: Author.

Shur, P., Maini, R., & Gibofsky, A. (2012, April 17). Nonpharmacologic and preventive therapies of rheumatoid arthritis. *UpToDate®*. Philadelphia: Wolters Kluwer Health., Retrieved from http://www.uptodate.com/contents/nonpharmacologic-and-preventive-therapies

Symmons, D.P., Barret, E.M., Bankhead, C.R., Scott, D.G., & Silman, A. (1994). The incidence of rheumatoid arthritis in the United Kingdom: Results from the Norfolk Arthritis Register. *British Journal of Rheumatology,* 33(8),735-739.

UCB. (2012). *Cimzia®*: Prescribing information. Smyrna, GA: Author.

Vermeer, M., Kuper, H.H., Hoekstra, M., Haagsma, C.J., Posthumus, M.D. Brus, H.L.M., ... van de Laar, M.A.F.J. (2011). Implementation of a treat-to-target strategy in very early rheumatoid arthritis. Results of the Dutch rheumatoid arthritis monitoring remission induction cohort study. *Arthritis & Rheumatism, 63*(10), 2865-2872. DOI 10.1002/art.30494

Whelan, P., & Stone, J.H. (2011, December 1). Clinical manifestations and diagnosis of rheumatoid vasculitis. *UpToDate®*. Philadelphia: Wolters Kluwer Health. Retrieved from http://www.uptodate.com/contents/clinical-manifestations-and-diagnosis-of-rheumatoid-vasculitis

4
4.1
4.2
4.3
4.4
4.5
4.6
4.7
4.8
4.9
4.10

Section 4.4
Spondyloarthropathies

Elizabeth Kirchner, CNP, Sheree C. Carter, PhD, RN, and Victor Mo, MSN, RN

Introduction

The spondyloarthropathies (SpA) are a group of multisystem inflammatory disorders affecting various joints and extra-articular structures: The eye, skin, gastrointestinal (GI), and genitourinary (GU) systems, among others. The SpA are linked by common genetics (the human leukocyte antigen [HLA] class-I gene HLA B27 being the most prevalent) and a common pathology.

The spondyloarthropathies include ankylosing spondylitis (AS), reactive arthritis (ReA) (formerly known as Reiter's Syndrome), psoriatic arthritis (PsA), enteropathic arthropathy - spondyloarthropathy associated with inflammatory bowel disease (IBD) such as Crohn's disease and ulcerative colitis - and undifferentiated SpA (uSpA) for those disorders that do not fulfill individual criteria but have overlapping features. (See Figure 1 for a diagram showing the overlapping nature, relationships and clinical presentations of the spondyloarthropathies; see Table 1 for a snapshot view of subtype classifications.)

Between 2009 and 2011 important updates were made in the classifications of SpA which divided the spondyloarthropathies into either predominantly axial or peripheral (Rudwaleit, 2009) (Figure 2). The main reason for these new classifications was that the existing criteria used in clinical practice were limited to diagnosing SpA only when the disease was fairly advanced. With new research into SpA epidemiology, genetics and pathophysiology, as well as advances in radiographic identification of SpA, it was important to develop a new system of classification that would allow for earlier identification and treatment of the spondyloarthropathies.

Learning Objectives

Upon completion of this chapter, the nurse will be able to:

1. Describe the spondyloarthropathies and their typical manifestations.

2. Discuss the commonalities, differences, and unique features among AS, ReA, PsA, and IBD-associated spondyloarthropathy.

3. Review the proposed etiologies and prevalence among these conditions.

4. Describe realistic treatments (pharmacologic and non-pharmacologic) and patient functional goals.

Content Outline

I. Ankylosing Spondylitis (AS):

Prototype of Spondyloarthritis. Ankylosing spondylitis (AS) is a chronic, painful, multisystem inflammatory joint disease characterized by fibrosis, ossification, and fusion (ankylosis) of the spine and sacroiliac joints. The 2009 recharacterization of SpA broadens the spectrum of AS to include not just the classic type but earlier (sometimes referred to as "nonradiographic" or "preradiographic") forms as well (Braun, 2011).

A. Epidemiology.

1. Total population.

    a. The weighted, age-adjusted prevalence of HLA B27 positivity in persons age 20-69 in the United States is 6.1% (Reveille, 2012).

    b. AS affects approximately 0.1% to 2% of the general population (Reveille, 2012).

2. Race.

    a. Prevalence of both HLA B27 positivity and AS varies greatly between different ethnicities.

    b. Highest prevalence in northern European countries; lowest in sub-Saharan Africa.

    c. More common in certain Native American tribes than in African Americans, Asians, and other nonwhite ethnic groups.

3. Gender.

    a. There is no statistically significant difference between the genders in terms of HLA B27 positivity (Reveille, 2012).

Figure 1: The family of spondyloarthropathies.

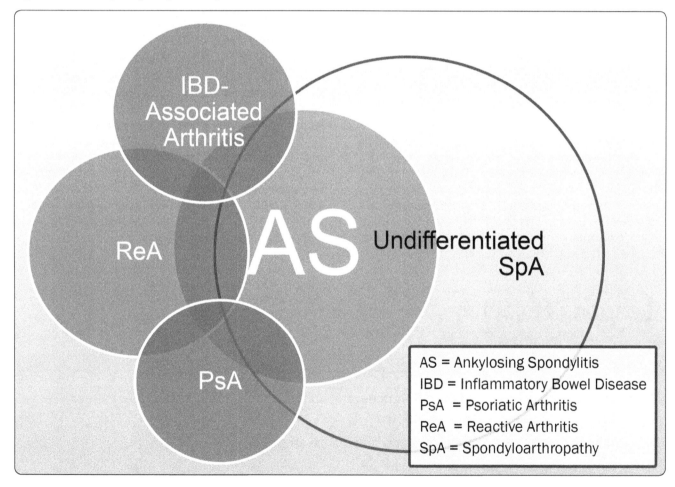

AS = Ankylosing Spondylitis
IBD = Inflammatory Bowel Disease
PsA = Psoriatic Arthritis
ReA = Reactive Arthritis
SpA = Spondyloarthropathy

Source: Reprinted by permission from Leonard H. Calabrese, DO. History of spondyloarthritis. Copyright 2014.

b. AS is more common in males than females (ratio is about 2:1 to 3:1) (Yu, 2014).

4. Age of onset.

   a. Usually develops in late adolescence or young adulthood, with a peak incidence at about 20 years of age (McCance, 2006).

   b. Approximately 10%-20% of all patients experience symptom onset before age 16 years (Linden, 1998).

   c. There is often a significant delay in diagnosis, usually occurring several years after the onset of inflammatory rheumatic symptoms (Rudwaleit, 2012).

B. Pathophysiology.

1. Targets of inflammation in AS.

   a. The primary pathologic process in AS is inflammation.

   b. Inflammation begins at the entheses.

     (1) Insertion site of ligaments and tendons into bones.

     (2) Found throughout the skeletal system.

     (3) Predominantly involve the axial skeleton and lower extremities.

     (4) Locations of entheses help explain the clinical manifestations of AS.

   c. Inflamed tendons and ligaments are located in the peri-articular joint space.

     (1) Associated redness, swelling, and warmth commonly extend above and/or below the involved joint.

   d. Extra-articular structures such as the gut, skin, eye, and aortic valve can also be affected by inflammation in AS (Khan, 2002).

2. Relationship of inflammation to fusion.

   a. Inflammation of fibrocartilage in the vertebrae includes:

     (1) Fibrous tissue of the joint capsule.

     (2) Cartilage surrounding the inter-vertebral disks.

     (3) Entheses.

     (4) Periosteum.

Table 1: Spondyloarthropathies: Subtype classification.

Ankylosing Spondylitis (AS)	Psoriatic Arthritis (PsA)	Enteropathic (IBD – associated)	Reactive Arthritis (ReA)	Undifferentiated SpA (uSpA)
Most common subtype along with uSpa. 2.5:1 male:female. Gradual onset of IBP. Acute anterior uveitis most common extra-articular manifestation. Can lead to sacroiliac fusion and spinal syndesmophyte formation.	Between 10% and 40% of patients with psoriasis (PS) develop PsA, depending on study population and PS severity. Most phenotypically diverse SpA with 5 subtypes. Skin disease precedes joint disease in approximately 70% of cases.	5% to 29% of patients with IBD develop arthritis. Peripheral arthritis (not axial) can parallel bowel inflammation and can occur in up to 20% of patients. Spondylitis occurs in 3% to 6%.	Acute asymmetric oligoarticular (<4 joints) arthritis 1-3 months after gastrointestinal and genitourinary infection. Characteristic triad of urethritis, conjunctivitis, and arthritis seen in < 35% of patients. Keratoderma blennorrhagica and circinate balanitis may be seen.	Most common subtype along with AS. Typically used to describe patients not fulfilling criteria of any one SpA but presenting with IBP and other extra-articular SpA manifestations. Up to 50% of uSpA will develop into AS.

» AS = Ankylosing Spondylitis
» IBP = Inflammatory Back Pain
» IBD = Inflammatory Bowel Disease

» PS = Psoriasis
» PsA = Psoriatic Arthritis
» ReA = Reactive Arthritis

» SpA = Spondyloarthropathy
» uSpA = Undifferentiated SpA

Source: Reprinted by permission from Anthony M. Turkiewicz, M.D. *Spondyloarthropathies: subtype classification*, Copyright 2015.

4
4.1
4.2
4.3
4.4
4.5
4.6
4.7
4.8
4.9
4.10

b. These areas all can be infiltrated by inflammatory cells.

   (1) Mainly macrophages and lymphocytes.

   (2) Inflammatory cells infiltrate and erode the bone and fibrocartilage of the joints.

   (3) Process of repair begins (Figure 3c).

c. Repairing of the cartilaginous structures.

   (1) Begins with the proliferation of fibroblasts.

   (2) Fibroblasts synthesize and secrete collagen.

   (3) Collagen becomes organized into fibrous scar tissue.

   (4) Scar tissue eventually undergoes calcification and ossification.

   (5) With time, all the cartilaginous structures of the joint are replaced by ossified scar tissue, causing the joint to fuse and lose flexibility (Figure 3d).

d. Repair of eroded bone.

   (1) Begins with osteoblast activation and proliferation.

   (2) Osteoblasts lay down new bone (callus).

   (3) Callus is remodeled and replaced by compact, lamellar bone.

   (4) Bone repair changes the contour of the surface of the bone.

   (5) Abnormal structures called syndesmophytes are formed which are basically a new enthesis grown on top of an old one.

e. Progression of calcification of the spinal ligaments.

   (1) Vertebral bodies lose their concave anterior contour and become square.

   (2) Radiographically, these vertebral bodies have a distinct appearance referred to as a "bamboo spine."

   (3) Bamboo spine is generally seen at the end-stage of the disease in AS (McCance, 2006).

C. Etiology.

   1. Genetic predisposition.

      a. The cause of AS is still largely unknown.

         (1) Generally thought to be a combination of genetic and environmental factors.

Figure 2: ASAS classification criteria for axial and peripheral SpA (van Tubergen, 2014).

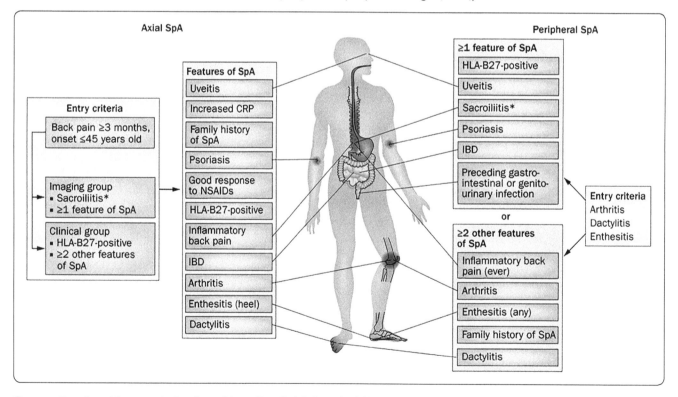

b. AS has been strongly associated with the presence of the gene for the major histocompatibility human leukocyte antigen (HLA) B27 on the chromosomes of the affected individuals.

    (1) Suggests a genetic predisposition to the disease (Khan, 2002).

c. Not all HLA B27 positive individuals develop AS.

    (1) 90-95% of those with AS are HLA B27+

    (2) Only 5% of those who are HLA B27+ will develop any spondyloarthropathy (including AS) (Reveille, 2012).

2. Environmental factors.

a. It has been postulated that an infectious agent (possibly *Klebsiella, Shigella, Salmonella, Yersinia,* or *Chlamydia*-delivered peptides) interacts with HLA B27.

    (1) Interaction triggers and perpetuates the inflammatory response in the entheses (Khan, 2002; Linden, 1998).

3. Autoimmune inflammation.

a. Typical inflammatory response in AS is exuberant and chronic.

    (1) Characterized by an elevation of the pro-inflammatory cytokine tumor necrosis factor-alpha (TNF-α) (Gorman, 2002).

Figure 3: The progression of inflammatory back pain in spondyloarthritis.

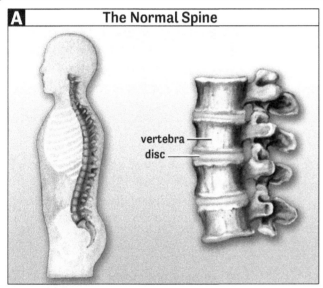
A The Normal Spine

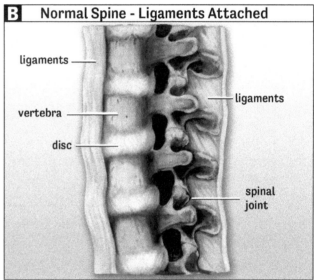
B Normal Spine - Ligaments Attached

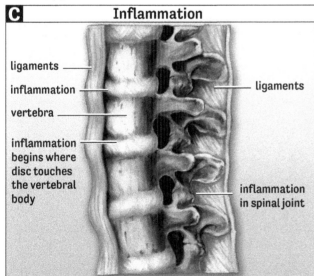
C Inflammation

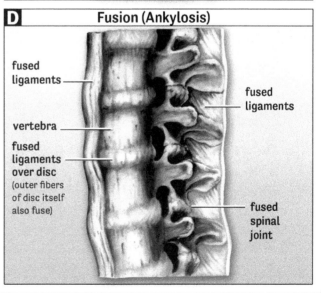
D Fusion (Ankylosis)

4
4.1
4.2
4.3
4.4
4.5
4.6
4.7
4.8
4.9
4.10

(2) TNF-α has been shown to be elevated in the serum, synovium, and sacroiliac joints of patients with AS (Gorman, 2002).

D. Clinical Features.

1. Axial skeletal involvement.

   a. Persistent symptoms of "inflammatory low back pain" for at least three months.

   b. Insidious onset of back pain, stiffness (in the morning or after periods of inactivity), or tenderness to palpation of the spine, peripheral joints, or entheses.

   c. Intermittent, dull in character, and difficult to localize.

   d. Starts with SI joint or mid-thoracic spine.

   e. Initially also involves asymmetric peripheral joint.

2. Lumbar morning stiffness.

   a. Improves with exercise and stretching and worsens with inactivity.

   b. Patient often needs to take a warm shower, or stretch, to loosen up in the morning.

   c. Low back pain may awaken patient at night. Patient commonly reports awakening several times a night.

   d. Decreased lumbar lordosis – increased thoracic kyphosis.

3. Dactylitis.

   a. Inflammation of the peri-articular ligaments, causing "sausage digits" of the fingers and toes.

   b. Not typically painful.

4. Enthesitis.

   a. Pain and tenderness due to inflammation at the site where tendon or ligament attaches to bone.

5. General.

   a. Fatigue.

   b. Weight loss.

   c. Low-grade fever.

6. Extra-articular involvement.

   a. Acute anterior uveitis is the most common extra-articular manifestation of AS.

      (1) More commonly unilateral but may be bilateral.

      (2) Attacks may last up to 6 weeks.

      (3) Recurrence of attacks is common.

      (4) Associated with HLA B27 (Stolwijk, 2013).

      (5) Painful red eye, photophobia, blurred vision, and increased tearing.

      (6) AS can also be associated with cataracts and glaucoma.

   b. Dermatologic.

      (1) Psoriasis is found in approximately 9.3% of AS patients (Stolwijk, 2015).

      (2) Presence of psoriasis may predict a more severe AS course (Edmunds, 1991).

   c. Gastrointestinal.

      (1) Crohn's disease.

      (2) Ulcerative colitis.

      (3) Both require endoscopic evaluation with biopsies for accurate diagnosis.

      (4) Mild forms may be present on biopsies in asymptomatic patients with spondyloarthritis.

   d. Cardiac.

      (1) AS is associated with an increased incidence of aortic regurgitation and conduction disturbances.

      (2) Increased risk of cardiovascular disease in general, heart failure, and peripheral vascular disease (Han, 2006).

   e. Pulmonary.

      (1) Mechanical restrictive changes may develop related to diminished chest wall mobility.

      (2) Apical pulmonary fibrosis.

         i) Usually asymptomatic.

         ii) Associated with longer duration of the disease.

   f. Amyloidosis.

      (1) Very rarely associated with AS.

      (2) Deposition of inflammatory protein (amyloid) in the heart, kidney or liver.

E. Treatments (Braun, 2011).

1. Treatment measures should include both pharmacologic and non-pharmacologic interventions.

2. Treatment should be individualized based on:

4
4.1
4.2
4.3
4.4
4.5
4.6
4.7
4.8
4.9
4.10

a. The current manifestations of the disease.

b. Severity of symptoms.

c. General clinical status of the patient.

3. Regular exercise is a cornerstone of non-pharmacologic treatment.

a. Structured physical therapy is preferred.

b. Home exercises are also effective.

4. First-line pharmacologic treatment includes NSAIDs (including Cox-2s).

5. Glucocorticoids.

a. Systemic glucocorticoid use for axial disease is not supported by evidence and therefore not recommended.

b. Steroid injections directly into the affected local site of inflammation may be considered.

6. There is no evidence that any DMARD works effectively against axial disease.

a. Sulfasalazine (SSZ) may be effective for the peripheral arthritis sometimes associated with AS.

7. Anti-TNF medications are effective in patients with AS and should be given to patients who fail first-line (*i.e.* NSAID) therapy.

8. Other biologics have been or are currently being investigated for the treatment of AS with varying results (Kiltz, 2012).

F. Nursing Management.

1. As with any chronic disease, patient education is vital to familiarize the patient with the symptoms, course, and treatment of the disease.

2. Patients should be asked about medication adherence and adherence to exercise programs at every visit and barriers to adherence should be addressed.

3. Monitoring for side effects of medication is crucial; patients on chronic NSAIDs are at higher risk for multiple complications and patient on anti-TNFs are at higher risk for infection.

4. Patients on chronic medications (including NSAIDs, DMARDs or biologics) require routine monitoring of labs including CBC, renal function and hepatic function.

5. Encourage patients to receive all recommended vaccinations.

II. Reactive arthritis:

Reactive arthritis (previously called Reiter's Syndrome) is a sterile synovitis which develops after an infection; it is characterized by inflammation of the joints, and in some cases is accompanied by inflammation of the urethra and eyes.

A. Epidemiology.

1. Data on the incidence and prevalence are scarce, partly because of a lack of a disease definition and diagnostic criteria.

a. Estimated about 30-40 cases per 100,000 adults (Hannu, 2011).

b. Race: More common in Caucasians.

c. Gender: Equally common in males and females.

d. Age: 20-40 years more common.

B. Pathophysiology.

1. Reactive arthritis usually develops days to weeks after a genitourinary or gastrointestinal infection.

2. Inflammation of joints, entheses, axial skeleton, skin, mucous membranes, gastrointestinal tract, and eyes may occur.

3. Results for HLA B27 are positive in 30-50% of patients with reactive arthritis (Hannu, 2011).

4. The mechanism of the interaction of the inciting organism with the host leading to the development of reactive arthritis is not known.

5. Synovial fluid cultures are negative for enteric organisms.

6. A systemic and intrasynovial immune response to infectious organisms has been found.

a. Intra-articular antibody and bacterial reactive T cells.

b. Bacterial antigen has been found in the synovial fluid of patients with ReA.

7. Reactive arthritis can occur in patients infected with HIV.

a. Incidence of ReA in this population is anywhere from approximately 1.5-11% (Cuellar, 2000).

4
4.1
4.2
4.3
4.4
4.5
4.6
4.7
4.8
4.9
4.10

b. Presentation is often different from ReA in non-HIV infected individuals.

   (1) Axial involvement and uveitis are uncommon.

   (2) Dermatologic manifestations are seen more frequently.

8. Diagnosis of ReA may include.

   a. Inflammatory changes in synovial fluid (turbid, poor viscosity, WBC 5,000-50,000, increased protein, normal glucose).

   b. Increased ESR.

   c. RF/CCP/ANA negative.

   d. Normochromic/normocytic anemia.

   e. Positive HLA B27.

   f. Radiographic changes may or may not be present.

C. Etiology.

   1. Triggered by infection, such as *Campylobacter, Chlamydia (trachomatis and pneumoniae), C. difficile, Salmonella, Shigella, Yersinia, E. Coli.*

2. Associated with HIV infection.

D. Clinical Manifestations.

   1. Arthritis.

      a. Typically asymmetric.

      b. Oligoarticular.

         (1) Average of four joints.

         (2) Lower extremities more commonly affected than upper extremities.

   2. Dactylitis (see Figure 4).

      a. Sausage digits.

      b. Pain on range of motion.

   3. Dermatologic.

      a. Skin.

         (1) Hypertrophic skin lesions on palms and soles.

      b. Nails.

         (1) Thickened and opacified, crumbling, non-pitting (see Figure 4).

Figure 4: Clinical manifestations of arthritis, dactylitis (sausage digits), and nail changes.

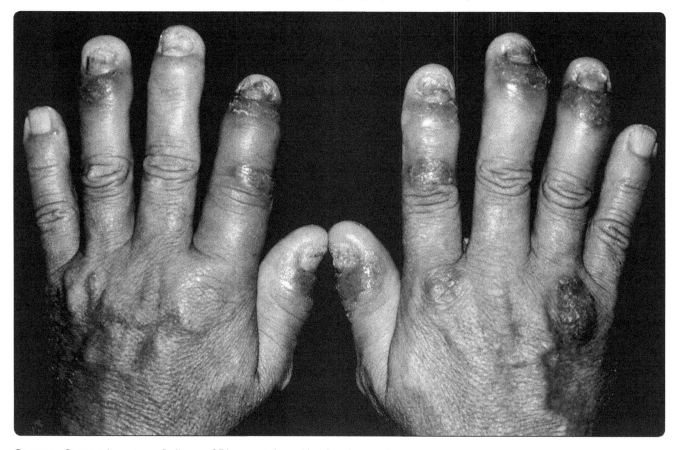

Source: © 2014 American College of Rheumatology. Used with permission.

4
4.1
4.2
4.3
4.4
4.5
4.6
4.7
4.8
4.9
4.10

4. Enthesopathies.

   a. Swelling at the insertion of tendons and ligaments.

   b. Often seen in the Achilles tendon.

5. Sacroiliitis.

   a. Low back pain.

6. Ocular.

   a. Conjunctivitis.

   b. Iritis.

   c. Uveitis.

   d. Episcleritis.

   e. Corneal ulceration.

7. Genitourinary.

   a. Urethritis.

   b. Meatal erythema and edema.

8. Cardiac.

   a. Pericarditis (especially during the acute phase of ReA).

   b. Valve disease.

   c. Conduction defects.

9. General.

   a. Weight loss.

   b. Fever.

E. Treatment.

   1. Acute infection.

      a. Antibiotics are indicated for the treatment of an identifiable underlying infection when there is evidence of ongoing pathogenic replication.

         (1) Enteric infection: Antibiotics rarely used.

         (2) Genitourinary infection: Antibiotics generally indicated.

   2. Acute ReA.

      a. NSAIDs.

         (1) Must give at least two weeks before assessing efficacy.

         (2) May need to try multiple NSAIDs before finding one that is effective.

         (3) No evidence that NSAIDs affect the course of ReA.

      b. Intraarticular glucocorticoids.

         (1) May be used if NSAIDs fail.

      (2) Although ReA is associated with an infectious etiology there are no reports of intra-articular glucocorticoids worsening the disease.

      c. Systemic glucocorticoids.

         (1) May be used when there is an inadequate response (or intolerance) to NSAIDs.

         (2) Generally start at 20 mg per day, then gradually taper.

         (3) There are no randomized trials of the use of systemic glucocorticoids for the treatment of ReA.

      d. DMARDs.

         (1) Only used when above therapies have failed.

         (2) Once the patient achieves remission the DMARD should be continued an additional 3-6 months, then stopped.

         (3) Relapses should be treated with the previously effective therapy.

         (4) Sulfasalazine (SSZ).

            i) Very limited data.

            ii) Recommendations for use are based mainly on meta-analyses of studies in other autoimmune inflammatory diseases.

         (5) Methotrexate (MTX).

            i) No randomized controlled data.

            ii) Recommendations for use are based on expert opinion.

      e. Treatment of extra-articular manifestations of acute ReA.

         (1) Topical steroids may be indicated for dermatologic manifestations of ReA.

         (2) Ophthalmic involvement requires a referral to a specialist.

   3. Chronic ReA.

      a. Patients are considered to have chronic ReA if they are still symptomatic after 6 months of treatment with NSAIDs or systemic glucocorticoids.

      b. If DMARDs have not yet been initiated for acute ReA they may be utilized for treatment of chronic ReA as above.

      c. Anti-TNFs.

4
4.1
4.2
4.3
4.4
4.5
4.6
4.7
4.8
4.9
4.10

(1) Recommendations for the use of anti-TNFs in chronic ReA are based on case reports only.

(2) Once the patient achieves remission the anti-TNF should be continued an additional 3-6 months, then stopped.

(3) Relapses should be retreated with the previously effective therapy.

F. Nursing Management.

1. As with any chronic disease, patient education is vital to familiarize the patient with the symptoms, course, and treatment of the disease.

2. Since ReA is closely associated with an infectious trigger, issues such as infection avoidance and safer sex practices should be addressed.

3. Patients should be asked about medication adherence at every visit and barriers to adherence must be addressed.

4. Monitoring for side effects of medication is crucial; patients on chronic NSAIDs are at higher risk for multiple complications and patients on anti-TNFs are at higher risk for infection.

5. Patients on chronic NSAIDs or systemic glucocorticoids require routine monitoring of labs including CBC, renal function and hepatic function.

6. Unless there is an urgent need, vaccinations should be held until after the initial infection has cleared and the acute phase of ReA has passed.

III. Psoriatic arthritis (PsA):

Psoriatic Arthritis is a chronic, systemic inflammatory arthritis associated with psoriasis. In most cases, but not all, skin manifestations are present before the arthritis.

A. Epidemiology.

1. Incidence 6 per 100,000 per year.

2. Prevalence 1-2 per 1,000.

3. Race.

a. Prevalence rates vary widely between studies.

b. More common in Caucasians than African American and Native American populations.

4. Gender.

a. Male-to-female ratio is 1:1.

5. Age.

a. Most often develops in persons aged 35-55 years.

b. The most typical age of onset for the juvenile form is 9-11 years.

c. Can occur in persons of almost any age.

B. Pathophysiology.

1. Inflammation.

a. Leads to joint erosion and resorption of cortical bone.

b. Formation of enthesiophytes: Bony spurs at the insertion sites of entheses (Schett, 2011).

2. Predictors of severity of destruction.

a. High erythrocyte sedimentation rate at diagnosis.

b. Synovitis at diagnosis.

c. Presence of axial disease correlates with more severe peripheral disease (Schett, 2011).

C. Etiology.

1. The precise cause of PsA has not been identified, but is likely a combination of genetic, environmental and immunologic factors.

a. Genetic.

(1) ~40% of patients have a 1st degree relative with PsA.

(2) Identical twins are more likely to both have PsA than fraternal twins.

(3) Several HLA antigens are found more frequently in PsA patients than in the general population (HLA B13, HLA B17, HLA B57, and HLA-Cw*0602) (Ritchlin, 2005).

b. Environmental.

(1) Infection – possible link.

(2) Trauma – possible link.

(3) Obesity – known increase in incidence.

c. Immunologic.

(1) In the early phase there is evidence of activity of tissue-specific and innate immune activation.

(2) In the established phase of PsA there is evidence for a widespread immunologic response.

   i) Elevated levels of immunoglobulins.

   ii) Increased levels of TNF-α, Il-1, Il-2, Il-6, and others (van Kuijk, 2006).

D. Clinical features.

1. General clinical features.

  a. Pain and stiffness in affected joints.

  b. Morning stiffness > 30 minutes in ~50% of patients.

  c. Stiffness associated with prolonged immobility.

  d. Pain and stiffness improve with physical activity.

2. Five clinical phenotypes of PsA (Wright, 1971). May occur individually or in combination; one subtype may evolve over time into a different type.

  a. Asymmetrical oligoarthritis.

    (1) PsA typically starts off with this presentation.

    (2) A few (<4 joints) asymmetric joints.

    (3) Can later progress to a "rheumatoid arthritis-like" symmetric presentation.

  b. Symmetrical polyarthritis.

    (1) 30-50% of cases.

    (2) The most common phenotype of PsA.

    (3) May be confused with rheumatoid arthritis, especially if patient has low titer positive RF.

    (4) Key differentiating feature is found on joint X-rays.

      i) RA = periarticular osteopenia with or without erosions.

      ii) PsA = new bone formation with or without erosions.

  c. Distal interphalangeal (DIP) joint involvement.

    (1) Associated with nail psoriasis.

      i) Onychodystrophic changes.

      ii) Not onychomycosis; no nail fungus.

  d. Arthritis mutilans.

(1) Characterized by resorption of the phalanges.

  e. Axial arthritis.

    (1) Prototypical HLA B27-associated spondyloarthritis.

3. Skin and nails.

  a. Psoriatic skin lesions.

    (1) Erythematous based rash with silvery scales.

    (2) Auspitz sign (gentle scraping of the lesions results in pinpoint bleeding).

    (3) Located over the extensor surfaces.

  b. Nail pitting.

4. Arthritis.

  a. Stiffness of the spine lasting 30 minutes or longer.

  b. Asymmetric.

  c. Enthesitis (oligoarticular and monoarticular).

  d. Large joints (esp knee).

  e. DIP joint involvement.

  f. Dactylitis.

    (1) Swelling of an entire finger or toe.

    (2) "Sausage digit"

    (3) Occurs in about 50% of patients with PsA.

    (4) Associated with more destructive course.

  g. Arthritis mutilans.

    (1) "Telescoping of the finger"

  h. Enthesopathy.

    (1) Inflammation of the enthesis (insertion of ligament, tendon, joint capsule, and bone).

  i. Spondylitis, sacroiliitis.

  j. Tenosynovitis.

    (1) Flexor tendons of hands.

    (2) Extensor carpi ulnaris.

    (3) Other sites.

5. Others.

  a. Conjunctivitis.

  b. Iritis.

  c. Aortic insufficiency.

4
4.1
4.2
4.3
4.4
4.5
4.6
4.7
4.8
4.9
4.10

E. Treatment.

1. Treatment measures should include both pharmacologic and non-pharmacologic interventions.

2. Non-pharmacologic.

   a. Exercise.

   b. Physical therapy.

   c. Heat for stiffness.

   d. Ice for swelling.

   e. Surgery may be necessary for those with severe joint damage.

3. Oral corticosteroids.

   a. Have not been proven to be effective.

   b. May cause a flare of psoriasis when tapered.

4. NSAIDs.

   a. Non-selective and selective (COX-2).

   b. First-line therapy.

   c. For mild PsA symptom management.

   d. NSAIDs do not affect disease progression.

5. DMARDs.

   a. DMARDs have not been proven to affect disease progression but may alleviate symptoms.

   b. Reasonable choice for patients who do not have access or are intolerant to anti-TNFs.

   c. Choice of DMARDs depends on severity of skin involvement.

   d. Some DMARDs have been shown to improve both joint and skin manifestations (but not slow progression of disease).

      (1) Methotrexate (MTX).

         i) Most commonly prescribed DMARD for PsA.

         ii) Few randomized trials show efficacy.

         iii) 7.5 – 25 mg per week.

         iv) Oral or parenteral.

         v) Patients who do not respond to MTX after 6-8 weeks of maximum dose are unlikely to see any benefit.

         vi) MTX should be tapered rather than stopped suddenly to prevent rebound flare.

      (2) Psoralen and ultraviolet light (PUVA).

         i) Used mainly in patients with severe skin disease.

         ii) Often combined with an oral DMARD.

      (3) Retinoic acid derivatives.

         i) Value of use in PsA is uncertain.

         ii) Takes 4 months to produce a response.

         iii) Can produce extraskeletal bone deposition leading to worsening of joint pain.

      (4) Cyclosporine A.

         i) 2.5 – 5 mg/kg/day (divided doses).

         ii) Time to response is usually 3-4 months.

         iii) May be added to MTX (dual-DMARD therapy).

   e. Some DMARDs are appropriate for patients in whom skin manifestations are minimal.

      (1) Sulfasalazine (SSZ).

         i) "Niche" role in the treatment of extra-axial arthritis.

         ii) Level of benefit is modest.

         iii) Requires higher dosing than in RA; therefore GI side effects are more common.

      (2) Antimalarials.

         i) Used in the past, but no longer recommended for treatment of PsA.

      (3) Gold.

         i) Used in the past, but no longer recommended for treatment of PsA.

         ii) IM more effective than oral.

      (4) Penicillamine.

         i) Used in the past.

         ii) Multiple GI side effects.

      (5) Azathioprine.

         i) Very limited data but anecdotally effective.

         ii) Generally well-tolerated.

      (6) Leflunomide.

         i) Appropriate for use in MTX non-responders.

         ii) Unknown whether leflunomide prevents progression of joint damage.

4
4.1
4.2
4.3
4.4
4.5
4.6
4.7
4.8
4.9
4.10

6. Biologics.

    a. Anti-TNFs.

        (1) All five are FDA approved for the treatment of PsA.

            i) Etanercept (subcutaneous).

            ii) Infliximab (intravenous).

            iii) Adalimumab (subcutaneous).

            iv) Golimumab (subcutaneous).

            v) Certolizumab pegol (subcutaneous).

        (2) Improve clinical signs and symptoms.

        (3) Slow radiographic progression.

    b. PDE4 Inhibitor.

        (1) Apremilast.

            i) Improves clinical signs and symptoms.

            ii) Ability to slow radiographic progression is unknown.

            iii) Oral.

            iv) Dose titration recommended to minimize GI side effects.

    c. Anti-IL12/Anti-IL23.

        (1) Ustekinumab.

            i) Improves clinical signs and symptoms.

            ii) Slows radiographic progression.

            iii) Subcutaneous injection.

F. Nursing Management.

    1. As with any chronic disease, patient education is vital to familiarize the patient with the symptoms, course, and treatment of the disease.

    2. Patients should be asked about medication adherence at every visit and barriers to adherence must be addressed.

    3. Monitoring for side effects of medication is crucial.

    4. Patients on many of the medications used to treat PsA require routine monitoring of labs including CBC, renal function and hepatic function. Patients on antimalarials need annual eye exams.

    5. Vaccinations should be up to date as per ACR and/or EULAR guidelines.

IV. Enteropathic (IBD) associated arthritis:

(aka: SpA associated with inflammatory bowel disease [IBD] Crohn's Disease Associated Arthritis, Ulcerative Colitis Associated Arthritis, Colitic Arthritis, Arthritis associated with Ulcerative Colitis, Inflammatory Bowel Disease with Spondyloarthropathy, Arthropathy of Inflammatory Bowel Disease, and Enteropathic arthropathy [EA]).

The relationship between SpA and gut inflammation has been substantiated in several studies (Mielants et al., 1991; and Schatteman, et al., 1995). Bacterial gut infections such as *Salmonella typhimurium, Yersinia enterocolitica, Shigella, Klebsiella,*and *Campylobacter jejuni* may induce reactive peripheral arthritis and 20% of these patients could develop chronic spondyloarthropathy. Clinical articular manifestations compatible with spondyloarthropathy are present in 10% to 40% of patients with inflammatory bowel diseases (Karimi and Peña, 2008). In the past decade, attention to this set of diseases, research, diagnostic options and treatment options have expanded significantly. However, there is much more to uncover with the assistance of genetic research.

4
4.1
4.2
4.3
4.4
4.5
4.6
4.7
4.8
4.9
4.10

A. Epidemiology.

    1. De Vos, et al. (1996) reported intestinal tract involvement as a feature of SpA in 25%-75% of patients studied with ulcerative colitis (UC and Crohn's disease (CD) as the most frequent types of IBD associated with SpA.

    2. Rheumatic manifestation such as arthralgias, and enthesitis, are the most frequent extraintestinal findings of IBD with a prevalence between 17% and 39% (Peluso, et al., 2013).

B. Pathophysiology.

    1. The precise cause of EA is unknown.

    2. Genetic factors such as a positive HLA-B27 gene expression have been observed in a predisposing role as well as environmental

factors such as infectious organisms observed in a causative role in this complex pathology (Peluso, et al., 2013; and van Tubergen, 2014).

3. Other HLA genes associated have been: HLA-B24, HLA-B35, HLA-B44, and HLA-DrB10103 along with associations with IL-23R signaling Th17-mediated inflammation (Peluso, et al., 2013).

C. Clinical Features.

1. Arthritic manifestations in EA are divided into axial or peripheral joint involvements including sacroiliitis with or without spondylitis (Jadon & McHugh, 2014; and Peluso et al., 2013).

2. Peripheral arthritis is 17%-20% more common in both CD and UC, with the frequency higher in CD, equally effects both sexes, has an onset age between 25 and 45 years of age and can be diagnosed before, simultaneously, or after a diagnosis of IBD (Peluso, et al., 2013).

3. Features of the three types of classification in EA are noted in Table 2.

4. Extra-articular manifestations and Extra-intestinal manifestations (EIMs).

   a. About 25%-35% of patients with EA have extra-intestinal EIMs. The most common ones are ophthalmologic (iritis/uveitis), mucocutaneous manifestations, and hepatobiliary disease (Wilson & Folzenlogen, 2012).

   b. Erythema nodosa, uveitis, and pyoderma gangrenosum occur more often in patients with spondyloarthritis with Crohn's disease (Jadon & McHugh, 2014).

D. Treatments.

1. The treatment approach is based on the severity of the disease, symptoms, clinical findings, associated extra-articular findings, and specific patient wishes and

Table 2: Classification and features of articular involvement subsets in inflammatory bowel disease (IBD).

Peripheral			Axial	
Type 1	Type 2	Type 3	Isolated sacroiliitis	Spondylitis
i. Pauciarticular (less than 5 joints). ii. Asymmetric involvement. iii. Acute, self-limiting attack (<10 weeks). iv. Usually coincides with relapse of IBD. v. Strongly associated with other extra-intestinal manifestations. vi. Lower limbs more affected. vii. Associated with HLA DRB1, B35, B27.	i. Polyarticular (5 or more joints). ii. Symptoms persist for months or even years. iii. May be erosive. iv. Runs a course independent of IBD. v. Affects both large and small joints. vi. Strongly associated with uveitis. vii. Associated with HLA B44.	i. Both axial and peripheral involvement.	i. Asymptomatic. ii. Usually non progressive disease.	i. Usually precedes the onset of IBD. ii. Runs a course independent of IBD. iii. Clinical course is similar to idiopathic ankylosing spondylitis. iv. Disease progression leads to increasing immobility and ankylosis. v. Associated with uveitis. vi. Strongly associated with HLA B27.

Source: Rosario Peluso, Matteo Nicola Dario Di Minno, Salvatore Iervolino, et al., "Enteropathic Spondyloarthritis: From Diagnosis to Treatment," Clinical and Developmental Immunology, vol. 2013, Article ID 631408, 12 pages, 2013. doi:10.1155/2013/631408

4
4.1
4.2
4.3
4.4
4.5
4.6
4.7
4.8
4.9
4.10

expectations. Although, there is no known cure, medications and various treatments can be used to reduce symptoms, pain, and stiffness, improve physical function, and prevent disability. In general, both non-pharmacologic and pharmacologic treatments are used simultaneously.

2. Nonsteroidal anti-inflammatory drugs (NSAIDS) can increase gut permeability and flare colitis (Jadon & McHugh, 2014; Wilson & Folzenlogen, 2012).

3. Corticosteroid injection of affected joints used in combination with SSZ has been useful in persistent synovitis (Jadon & McHugh, 2014).

4. Methotrexate (MTX), azathioprine, and 6-mercaptopurine are used for patients unable to take SSZ (Jadon & McHugh, 2014).

5. For patients with associated Crohn's disease, appropriate TNF-alpha inhibitors are effective to treat the disease as well as the joint involvement (Jadon and McHugh, 2014).

6. Therapeutic ultrasound and physical therapy can ameliorate peripheral arthritis in some cases (Wilson & Folzenlogen, 2012).

7. Voulgari (2011) reported mesalamine used for IBD may decrease peripheral arthritis symptoms.

8. In severe UC cases, surgical removal of the diseased colon has been known to have the added benefit to improve peripheral but not axial arthritis. By contrast, removal of diseased colon in CD does not affect peripheral arthritis (Ehrenfeld, 2012; Podswiadek, D'Incà, Sturniolo, Oliviero, & Punzi, 2007; and Wilson & Folzenlogen, 2012).

E. Nursing Management.

1. Education.

   a. Patient education is very important to increase active participation in a therapeutic program.

   b. Encourage self-help education programs – Generally well accepted by patients to improve behavioral and health status outcomes.

   c. Early diagnosis and treatment is very important because failure to control initially can result in more persistent or chronic disease.

   d. Initiate or collaborate in a multidisciplinary approach for the well-being of the patient.

   e. Maintain good posture. Maintaining skeletal mobility and preventing natural contractures that lead to deformity.

   f. Firm mattress, sleep in supine or prone position. Prevent flexion contractures especially of shoulders and knees. Do not sleep or rest with pillows under knees.

   g. Driving safety. Get long rear view mirror to see blind spots easier, especially with limited cervical range of motion.

   h. Spine mobility. Perform extension exercises, preventing natural contractures that lead to deformity. Swimming is ideal as it involves all joints and muscles in a low gravity environment. Weight bearing exercises to prevent spinal osteoporosis. Slow movement exercises like tai chi, Pilates, yoga, and stretching have been shown to increase range of motion and improve posture while minimizing deformities.

   i. Splints, braces, and corsets are not helpful and should be avoided as these devices restrict motion and contribute to contracture formation.

   j. Massages and other physical manipulations of the joints should only be done by therapists familiar with SpA.

   k. Pulmonary. Maintain chest expansion with deep breathing exercises. Encourage cessation of smoking.

2. Psychosocial.

   a. Genetic counseling is useful in assisting patients with questions regarding the risks (to them and their family members) of developing other spondyloarthropathies. (Boonen, 2002).

   b. Vocational counseling may help to decrease the risk of employment disability.

   c. Depression screening is useful due to the high potential negative effect on patient's personal and professional life.

   d. Emotional stress. Be alert for signs for potential withdrawal from the workforce.

   e. Financial stress. The high costs associated with diagnosis and treatment adds to patient's socioeconomic burden.

4
4.1
4.2
4.3
4.4
4.5
4.6
4.7
4.8
4.9
4.10

3. Alternative therapies.

   a. Some patients find relief with acupuncture treatments and herbal medicines.

   b. Acupuncture treatment applied on various points of the body, especially where the pain is located.

   c. Herbal medicine may also help relieve pain, reduce inflammation, or provide natural supplements to strengthen muscles, tendons, or even bones. The most important aspect of the use of alternative therapies is an open discussion between the healthcare provider and patient to ensure that the treatment is safe and side effects are minimized and caught early.

F. Recent issues.

1. Due to a significant lack of studies on EA related SpA, most of what we know are derived from studies on IBD or other types of spondyloarthritis studies. More research is needed in this area.

V. Undifferentiated (aka Unclassified) Spondyloarthropathy (uSpA):

uSpA is a subtype of SpA. It is very difficult to diagnose and consequently may be underdiagnosed because it does not fulfill the criteria of some of the other specific forms of SpA like AS, PsA, or SpA with IBD (Burgeos-Vargus, 2013). Contributing to the difficulty of a definitive diagnosis is that some patients become depressed and anxious and have time and money invested in the healthcare system only to be assigned an incorrect diagnosis of fibromyalgia. Additionally, some patients may not experience spinal involvement, yet report a seemingly disparate mix of symptoms such as heel pain, edematous fingers and/or toes or, on occasion, iritis. More evidence is needed to further define uSpA from an early manifestation of AS or PsA versus classification as a separate and distinct clinical condition (Baeten, Breban, Lories, Schett, & Sieper, 2013; Burgeos-Vargus, 2013; and Paramarta, De Rycke, Ambarus, Tak & Baeten, 2013).

A. Epidemiology.

1. There is a female predominance of 1:3 (Ehrenfeld, 2012).

B. Pathophysiology.

1. There is a genetic link to HLA-B27 and other HLA alleles (Ehrenfeld, 2012). However, HLA B-27 positivity may be lower (20-25% positivity in uSpA) as compared to other Spa's such as AS (Burgeos-Vargus, 2013).

C. Clinical features.

1. Clinical manifestations are similar to other SpA features but with fewer extra-articular manifestations (Ehrenfeld, 2012).

2. Patients tend to have peripheral rather than axial involvement at onset with progression to a combination of axial and peripheral involvement throughout the course of the disease (Burgeos-Vargus, 2013).

3. The disease is insidious, can remain chronic yet undifferentiated (absent or mild) on routine radiographs (Ehrenfeld, 2012; Burgeos-Vargus, 2013; and Paparo, et al., 2014).

4. The Spondylitis Association of America (SSA, n.d.) lists symptoms of uSpA as having one or more the following:

   a. Inflammatory back pain.

   b. Unilateral or alternating buttock pain.

   c. Enethesitis.

   d. Peripheral arthritis.

   e. Arthritis in the small joints.

   f. Edematous fingers or toes.

   g. Heel pain.

   h. Iritis.

   i. Fatigue.

D. Treatments.

1. Medical treatment is generally a combination of NSAIDS or DMARDS.

2. Physical therapy and regular exercise.

3. Application of heat and/or cold packs to affected joints.

4. Use of a transcutaneous electrical nerve stimulator (TENS).

5. Practicing good posture.

4
4.1
4.2
4.3
4.4
4.5
4.6
4.7
4.8
4.9
4.10

E. Nursing Management.

1. Difficulty in diagnosis highlights issues with suboptimal treatment as well as financial burden on the individual in lost wages and healthcare costs.

2. Being alert for depression and anxiety and obtaining proper referrals.

3. Educating use of proper body mechanics and other forms of supportive exercise.

F. Recent Issues.

1. Utilization of the Assessment of SpondyloArthritis International Society (ASAS) spectrum of axial and peripheral SpA could result in a more timely identification of SpA which leads to a positive impact on the healthcare budget, but more importantly, to the new treatment options and quality of life for patients suffering with some form of SpA (van Tubergan, 2014).

2. Burgos-Vargus (2013) postulates uSpA can represent the early stages of AS before meeting definitive criteria for classification. Information on remission rates or transition to other SpA's is needed.

3. Conventional radiography, which is often the first-step imaging modality in SpA, does not allow an early diagnosis. Computed tomography (CT) demonstrates with a very high spatial resolution the tiny structural alterations of cortical and spongy bone before they become evident on plain film radiographs. Magnetic resonance imaging (MRI) is the only modality that provides demonstration of bone marrow edema, which reflects vasodilatation and inflammatory hyperemia (Paparo, et al., 2014). There are restrictive issues with MRI due to cost.

VI. Juvenile-onset Spondyloarthropathy (JoSpA or JSpA).

A. JSpA is characterized by arthritis in the lower limbs, enthesitis, and in some cases, inflammatory back pain (Jadon, Sengupta, & Ramanan, 2013). Patients experiencing symptoms of spondyloarthropathy before the age of 16 years of age may be diagnosed with some form of the juvenile idiopathic arthropathies (JIA) like enthesitis-related arthritis, psoriatic arthritis, and

undifferentiated arthritis (Colbert, 2010; and Scofield & Sestak, 2012).

A couple of major challenges to detecting, diagnosing, and successful early treatment of JSpA have to do with overlapping features of the disease but more importantly is which set of classification and diagnostic criteria is used. For example, the Assessment SpondyloArthritis International Society (ASAS) criteria classifies JSpA as a single classification with HLA-B27 associated pediatric rheumatic disease, enthesitis, lower extremity arthritis with eventual involvement [in many cases] of the spine and sacroiliac (Scofield & Sestak, 2012). While the International League of Associations for Rheumatology (ILAR) classification proposes the term enthesitis-related arthritis (ERA) for children with arthritis and enthesitis, or arthritis plus several of the features noted as characteristic of SpA (Scofield & Sestak, 2012; and Jadon, Sengupta, & Ramanan, 2013).

1. Pagini, et al., (2010) report 30% of children with ERA/JIA develop clinical and dynamic MRI evidence of sacroiliitis within one year of disease onset.

2. Stoll, Bhore, Dempsey-Robertson, and Punaro, (2010) found JSpA patients are at risk for silent (undiagnosed) sacroiliitis without clinical signs or symptoms as early childhood SpA may take 5-10 years to develop axial manifestations.

3. Left unchecked, underdiagnosed, and improperly treated children with JSpA could experience serious impacts with school performance, social, as well as psychological development. Likewise, impairment of function could have serious economic consequences.

4. JSpA subsets can easily overlap with several categories of JIA. Difficulty identifying JSpA with certainty created difficulty in establishing prevalence.

5. Inflammatory back pain is less common in children with JSpA, instead hip arthritis is the predominant feature and the disease presents as more severe affecting functional status worse in children than adults (Scofield & Sestak, 2012).

6. Treatment of JSpA involves a team approach with the patient, parents, rheumatology nurse, doctor, physical and occupational therapists.

4
4.1
4.2
4.3
4.4
4.5
4.6
4.7
4.8
4.9
4.10

7. Exercises to maintain range of motion are a critical aspect of care and treatment (Scofield & Sestak, 2012).

B. The subset of JSpA in JIA can further be differentiated to juvenile-onset ankylosing spondylitis (JoAS).

1. Males more likely than females but there is little data on prevalence and incidence (Ehrenfeld, 2012; and Jadon, Sengupta, & Ramanan, 2013).

2. May account for approximately 1/5th of JSpA cases (Jadon, Sengupta, & Ramanan, 2013).

3. Arthritis mainly in the lower limbs, an association with HLA-B27, and extra-articular manifestations such as uveitis, enthesitis, and cutaneous psoriasis (Jadon, Sengupta, & Ramanan, 2013).

4. In some countries, such as those with a national prescribing healthcare framework, JoAS patients with predominately peripheral disease may not qualify for biologic therapy which in the long term contributes to poor clinical outcome (Jadon, Sengupta, & Ramanan, 2013).

5. JoAS patients are more likely to require hip arthroplasty than adults with AS. Standardized classification criteria, earlier diagnosis, management and treatment of JoAS could prevent surgeries, reduce the social and economic impact, as well as result in less absence from school or work productivity. (Gensler, et al., 2008; Jadon, Hunt, Arumugam, Ramanan, & Sengupta, 2013; and Jadon, et al., 2013).

VII. Other Syndromes associated with Spondyloarthrotides.

A. Synovitis, acne, pustulosis, hyperostosis, and osteitis (SAPHO) syndrome.

1. SAPHO syndrome affects both children and adults but rarely adults over 60 years of age. It shares many clinical and radiographic features with SpA such enthesitis, sacroiliitis, paraevertebral ossifications, and ankyloses. SAPHO is also associated with psoriasis, PsA, IBD, and EA with IBD (Carneiro & Sampaio-Barros, 2013). SAPHO is a condition primarily seen in Europe with an estimated prevalence of 1 in 10,000 (Carneiro & Sampaio-Barros, 2013). The diagnosis of SAPHO is difficult in the absence of skin disease and the overlap of SpA features. Radiographic and MRI findings are critical to proper diagnosis.

B. Behçet's disease.

1. Sacroiliitis and/ or inflammatory lumbosacral pain, an association with the HLA-B27 allele, or anterior uveitis could be diagnosed as Behçet's disease or JSpA as enthesitis-related arthritis (ERA) under ILAR criteria (Scofield & Sestak, 2012).

C. Whipple's disease.

1. The hallmark long-term, unexplained, sero-negative oligo or polyarthritis with spondyloarthropathic features as a precursor to the identification of the Whipple bacterium in the gut can create an incorrect initial diagnosis in adult SpA (Puéchal, 2001).

Summary

Ankylosing spondylitis, psoriatic arthritis, reactive arthritis, and enteropathic arthropathy fall under the heading of spondyloarthropathies. Spondyloarthropathies are divided into axial and peripheral. All of these conditions may mimic each other as well as multiple other arthritides. Treatment options are complex. Nursing interventions are imperative for positive patient outcomes.

References

Baeten, D., Breban, M., Lones, R., Schett, G. & Sieper, J. (2013). *Are spondylarthritides related but distinct conditions or a single disease with a heterogeneous phenotype?* Arthritis & Rheumatism. 65, 12-20.

Boonen, A. (2002). Socioeconomic consequences of ankylosing sppondylitis. *Clinical and Experimental Rheumatology, 20*(6), 23-26.

Braun J. et al. (2010). Update of the ASAS/EULAR recommendations for the management of ankylosing spondylitis. *Ann Rheum Dis* 2011;70:896-904.

Burgeos-Vargas, R. (2013). From undifferentiated SpA to ankylosing spondylitis. *Nature Reviews Rheumatology, 9, 639+*

Carneiro, S., & Sampaio-Barros, P. D. (2013). SAPHO Syndrome. *Rheumatic Disease Clinics of North America*, 39(2), 401-418. doi:10.1016/j.rdc.2013.02.2009.

Colbert, R.A., (2010). Classification of juvenile spondyloarthritis: Enthesitis related arthritis and beyond. *Nature Reviews Rheumatology.* 6:477–85. doi: 10.1038/nrrheum.2010.103.

Cuellar ML, Espinoza LR. (2000) Rheumatic manifestations of HIV-AIDS. Baillieres Best Pract Res Clin Rheumatol. 14(3):579–593.

De Vos M, Mielants H, Cuvelier C, et al., (1996). Long-term evolution of gut inflammation in patients with spondyloarthropathy. *Gastroenterology.* 110, 1696–1703.

Edmunds L. et al. (1991). Primary ankylosing spondylitis, psoriatic and eteropathic spondyloarthropathy: a controlled analysis. *J Rheumatol.* May;18(5):696-8.

Ehrenfeld, M. (2012). Spondyloarthropathies, *Best Practice & Research Clinical Rheumatology,* 26, (1). February 2012,135-145.

Gensler LS, Ward MM, Reveille JD, Learch TJ, Weisman MH, Davis JC Jr., (2008). Clinical, radiographic and functional differences between juvenile-onset and adult-onset ankylosing spondylitis: Results from the PSOAS cohort. *Annals of the Rheumatic Diseases.* 67(2), 233-237.

Gorman, J. D., Sack, K., & Davis, J. C. (2002). Treatment of ankylosing spondylitis by inhibition of tumor necrosis factor alpha. *The New England Journal of Medicine, 346*(18), 1349-1400.

Han C. et al. (2006) Cardiovascular disease and risk factors in patients with rheumatoid arthritis, psoriatic arthritis and Ankylosing spondylitis. *J Rheumatol.* ;33(11);2167.

Hannu T. (2011). Reactive Arthritis. *Best Pract Res Clin Rheumatol.* 25(3):347.

Jadon DR, Hunt LP, Arumugam R, Ramanan AV, Sengupta R., (2013) Prognostic markers in juvenile vs. adult onset ankylosing spondylitis. Presented at: Programs and Abstracts of the European League Against Rheumatism Congress 2013 . Madrid, Spain, 12-15 June 2013 (Abstract FRI0435).

Jadon DR, Shaddick G, Arumugam R, Nightingale A, Ramanan V, Sengupta R. (2013) Primary and subsequent orthopedic surgeries more common in juvenile vs. adult-onset ankylosing spondylitis. Presented at: Programs and Absracts of the ACR Congress Annual Meeting 2013 . San Diego, CA, USA, 25-30 October 2013 (Abstract 1537).

Jadon, D. R., & McHugh, N. J. (2014). Other seronegative spondyloarthropathies. *Medicine* (United Kingdom), 42(5), 257-261.

Jadon, D. R., Sengupta, R., & Ramanan, A. V. (2013). Challenges in the management and research of juvenile-onset ankylosing spondylitis. *International Journal of Clinical Rheumatology, 8,* 615+. doi: 10.2217/ijr.13.60.

Karimi, O., & Peña, A. S. (2008). Indications and challenges of probiotics, prebiotics, and synbiotics in the management of arthralgias and spondyloarthropathies in inflammatory bowel disease. *Journal of clinical gastroenterology,* 42 Suppl 3 Pt 1, S136-141.

Khan, M. A. (2002). Update on spondyloarthropathies. *Annals of Internal Medicine, 136*(12), 896-907.

Kiltz U et al. Treatment of Ankylosing Spondylitis in Patients Refractory to TNF-Inhibition. *Curr Opin Rheumatol.* 2012;24(3),252-260.

Linden, S. V., & Heijde, D. V. (1998). Ankylosing spondylitis clinical features. *Rheumatic Disease Clinics of North America, 24*(4), 663-676.

McCance, K. L., & Huether, S. E. (2006). Alterations of musculoskeletal function. In Crowthier, L., & McCance, K. L. (Eds.), *Pathophysiology: The biologic basis of disease in adults and children* (pp. 1529-1531). St. Louis, MO: Elsevier Mosby.

Mielants H, Veys EM, Goemaere S, et al., (1991). Gut inflammation in the spondyloarthropathies: Clinical, radiologic, biologic and genetic features in relation to the type of histology. A prospective study. *Journal of Rheumatology,18,* 1542–1551.

Pagnini I, Savelli S, Matucci-Cerinic M, Fonda C, Cimaz R, Simonini G., (2010). Early predictors of juvenile sacroiliitis in enthesitis-related arthritis. *Journal of Rheumatology.* 37(11), 2395-2401.

Paparo, F., Revelli, M., Semprini, A., Camellino, D., Garlaschi, A., Cimmino, M. A., . . . Leone, A. (2014). Seronegative spondyloarthropathies: What radiologists should know. *Radiologia Medica, 119(3)*, 156-163.

Paramarta, J. E., De Rycke, L., Ambarus, C. A., Tak, P. P., & Baeten, D. (2013). Undifferentiated spondyloarthritis vs ankylosing spondylitis and psoriatic arthritis: A real-life prospective cohort study of clinical presentation and response to treatment. *Rheumatology* (Oxford), *52(10)*, 1873-1878. doi: 10.1093/rheumatology/ket239.

Peluso, D. M., Iervolino, Manguso, Tramontano, Ambrosino, Esposito, Scalera, Castiglione, and Scarpa. (2013). Enteropathic spondyloarthritis: From diagnosis to treatment. *Clinical and Developmental Immunology, March 2013.* doi: 10.1155/2013/631408.

Podswiadek, M., D'Incà, R., Sturniolo, G. C., Oliviero, F., & Punzi, L. (2007). Rheumatic manifestations associated with inflammatory bowel diseases. *Current Rheumatology Reviews, 3(1)*, 47-56.

Puéchal, X. (2010). Whipple's disease and arthritis. *Current Opinions in Rheumatology, 13* (1) 74-79. doi:11148719/2010/cor719.

Reveille JD. (2012) Genetics of spondyloarthritis – beyond the MHC. *Nat Rev Rheumatol* 8(5):296-304.

Ritchlin CT. (2005) Pathogenesis of psoriatic arthritis. *Curr Opin Rheumatol* 17:406-412.

Rudwaleit M et al. (2009) The development of assessment of spondyloarthritis international society classification criteria for axial spondyloarthritis (part II): validation and final selection. *Ann Rheum Dis*; 68,777-783.

Rudwaleit, M. & Sieper, J. (2012) Referral strategies for early diagnosis of axial spondyloarthritis. *Nat. Rev. Rheumatol.* 8, 262–268.

Schatteman L, Mielants H, Veys EM, et al., (1995). Gut inflammation in psoriatic arthritis: A prospective ileocolonoscopic study. *Journal of Rheumatology. 22*, 680–683.

Schett G et al. (2011). Structural damage in rheumatoid arthritis, psoriatic arthritis, and ankylosing spondylitis: traditional views, novel insights gained from TNF blockade, and concepts for the future. *Arthritis Res Ther.*; 13(Suppl 1): S4.

Scofield, R. H., & Sestak, A. L. (2012). Juvenile spondyloarthropathies. *Current Rheumatology Reports, 14(5)*, 395-401. doi: 10.1007/s11926-012-0273-3.

SSA. Spondylitis Association of America (n.d.). Undifferentiated spondyloarthropathy. Spondylitis. org/about/undif.aspx.

Stoll ML, Bhore R, Dempsey-Robertson M, Punaro M., (2010). Spondyloarthritis in a pediatric population: Risk factors for sacroiliitis. *Journal of Rheumatology. 37*(11), 2402-2408.

Stolwijk C et al. (2015). Prevalence of extra-articular manifestations in patients with Ankylosing spondylitis: a systematic review and meta-analysis. Ann Rheum Dis.; 74:65-73.

van Kuijk AW, et al. (2006). Detailed analysis of the cell infiltrate and the expression of mediators of synovial inflammation and joint destruction in the synovium of patients with psoriatic arthritis: implications for treatment. Ann Rheum Dis.; 65(12):1551.

van Tubergen A. (2014). The changing clinical picture and epidemiology of spondyloarthritis. *Nat Rev Rheumatol advance online publication.*

Voulgari, P., (2011). Rheumatological manifestations in inflammatory bowel disease. *Annals of Gastroenterology*, 24(3): 173-180.

Wilson, G., & Folzenlogen, D. D. (2012). Spondyloarthropathies: New directions in etiopathogenesis, diagnosis and treatment. *Missouri medicine, 109(1)*, 69-74.

Wright V, Moll JM. (1971). Psoriatic Arthritis. *Bull Rheum Dis.* 21(5):627.

Yu, D et al. (2014). Clinical Manifestations of Ankylosing Spondylitis in Adults. In: UpToDate, Schur P (Ed), UpToDate, Waltham, MA.

4

4.1
4.2
4.3
4.4
4.5
4.6
4.7
4.8
4.9
4.10

Section 4.5
Nursing Management of Systemic Lupus Erythematosus

Dawn E. Isherwood, MSIR, BSN, RN

Introduction

Because of the heterogeneity of lupus, as well as its ability to mimic other autoimmune diseases in physical presentation and laboratory findings, the diagnosis of lupus can be a prolonged and frustrating experience for both the patient and healthcare provider. To care effectively for a patient with lupus, the healthcare provider needs an up-to-date understanding of the disease, its many manifestations, and its changing and often unpredictable course (Lupus Foundation of America [LFA], 2011).

Our understanding of the pathogenesis and treatment of lupus has grown considerably in this century, especially over the past fifty years (Helmick et al., 1998). And while the healthcare professional's knowledge about lupus has increased dramatically, there is still much to be learned. Research to better diagnose and treat this disease process continues.

The purpose of this chapter is to review the pathophysiology, diagnostic criteria, physical socioeconomic impact, and standards of care in patients with systemic lupus erythematosus (SLE).

Learning Objectives

Upon completion of this chapter, the nurse will be able to:

1. Define and classify the various forms of lupus.

2. Describe the epidemiology and pathogenesis of lupus.

3. Identify the American College of Rheumatology symptoms and laboratory criteria which support the diagnosis of lupus.

4. Identify the potential impact of lupus on the various parts of the body.

5. Describe current drug therapy and disease management of the patient with lupus.

6. Recognize potential co-morbid conditions that may develop from the disease and the medications used to control disease and its symptoms.

7. Identify short and long term impact on life style and develop a management plan to meet the individual patient's needs.

Content Outline

I. Pathophysiology of systemic lupus erythematosus.

A. Systemic lupus erythematosus (SLE) is an autoimmune inflammatory disease that can progressively damage multiple organs. The pathophysiology of SLE involves antibody formation against self-molecules, including those directed against RNA and DNA.

B. The pathogenesis of lupus is thought to be a combination of predisposing genetic factors and environmental factors such as medication or infectious agents that trigger an abnormal immune response (see Figure 1).

C. This occurs when:

1. Suppressor T cells fail to suppress; in other words, there are defects in cell signaling (Wallace, 2008).

2. There are defects in immune tolerance.

3. Apoptotic cells (cells going through the normal dying process) promote the creation of autoantibodies (Wallace, 2008).

4. And/or there is loss of T regulatory cells that control auto- reactivity. This leads to the formation of autoantibodies and immune complexes, which promote inflammation and tissue damage (Wallace, 2008).

II. Etiology / epidemiology of systemic lupus erythematosus.

A. There are an estimated 1.5 to 2 million individuals diagnosed with SLE in the United States.

1. The reported prevalence of systemic lupus erythematosus (SLE) in the United States is 20 to 150 cases per 100,000 (Lawrence et al., 1998; Pons-Estel et al., 2010).

2. In women, prevalence rates vary from 164 (white) to 406 (African American) per 100,000 (Chakravarty, 2007).

3. The prevalence of SLE is higher among Asians, Afro-Americans, Afro-Caribbeans, Hispanic Americans, and Native Americans compared with Americans of European decent in the United States (Rus et al., 2002).

4. SLE is more prevalent in women than men.

a. The increased frequency of SLE among women has been attributed in part to an estrogen hormonal effect (see 'Hormonal factors' below) (Cooper et al., 1998; Costenbader et al., 2007).

b. An estrogen effect is suggested by a number of observations including the female-to-male ratio of SLE in different age groups:

(1) In children, in whom sex hormonal effects are presumably minimal, the female-to-male ratio is 3:1 (Lahita, 2004).

(2) In adults, especially in women of child-bearing years, the ratio ranges from 7:1 to 15:1 (Chakravarty et al., 2007; Lahita, 2004).

(3) In "older" individuals, especially post-menopausal women, the ratio is approximately 8:1 (Chakravarty et al., 2007; Lahita, 2004).

(4) The ratio approaches 1:1 in very young children under 2 (Ilowite, 2011).

B. Investigators have found evidence to support several likely possibilities in the etiology of SLE.

1. Some believe there may be more than one type of SLE and that its etiology may vary from one person to the next.

C. Current studies are focusing on the following elements:

1. Immune system dysfunction – (see pathophysiology above).

2. Genetics.

a. Studies to date suggest that many different genes contribute to lupus susceptibility and that no single genetic abnormality causes the disease.

b. It also appears that genes may be influential in determining the type or severity of lupus.

c. Genes that have been associated with lupus in humans include:

(1) The immune system genes human leukocyte antigen HLA-DR3 (and B8 in

older data), HLA-DR2, and complement C4 genes; other HLA-DR alleles; and alleles at HLA-DQ (National Institute of Arthritis and Musculoskeletal and Skin Diseases [NIAMS], 2006).

(2) Genes that ensure cells die at an appropriate time (apoptosis genes).

  i) Defective fas gene which contributes to apoptosis.

(3) Genes that regulate key inflammatory molecules, the cytokines.

3. Environmental influences (LFA, 2011).

  a. Ultraviolet rays from the sun.

  b. Ultraviolet rays from fluorescent light bulbs.

  c. Sulfa drugs, which make a person more sensitive to the sun, such as: Bactrim® and trimethoprim-sulfamethoxazole (Septra®); sulfisoxazole (Gantrisin®); tolbutamide (Orinase®); sulfasalazine (SSZ) (Azulfidine®); diuretics.

  d. Sun-sensitizing tetracycline drugs such as minocycline (Minocin®).

  e. Penicillin or other antibiotic drugs such as: Amoxicillin (Amoxil®); ampicillin (Ampicillin Sodium ADD-Vantage®); cloxacillin (Cloxapen®).

  f. An infection.

  g. A cold or a viral illness.

  h. Exhaustion.

  i. An injury.

  j. Emotional stress, such as a divorce, illness, death in the family, or other life complications.

  k. Anything that causes stress to the body, such as surgery, physical harm, pregnancy, or giving birth.

  l. Silica exposure.

Figure 1: A Model of the Pathogenesis of Systemic Lupus Erythematosus (SLE) That Implicates the Products of Disease-Associated Polymorphic Genes

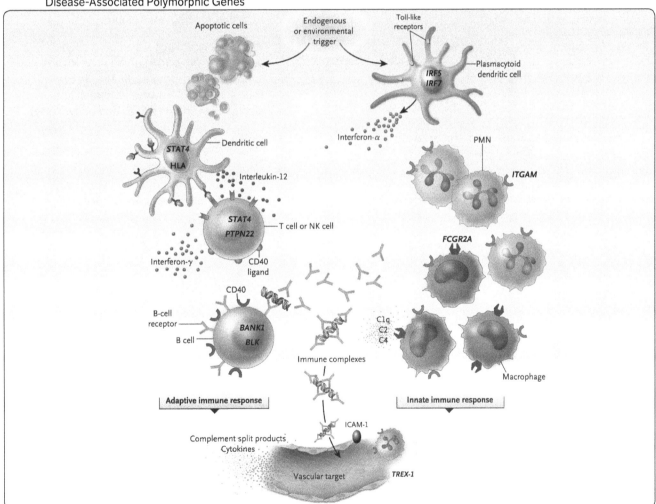

Source: Crow, Mary K. (2008). Collaboration, Genetic Associations, and Lupus Erythematosus. *New England Journal of Medicine*, 358, 956-961. doi: 10.1056/NEJMe0800096. Reprinted with permission.

4. Hormones.

    a. Hormones which are the body's messengers that regulate many of the body's functions.

    b. The hormone estrogen appears to play a role in lupus.

        (1) Female sex hormones have the ability to stimulate the helper T lymphocytes, so-called because they help B lymphocytes to produce antibodies (Isenberg et al., 2008).

        (2) Male hormones encourage suppressor T lymphocytes, which tend to block the production of antibodies (Isenberg et al., 2008).

III. Nursing assessment.

A. Asses flares.

    1. Number of flares since last visit.

    2. Severity of flare (impact on activities of daily living).

    3. Symptoms associated with flare.

    4. Triggers that bring on or are associated with flare.

B. Psychosocial history to include stress, work, social activities, and ability to accomplish activities of daily living.

    1. Discuss with patient the possible need for evaluation and intervention of a social worker, mental health counselor, or psychologist.

C. Current medication and supplements.

    1. Adherence to treatment plan.

IV. Diagnosis.

A. The diagnosis of lupus is based on a combination of physical symptoms and laboratory results.

B. It is usually a diagnosis that evolves over time either toward more certainty or to the conclusion that the person does not have lupus.

C. The diagnosis of SLE is made by a careful review of:

1. Current symptoms.

2. Laboratory test results.

3. Medical history.

4. Medical history of close family members.

D. The American College of Rheumatology (ACR) established criteria for SLE in 1982, which were most recently revised in 1997.

    1. These criteria establish guidelines for diagnosis and consist of 4 cutaneous, 4 systemic, and 3 laboratory criteria.

V. American College of Rheumatology Criteria for Classifying SLE for Research Purposes.

A. Malar rash (LFA, 2011).

    1. Lesions occur when systemic lupus is active.

    2. Flattened areas of red skin on the face that resemble a sunburn.

    3. When the rash appears on both cheeks and across the bridge of the nose in the shape of a butterfly, it is known as the "butterfly rash." However, the rash can also appear on arms, legs, and body.

B. Discoid rash (LFA, 2011).

    1. Appears as disk-shaped, round lesions. The sores usually appear on scalp and face, but sometimes they will occur on other parts of the body as well.

    2. Discoid lupus lesions are often red, scaly, and thick.

    3. Usually they do not hurt or itch.

C. Photosensitivity.

D. Oral ulcers.

E. Arthritis.

    1. Polyarthralgia and polyarthritis, defined as arthralgias or arthritis affecting 5 or more joints, are the most common joint problems seen in people with SLE.

    2. Over 50% of lupus patients manifest arthralgias upon their initial diagnosis.

4
4.1
4.2
4.3
4.4
4.5
4.6
4.7
4.8
4.9
4.10

3. Both large joints, such as the knees, shoulders, and elbows, and small joints, such as the toe and finger joints, can be affected by lupus arthritis.

F. Serositis (pleuritis or pericarditis).

1. Pleuritis and pericarditis are the most frequent pulmonary and cardiac manifestations of SLE. A prevalence of serositis at disease onset of 17% with a cumulative incidence of 36% (Kean et al., 2000).

2. Pleuritic chest pain may occur during the course of lupus in up to 60% (Kean et al., 2000).

3. Manifestations of serositis (Kean et al., 2000; Tincani et al., 2006).

   a. Chest pain may be unilateral or bilateral and usually is located at the costophrenic margins, either anterior or posterior.

   b. Cough and dyspnea.

   c. Pericarditis usually manifests as precordial pain aggravated by deep breathing and decubitus, typically improving with sitting up.

   d. Friction rubs may be heard.

G. Renal disorder (persistent proteinuria or cellular casts).

1. Manifestations of lupus nephritis (John Hopkins, 2013).

   a. High blood pressure.

   b. Dark urine.

   c. Flu-like symptoms.

   d. Joint pains and aches.

   e. Swelling (edema) of the legs, ankles, eyes, and hands.

   f. Weight gain, caused by water retention when the kidneys do not filter properly.

2. Some patients may have few and subtle symptoms or none at all in the early stages of the disease.

H. Neurological disorder (seizures or psychosis).

1. Neuropsychiatric systemic lupus erythematosus (NPSLE) is arguably the least understood manifestation of SLE,

as it is associated with a complicated and often baffling range of clinical presentations (Hermosillo-Romo et al., 2002).

2. NP-SLE can involve the central nervous system (CNS), peripheral nervous system, and/or the autonomic nervous system.

3. Manifestations can include (ACR Ad Hoc Committee, 1999; Bertsias, et al., 2010):

   a. Central nervous system.

      (1) Acute confusional state.

      (2) Cognitive dysfunction.

         i) Mild to moderate.

         ii) Severe (dementia).

      (3) Headache.

      (4) Aseptic meningitis.

      (5) Myelopathy.

      (6) Movement disorders.

      (7) Demyelinating syndromes.

      (8) Seizures.

   b. Psychiatric disturbances.

      (1) Psychosis.

      (2) Mood and anxiety disorders.

         i) Severe depression.

         ii) Anxiety.

   c. Peripheral nervous system.

      (1) Cranial neuropathy.

      (2) Guillain-Barrè syndrome.

      (3) Plexopathy.

      (4) Autonomic neuropathy.

      (5) Myasthenia gravis.

4. Cognitive impairment from NPSLE can affect any or all of the following cognitive functions (Brunner et al., 2009):

   a. Simple or complex attention.

   b. Reasoning.

   c. Executive skills (e.g., planning, organizing, sequencing).

   d. Memory (e.g., learning, recall).

   e. Visual-spatial processing.

   f. Language (e.g., verbal fluency).

   g. Psychomotor speed.

4
4.1
4.2
4.3
4.4
4.5
4.6
4.7
4.8
4.9
4.10

I. Hematologic disorder (anemia, leukopenia, or lymphopenia on two or more occasions, thrombocytopenia).

1. Immunologic disorder (abnormal anti-dsDNA or anti-Sm, positive antiphospholipid antibodies).

2. Abnormal anti-nuclear antibody (ANA) titer.

   a. Auto-Antibody Testing.

      (1) Anti-nuclear antibody test (ANA).

         i) Antinuclear antibodies (ANA) are antibodies that connect, or bind, to the nucleus -- the "command center" -- of the cell.

         ii) This process damages and can destroy the cells.

         iii) The ANA blood test is a sensitive test for lupus since these antibodies are found in 97 percent of people with the disease.

         iv) When three or more typical features of lupus are present -- such as involvement of the skin, joints, kidneys, lungs, heart, blood, or nervous system -- a positive ANA test can help confirm a diagnosis of lupus.

         v) A positive ANA test result does not always mean an individual has lupus.

            1) The ANA can be positive in people with other illnesses or positive in people with no illness.

            2) The ANA can also change from positive to negative or negative to positive in the same person.

            3) The ANA may show a negative reading in some patients who have received immunosuppressant therapy only to later return to a positive reading.

            4) Immune fluorescence pattern can help distinguish different auto-immune disease:

               (a) Homogeneous or rimmed patterns are suggestive of SLE.

               (b) Speckled pattern is the most common but least specific. Suggestive of:

                  (i) SLE.

                  (ii) Sjögren's syndrome.

                  (iii) Mixed connective tissue disease.

                  (iv) Scleroderma.

               (c) Nucleolar pattern is suggestive of scleroderma or CREST syndrome.

      (2) Antibodies to double-stranded DNA.

         i) Anti-dsDNA antibodies are found in 50 percent of the people with SLE.

            1) The antibodies form in response to DNA exposed during apoptosis and can bind to proteins and deposit in tissues (such as in the kidney) and damage the organ.

         ii) The disease can still be present even if these antibodies are not detected.

      (3) Anti-Sm antibodies.

         i) Target Sm proteins in the cell nucleus.

         ii) Found in 30-40 percent of people with SLE.

         iii) The presence of this antibody almost always confirms the diagnosis of SLE.

      (4) Antibodies to phospholipids (aPLs).

         i) Nearly 30 percent of people with lupus will test positive for antiphospholipid antibodies.

         ii) The most commonly measured aPLs are lupus anticoagulant, anticardiolipin antibody, and anti-beta2 glycoprotein I.

         iii) Can cause narrowing of blood vessels, leading to blood clots in the legs or lungs, stroke, heart attack, or miscarriage.

      (5) Antibodies to Ro/SS-A and La/SS-B.

         i) Ro and La are the names of proteins in the cell nucleus.

            1) Often found in people with Sjögren's syndrome.

      (6) Antibodies to RNP target ribonucleoproteins.

         i) Help to control chemical activities of the cells.

         ii) Anti-RNPs are found in many autoimmune conditions and will be

4
4.1
4.2
4.3
4.4
4.5
4.6
4.7
4.8
4.9
4.10

at very high levels in patients whose symptoms combine features of several diseases, including lupus.

(7) Antibodies to histone.

    i) A protein that surrounds the DNA molecule.

    ii) Sometimes found in people with systemic lupus but more often seen in people with drug-induced lupus.

(8) Complements.

    i) A group of proteins that protect the body against infections.

    ii) Complement proteins are used up by the inflammation caused by lupus.

      1) People with inflammation due to active lupus often have decreased complement levels.

    iii) There are nine protein groups of complement, so complement is identified by the letter C and the numbers 1 through 9.

      1) The most common complement tests are CH50, C3, and C4.

      2) CH50 measures the overall function of complement in the blood. Low levels of C3 or C4 may indicate active lupus.

b. Other laboratory testing.

(1) CRP (C-reactive protein) binding.

    i) A protein produced by the liver.

    ii) High levels may indicate inflammation due to lupus.

(2) Erythrocyte sedimentation rate (ESR or "sed" rate).

    i) Indicator of inflammation in the body.

    ii) Measures the amount of a protein that makes the red blood cells clump together.

    iii) May be elevated in people with active lupus, but it can also be high due to other reasons, such as an infection.

(3) Complete Blood Count.

    i) Anemia.

      1) About 40 percent of individuals with lupus experience anemia.

      2) May be caused by iron deficiency, gastrointestinal (GI) bleeding, medications, and autoantibody

formation to RBCs, or "chronic disease" (National Institute of Arthritis and Musculoskeletal and Skin Diseases [NIAMS], 2006).

    ii) Leukopenia and thrombocytopenia.

      1) Abnormalities in the white blood cell (WBC) and platelet counts are an important indicator of SLE.

      2) Around 40 percent of lupus patients have a low level of total white cells (Isenberg et al., 2008).

      3) Approximately 80 percent of lupus patients have low levels of lymphocytes (Isenberg et al., 2008).

      4) Occurs in 25 to 35 percent of patients with SLE (NIAMS, 2006).

VI. Treatment.

A. Treatment varies depending on the symptoms, severity, and organ systems involved in the individual's disease.

B. Developing new treatments for lupus that are safe, effective, and tolerable has been particularly challenging given certain steep barriers to drug development and approval in lupus. Among these barriers, some of the most prominent are (Lewin Group, 2009):

1. The poorly understood biology of the disease.

2. Difficulties in clinical trial participant selection.

3. Challenges to selection of appropriate clinical trial endpoints.

4. Adapting instruments and tools for measuring disease activity in clinical trials.

5. The confounding role of background medications.

C. Goal of treatment:

1. Reduce inflammation caused by lupus.

2. Suppress overactive immune system.

3. Prevent flares, and treat them when they occur.

4. Control symptoms such as joint pain and fatigue.

5. Minimize damage to organs.

4
4.1
4.2
4.3
4.4
4.5
4.6
4.7
4.8
4.9
4.10

D. Medications used to treat SLE.

1. Anti-inflammatories.

   a. Aspirin has pain-reducing, anti-inflammatory, and anticoagulant properties that can control some of the symptoms of lupus.

   b. Non-steroidal antiinflammatory drugs (NSAIDs).

      (1) Suppress inflammation.

      (2) Decrease joint pain and stiffness.

      (3) Types of NSAIDs:

         i) Ibuprofen (Motrin®)

         ii) Naproxen (Naprosyn®)

         iii) Indomethacin (Indocin®)

         iv) Nabumetone (Relafen®)

         v) Celecoxib (Celebrex®)

   c. Side effects (NIAMS, 2006).

      (1) Gastrointestinal (GI): Dyspepsia, heartburn, epigastric distress, and nausea; less frequently, vomiting, anorexia, abdominal pain, GI bleeding, and mucosal lesions. Misoprostol (Cytotec®), a synthetic prostaglandin that inhibits gastric acid secretion, may be given to prevent GI intolerance. It prevents gastric ulcers and the associated GI bleeding in patients receiving NSAIDs. Another product, Arthrotec®, combines misoprostol with the NSAID diclofenac sodium in a single pill.

      (2) Genitourinary: Fluid retention, reduction in creatinine clearance, and acute tubular necrosis with renal failure.

      (3) Hepatic: Acute reversible hepatotoxicity.

      (4) Cardiovascular: Hypertension and moderate to severe noncardiogenic pulmonary edema. All NSAIDS now carry a warning that they may increase the risk of myocardial infarction.

      (5) Hematologic: Altered hemostasis through effects on platelet function.

      (6) Other: Skin eruption, sensitivity reactions, tinnitus, and hearing loss.

2. Antimalarial (NIAMS, 2006).

   a. Anti-inflammatory action of these drugs is not well understood.

   b. Anti-coagulant properties platelets to reduce the risk of blood clots.

   c. Decrease in plasma levels.

   d. Types of antimalarial medications.

      (1) Hydroxychloroquine sulfate (Plaquenil®)

      (2) Chloroquine (Aralen®)

   e. Side effects.

      (1) Central nervous system: Headache, nervousness, irritability, dizziness, muscle weakness, and tinnitus.

      (2) Gastrointestinal: Nausea, vomiting, diarrhea, abdominal cramps, and loss of appetite.

      (3) Ophthalmologic: Visual disturbances and retinal changes manifested by blurring of vision and difficulty in focusing. A very serious potential side effect of antimalarial drugs is damage to the retina. Because of the relatively low doses used to treat SLE, the risk of retinal damage is quite small; however, patients should have a thorough eye examination before starting this treatment and yearly thereafter. The risk of retinal toxicity with chloroquine is higher than with hydroxychloroquine and occurs at lower doses (>3 mg/kg/day). After taking hydroxychloroquine for five years or longer, 1% of users had evidence of retinal toxicity (Wolfe, 2010).

      (4) Dermatologic: Dryness, pruritus, alopecia, skin and mucosal pigmentation, skin eruptions, and exfoliative dermatitis.

      (5) Hematologic: Blood dyscrasia and hemolysis in patients with glucose 6-phosphate dehydrogenase (G6PD) deficiency.

3. Corticosteroids (NIAMS, 2006).

   a. Hormones secreted by the cortex of the adrenal gland.

   b. Highly effective in reducing inflammation and suppressing the immune response.

   c. These drugs may be used to control exacerbation of symptoms and to control severe forms of the disease.

   d. Types of corticosteroids.

      (1) Prednisone (Orasone®, Meticorten®, Deltasone®, Cortan®, Sterapred®)

4
4.1
4.2
4.3
4.4
4.5
4.6
4.7
4.8
4.9
4.10

(2) Hydrocortisone (Cortef®, Hydrocortone®)

(3) Methylprednisolone (Medrol®)

(4) Dexamethasone (Decadron®)

e. Side effects (* long-term effects).

(1) Central nervous system: Depression, mood swings, and psychosis.

(2) Cardiovascular: Congestive heart failure (CHF) and hypertension.

(3) Endocrine: Cushing's syndrome, menstrual irregularities, and hyperglycemia.

(4) Gastrointestinal: GI irritation, peptic ulcer, and weight gain.

(5) Dermatologic: Thin skin, petechiae, ecchymoses, facial erythema, poor wound healing, hirsutism, urticaria, and acne.

(6) Musculoskeletal: Muscle weakness, loss of muscle mass, and osteoporosis*.

(7) Ophthalmologic: Increased intraocular pressure, glaucoma, exophthalmos, and cataracts.

(8) Other: Immunosuppression and increased susceptibility to infection.

4. Immunosuppressive (NIAMS, 2006).

a. Although they have different mechanisms of action, each type functions to decrease or prevent an immune response.

b. Types of immunosuppressive medications.

(1) Azathioprine (Imuran®): Azathioprine, one of the most widely used immunosuppressives for lupus, is an antimetabolite. Antimetabolites work by blocking metabolic steps within immune cells and then interfering with immune function. Used to control the underlying disease process, azathioprine has fewer serious side-effect risks than some other drugs used to control lupus.

(2) Cyclophosphamide (Cytoxan®): An alkylating agent and strong immunosuppressive, cyclophosphamide is reserved for treating lupus with kidney disease or other internal organ involvement. It works by targeting and damaging autoantibody-producing cells, thereby suppressing the hyperactive immune response and reducing disease activity. It has the potential for severe side effects, including risk of serious infection.

(3) Methotrexate (MTX) (Rheumatrex®): Originally developed as a cancer treatment and later approved for rheumatoid arthritis, MTX, like azathioprine, is an antimetabolite. It is predominantly used for lupus arthritis. It requires monitoring of the CBC and liver function tests. To reduce toxicity, daily folic acid is prescribed.

(4) Cyclosporine (Neoral®): Originally developed to prevent the body from rejecting transplanted organs, cyclosporine is now commonly used to treat rheumatic diseases, including lupus. Cyclosporine is an antimetabolite.

(5) Mycophenolate mofetil (CellCept®): A strong immunosuppressive drug developed to prevent the rejection of transplanted organs, mycophenolate is sometimes used as an alternative to cyclophosphamide for lupus with kidney involvement. Mycophenolate works by keeping T and B lymphocytes from replicating.

c. Side effects.

(1) Immunosuppressives can have serious side effects.

(2) Patients need to understand, however, that side effects are dose-dependent and are generally reversible by reducing the dose or stopping the medication.

(3) Immunosuppression (resulting in increased susceptibility to infection).

(4) Bone marrow suppression (resulting in decreased numbers of RBCs, WBCs, and platelets).

(5) Development of malignancies.

(6) Dermatologic: Alopecia (cyclophosphamide and MTX).

(7) Gastrointestinal: Nausea, vomiting, stomatitis, esophagitis, and hepatotoxicity.

(8) Genitourinary: Hemorrhagic cystitis, hematuria, amenorrhea, impotence, and gonadal suppression (cyclophosphamide only).

(9) Hematologic: Thrombocytopenia, leukopenia, pancytopenia, anemia, and myelosuppression.

4
4.1
4.2
4.3
4.4
4.5
4.6
4.7
4.8
4.9
4.10

(10) Respiratory: Pulmonary fibrosis.

(11) Other: Increased risk of serious infections.

5. Monoclonal antibody (mAbs).

   a. The monoclonal antibody approach has been used to target both B and T lymphocytes, the white blood cells responsible for autoantibody production in lupus (LFA, 2011).

   b. While several monoclonal antibody therapies are used in the treatment of SLE, only BENLYSTA® has been approved by the FDA.

   c. Types of monoclonal antibody medications.

      (1) Belimumab (*BENLYSTA®*): Specifically recognizes and blocks the biological activity of B-lymphocyte stimulator, or BLyS® (pronounced bliss), a naturally occurring protein which was discovered by scientists at Human Genome Sciences (HGS). Elevated levels of BLyS prolong the survival of B cells which can contribute to the production of autoantibodies – antibodies that target the body's own tissues. Studies have shown that BENLYSTA® can reduce autoantibody levels and help control autoimmune disease activity (LFA, 2011).

      (2) Rituximab (Rituxan®, anti-CD20): Targets a specific protein known as CD20 that appears on the surface of B cells. Rituxan® binds to CD20 and is believed to work with the body's own immune system to attack and kill the marked B cells (LFA, 2011).

      (3) Epratuzumab: An anti-CD22 antibody designed to bind to the CD22 antigen on B cells and may control lupus disease by depleting B cells and by controlling or modulating B cell function (LFA, 2011).

      (4) Anti-IL6: Elevated levels of Interleukin 6 (IL-6) in blood, urine, and kidneys have been seen in people with active lupus. Treatment with anti-IL-6 may be able to suppress inflammation induced by autoreactive B cells and autoreactive T cells (LFA, 2011).

      (5) MEDI-545 (anti-interferon-alpha): Targets interferon-alpha by binding to multiple INF-alpha subtypes seen in the serum of people with lupus. Levels of interferon-alpha are elevated in active lupus and other autoimmune disorders, and may be associated with disease activity (LFA, 2011).

      (6) Eculizumab (anti C5a): Was developed to inhibit the complement component C5. Complement is a collection of proteins that can become overactive or misdirected by autoantibodies in a disease like lupus (LFA, 2011).

      (7) Anti-TNF therapies (Enbrel®, Humira®, Remicade®): Are primarily used in RA. Although these drugs have been found to cause drug-induced lupus in some people (reversible when the medicine is stopped), they have also been shown to be effective in treating the arthritis that can occur in lupus (LFA, 2011).

      (8) Anti-IL10: An antibody that blocks the activity of IL10, which is important in the activation of B cells in lupus (LFA, 2011).

   d. Side effects (Mayo Clinic, 2011).

      (1) In general, monoclonal antibody medications have fewer side effects than do other immunosuppressive therapies.

      (2) The more-common side effects caused by monoclonal antibody drugs include:

          i) Allergic reactions, such as hives or itching.

          ii) Flu-like signs and symptoms, including chills, fatigue, fever, and muscle aches and pains.

          iii) Nausea.

          iv) Diarrhea.

          v) Skin rashes.

      (3) Serious, but rare, side effects of monoclonal antibody therapy may include:

          i) Infusion reactions. Severe allergy-like reactions can occur and, in very few cases, lead to death.

          ii) Dangerously low blood cell counts. Low levels of red blood cells, white blood cells, and platelets may lead to serious complications.

          iii) Heart problems. Certain monoclonal antibodies may cause heart problems, including heart failure and a small risk of heart attack.

4
4.1
4.2
4.3
4.4
4.5
4.6
4.7
4.8
4.9
4.10

VII. Co-morbid conditions.

A. Osteoporosis.

1. A high prevalence of osteoporosis and osteopenia is present in SLE (Pineau et al., 2007).

2. Although part of this increase in risk is due to recognized risk factors (e.g., corticosteroid use, decreased physical activity, decreased sun exposure), lupus activity may also play a role (Pineau et al., 2007).

B. Cardiovascular disease.

1. Lupus patients have a significant increased risk of cardiovascular events (Pineau et al., 2007).

2. This increase in risk is related to an increased number traditional risk factors (e.g., hypertension, hyperlipidemia) but lupus-related factors (e.g. steroid exposure, SLE activity) may also be important (Pineau et al., 2007).

3. Because patients with lupus are at high risk of cardiovascular disease (CVD), they should have regular screening for the presence of traditional risk factors, and aggressive risk reduction (Pineau et al., 2007).

C. Malignancy and SLE.

1. SLE is associated with an increased risk of malignancies, particularly lymphoma and lung cancer (Pineau et al., 2007).

2. Although immunosuppressive therapy may not be the principal driving factor for overall cancer risk in autoimmune diseases such as SLE, it may contribute to an increased risk of some hematological malignancies (Pineau et al., 2007).

3. Lymphoma risk in SLE may in part be driven by disease activity, but work in progress aims to differentiate the effects of lupus treatment from lupus activity (Pineau et al., 2007).

VIII. Nursing implications.

A. Osteoporosis.

1. Screening for osteoporosis with bone mineral densitometry should be considered in all patients with SLE, especially in the presence of osteoporosis risk factors (Pineau et al., 2007).

2. Early and aggressive measures for bone preservation should be considered in all patients treated with corticosteroids (Pineau et al., 2007).

B. Cardiovascular disease.

1. Because patients with lupus are at high risk of CVD, they should have regular screening for the presence of traditional risk factors, and aggressive risk reduction (Pineau et al., 2007).

C. Medication adherence (LFA, 2011; NIAMS, 2006).

1. Create rapport with patients.

2. Fully explain all medications to the patient to include possible side effects and potential problems that may result from non-adherence with medication regimens.

3. Provide the patient with strategies on how to integrate medication treatment plan into daily activities of living.

4. Prepare medications in advance by using a pill box to help organize one or even two weeks' worth of medications.

5. Use alarm clock or cell phone alarm to alert patient when it is time to take medication.

6. Encourage family and friends to form a support system with the patient (particularly for teens and young adults), who will help reinforce medication adherence.

7. Verify adherence with medication treatment plan during follow-up appointments.

8. Remain vigilant for signs of non-adherence, as the patient may be embarrassed and not admit to being non-adherent.

9. Consider intravenous medications when concerns about non-adherence affect disease management.

D. Photosensitivity (LFA, 2011; NIAMS, 2006).

1. Teach the patient to minimize direct exposure to UV from sun and/or fluorescent and halogen light bulbs. (Glass does not provide complete protection from UV rays) (NIAMS, 2006).

2. Instruct the patient to use sunscreen of SPF 30 or greater and encourage the use of broad-brimmed hats and tightly-woven, loose-fitting clothing with long sleeves and long pants.

4
4.1
4.2
4.3
4.4
4.5
4.6
4.7
4.8
4.9
4.10

3. Teach patients about the benefits of shields that cover fluorescent bulbs to minimize indoor exposure. Recommend shields with nanometer readings of 380 to 400.

4. Assess the need for window films on the patient's car.

5. Instruct the patient that certain drugs can increase sensitivity to the sun, including antihistamines, diuretics, non-steroidal antiinflammatory drugs (NSAIDs), and antibiotics, including tetracycline or "sulfa" antibiotics. Extra precautions should be made if taking these medications.

   a. Special emphasis on the effects of photosensitivity is necessary if the patient is taking any of these medications.

6. Special emphasis on the effects of photosensitivity should be given to people of color (e.g., African American, Hispanic, Asian, and Native American).

E. Extreme fatigue (LFA, 2011; NIAMS, 2006).

   1. Assess the patient's general fatigue level.

   2. Assess for the presence of depression, anxiety, and other stressors.

   3. Conduct an assessment to determine the patient's daily activities that contribute to fatigue.

   4. Help the patient to develop an energy-conserving plan for completing daily and other activities and work. Many people with lupus need to take a daily nap. Encourage a nap earlier in the day to prevent any issues with insomnia.

   5. Encourage the patient to get 8 to 10 hours of sleep at night.

   6. Encourage exercise as tolerated.

F. Diet and nutrition (LFA, 2011; NIAMS, 2006).

   1. Assess the patient's prescription and nonprescription drug regimen and dosages for medications that may affect patient's nutritional status.

   2. Assess the patient's usual daily dietary intake by recommending that the patient keep a food diary.

   3. Educate patient about which medications to take with food.

4. Develop a dietary plan with the patient that encourages healthful eating. If the patient has nutrition-related lupus complications, refer to a dietician for counseling.

5. Encourage exercise as tolerated.

6. Record the patient's weight at each visit.

7. Instruct the patient to weigh at home once a week, record it, and bring to all patient visits.

G. Pregnancy.

   1. SLE primarily affects women of childbearing age; pregnancy is therefore a dilemma frequently encountered in this patient population that requires prudent clinical guidance. The majority of pregnancies in women with SLE result in a healthy infant and mother (Clark et al., 2005).

   2. An estimated 50% of women with SLE will experience a flare during pregnancy (Carmona et al., 1990; Clowse et al., 2005).

   3. In most women, the flare will be mild, involve the skin or joints, and will not have a major impact on the pregnancy outcome or fetus.

   4. Up to 20% of women with SLE will have a more severe flare, involving the kidneys, hematologic disease, serositis, and/or severe arthritis, which can increase the risks for pregnancy loss, preterm birth, and preeclampsia (Chakravarty et al., 2005; Clowse et al., 2005; Rubbert et al., 1992),

   5. Cyclophosphamide, mycophenolate Mofetil (MMF) – and probably mycophenolic acid – pose significant risks for pregnancy loss and for teratogenic effects on the fetus (Østensen et al., 2006).

   6. Azathioprine, hydroxychloroquine, and cyclosporine are associated with no or minimal increase in pregnancy loss, preterm birth, and teratogenicity (Østensen et al., 2006).

   7. If possible, MMF or cyclophosphamide should be switched to azathioprine or cyclosporine at least 3 to 6 months before conception to determine whether a SLE flare will occur on the revised regimen (Østensen et al., 2006).

   8. Corticosteroid use is relatively safe in pregnancy.

      a. Prednisone and prednisolone are recommended; less than 10% of the

4
4.1
4.2
4.3
4.4
4.5
4.6
4.7
4.8
4.9
4.10

dose will cross the maternal-fetal membranes (Østensen et al., 2006).

9. Anti-Ro (SS-A) and anti-La (SS-B) antibodies are risk factors for neonatal lupus erythematosus (NLE), a condition in the newborn that may include low blood counts, rash, liver test abnormalities, and congenital heart block (CHB). The only permanent complication is CHB and this is rare, occurring in about 2% of babies of mothers who are anti-Ro (SS-A)/La (SS-B) positive (LFA, 2011).

H. Smoking (LFA, 2011; NIAMS, 2006).

1. Assess smoking habits of the patient.

2. Provide support, guidance, and instruction on the safest techniques of smoking cessation.

3. Provide contacts for local smoking cessation classes.

I. Infection (LFA, 2011; NIAMS, 2006).

1. Assess the patient's current medications, particularly those that promote susceptibility to infection such as corticosteroids and immunosuppressive medications.

2. Teach the patient to use good hand-washing and personal-hygiene techniques.

3. Teach the patient the signs and symptoms of infection and reinforce the importance of reporting them to the healthcare provider.

4. Encourage the patient to eat a balanced diet with adequate calories to help preserve the immune system.

5. Teach the patient to minimize exposure to crowds and people with infections or contagious illnesses.

6. Check the patient's current immunization status.

7. Teach the patient that infections can be minimized with immunizations.

8. Encourage the patient to consult the healthcare provider about vaccines and/ or allergy shots that are being considered.

J. Stress (LFA, 2011; NIAMS, 2006).

1. Assess for presence and degree of anxiety or life stressor.

2. Encourage patient to find positive coping mechanisms for stressor.

3. Encourage the patient to accept help from others, such as counseling or a support group.

4. Discuss complementary coping activities such as biofeedback, yoga, and/or acupuncture.

5. Encourage development of a consistent exercise regime.

K. Depression (LFA, 2011; NIAMS, 2006).

1. Assess the patient for the signs and symptoms of depression.

2. Assess the patient's interpersonal and social support systems.

3. Encourage the patient to express feelings.

4. Initiate a referral to a social worker, mental health counselor, psychologist or psychiatrist.

L. Neuropsychiatric issues (LFA, 2011; NIAMS, 2006).

1. Assess the patient for any changes in cognition, memory, and/or mental status.

2. Provide tips that may help ease the frustrations of cognitive impairment caused by lupus.

   a. Patient should focus attention when receiving new information. Repeat information back to the provider, ask for clarification, ask for memory tools, and/or write the information down. Verify any details.

   b. Focus on one task at a time.

   c. Encourage exercise, heart healthy diet, and sufficient sleep.

   d. Learn and use memory techniques, such as associating a person's name with an image, or repeating the name several times in conversation.

   e. Try to stay organized. One helpful hint is to use a year-long calendar notebook so that all appointments, plans, contact information, and reminders can be kept in one place.

3. Initiate a referral for neuropsychiatric evaluation if ordered by the healthcare provider.

4
4.1
4.2
4.3
4.4
4.5
4.6
4.7
4.8
4.9
4.10

Summary

Lupus is an autoimmune disease of varying forms. When not well controlled, lupus impacts various body parts including the skin, heart, joints and most especially the kidneys. Disorders of the central nervous system, psychiatric disorders, and cognitive impairment are also seen in those with lupus. Nurses should apply various techniques in assisting patients with this diagnosis..

References

ACR Ad Hoc Committee on Neuropsychiatric Lupus Nomenclature. (1999). The American College of Rheumatology Nomenclature and Case Definitions for Neuropsychiatric Lupus Syndromes. *Arthritis and Rheumatism, 42*, 599-608.

Bertsias G.K., Ioannidis, J.P.A., Aringer, M., Bollen, E., Bombardieri, S., Bruce, I.N., ... Boumpas, D.T. (2010). EULAR recommendations for the management of systemic lupus erythematosus and neuropsychiatric manifestations: Report of a task force of the EULAR standing committee for clinical affairs. *Annals of Rheumatic Disease, 69*, 2074-2082.

Brunner, H., & Klein-Gitelman M. (2009, March). Lupus in the child's mind: Unique neuropsychiatric problems require a unique approach. The Rheumatologist. Retrieved from Unique neuropsychiatric problems require a unique approach.

Carmona F., Font J., Cervera R., Muñoz, F., Cararach, V., & Balasch, J. (1990. Obstretrical outcome of pregnancy in patients with systemic lupus erythematosus. A study of 60 cases. *European Journal of Obstetrics, Gynecology, and Reproductive Bilogy, 83*(2), 137-142.

Chakravarty, E.F., Bush, T.M., Manzi, S., Clarke, A.E., & Ward, M.M. (2007). Prevalence of adult systemic lupus erythematosus in California and Pennsylvania in 2000: Estimates obtained using hospitalization data. *Arthritis and Rheumatism, 56*(6), 2092-2094.

Chakravarty, E.F., Colòn, I., Langen, E.S., Nix, D.A., El-Sayed, Y.Y., Genovese, M.C., & Druzin, M.L. (2005). Factors that predict prematurity and preeclampsia in pregnancies that are complicated by systemic lupus erythematosus. *American Journal of Obstetrics and Gynecology, 192*(6), 1897-1904,

Clark, C.A., Spitzer, K.A., & Laskin, C.A. (2005). Decrease in pregnancy loss rates in patients with systemic lupus erythematosus over a 40 year period. *Journal of Rheumatology, 32*(9), 1709-1712.

Clowse, M.E., Magder, L.S., Witter, F., Petri, M. (2005). The impact of increased lupus activity on obstetric outcomes. *Arthritis and Rheumatism, 52*(2), 514-521.

Cooper, G.S., Dooley, M.A., Treadwell, E.L., St. Clair, E.W., Parks, C.G., & Gilkeson, G.S. (1998). Hormonal, environmental, and infectious risk factors for developing systemic lupus erythematosus. Arthritis and Rheumatism, 41(10), 1714-1724.

Costenbader, K.H., Feskanich, D., Stampfer, M.J., & Karlson, E.W. (2007). Reproductive and menopausal factors and risk of systemic lupus erythematosus in women. Arthritis and Rheumatism, 56(4), 1251-1262.

Francès, C., Papo, T., Wechsler, B., Laporte, J.L., Biousse, V., & Piette, J.C. (1999). Sneddon syndrome with or without antiphospholipid antibodies. A comparative study in 46 patients. Medicine (Baltimore), 78(4), 209-219.

Hermosillo-Romo, D., & Brey, R.L. (2002). Neuropsychiatric involvement in systemic lupus erythematosus. Current Rheumatology Reports, 4, 337-344.

Isenberg, D., & Manzi, S. (2008).Lupus: The facts (2nd ed.). New York: Oxford University Press.

Ilowite, N. T. (2011). 15 questions with Dr. Norman Ilowite – pediatric lupus. Retrieved from http://www.lupus.org/webmodules/webarticlesnet/templates/new_learnclinical.aspx?articleid=4139&zoneid=531

John Hopkins Children's Hospital. (2013), Lupus nephritis. Retrieved from https://www.hopkinschildrens.org/Lupus-Nephritis.aspx

Kean, M.P., & Lynch, J.P. (2000). Pleuropulmonary manifestations of systemic lupus erythematosus. Thorax, 55, 159-166.

Lahita, R.G. (2004). *Systemic lupus erythematosus* (4th ed.). San Diego, CA: Academic Press.

Lawrence, R.C., Helmick, C.G., Arnett, F.C., Deyo, R.A., Felson, D.T., Giannini, E.H., ...Wolfe, E. (1998). Estimates of the prevalence of arthritis and selected musculoskeletal disorders in the United States. *Arthritis and Rheumatism, 41*(5), 778-799.

The Lewin Group, Inc. (2009). *Overcoming barriers to drug development in lupus.* Washington, DC: The Lupus Foundation of America, Inc.

Lupus Foundation of America, Inc. (2011). *Learn about lupus.* Retrieved from www.lupus.org

4
4.1
4.2
4.3
4.4
4.5
4.6
4.7
4.8
4.9
4.10

Monoclonal antibody drugs for cancer treatment: How they work. (2011, November 29). 2011. Retrieved from http://www.mayoclinic.com/health/monoclonal-antibody/CA00082

National Institute of Arthritis and Musculoskeletal and Skin Diseases (NIAMS). (2006). *Lupus: A patient care guide for nurses and other health professionals* (3rd ed.). Bethesda, MD: Author.

Østensen, M., Khamashto, M., Lockshin, M., Parke, A., Brucato, A., Carp, H., ...Tincani, A. (2006). Anti-inflammatory and immunosuppressive drugs and reproduction. *Arthritis Research and Therapy, 8*(3), 209.

Pineau, C. A., Lee, C., Ramsey-Goldman, R., Clarke, A.E., & Bernatsky, S. (2007). The second hit: Co-morbidities in systemic lupus erythematosus. *Future Rheumatology, 2*(5), 497-506.

Pons-Estel, G.J., Alarcón, G.S., Scofield, L., Reinlib, L., & Cooper, G.S. (2010). Understanding the epidemiology and progression of systemic lupus erythematosus. *Seminars in Arthritis and Rheumatism, 39*(4), 257-268.

Rubbert, A., Pimer, K., Wildt, L., Kalden, J.R., & Manger, B. (1992). Pregnancy course and complications in patients with systemic lupus erythematosus. *American Journal of Reproductive Immunology, 28*(3-4), 205-207.

Rus, V., Maury, E.E., & Hochberg, M.C. (2002). The epidemiology of systemic lupus erythematosus. In D.J. Wallace & B.H. Hahn (Eds.), *Dubois' lupus erythematosus* (pp. __). Philadelphia: Lippincott Williams and Wilkins.

Tincani, A., Rebaioli, C.B., Taglietti, M., & Shoenfeld, Y. (2006). Heart involvement in systemic lupus erythematosus, anti-phospholipid syndrome and neonatal lupus. *Rheumatology* (Oxford), *45*(Suppl 4), 8-13.

Wallace, D. J. (2008). *Lupus: The essential clinician's guide*. New York: Oxford American Rheumatology Library.

Wolfe, R., & Marmor, M.F. (2010). Rates and predictors of hydroxychloroquine retinal toxicity in patients with rheumatoid arthritis and systemic lupus erythematosus. *Arthritis Care and Research* (Hoboken), *62*, 775-784.

Suggested Readings

Hochberg, M.C. (1985). The incidence of systemic lupus erythematosus in Baltimore, Maryland, 1970-1977. *Arthritis and Rheumatism, 28*(1), 80-86.

Krajewski, D. (2011, May 7). *Endocrine manifestationsin systemic lupus erythematosus*. Department of Endocrinology Georgetown University Hospital. [Power Point Slides]. Retrieved from http://www.lupus.org/webmodules/webarticlesnet/articlefiles/3918-Endocrine%20Manifestations%20in%20Lupus%20May%202011.pdf

Serdula, M.K., & Rhoads, G.G. (1979). Frequency of systemic lupus erythematosus in different ethnic groups in Hawaii. *Arthritis and Rheumatism, 22*(4), 328-333.

4
4.1
4.2
4.3
4.4
4.5
4.6
4.7
4.8
4.9
4.10

Section 4.6
Gout

Sheree C. Carter, PhD, RN

Introduction

Gout is perhaps one of the oldest documented diseases of humankind known worldwide appearing in works of art and literature. Helfgott (2013) recently referred to an evolutionary rheumatology "Big Bang" where gout is associated around 11 to 16 million years ago when hominids lost the ability to create the enzyme uricase used to breakdown uric acid to allantoin. Humans and Great Apes share that fate today.

It was the Egyptians in 2640 B.C. who identified gout in the first metatarsal joint as podagra (Hill, 2006; Nuki & Simkin, 2006). There are Egyptian mummies with evidence of uric acid deposits in joints which date back 4,000 years (Helfgott, 2013). However, most credit Hippocrates as identifying the disease in the fifth century B.C. as he defined the affliction as 'the unwalkable disease'. Hippocrates recognized the common pathway of rich foods and wines in the development of the disease and in keeping with the common treatments of the era selected the meadow saffron, Colchicum autumnale, as a treatment to induce a laxative effect to purge the system in an acute attack (Helfgott, 2013). In the case of Colchicine, what was once old is now new again. The Romans were particularly fond of their wines in copious amounts, but it was with the presence of highly toxic amounts of lead in the materials used to prepare and serve the wine that insoluble purine, quinine, was formulated which caused gout to be widespread (Helfgott, 2013). Thus the pandemic saturnine gout of the Roman Empire took its place in history. In medieval times, gout was known as the 'disease of kings' largely because of the association of a gluttonous lifestyle of rich foods and alcohol consumption. However, it wasn't until the early 1200s when Dominican monk, Randolphus of Bocking, used the term we know today as 'gout' to describe podagra (Nuki & Simkin, 2006). The word 'gout' in Latin is 'gutta,' meaning "a drop" because the disease was thought to be caused by drops of the humors seeping from the blood to the joints (Greener, 2011).

Learning Objectives

Upon completion of this chapter, the nurse will be able to:

1. Describe risk factors that contribute to the development of hyperuricemia and gout.

2. Provide examples of patient conditions (e.g., obesity, hypertension, hyperlipidemia, diabetes) associated with clinical manifestations of gout.

3. Describe appropriate treatment for the three stages of the disease.

4. Advise patients about lifestyle interventions for the prevention and management of gout, focusing on the importance of weight loss and dietary modifications.

5. Counsel patients about the appropriate medications to be used for acute and chronic gout, with a special focus on co-morbidities, medication contraindications, and drug interactions.

6. Implement a patient education program for gout to improve knowledge about the disease state, the importance of adherence to medications, and patient commitment to treatment.

Introduction (Continued)

Today we know gout to be an inflammatory condition caused by excessive production of monosodium urate crystals, a by-product of purine metabolism being deposited in synovial fluid and other tissues (Greener, 2011; Neogi, 2011). Gout is a disease that primarily affects males most commonly during the peak years of 30-50 and, less frequently, post-menopausal females (Vannucchi, 2012). Studies have shown patients with gout to have multiple co-morbidities, experience extensive loss of work, are often inadequately treated, and have higher mortality rates (Crittenden et al., 2012; Crittenden & Pillinger, 2013; Keenan et al., 2012; Zhang et al., 2006). It has been suggested that because of the worldwide notoriety, gout is frequently underestimated as a public health problem (Crittenden & Pillinger, 2013; Keenan et al., 2011). Moreover, the National Health and Nutrition Examination survey (NHANE) has listed gout as the most common form of inflammatory arthritis in the U.S (Crittenden & Pillinger, 2013).

Content Outline

I. Incidence.

A. A Rochester Epidemiology Project study showed an increase in the incidence of gout from 45.0 per 100,000 in 1977-1978 to 63.3 per 100,000 in 1995-1996. Male to female ratios were 3.3 to 1 at both time periods. Considering primary gout (excluding people with gout on diuretics), the incidence of gout increased from 20.2 to 45.9 per 100,000 (Arromdee, Michet, Crowson, O'Fallon, & Gabriel, 2002).

   1. The economic burden of gout in the U.S. has increased over the past 40 years as humans live longer; with each added decade of life, the incidence of gout reaches a rising population burden. The cost of newer treatments and even the inappropriate use of such medications add to the economic cost (Crittenden & Pillinger, 2013).

B. Prevalence.

   1. Prevalence of tophaceous gout varies among populations but increases with age and is higher in men than women with an estimated ratio of 4:1. The disparity of sex decreases in older aged women where declining levels of estrogen can have a negative effect on the excretion of uric acid in the urine.

   2. Asian populations and people of the Pacific Islands have a much higher prevalence and more severe disease.

   3. Gout affects 1-2% of adults in developed countries. The rate of gout has increased in recent decades, not only in America but in other developed countries. The increase is most likely due to dietary and lifestyle changes, greater use of medications, such as diuretics, that boost uric acid levels, and aging populations. Gout is very uncommon in underdeveloped countries.

   4. An estimated 8.3 million adults in the U.S. have experienced gout, a self-reported prevalence of 3.9% of adults (Arromdee et al., 2002; Khanna et al., 2012).

II. The rise of gout in women.

A. The frequency of gout has risen steadily in post-menopausal women.

   1. The Third National Health and Nutrition Examination Survey (NHANES III) reported a prevalence of gout in women as 3.5% in ages 60-69, 4.6% in ages 70-79, and 5.6% for ≥ 80 years old.

   2. The Rochester Epidemiologic project study reported that the incidence of gout in women has doubled over the past 20 years.

   3. Risk factors in women include higher mean levels of serum uric acid than in men with gout (women with ≥8 mg/dl were 46 times higher to develop gout), increased age, obesity, hypertension, use of diuretics, and alcohol consumption ≥ 7 ounces of pure alcohol per week.

   4. Long-term coffee consumption is associated with a lower risk of incident of gout in women.

   5. In one cohort of women (Nurses' Health Study) increased intake of sugar-sweetened soda was independently associated with an increasing risk of gout.

   6. Elderly women (≥ 65) with gout have an increased risk for acute myocardial infarction.

   7. Menopause increases the risk of gout whereas post-menopause hormone replacement therapy modestly reduces gout risk. (Bhole, de Vera, Tahman, Krishnan, & Choi, 2010; Choi & Curhan, 2010; De Vera,

4
4.1
4.2
4.3
4.4
4.5
4.6
4.7
4.8
4.9
4.10

Rahman, Bhole, Kopec, & Choi, 2010;
Hak, Curhan, Grodstein, & Choi, 2010).

III. Gout in the rheumatologist's office.

A. In the U.S., it is estimated that
rheumatologists perform fewer than 2%
of all office visits for gout, compared
with primary care physicians who see
70% and cardiologists who manage 10%
of gout sufferers (Helfgott, 2013).

IV. The economic burden of gout.

A. The rise of incidence and prevalence of gout
in the United States brings with it an increase
in the economic burden of the disease. Gout
can be expensive. Wu, Forsythe, Guerin,
Yu, Latremouille-Viau, and Tsaneva (2012)
estimated the cost of the patient with severe
treatment failure gout (characterized as six
or more gout attacks per year) as more than
$25,000/year as compared with less than
$5,000/year for patients without the disease.

B. The median number of loss of work
days for gout flares for patients less
than 65 years of age for one year was
between 30 and 60 days. Additionally,
the patient with gout experiences more
loss in days related to social activities
and self-care activities (Edwards, Sundy,
Forsythe, Blume, Pan, & Decker, 2011).

V. Gout – An inflammatory arthritis.

A. Gout is a very common form of inflammatory
arthritis predominantly seen among men
caused by an uncontrolled metabolic disorder
known as hyperuricemia. Gout can be
dormant, acute, remit for prolonged periods,
or become chronic. Generally speaking
there are three to four stages associated
with the onset and disease of gout.

1. Asymptomatic tissue deposition stage – the
asymptomatic deposition of urate crystals in
the tissues resulting from hyperuricemia. It
is important to note that hyperuricemia is an
imbalance in the production and excretion
of urate (a salt of the end byproduct of
the breakdown of purine) which can be an
overproduction, underexcretion, or both.

However, underexcretion is predominately
the cause. Additionally, hyperuricemia is
not the same as gout and asymptomatic
hyperuricemia does not need to be treated.
It is the deposition of crystals in the soft
tissues that causes the damage.

2. Acute gout flares/acute gout attacks – is the
stage where the crystals accumulate in the
joint(s). This causes the characteristic acute
redness, inflammation, intense pain, swelling,
and warmth in the joint(s), most commonly the
metatarsophalangeal joint of the big toe. Gout
attacks often begin at night. Patients will relate
they cannot stand even a light sheet over
their toe in bed. Flares or attacks can last up
to 10 days. Of particular note: Uric acid levels
in the blood stream may be normal in at least
half of patients suffering from an acute flare.
Gaffo et al., (2012) have described an empirical
definition for a gout flare from patient-
reported features as: Any patient–reported
warm joint, swollen joint, patient-reported
pain at rest score of >3 on a 0-10 scale, and
patient-reported flare symptoms validated
by a rheumatologist as a gout flare.

3. Intercritical gout – is a stage after the acute
flare where the patient may be asymptomatic
and the disease is at a clinically inactive state
before the next flare might occur. The patient
will still have hyperuricemia and continue to
deposit urate crystals in the soft tissues until
such time a flare will develop. The Intercritical
stages are known to become shorter in
duration as the disease progresses in severity.

4. Chronic gout/ chronic tophaceous gout –
chronic gout is characterized by a generalized
chronic arthritis with tender and aching joints.
Patients may develop solid deposits of urate
crystals in the joints (tophi) in the elbows, ears,
and distal finger joints. Tophi may take up to
10 years to develop after the onset of acute
gouty arthritis and have the potential to cause
permanent damage to the joints as well as
the kidneys (Crittenden & Pillinger, 2012; Hill,
2006; Schub, 2012; Teng, Nair, & Saag, 2006).

B. Risk factors/Co-morbidities.

1. Age: Usually in people over 45.

2. Gender: Affects men more often than women.

3. Obesity.

4. High blood pressure.

4
4.1
4.2
4.3
4.4
4.5
4.6
4.7
4.8
4.9
4.10

5. Consuming excessive amounts of alcohol (especially beer and hard liquor).

6. Frequent consumption of high-fructose corn syrup.

7. Eating large amounts of meat and seafood.

8. Taking medications that affect blood levels of uric acid (some diuretics).

9. Kidney disease: Hyperuricemia is a marker of worsening function.

10. Cardiovascular disease: Hyperuricemia is a marker of worsening function.

11. Diabetes.

12. Metabolic Syndrome: Hyperuricemia is a marker of worsening function.

13. Congestive heart failure.

14. Genetics: 25% of people with gout have relatives who also have gout.

15. Transplant recipients (allograft) on calcineurin antagonists (i.e., cyclosporin and tacrolimis) become hyperuricemic and 10% may develop gout.

(Choi, Willett, & Curhan, 2010; Crittenden & Pillinger, 2012; De Vera, Rahman, Bhole, Kopec, & Choi, 2010; Gibson, 2013; Neogi, 2011; Teng, Nair, & Saag, 2006; West, 2002).

C. Theories and new research related to gout.

1. Is there a neuroprotective association of gout? Gout has never been reported in patients with multiple sclerosis and very low incidence in patients with Parkinson's, amyotrophic lateral sclerosis, and Alzheimer's (Helfgott, 2013).

2. Homocysteine (a marker of cardiovascular disease) was highly prevalent in a European survey of patients with gout along with low levels of folate and cobalamine and high levels of urate (Slot, 2013).

3. Colchicine use in patients with gout may have an associated lower C-reactive protein levels, lower prevalence of myocardial infarctions, and overall mortality rates as compared to patients with gout not on colchicine. The exact mechanism of action of colchicine in this cardio-protective effect requires further study (Crittenden et al., 2012).

4. Uric acid may play a role in the development and progression of osteoarthritis. Interleukin -1beta (IL -1β) is one of the cytokines most strongly associated with osteoarthritis. This association has yet to be completely validated and more research is warranted (Denoble et al., 2011).

5. There are three new modalities of interest for gout imaging currently in research. These are MRI, ultrasound, and dual energy CT. While this technology may be used for research and not play a routine role in clinical care currently there are open options for diagnostic and treatment decisions for the future (Crittenden & Pillinger, 2012).

6. Research has shown IL -1β antagonists as a key cytokine influencing the inflammation of acute gout. Active studies are testing agents that either block IL -1β directly or interfere with the signal/receptor in order to decrease the IL -1β effects (Crittenden & Pillinger 2013).

7. Humans lack the ability to create uricase in order to metabolize and excrete urate and its metabolites. Another area of current research is on the development of more effective uricosuric agents (Crittenden & Pillinger, 2013).

8. New research has shown erectile dysfunction (ED) is present with men diagnosed with gout at a significantly greater proportion to men without gout (Schlesinger, Radvanski, Fischkoff , Kostis, 2014).

D. Diagnosis of gout.

1. Key laboratory tests that may be ordered:

   a. CBC may show leukocytosis during an acute attack.

   b. Serum levels of uric acid may be elevated >6.8 mg/dL.

   c. Urinalysis may show elevated levels of uric acid and creatinine.

   d. Synovial fluid aspirated from the infected joint will have a cytologic examination that reveals presence of needle shaped urate crystals (Schub, 2012).

E. Drugs associated with causing hyperuricemia due to decreased renal excretion of urate.

4
4.1
4.2
4.3
4.4
4.5
4.6
4.7
4.8
4.9
4.10

1. Use the mnemonic "can't leap":

   C - Cyclosporine   **L** - Lasix
                                     (furosemide and
                                     other loop diuretics)
   A - Alcohol   **E** - Ethambutol
   N - Nicotinic Acid   **A** - Aspirin (low dose)
   T - Thiazides   **P** – Pyrazinamide
   (Janson, 2002).

F. Pharmacological treatment.

1. Pharmacological treatment for gout has changed considerably in the past several years. Old standards of NSAIDs, corticosteroids, and the standbys of colchicine, allopurinol, and probenecid were once all that was available. Increased understanding of gout pathogenesis has led to newer compounds acting on the inhibition of xanthine oxidase, interference of ligand-ligand receptor interactions, as well as the introduction of genetically engineered uricase. Yet, the arsenal for treatment of gout remains severely limited especially where co-morbidities further complicate effective treatment options due to contraindications of drug-to-drug and disease-to-drug interactions. Urate lowering therapy has been recommended as prophylaxis against acute gout attacks for about six months (Gaffo et al., 2012). Clinical studies are ongoing for new targets such as the IL-1β blockade, urate lowering agents, and uricosuric agents. The following is a current list of approved pharmacological treatments (see Table 1).

2. Potential gout medication.

a. Table 1 was created by the Gout & Uric Acid Education Society. Prescribing gout medications in the presence of co-morbidities with potential contraindications is a challenge. Decisions are made based on the limited array of gout treatments, individual clinical findings, and an educated decision weighing the risks/benefits of treatment. Monitoring of gout treatment from a rheumatologist's office is optimal (Gelber & Soloman, 2012; Keenan et al., 2011).

VI. Nursing implications.

A. Although different patients experience similar clinical manifestations of gout, the nurse should provide individualized care to fit the needs of each patient. Some of the nursing implications that should be taking into consideration are as follows:

1. Good communication.

a. Inform the patient about the disease process. Gout is potentially remediable, especially by lifestyle interventions and proper drug therapies.

b. The patient should understand the target and practicalities of any drug therapy.

c. The patient should understand how to prevent and manage flares and most importantly, recognize dietary factors and lifestyle changes as vitally important to the management of the disease.

2. Acute gout attacks.

a. Reassure the patient that he or she will recover from an acute gout attack, even without treatment, typically within seven days.

b. Management of the gout attack itself includes resting the afflicted joint for one to two days and applying cold packs to help alleviate some pain. Instruct patient always to use ice, never heat, because heat can exacerbate the inflammation and pain.

c. Drug therapy during the acute phase - instruct the patient that taking high doses of rapid acting oral nonsteroidal anti-inflammatory drugs will put them at an increased risk for peptic ulcers, and other GI bleeds. Encourage the use of gastro-protective agents in conjunction with this type of therapy.

3. Nutritional Approaches to Gout Prevention and Treatment.

a. If obese, prevent recurrence of gout attacks begin by gradually losing weight. However, caution patients with gout to avoid crash dieting and diets that are high in protein and low in carbohydrate.

b. Encourage patients to switch to skim milk and low-fat yogurt, to increase use of soybeans and vegetable sources of proteins in their diet, to limit consumption of foods rich in purines like red meats and game, to avoid liver and shellfish, and to restrict an overall large dietary percentage of protein intake. Other foods high in purines to limit are mushrooms, yeast, oatmeal, spinach, asparagus, other beans, peas, and lentils.

4
4.1
4.2
4.3
4.4
4.5
4.6
4.7
4.8
4.9
4.10

Table 1. Urate Lowering Therapies – These are life-long therapies

Name	Dosage	Special Instructions	Possible Side Effects	Be Aware
Allopurinol *Lopurin®, Zyloprim®*	100 to 800 mg per day in a single dose. The dose is started and adjusted by 100 mg every two to four weeks to achieve a serum uric acid level lower than 6.0/dL.	Take immediately after a meal. Stop taking medication at the first sign of a rash, which may indicate an allergic or hypersensitivity reaction. May need to give as BID in doses over 300 mg/day to avoid nausea.	Rash, hives or itching; nausea; transaminase elevation, rare severe cutaneous reactions occur in approximately 1 in 250-300 patient starts.	Never start or stop allopurinol during a gout attack. **Minimize attacks by initially prescribing lower doses along with colchicine or NSAIDs and until goal of a uric acid level of ≤ 6.0 mg. is reached.** Caution with azothioprine, 6-mercaptopurine and theophylline.
Febuxostat *Uloric®*	40 mg per day initially then increase to 80 mg per day in two weeks if serum uric acid level not lower than 6.0 mg.	Take any time of day without regard to food or antacid use.	Elevated liver enzymes (liver irritation); nausea; joint pain; rash.	Never start or stop febuxostat during a gout attack. **Minimize attacks by prescribing colchicine or NSAIDs at the time of initiating treatment and until goal of a uric acid level of ≤ 6.0 mg. is reached.** Contraindicated with azothioprine, 6-mercaptopurine and theophylline.
Pegloticase *Krystexxa®*	8 mgs given IV every 2 weeks.	For use in difficult to control hyperuricemia and chronic gout.	Infusion reactions including fever, nausea, and hypotension.	This drug should be given in a monitored infusion center.
Probenecid *Benemid®, Probalan®*	500 to 3,000 mg per day in two or three divided doses.	Take with food or an antacid. Drink plenty of fluids. Do not take with aspirin or other NSAIDs. Avoid alcohol.	Headache; loss of appetite; nausea or vomiting.	Ineffective in patients with GFR less than 50. Should not be used with history of kidney stones.
Probenecid and colchicine *ColBenemid®, Col-Probenecid®, Proben-C®*	One tablet (contains 500 mg probenecid and 0.5 mg colchicine) twice per day.	Take with food or an antacid. Drink plenty of fluids. Do not take with aspirin or other NSAIDs. Avoid alcohol.	Diarrhea; headache; loss of appetite; nausea or vomiting; stomach pain; rash.	Ineffective in patients with GFR less than 50. Should not be used with history of kidney stones.

4
4.1
4.2
4.3
4.4
4.5
4.6
4.7
4.8
4.9
4.10

Therapies to Relieve Pain and Reduce Swelling of Acute Gout

Name	Dosage	Special Instructions	Possible Side Effects	Be Aware
Colchicine *Colcrys®*	Two tablets (1.2 mg) immediately then one tablet (0.6 mg) after one hour. Then one tablet twice or three times daily for one week.	Take with food if stomach upset occurs. Drink plenty of fluids.	Diarrhea; nausea or vomiting; stomach pain.	High dose colchicine for acute flares is inappropriate. Colchicine should be used with caution in people with renal disease and those with bone marrow suppression.
Glucocorticosteroids Methylprednisolone *(Medrol®)*;Prednisone *(Deltasone®)*; Triamcinolone *(Kenalog®)*	Kenalog 60 mgs x1, followed by low dose steroids or oral prednisone given at 30 mg with a taper to 0 mg over 10 days.		Retention of sodium (salt) and fluids; weight gain; high blood pressure; loss of potassium; poor glucose control; and headache.	Particularly useful for those with chronic kidney disease. Use with caution in patients with diabetes.
Nonsteroidal anti-inflammatory drugs (NSAIDs) Celecoxib *(Celebrex®)*; Ibuprofen *(Advil®)*; Indomethacin *(Indocin®)*; Naproxen *(Aleve®, Naprosyn®)*.	High dose of any non-steroidal given for first 3 days, followed by moderate doses for an additional 7 days.		Nausea; stomach discomfort; retention of sodium; and fluids; dyspepsia; gastric ulcers; and headache.	May interact with blood pressure and heart medications, especially in the elderly. Use caution in patients with a history of GI ulcers, kidney disease, and the elderly.

Anti-Inflammatory Prophylaxis for Prevention of Gout Flares

Name	Dosage	Special Instructions	Possible Side Effects	Be Aware
Colchicine *Colcrys®*	One or two tablets (0.6 mgs) per day. 1.2 mgs maximum per day. Patients with severe kidney disease may only need one tablet every other day or every third day, depending on creatinine clearance.	Take with food if stomach upset occurs. Drink plenty of fluids.	Diarrhea; nausea or vomiting; stomach pain.	Some people are very sensitive to colchicine. If diarrhea or abdominal pains occur, dosage should be reduced.
Nonsteroidal anti-inflammatory drugs (NSAIDs)	Low dose of any non-steroidal may be used prophylactically following the first six months of urate lowering therapy.		Nausea; stomach discomfort; retention of sodium; and fluids; dyspepsia; gastric ulcers; and headache.	May interact with blood pressure and heart medications, especially in the elderly. Use caution in patients with a history of GI ulcers, kidney disease, and the elderly. Ulcers may occur without any preceding symptoms.

4
4.1
4.2
4.3
4.4
4.5
4.6
4.7
4.8
4.9
4.10

c. Encourage drinking more than 2 liters of water daily and avoiding dehydration.

d. Limit alcohol consumption. Teach patients to avoid hard liquor, beer (or limit to 1-2 glasses per day), stout, port, and other fortified wines.

e. Recent studies have shown some benefit to the reduction and recurrence of gout attacks in some animal models and in a very few human models with the consumption of fresh cherries and/or cherry extract. The high levels of anthocyanin in cherries have anti-inflammatory as well as antioxidant properties. Cherries, specifically the tart Montmorency cherries, also contain high levels of Vitamin C. More research is needed on this interesting complimentary therapy.

f. Fructose, most commonly found with the additive corn syrup in processed foods and beverages, has been associated with an increased risk of incidental gout. The pathways believed because by increasing adenosine triphosphate degradation to uric acid precursor adenosine monophosphate. More research is needed in this area. (Greener, 2011; Gelber & Soloman, 2012; Zhang, Neogi, Chen, Chaisson, Hunter, & Choi, 2012).

Summary

Gout or gouty arthritis is one of the oldest documented diseases in human history. As a piercingly painful inflammatory arthritis, gout, in the US is on the rise in men and women. Gout is typically diagnosed and treated in the general practitioner's/primary physician's office rather than the rheumatologist. However, being a more common inflammatory arthritis, the importance for the rheumatology nurse to understand the mechanism of disease and actions of medications for treatment are not only necessary for daily practice but useful in consultations to provide the best practice and evidence-based treatment and care.

References

Arromdee, E., Michet, C.J., Crowson, C.S., O'Fallon, W.M., & Gabriel, S.E. (2002). Epidemiology of gout: Is the incidence rising? *Journal of Rheumatology,* 29 2403–2406.

Choi, H. K., & Curhan, G. (2010). Coffee consumption and risk of incident gout in women: The Nurses' Health Study. *American Journal of Clinical Nutrition,* 92(4), 922-927. doi: 10.3945/ajcn.2010.29565.

Choi, H. K., Willett, W., & Curhan, G. (2010). Fructose-rich beverages and risk of gout in women. *Journal of the American Medical Association,* 304(20), 2270-2278. doi: 10.1001/jama.2010.1638.

Crittenden, D. B., Lehmann, R. A., Schneck, L., Keenan, R. T., Shah, B., Greenberg, J. D., . . . Pillinger, M. H. (2012). Colchicine use is associated with decreased prevalence of myocardial infarction in patients with gout. *Journal of Rheumatology,* 39(7), 1458-1464. doi: 10.3899/jrheum.111533.

Crittenden, D. B., & Pillinger, M. H. (2012). The year in gout: 2011-2012. *Bulletin of the NYU Hospital for Joint Diseases,* 70(3), 145-151.

Crittenden, D. B., & Pillinger, M. H. (2013). New therapies for gout. *Annual Review of Medicine,* 64, 325-337. doi: 10.1146/annurev-med-080911-105830.

Denoble, A. E., Huffman, K. M., Stabler, T. V., Kelly, S. J., Hershfield, M. S., McDaniel, G. E., . . . Kraus, V. B. (2011). Uric acid is a danger signal of increasing risk for osteoarthritis through inflammasome activation. *Proceedings from the National Academy of Science U S A,* 108(5), 2088-2093. doi: 10.1073/pnas.1012743108.

De Vera, M. A., Rahman, M. M., Bhole, V., Kopec, J. A., & Choi, H. K. (2010). Independent impact of gout on the risk of acute myocardial infarction among elderly women: A population-based study. *Annals of the Rheumatic Diseases,* 69(6), 1162-1164. doi: 10.1136/ard.2009.122770.

Edwards, N. L., Sundy, J. S., Forsythe, A., Blume, S., Pan, F., & Becker, M. A. (2011). Work productivity loss due to flares in patients with chronic gout refractory to conventional therapy. *Journal of Medical Economics,* 14(1), 10-15. doi: 10.3111/13696998.2010.540874.

Gaffo, A. L., Schumacher, H. R., Saag, K. G., Taylor, W. J., Dinnella, J., Outman, R., . . . Singh, J. A. (2012). Developing a provisional definition of flare in patients with established gout. *Arthritis & Rheumatism,* 64(5), 1508-1517. doi: 10.1002/art.33483.

4
4.1
4.2
4.3
4.4
4.5
4.6
4.7
4.8
4.9
4.10

Gelber, A. C., & Solomon, D. H. (2012). If life serves up a bowl of cherries, and gout attacks are "the pitts": Implications for therapy. *Arthritis & Rheumatism*, 64(12), 3827-3830. doi: 10.1002/art.34676.

Gibson, T. J. (2013). Hypertension, its treatment, hyperuricaemia and gout. *Current Opinions in Rheumatology*, 25(2), 217-222. doi:10.1097/BOR.0b013e32835cedd4.

Greener, M. (2011). For an effective management of gout. *Nurse Prescribing, 9*(7), 342-346.

Hak, A. E., Curhan, G. C., Grodstein, F., & Choi, H. K. (2010). Menopause, postmenopausal hormone use and risk of incident gout. *Annals of the Rheumatic Diseases*, 69(7), 1305-1309. doi: 10.1136/ard.2009.109884.

Helfgott, S. M. (2013, January). Was gout rampant among the Romans? *The Rheumatologist*.

Hill, J. (2006). *Rheumatology nursing: A creative approach* (2nd ed.). Chichester, UK: John Wiley & Sons.

Janson, R. W. (2002). Gout. In S.G. West (Ed.), *Rheumatology secrets* (2nd ed., pp.325-333). Philadelphia: Hanley & Belfus.

Keenan, R. T., O'Brien, W. R., Lee, K. H., Crittenden, D. B., Fisher, M. C., Goldfarb, D. S., . . . Pillinger, M. H. (2011). Prevalence of contraindications and prescription of pharmacologic therapies for gout. *American Journal of Medicine*, 124(2), 155-163. doi: 10.1016/j.amjmed.2010.09.012.

Khanna, D., Fitzgerald, J. D., Khanna, P. P., Bae, S., Singh, M. K., Neogi, T., . . . Terkeltaub, R. (2012). 2012 American College of Rheumatology guidelines for management of gout. Part 1: Systematic nonpharmacologic and pharmacologic therapeutic approaches to hyperuricemia. *Arthritis Care & Research (Hoboken), 64*, 1431-1446. doi:10.1002/acr.21772.

Neogi, T. (2011). Gout. *New England Journal of Medicine, 364*(5), 443-452. doi: 10.1056/NEJMcp1001124.

Nuki, G., & Simkin, P. A. (2006). A concise history of gout and hyperuricemia and their treatment. Arthritis Research & Therapy, 8(Suppl 1:S1). doi: 10.1186/ar1906.

Schlesinger, N., Radvanski, D.C., Fischkoff, J., & Kostis, J.B., (2014) Erectile dysfunction is common among gout patients. Paris, France: EULAR; Abstract Number OP0135.

Schub, T. (2012). Gout. In D. Pravikoff (Ed.), (pp. 2p). Glendale, California: Cinahl Information Systems.

Slot, O. (2013). Homocysteine, a marker of cardiovascular disease risk, is markedly elevated in patients with gout. *Annals of the Rheumatic Diseases*, 72(3), 457. doi: 10.1136/annrheumdis-2012-202023.

Teng, G. G., Nair, R., & Saag, K. G. (2006). Pathophysiology, clinical presentation and treatment of gout. *Drugs*, 66(12), 1547-1563.

Vannucchi, P. (2012). Understanding, diagnosing, and treating gout. *Podiatry Management, 31*(4), 191-200.

West, S. G. (2002). *Rheumatology secrets* (2nd ed.). Philadelphia: Hanley & Belfus.

Wu, E. Q., Forsythe, A., Guerin, A., Yu, A. P., Latremouille-Viau, D., & Tsaneva, M. (2012). Comorbidity burden, healthcare resource utilization, and costs in chronic gout patients refractory to conventional urate-lowering therapy. *American Journal of Therapeutics*, 19(6), e157-166. doi: 10.1097/MJT.0b013e31820543c5.

Zhang, Y., Neogi, T., Chen, C., Chaisson, C., Hunter, D. J., & Choi, H. K. (2012). Cherry consumption and decreased risk of recurrent gout attacks. *Arthritis & Rheumatism*, 64(12), 4004-4011. doi: 10.1002/art.34677.

Zhang, W., Doherty, M., Bardin, T., Pascual, E., Barskova, V., Conaghan, P., . . . Zimmermann-Gorska, I. (2006). EULAR evidence based recommendations for gout. Part II: Management report of a task force of the EULAR Standing Committee for International Clinical Studies Including Therapeutics (ESCISIT). *Annals of Rheumatic Disease, 65*(10), 1312-1324. doi: 10.1136/ard.2006.055269

4
4.1
4.2
4.3
4.4
4.5
4.6
4.7
4.8
4.9
4.10

Section 4.7
Vasculitis

Ruth Busch, MSN, APRN, BC

Introduction

Vasculitis refers to a group of conditions characterized by inflammation of the blood vessel walls. This condition is often considered in patients who present with malaise, fever, and joint or muscle pain as well as organ system dysfunction (Firestein, Budd, Gabreil, McInnes, & O'Dell, 2012).

Classification of this disease is associated with the size of the vessel that is affected. For example, temporal arteritis and Takayaksu's Arteritis are considered large vessel vasculidities. Behçet's Syndrome is unique in that it can affect blood vessels of any size (Latinis, Dao, Gutierrez, Shepherd, & Velazquez, 2004). Diagnosis begins with assigning a vessel size based on the patient's presentation with signs and symptoms and compared with lab data. Other testing may include urinalysis, renal biopsy, abdominal ultrasound, pulmonary function tests, and high resolution CT of lungs. Once vessel size is determined, all characteristics of conditions in that classification should be analyzed (Firestein et al., 2012).

Vessel involvement can be determined by presentation at history and physical exam. Small vessel vasculitis is seen as palpable purpura, mononeuritis multiplex, superficial ulcerations, and RBC casts in the urine. Medium vessel disease is observed in individuals who have cutaneous nodules, papilonecrotic lesions, digital infarction, and livedo reticularis. Pulse discrepancies and bruits are seen in large vessel vasculitis (Latinis et al., 2004).

Organ dysfunction helps in the diagnosis as well. In renal failure, glomerulonephritis can be small vessel. Renal infarct or chronic renal ischemia can occur with medium or large vessel disease. Pulmonary disease, generally presents with hemoptysis, can affect small vessels in alveolar hemorrhage and medium vessels in bronchial artery aneurism rupture (Firestein et al., 2012).

The average time from onset of symptoms to diagnosis is 19 months (Latinis et al., 2004). At this time, there is no cure. Patients may achieve remission, but relapse is common. The purpose of this chapter is to describe the pathophysiology, diagnostic criteria, treatment, and nursing care of the patient with vasculitis (Firestein et al., 2012).

Learning Objectives

Upon completion of this chapter, the nurse will be able to:

1. Define and classify the various forms of vasculitis.

2. Describe the epidemiology and pathogenesis of vasculitis.

3. Identify the American College of Rheumatology symptoms and laboratory criteria that support the diagnosis of vasculitis.

4. Identify the potential impact of vasculitis on various areas of the body.

5. Describe current drug therapy and disease management of the patient with vasculitis.

6. Describe potential co-morbid conditions that may develop from the disease and the medications used to control the disease and its symptoms.

7. Develop a management plan to meet the individual patient's needs.

Content Outline

I. Giant cell arteritis (GCA).

A. Pathophysiology.

1. Both humeral (macro-molecule) and cellular (cell-mediated) immunity involved.

2. Endothelial leukocyte adhesion molecules (IL-6) and other immune complexes have been observed in patients with GCA and polymyalgia rheumatica. Whether an individual develops polymyalgia rheumatica (PMR) or GCA may depend on activation of certain cytokines.

3. Cytotoxic T cells may occur in some patients. Associated with HLA-DRB1 gene.

4. Temporal, vertebral, ophthalmic, and ciliary arteries are most likely to be affected. The intima of the vessel wall is thickened; cellular infiltration with lymphocytes and multinucleated giant cells are present (Firestein et al., 2012).

B. Granulomas, necrosis of the vessel wall may be present (Latinis et al., 2012). Etiology/epidemiology of giant cell arteritis.

1. Occurrence varies widely, most common in individuals >50 years of age (Coblyn, Bermas, Weinblatt, & Helfgott, 2011; Firestein et al., 2012).

2. Highest incidence in people of Scandinavian and in Americans of Scandinavian descent Incidence much lower in African-Americans, northern Indians, and the Japanese.

3. More common in the northern portion of Europe than southern. Increased provider awareness may have caused increase in numbers of individuals with GCA because of recognition and early diagnosis.

4. Association with human leukocyte antigen (HLA) class II region.

5. Women who smoke have a six-fold risk of developing GCA. Some evidence for link with Mycoplasma pneumonia, varicella zoster virus, parainfluenza virus type 1, parvovirus B19, or herpes virus DNA, and Clamydia peumoniae, but has not been consistent.

6. Occurs more frequently in women than men (2:1). Diabetes increases the risk.

7. May have greater chance of developing thoracic aneurisms; mortality rate similar.

8. PMR and GCA both associated with same HLA DR4 genes.

9. PMR is more common than GCA (Firestein et al., 2012).

C. Nursing assessment.

1. Understand the need to confirm the diagnosis and begin appropriate therapy when life altering disease is present.

2. Implement appropriate laboratory studies and imaging, and interpret the results to verify or rule out a diagnosis of vasculitis.

3. If a biopsy has been performed, assess site and instruct the patient on appropriate wound care.

4. When treatment has begun.

   a. Assess for tolerance and compliance with medications.

   b. Assess for flares: Number since last office visit (if patient being seen in rheumatologist's office), severity (did it interfere with work, family life?).

   c. What triggered the flare, what relieved symptoms?

   d. Specific symptoms associated with the flare.

5. Assess ability to accomplish activities of daily living, manage stress, participate in work, family, and social life activities.

6. Physical assessment with additional focus on systems affected by the disease to determine improvement or worsening of condition.

D. Diagnosis.

1. Occurs primarily in people between the ages of 50-90 (Coblyn et al., 2011); more common in women.

2. Sudden onset or may develop over time (Firestein et al., 2012).

3. Most common symptom is headache, which can be accompanied by jaw claudication, and visual symptoms (Firestein et al., 2012).

4
4.1
4.2
4.3
4.4
4.5
4.6
4.7
4.8
4.9
4.10

4. Scalp pain as well as presence of PMR constitutional symptoms such as fever, fatigue, anorexia, weight loss (Fauci & Langford, 2006).

5. Rated at moderate severity, not a typical headache, and located in the temporal area.

6. Some headaches are so severe that the patient presents to the emergency room for treatment.

7. Changes in the temporal artery such as nodules, swelling, tenderness with palpation or loss of pulse (Coblyn et al., 2011) only occur in about one half of those with GCA (Firestein et al., 2012).

8. Visual symptoms can affect one eye or both, cause double or blurred vision or double vision.

9. Vision changes that last greater than 4 hours generally do not reverse. Occlusion of the posterior ciliary artery can cause ischemic neuropathy resulting in loss of vision. May also occur with inflammation of the retinal artery or an occlusion. Pallor and edema of the optic disc can be seen on physical exam. Cotton wool spots and small hemorrhages with edema can be present, leading to optic nerve degeneration. Ophthalmoplegia, weakness of the muscles controlling eye movement, is another complication of GCA. Diplopia from ischemia and ocular motor nerve palsies generally improve after therapy has begun.

10. Claudication in the muscles of the jaw or in muscles of the extremities may be present.

11. May involve one side of the mandible more than the other (Firestein et al., 2012).

E. Laboratory studies.

1. Lab results in PMR similar to GCA.

   a. Typically sedimentation rates are greater than 100mm/hr.; C-reactive protein is elevated as well. A normal sedimentation rate does not rule out GCA, especially in the presence of classic symptoms.

   b. Other lab results:

      (1) Rheumatoid factor and anti-nuclear antibody are usually negative.

      (2) Plasma proteins are nonspecific if present. There can be increase in complement.

(3) Renal and hepatic function tests are generally normal. Enzymes associated with muscle pain or damage are typically normal (Firestein et al., 2012).

F. Temporal artery biopsy.

1. Not always predicted by lab values (Coblyn et al., 2011).

2. Preferred method for diagnosing GCA (Coblyn et al., 2011).

3. Biopsy should include a palpable abnormality or a section that measures several centimeters long (Latinis et al., 2004).

4. If biopsy on the symptomatic side is negative, and GCA continues to be suspected, a biopsy on the other side should be performed (Coblyn et al., 2011).

5. Temporal artery biopsies very important in determining the need for steroid therapy.

6. Biopsy occipital artery if the patient complains of headache in the occipital area.

7. If both biopsies are negative, may need to look for large vessel disease with imaging studies. Aortic or abdominal aneurisms are best evaluated by MRI or CT (Firestein et al., 2012).

G. Treatment.

1. Begin glucocorticoid therapy in presumed diagnosis of GCA (Coblyn et al., 2011).

   a. Prevent loss of vision.

H. Biopsy is typically not altered by steroids for two weeks (Firestein et al., 2012).

1. Prednisone 40-60 mg daily (Coblyn et al., 2011).

   a. Use divided doses for the first 1-2 weeks to hasten improvement.

   b. With vision loss, 1000 mg/day IV methylprednisolone x 3 days has been used, but not always successful. Reduce by 10% of the total dose every one to two weeks after four weeks of initial therapy; however, 2 months of initial levels of therapy may be required (Firestein et al., 2012).

I. Based on symptoms and laboratory values.

J. Most require treatment for one to two years.

4
4.1
4.2
4.3
4.4
4.5
4.6
4.7
4.8
4.9
4.10

1. Common side effects include depression, psychosis, and mood swings.

    a. Hypertension, congestive heart failure.

    b. Hyperglycemia.

    c. Weight gain, peptic ulcer disease.

    d. Masks infections, slows wound healing, triggers acne, thins the skin, causes skin to bruise easily.

    e. Muscle weakness in long term use, osteoporosis.

    f. May cause cataracts or will worsen existing cataracts, glaucoma.

    g. Contraindications: Active infections (Doherty, 2010).

K. Methotrexate (MTX) in combination with prednisone has been studied, but no convincing evidence that this is effective (Fauci & Langford, 2006).

L. TNF agents have been studied and demonstrated no effectiveness in this disease.

M. Treat other vessels affected by GCA.

    1. Subclavian and axillary arteries improve upper extremity claudication with corticosteroids.

    2. Thoracic aortic aneurism is in increased in GCA, most commonly seen an average of 7 years after diagnosis. Chest X-ray used to detect thoracic aortic aneurisms (Firestein et al., 2012).

    3. Treat chronic diseases such as osteoporosis, hypertension, diabetes, and hyperlipidemia, if present.

    4. Encourage smoking cessation.

        a. Decrease alcohol consumption if excessive.

        b. Recommend daily physical activity, preferably weight bearing.

        c. Suggest weight reduction, if appropriate.

II. Takayasu's Arteritis.

A. Pathology.

    1. Large vessel disease (Fauci & Langford, 2006).

    2. Affects aorta and the major branches, as well as pulmonary and coronary arteries (Fauci & Langford, 2006).

B. Vessels are found to be thickened and fixed. Occlusion, thrombosis, or aneurisms.

C. Alternating normal lumen, with occlusions or aneurisms.

D. Involvement in all 3 layers of the blood vessel:

    1. Vasa vasorum (outer layer) linked with lymphocytes and plasma cells.

        a. Media neovascularization.

        b. Intima fibroblast and smooth muscle cell proliferation.

    2. Aortitis: Fibrosis in all layers and occurs with above, demonstrating a repeated pattern (Firestein et al., 2012).

    3. TAK occurs as a result of systemic chronic inflammation or occlusion or aneurism formation (Latinis et al., 2004).

E. Etiology and epidemiology.

    1. Usually <50 years of age, peak onset at 3rd decade.

    2. Women > men (8:1 ratio) (Firestein et al., 2012); women ages 15-25 (Coblyn et al., 2011).

    3. Average time between symptom onset and diagnosis is 19 months (Latinis et al., 2004).

    4. Most commonly found in Japan (150 cases / million/year), China, India, and Southeast Asia.

    5. Also prevalent in Mexico.

    6. Europe and America (0.2-2.6 cases per million/year).

    7. Onset of disease is generally 25 years, although 25% of cases were diagnosed before the age of 20 and 20% occurred after the age of 40.

    8. Japanese studies have shown a possible association with several HLAs.

    9. Koreans and Indians have associated different HLAs.

    10. There is no HLA association in people with TAK in North America (Firestein et al., 2012).

    11. The population with TAK in Mexico has been associated with Mycobacterium tuberculosis exposure (Firestein et al., 2012).

4
4.1
4.2
4.3
4.4
4.5
4.6
4.7
4.8
4.9
4.10

F. Nursing assessment.

1. Understand the need to confirm the diagnosis and begin appropriate therapy when life altering disease is present.

2. Implement appropriate laboratory studies and imaging, and interpret the results to verify or rule out a diagnosis of vasculitis.

3. If a biopsy has been performed, assess site and instruct the patient on appropriate wound care.

4. When treatment has begun.

   a. Assess for tolerance and compliance with medications.

   b. Assess for flares.

   c. Number since last office visit (if patient is being treated in rheumatologist's office), severity (did it interfere with work, family life?).

5. What triggered the flare, what relieved symptoms?

6. Specific symptoms associated with the flare.

7. Assess ability to accomplish activities of daily living, manage stress, participate in work, family, and social life activities.

8. Physical assessment with additional focus on systems affected by the disease to determine improvement or worsening of condition.

G. Diagnosis.

1. Based on history and physical.

2. Based on American College of Rheumatology (ACR) Classification Criteria for Takayasu's Arteritis (Arend et al., 1990), the presence of 3 or more of the following 6 criteria is 91% sensitive and 98% specific for the diagnosis of TAK.

   a. Age at disease onset < 40 years.

   b. Claudication of extremities.

   c. Decreased brachial artery pulse.

   d. BP difference >10mm Hg Difference of >10mm Hg in systolic blood pressure between arms.

   e. Bruit over subclavian arteries or aorta.

   f. Arteriogram abnormality: Arteriographic narrowing or occlusion of the entire aorta, its primary branches, or large arteries in the proximal upper or lower extremities, not due to arteriosclerosis, fibromuscular dysplasia, or similar causes; changes usually focal or segmental (Firestein et al., 2012).

3. Three phase disease process.

   a. Constitutional stage: Malaise, fever, weight loss.

   b. Vessel inflammation stage: Vessel tenderness or pain with palpation.

   c. Fibrotic stage: Burn out stage- ischemic signs and symptoms.

4. Limitations: Less than 16% of patients will have constitutional symptoms, but many will have inflammation and ischemic signs at the same time (Latinis et al., 2004).

5. Signs and symptoms.

   a. Most patients present with symptoms of vascular insufficiency (stenosis, occlusion, or aneurism).

   b. Claudication.

      (1) Weakness in arms, fatigue such as when raising arms to dry hair.

      (2) Occurs in the upper extremities twice as often as in the lower extremities.

      (3) Reduced or absent pulse.

   c. Carotid bruit.

      (1) Most common sign, usually in carotid, but also present in supraclavicular, infraclavicular, axillary, chest, flank, abdominal, and femoral areas.

      (2) May have more than one bruit.

      (3) Hypertension, carotidynia, lightheadedness. Stroke.

      (4) Asymmetrical blood pressure occurs in about ½ of the patients. Fewer than 10% of patients present with stroke, aortic regurgitation or visual abnormalities.

      (5) Visual abnormalities that lead to blindness are less common in TAK than in Temporal Arteritis. Claudication in the upper extremities occurs twice that of claudication in the lower extremities.

6. Constitutional symptoms are common.

   a. Fever, malaise, weight loss, night sweats.

   b. May have fever of unknown origin prior to TAK.

   c. Myalgia, arthralgia, mid-thoracic back pain.

4
4.1
4.2
4.3
4.4
4.5
4.6
4.7
4.8
4.9
4.10

7. Cardiac involvement.

   a. Aortic regurgitation, can lead to congestive heart failure.

   b. Can affect coronary arteries.

     (1) Myocarditis.

   c. Pulmonary arteries.

     (1) Chest wall pain, cough (persistent dry), dyspnea, and hemoptysis.

   d. Cutaneous.

     (1) Appears in fewer than 10% of patients.

     (2) Erythema nodosum, most common.

     (3) Purpura, ulcerations, livedo reticularis (Firestein et al., 2012).

8. Laboratory findings.

   a. Sedimentation rate and C reactive protein (CRP) are elevated.

   b. Mild anemia, hypergammaglobulinemia.

   c. White blood cell generally normal.

9. Platelet count is commonly elevated.

10. Serum creatinine and urinalysis are generally normal, unless there is renal involvement.

11. Abnormal renal function tests, if abnormal, are generally secondary to hypertension (glomerulonephritis is rare in TAK) (Firestein et al., 2012).

H. Imaging studies.

1. Conventional angiography.

   a. Gold standard for image quality, allows for dangerous (culprit) atheromatic plaque (CAP) measurement, allows angioplasty at the same time.

   b. Invasive, exposure to radiation, will not visualize cell wall thickness (Firestein et al., 2012).

2. Magnetic resonance angiography (MRA).

   a. Excellent image quality, noninvasive, no radiation exposure, can visualize vessel wall thickness.

3. Image quality less than angiography, cannot be used if the patient has a pacemaker; cannot perform CAP measurement (Firestein et al., 2012).

4. Ultrasonography.

   a. Noninvasive, no radiation exposure, vessel wall edema can be measured, can visualize vessel edema.

   b. Quality of images less than angiography, obesity affects visualization, operator dependent, unable to perform CAP measurement (Firestein et al., 2012).

5. Computed tomography angiography.

   a. Quality images obtained.

   b. Radiation exposure, CAP measurement not possible, intravenous (IV) contrast necessary (Firestein et al., 2012).

6. Positron emission tomography.

   a. Measures the intensity of vascular inflammation.

   b. Radiation exposure, unable to see vascular anatomy, unable to measure CAP and IV contrast is needed (Firestein et al., 2012).

I. Treatment.

1. Goal is to reduce symptoms and achieve remission.

2. Medical therapy.

   a. Steroids–foundation of treatment.

     (1) Prednisone 0.5-1 mg/kg/day for active disease (Coblyn et al., 2011; Firestein et al., 2012).

     (2) Continue for 4-12 weeks before beginning a slow taper.

     (3) Relapses common when prednisone is less than 20 mg daily (Firestein et al., 2012).

     (4) Common side effects include depression, psychosis, and mood swings.

       i) Hypertension, congestive heart failure.

       ii) Hyperglycemia.

       iii) Weight gain, peptic ulcer disease.

       iv) Masks infections, slows wound healing, triggers acne, thins the skin which bruises easily.

       v) Muscle weakness in long term use, osteoporosis.

       vi) May cause cataracts or will worsen existing cataracts, glaucoma.

       vii) Contraindications: Active infections (Doherty, 2010).

4
4.1
4.2
4.3
4.4
4.5
4.6
4.7
4.8
4.9
4.10

3. Disease-modifying antirheumatic drugs (DMARDs).

    a. Relapses can be treated with an increase in prednisone or adding a DMARD.

    b. MTX (oral) begin with 0.3 mg /kg/wk, can be increased to 25 mg weekly.

    c. Often requires combination of prednisone and MTX for adequate therapy.

    d. Common side effects of MTX include gastric intolerance, oral ulcers, alopecia, increase in liver function tests, bone marrow suppression, and possible pulmonary fibrosis.

    e. Contraindications: Acute renal failure, caution in pulmonary disease, caution in hepatic insufficiency.

    f. Anti-tumor necrosis factor (anti TNF) as etanercept and adilmubumab have been studied and may be effective in treating refractory TAK, but this is not a cure.

    g. Azothioprine (2 mg/kg/day) mycophenolate mofetil (2000 mg / day) and cyclophosphamide (2 mg/kg/ day) have been used (Doherty, 2010).

    h. Common side effects of azothiaprine include nausea, hepatic abnormalities, abdominal pain, leukopenia, infections, thrombocytopenia, pancreatitis (Cush & Kavanaugh, 2005).

4. Contraindications: Acute renal failure, caution in hepatic disease.

5. Common side effects of mycophenolate mofetil include alopecia, nausea, diarrhea, headache, hypertension, peripheral edema, rash, infection, and bone marrow suppression (Fauci & Langford, 2006).

    a. Contraindications: Pregnancy, bone marrow suppression, severe renal disease.

6. Common side effects of cyclophosphamide include nausea, vomiting during and after infusion, flu-like symptoms.

7. Alopecia.

8. Bone marrow suppression, increase in transaminases, changes in renal function.

9. Hemorrhagic cystitis and bladder cancers have been documented. Alert patient to report hematuria.

10. Ovarian failure in females and azoospermia in males (Colbyn, Bermas, Weinblatt, & Helfgott, 2011).

    a. Prophylaxis for Pneumocystis carii pneumonia with oral trimethoprim 160 mg/sulfamethoxazole 800 mg 3 x week.

11. Side effects for trimethoprim/sulfa include diarrhea that is watery or bloody; feeling light-headed, rapid heart rate, trouble concentrating; skin-easy bruising, unusual bleeding (nose, mouth, vagina, or rectum), purple or red pinpoint spots; nausea, upper stomach pain, itching, loss of appetite, dark urine, clay-colored stools, jaundice (yellowing of the skin or eyes); Steven's Johnson's Syndrome.

J. Treat chronic diseases such as osteoporosis, hypertension, diabetes, and hyperlipidemia, if present.

    1. Encourage smoking cessation.

    2. Decrease alcohol consumption if excessive.

    3. Recommend daily physical activity, preferably weight bearing.

    4. Suggest weight reduction, if appropriate.

K. Treat chronic diseases such as osteoporosis, hypertension, diabetes, and hyperlipidemia, if present.

    1. Encourage smoking cessation.

    2. Decrease alcohol consumption if excessive.

    3. Recommend daily physical activity, preferably weight bearing.

    4. Suggest weight reduction, if appropriate.

L. Surgical therapy.

    1. Frequently requires revascularization.

        a. Bypass surgery for stenosis.

        b. Aortic valve replacement for treatment of aortic regurgitation.

        c. Percutaneous transluminal angioplasty to treat stenotic renal arteries that are causing hypertension.

        d. Collateral circulation often protects against abdominal or extremity claudication (Firestein et al., 2012).

4
4.1
4.2
4.3
4.4
4.5
4.6
4.7
4.8
4.9
4.10

M. Prognosis.

1. Disease is self-limiting.

2. May be relapsing-remitting course or a progressive course requiring continuous steroid and other disease-modifying antirheumatic drugs (Firestein et al., 2012).

III. Cogan's Syndrome.

A. Pathology.

1. Rare, affects large blood vessels (aorta) (Firestein et al., 2012).

2. May be a type of systemic vasculitis linked to aortitis (Fauci & Langford, 2006).

B. Etiology and epidemiology.

1. Average age of onset is 25 years (Firestein et al., 2012).

C. Symptoms of red painful eyes and/or hearing loss (Firestein et al., 2012).

1. May occur at the same time or within 4 months in 75% of patients.

2. Vision loss is seldom permanent.

3. Aortitis and aneurism or aortic insufficiency.

IV. Atypical Cogan's syndrome
(Firestein et al., 2012).

A. Episcleritis, scleritis, iritis, uveitis, or chorioretinitis.

1. Poorer prognosis, aortic and systemic symptoms more prevalent.

2. Audio symptoms, partial or complete hearing loss that usually does not improve.

3. Vertigo and ataxia can improve.

4. Constitutional symptoms: Fever, lymphadenopathy, hepatomegaly, splenomegaly, weight loss, and purpura.

5. Most deaths occur because of aortic disease.

6. Changes in vision and hearing may occur prior to aortic involvement by months to years.

B. Nursing assessment.

1. Understand the need to confirm the diagnosis and begin appropriate therapy when life altering disease is present.

2. Implement appropriate laboratory studies and imaging, and interpret the results to verify or rule out a diagnosis of vasculitis.

3. If a biopsy has been performed, assess site and instruct the patient on appropriate wound care.

4. When treatment has begun.

   a. Assess for tolerance and compliance with medications.

   b. Assess for flares.

   c. Number since last office visit (if patient is being treated in rheumatologist's office), severity (did it interfere with work, family life?).

      (1) What triggered the flare, what relieved symptoms?

      (2) Specific symptoms associated with the flare.

5. Assess ability to accomplish activities of daily living, manage stress, participate in work, family, and social life activities.

6. Physical assessment with additional focus on systems affected by the disease to determine improvement or worsening of condition.

C. Diagnosis.

1. Lab results generally not helpful in diagnosis.

2. Echo and MRI reveal aortic insufficiency or aortic root dilation (Firestein et al., 2012).

D. Treatment.

1. Corticosteroids: Early initiation to prevent hearing loss (Fauci & Langford, 2006).

   a. Common side effects of steroids include depression, psychosis, and mood swings.

      (1) Hypertension, congestive heart failure.

      (2) Hyperglycemia.

      (3) Weight gain, peptic ulcer disease.

      (4) Masks infections, slows wound healing, triggers acne, thins the skin which bruises easily.

      (5) Muscle weakness in long term use, osteoporosis.

4
4.1
4.2
4.3
4.4
4.5
4.6
4.7
4.8
4.9
4.10

(6) May cause cataracts or will worsen existing cataracts, glaucoma.

(7) Contraindications: Active infections (Doherty, 2010).

(8) Other medications used: Cyclophosphamide, MTX, cyclosporine.

2. Variable: May only experience one episode of the disease; it may peak and remit for months to several years.

3. Cochlear implants, aortic valve replacement, repair of aortic aneurisms.

4. Treat chronic diseases such as osteoporosis, hypertension, diabetes, and hyperlipidemia, if present.

5. Encourage smoking cessation.

6. Decrease alcohol consumption if excessive.

7. Recommend daily physical activity, preferably weight bearing.

8. Suggest weight reduction, if appropriate.

V. Kawasaki Disease (KD).

A. Pathophysiology.

1. Monophasic inflammatory disease.

2. Buildup of monocytes and macrophages in medium size vessels.

3. Causes coronary artery damage (Firestein et al., 2012).

B. Etiology and epidemiology.

1. Greater incidence in Asian population, particularly Japanese children (Firestein et al., 2012).

   a. 1 in 100 Japanese children will develop KD before the age of 5.

   b. Boys to girls, 3:2.

      (1) Increase of 10 fold if a sibling has had the disease.

2. Increase of 2 fold if one of the parents has had the disease.

   a. This carries over to Japanese children who have embraced a Western lifestyle.

   b. Genetic factor likely present in KD.

3. Can occur in all ethnic and racial groups (Firestein et al., 2012).

4. Appearance of the child leads one to believe that KD has an infectious cause; however, no specific agent has been identified (Firestein et al., 2012).

5. Nursing assessment.

   a. Understand the need to confirm the diagnosis and begin appropriate therapy when life altering disease is present.

   b. Implement appropriate laboratory studies and imaging, and interpret the results to verify or rule out a diagnosis of vasculitis.

   c. If a biopsy has been performed, assess site and instruct the patient on appropriate wound care.

C. When treatment has begun.

1. Assess for tolerance and compliance with medications.

2. Assess for flares:

   a. Number since last office visit (if patient is being treated in rheumatologist's office), severity (did it interfere with work, family life?).

   b. What triggered the flare, what relieved symptoms?

   c. Specific symptoms associated with the flare.

D. Assess ability to accomplish activities of daily living, manage stress, participate in work, family, and social life activities.

E. Physical assessment with additional focus on systems affected by the disease to determine improvement or worsening of condition.

F. Diagnosis.

1. In children, this is the most common cause of acquired cardiac disease in developed nations (rheumatic fever most common in underdeveloped countries) (Firestein et al., 2012).

2. Medium vessels involved. Causes inflammation and aneurism formation, especially in the coronary vessels (Firestein et al., 2012).

3. Early diagnosis is critical, early treatment decreases/prevents coronary artery inflammation (Coblyn et al., 2011).

4
4.1
4.2
4.3
4.4
4.5
4.6
4.7
4.8
4.9
4.10

4. Within the first month of untreated disease, KD can cause life-long cardiac disease (Firestein et al., 2012).

5. On diagnosis of KD, an echocardiogram should be performed to detect early cardiac vessel involvement (Coblyn et al., 2011).

G. The child presents with.

1. Fever: Spiking and may last more than 5 days. This is intermittent and the child experiences normal temperature in between the fever. This occurs several times a day. Time frame of fever is best predictor for coronary artery damage.

2. Oral mucosal inflammation. Lips, mouth, tongue, and pharynx are erythematous. Dryness can cause bleeding. There are no oral ulcers and no exudate present in the pharynx. Strawberry tongue with enlarged papillae can be present.

3. Injection of the conjunctiva but no drainage or exudates. Involves the globe of the eye, not the eyelid or tear ducts. May be present for weeks. Photosensitivity may be present as anterior uveitis may occur in KD.

4. Redness and swelling of the hands and feet. The child may not walk or hold objects because of the pain. This symptom may assist in the diagnosis as this symptom does not occur in viral diseases. These changes are bilateral. After about 3-4 weeks of fever, desquamation of fingers and toes may occur; this is not a good diagnostic feature for KD as it occurs later in the disease.

5. Cervical lymphadenopathy. Difficult to assess in infants. Lymph node should be >1.5cm in diameter. Generally present in the anterior cervical and sternocleidomastoid muscle areas.

6. Rash: 3 forms.

   a. Erythematous maculopapular: Resent on the trunk and extremities.

   b. Scarlantiniform: On trunk initially thought to be group A streptococcal infection.

   c. Erythema multiforme: Target lesions (these lesions are usually associated with hypersensitivity, be careful not to confuse).

7. Groin rash can be confused with candidiasis, but desquamation also occurs and this is not typical for candida. Children who are toilet trained will develop the groin rash (Firestein et al., 2012).

8. Incomplete KD: Consider this diagnosis when the child presents with fever for at least 5 days or more and the child has at least 2 other symptoms for KD, as well as positive laboratory and echocardiographic findings (Firestein et al., 2012).

   a. Laboratory: No specific test is diagnostic.

      (1) CBC with differential: White count (WBC) is elevated, or the white count is elevated with an increase in absolute neutrophil count.

      (2) Acute phase reactants: C- reactive protein and/or sedimentation rate are elevated.

      (3) Urinalysis: Pyuria generally greater than 10 WBC per HPF.

   b. Laboratory values - C-reactive protein and sedimentation rate are monitored after discharge until in normal range. Post hospital visits at 2-3 and at 6-8 months should include CBC and at least CRP level (Firestein et al., 2012).

   c. Echocardiogram (echo): Baseline, determine presence of coronary artery dilation. At 2-3 weeks and at 6-8 weeks after fever onset. If no abnormal coronary artery abnormalities seen at the last echo, no further echo evaluations are necessary. If coronary artery disease is present, the child needs to be followed by a pediatric cardiologist (Firestein et al., 2012).

      (1) Differential Diagnosis: Measles, scarlet fever, toxic shock syndrome, drug reactions, and viral illnesses (Coblyn et al., 2011).

H. Treatment.

1. IV gammaglobulin (IV IgG) 2 gm/kg over 8-12 hours (Fauci & Langford, 2006).

   a. Side effects during infusion: Back ache, headache, joint pain, muscle pain, rash, leg cramping.

   b. Side effects post infusion: Dizziness, hives, chills, fever, hives, facial redness, weakness, nausea and vomiting.

   c. Sed rate can be affected by the IV IgG, so not a valuable tool for monitoring therapeutic response. Normalizes about 6-8 weeks after fever onset.

4
4.1
4.2
4.3
4.4
4.5
4.6
4.7
4.8
4.9
4.10

d. Side effects with gammaglobulin are very rare.

e. The majority of children with KD respond within 24-28 hours. About 15-20% require a second dose of IV IgG in addition to IV methylprednisolone at 30 mg/kg for one or two days (Firestein et al., 2012).

2. Oral aspirin 80-100 mg/kg/day for inflammation, reduced to a daily dose of 3-5 mg/kg on the 14th day or 2-3 days after fever subsides. Aspirin use is continued not just for its anti-inflammatory properties but for anti-thrombotic property as well. This dosing continues until the sedimentation rate is normal, and the echocardiograms have returned to normal for some time. Children with coronary artery aneurysms will require continued aspirin therapy, or long term anti-platelet therapy to decrease the opportunity for thrombosis (Firestein et al., 2012).

a. Side effects: Use caution if another viral illness is present (varicella or influenza) because of increased risk of Reye's Syndrome, gastrointestinal upset, increased bleeding, possible decrease in renal function.

3. IV methylprednisolone at 30 mg/kg for one or two days.

a. Common side effects of steroids include.

(1) Depression, psychosis, and mood swings.

(2) Hypertension, congestive heart failure.

(3) Hyperglycemia.

(4) Weight gain, peptic ulcer disease.

(5) Masks infections, slows wound healing, triggers acne, thins the skin which bruises easily.

(6) Muscle weakness in long term use, osteoporosis.

(7) May cause cataracts or will worsen existing cataracts, glaucoma.

(8) Contraindications: Active infections (Doherty, 2010).

b. IV infliximab 5 mg/kg is another option.

(1) Side effects: Risk of infection, infusion reactions, drug-induced lupus syndromes, cytopenias, and hepatotoxicity (Coblyn et al., 2011).

(2) Contraindicated: History of or in active TB, active hepatitis B, active infections, demyelinating conditions such as multiple sclerosis.

c. If still no response, refer to a medical center with KD expertise. May need additional steroids, infliximab or additional immunosuppressive therapies. These children are at great risk for coronary artery abnormalities.

VI. Polyarteritis Nodosa (PAN).

A. Pathophysiology.

1. Inflammation causing necrotizing of the small and medium wall vessels (Firestein et al., 2012).

2. Though relatively rare, one form is associated with Hepatitis B virus (HBV) ((Latinis et al., 2004).

3. Develops in 1-5% of individuals who have Hepatitis B (Firestein et al., 2012).

a. One form caused by Hepatitis B virus and decreased incidence is due to Hepatitis B vaccine (Latinis, Dao, Gutierrez, Shepherd, & Velazquez, 2004).

b. It is thought that in HBV-related PAN, the virus causes injury to the vessel by replicating the virus or by deposition of immune complexes. Compliment is activated which results in an inflammatory response to the endothelial cells.

c. Generally occurs within the first few months following the hepatitis infection, and can be the presenting symptom.

B. Hepatitis C virus (HCV)-associated PAN has more constitutional symptoms. In other patients with PAN, the cause is unknown.

1. Immunologic cause is suspicious as this type responds to immunosuppressive therapy.

2. Inflammatory lesions often occur at bifurcation sites of the vessels, followed by necrotizing inflammation of the vessels (medium and small). Proliferation, with thrombosis, can result in ischemia or infarct of the organ or tissue involved.

C. Biopsy shows necrotizing inflammation; organs affected typically provide the best yield. Medium blood vessel generally shows segmented and focal sites of inflammation. If

4
4.1
4.2
4.3
4.4
4.5
4.6
4.7
4.8
4.9
4.10

involvement of any small vessels is suspect, further examination needs to occur. Consider another type, microscopic polyangitis (MPA). Different stages present of scarring or inflammation, very typical. Inflammatory areas are combination of lymphocytes, neutrophils, macrophages, and eosinophils.

D. Active lesions are the location of most aneurisms; scarring results in narrowing of the vessel.

E. The appearance of the lesion is what gives the name "nodosa" (Firestein et al., 2012).

F. Etiology and epidemiology.

1. Occurs most often in people between the ages of 40-60. Men equal to women. Diagnosis difficult to make.

2. Clinical features similar to other conditions, joint pain, fever, weight loss, and muscle pain.

3. If more than one system is involved, raises the possibility of systemic vasculitis.

4. Organ systems maybe involved early, but have subtle involvement for months to years before symptoms occur. Only one organ may be involved or multisystem involvement.

5. Most frequent manifestations are the constitutional symptoms that occur at onset of disease in about 90% of patients.

G. Those with hepatitis B more likely had peripheral neuropathy, abdominal pain, orchitis, cardiomyopathy, and hypertension when compared to patients with PAN who do not have hepatitis B.

H. Relapse occurs in both HBV-PAN and in non-HBV-PAN; mortality rate is higher for people with non-HBV-PAN, especially in the elderly and is seen to be higher in individuals with skin involvement (Firestein et al., 2012).

I. Nursing assessment.

1. Understand the need to confirm the diagnosis and begin appropriate therapy when life altering disease is present.

2. Implement appropriate laboratory studies and imaging, and interpret the results to verify or rule out a diagnosis of vasculitis.

3. If a biopsy has been performed, assess site and instruct the patient on appropriate wound care.

4. When treatment has begun.
   a. Assess for tolerance and compliance with medications.
   b. Assess for flares.
      (1) Number since last office visit (if patient is being treated in a rheumatologist's office), severity (did it interfere with work, family life?).
      (2) What triggered the flare, what relieved symptoms?
      (3) Specific symptoms associated with the flare.

5. Assess ability to accomplish activities of daily living, manage stress, participate in work, family, and social life activities.

6. Physical assessment with additional focus on systems affected by the disease to determine improvement or worsening of condition.

J. Diagnosis.

1. Thorough history and physical (Latinis et al., 2004).

K. Based on the American College of Rheumatology 1990 criteria for the classification of polyarteritis nodosa (Lightfoot et al., 1990), the presence of 3 or more of the following 10 criteria is specific for the diagnosis of PAN:

1. Weight loss of equal to or greater than 4 kg.

2. Livedo reticularis.

3. Testicular pain or tenderness.

4. Myalgias, weakness or leg tenderness.

5. Mononeuropathy or polyneuropathy.

6. Diastolic blood pressure > 90 Hg.

7. Elevated serum nitrogen urea (>40 mg/dl) or creatinine (>1.5 mg dl).

8. Hepatitis B infection.

9. Arteriographic abnormality.

10. Biopsy of small or medium sized artery containing polymorphonuclear neutrophils.

L. There are no specific lab tests that will aid in the diagnosis of PAN, but many are useful in identifying the organ system involved (Firestein et al., 2012).

M. Angiogram is the most common test used in diagnosis. Will detect vessel defects, aneurisms, occlusive lesions present in medium size vessels (usually renal and mesenteric) (Firestein et al., 2012).

N. CTs and MRIs are less sensitive, unable to detect microaneurisms. If PAN is suspected, it is still necessary to follow CT and MRI with angiogram.

1. Doppler useful in identifying renal and hepatic aneurisms, although operator dependent.

2. Chest X-ray may detect other diseases or vasculidities that may affect the lungs. Useful in ruling out infection (Firestein et al., 2012).

O. PAN in children: A review of 110 children (Firestein et al., 2012).

1. Female to male equal, average age of 9.

2. Skin manifestation (cutaneous PAN) most common.

3. Less associated with hepatitis B.

4. Most were diagnosed with MPA (80%), associated with antineutrophil cytoplasmic antibodies ANCA) and 57% were diagnosed with systemic PAN (Firestein et al., 2012).

P. Microscopic polyangitis vs. polyangitis nodosum: A review of 410 patients.

1. Purpura more common in MPA.

2. Greater frequency of urticaria in PAN.

3. Presence or absence of HBV infection had moderate impact on the presence of skin disease.

4. Microscopic exam of tissue from MPA and PAN was the same (Firestein et al., 2012).

Q. Cutaneous polyarteritis nodosa.

1. Described as skin-limited PAN, considered separate from systemic PAN.

2. Questionable whether an early case of PAN, only cutaneous disease, or systemic PAN will follow.

3. Skin biopsy does not differentiate between cutaneous disease and early PAN. Hepatitis C virus has been associated with cutaneous PAN (Firestein et al., 2012).

R. Hepatitis B virus polyarteritis nodosa.

1. HBV vasculitis occurs in individuals with chronic disease who carry the hepatitis B surface antigen (antigemia) and most of these have active liver disease as well.

2. No specific presentation; signs and symptoms vary from small vessel disease with cutaneous findings to medium vessel disease (lesions) typical of PAN.

3. Symptoms range from purpura, to rash to renal disease, hypertension, stroke, and abdominal pain.

4. Less common because of vaccine programs (Firestein et al., 2012).

S. Treatment of polyarteritis nodosa.

1. Appropriate for the disease activity and the organs involved.

2. Treatment based on the Five Factor score: One point per item.

   a. The presence of raised serum creatinine.

   b. Proteinuria.

   c. Cardiac involvement.

   d. Central nervous system involvement.

   e. Gut involvement.

T. Outcome in small-vessel systemic vasculitis.

1. Treatment of HBV-PAN combines therapy for the hepatitis infection as well as the vasculitis.

2. IV methylprednisolone, pulse, only if there is severe vasculitis to manage.

3. Use in the first few weeks of the emergent situation and then stop to allow for viral clearance.

U. Plasma exchange to control symptoms of vasculitis after the steroids to treat the PAN.

1. Long-term use of steroids and immunosuppressants prolong or threaten viral clearance.

2. Consult of hepatologist is advised.

4
4.1
4.2
4.3
4.4
4.5
4.6
4.7
4.8
4.9
4.10

3. Treat hepatitis with standard therapy such as interferon alfa-2b or vidarabine.

V. Treatment of non-HBV-PAN.

1. Requires that none of the 5 factors are present at the time of diagnosis.

2. Treat with oral prednisone 1 mg/kg daily.

   a. Common side effects include depression, psychosis, and mood swings.

      (1) Hypertension, congestive heart failure.

      (2) Hyperglycemia.

      (3) Weight gain, peptic ulcer disease.

      (4) Masks infections, slows wound healing, triggers acne, thins the skin which bruises easily.

      (5) Muscle weakness in long term use, osteoporosis.

      (6) May cause cataracts or will worsen existing cataracts, glaucoma.

      (7) Contraindications: Active infections (Doherty, 2010).

W. If one or more of the 5 factors is present at diagnosis.

1. Pulse IV methylprednisolone at 1000 mg/daily for 3-5 days, followed with oral prednisone1 mg/kg/day.

   a. While the patient is on cyclophosphamide (see below), may taper prednisone slowly when the sedimentation rate has returned to normal (Latinis et al., 2004).

2. Pulse IV cyclophosphamide at 0.5-2.5 gram every week to every month.

   a. Depends on severity of disease, renal function, response to therapy and status of blood counts.

   b. Should not be given longer than a year (Latinis et al., 2004).

   c. Side effects include.

      (1) Nausea, vomiting during and after infusion, flu like symptoms.

      (2) Alopecia can occur.

      (3) Bone marrow suppression, increase in transaminases, changes in renal function.

      (4) Hemorrhagic cystitis and bladder cancers have been documented. Alert patient to report hematuria.

   (5) Ovarian failure in females and azoospermia in males (Colbyn, Bermas, Weinblatt, & Helfgott, 2011).

      i) Prophylaxis for Pneumocystis carii pneumonia with oral trimethoprim 160 mg/sulfamethoxazole 800 mg 3 x week.

      ii) Side effects include diarrhea that is watery or bloody; feeling light-headed, rapid heart rate, trouble concentrating.

      iii) Skin: Easy bruising, unusual bleeding (nose, mouth, vagina, or rectum), purple or red pinpoint spots.

      iv) Nausea, upper stomach pain, itching, loss of appetite, dark urine, clay-colored stools, jaundice (yellowing of the skin or eyes); Steven's Johnson's Syndrome.

3. Treat chronic diseases such as osteoporosis, hypertension, diabetes, and hyperlipidemia, if present.

   a. Encourage smoking cessation.

   b. Recommend daily physical activity, preferably weight bearing.

   c. Suggest weight reduction, if appropriate.

   d. Early diagnosis and treatment are essential to ensure positive outcomes.

      (1) Non-HBV-PAN, survival rate at 7 years is at 79%.

      (2) HBV-PAN survival at 5 years is 72.5%, relapse rate is low.

      (3) Delayed diagnosis does not increase relapse rate, but affects the mortality risk (Firestein et al., 2012).

   e. The Five Factor Score is useful in predicting outcomes; higher scores reflect reduced survival rate (Firestein et al., 2012).

   f. Nursing assessment.

      (1) Understand the need to confirm the diagnosis and begin appropriate therapy when life altering disease is present.

      (2) Implement appropriate laboratory studies and imaging, and interpret the results to verify or rule out a diagnosis of vasculitis.

      (3) If a biopsy has been performed, assess site and instruct the patient on appropriate wound care.

4
4.1
4.2
4.3
4.4
4.5
4.6
4.7
4.8
4.9
4.10

(4) When treatment has begun.

(5) Assess for tolerance and compliance with medications.

(6) Assess for flares.

g. Number since last office visit (if patient is being treated in a rheumatologist's office), severity (did it interfere with work, family life?).

(1) What triggered the flare, what relieved symptoms?

(2) Specific symptoms associated with the flare.

h. Assess ability to accomplish activities of daily living, manage stress, participate in work, family, and social life activities.

(1) Physical assessment with additional focus on systems affected by the disease to determine improvement or worsening of condition.

VII. Antineutrophil cytoplasm antibodies (ANCA)-associated vasculidities (AAVs).

A. These are small and medium vessel diseases that are considered autoimmune (Firestein et al., 2012) because of an association of autoantibodies, Antineutrophil Cytoplasm Antibodies (ANCA) that target neutrophils and monocytes (Fauci & Langford, 2006).

B. Conditions that are found in this category include Granulomatosis with Polyangiitis (GPA), formerly known as Wegener's Granulomatosis (Holle, Laudien, & Gross, 2010), allergic granulomatosis with polyangiitis (AGPA), formerly known as Churg-Strauss; microscopic polyangiitis (MPA); and renal limited pauci-immune necrotizing and cresentic glomerulonephritis (RLV) (Firestein et al., 2012). (Name changes were recommended by the ACR to put more focus on description of the disease.)

1. Pathology.

a. There are two types of these antibodies, c ANCA and p ANCA; they are named for their specific patterns: Cytoplasmic (c-ANCA) and perinuclear (p-ANCA) (Firestein et al., 2012).

2. Pathobiologic activities in the affected tissues (in AAVs), the neutrophils and monocytes,

attack blood vessel walls and an autoantigen is released influencing inflammation. Autoantibodies to endothelial cells are also manufactured and are associated with ANCA-associated vasculitis. During this inflammatory time frame, there is damage to the basal membrane of blood vessels and autoantibodies to the basement membrane of certain vessels (glomeruli and pulmonary) are produced, affecting function (Wiik, 2010).

3. Etiology/Epidemiology Peak onset is 65-74 years, rare in childhood, men to women 1.5:1.0.

a. Interesting relationship between GPA and MPA.

4. European ancestry, GPA, incidence of 2-10 per million, higher in the northern areas at 8-10 per million and lower (3-6.6 per million) in southern areas such as Spain and Greece. In the southern hemisphere, the relationship is the reverse: MPA more likely to be present. Current research studies focus on a relationship with ultraviolet exposure.

5. A study of Japanese population reported in Firestein et al. (2012) found that renal disease was more commonly associated with MPO-ANCA vasculitis and PR-3ANCA was not seen. No GPA or AGPA was seen clinically.

6. In China-MPA more common than GPA.

7. In Peru and Kuwait-MPA more common, 24/million.

8. In Finland, Norway, and Sweden GPA has increased over the past 2-3 decades; not so in Germany and United Kingdom.

9. The incidence of MPA alone has varied according to the research studies conducted. After the earthquake in Kobe, Japan, in 1995, there was increased incidence of MPA.

10. AGPA incidence is 1-3 /million. In those with asthma, increases to 34.6/million have been observed. Most rare. Affects similar population as GPA and MPA. More common in women than men.

a. Environmental factors related to AAVs.

b. Higher incidence in rural than urban. Not seasonal.

c. Infection found to be a likely trigger (Staphylococcus aureus and GPA).

d. Silica exposure seen in a few U.S. studies.

4
4.1
4.2
4.3
4.4
4.5
4.6
4.7
4.8
4.9
4.10

e. Exposure to drugs: Propylthiouracil.

f. Cocaine abuse, mimics GPA, linked to a midline destructive granulomatous disease.

C. Genetics.

1. Risk is mildly increased in first degree relatives.

2. Children of parents with GVA have increased risk of rheumatoid arthritis (RA).

3. Difficult to perform genetic testing because of the rarity of the disease.

4. PR3 seems to be genetically determined. Individuals with GPA have increased number of neutrophils that express PR3.

5. May be an association with HLA antigens (Firestein et al., 2012).

VIII. Microscopic polangiitis (MPA).

A. Pathology.

1. Different from polyarteritis nodosa: Segmental necrotizing glomerulonephritis and more apt to involve small vessels. Fibrinoid vasculitis, few or no immune deposits, affects small vessels such as capillaries, venules, and arterioles. Can spread to medium size vessels. Segmental necrotizing glomerulonephritis is common and may progress to crescentic glomerulonephritis. Given the sluggishness and insidious disease progression, there may already be permanent damage to the glomeruli and tubules with the first renal biopsy.

2. Pulmonary disease (inflammation of the capillaries) is followed by rupture of the capillaries. Blood spills into alveolar spaces and thrombus can form in the capillaries. Alveolar walls have marked neutrophilic infiltration, which leads to fibrinoid necrosis.

a. Usually associated with myeloperosicase (MPO) ANCA. There are a small percentage of patients who are associated with proteinase-3 (PR-3) ANCA.

B. Diagnosis.

1. Based on biopsy evidence of vasculitis or pauci-immune glomerulonephritis. If limited to the kidney, referred to as renal limited vasculitis. It can also be acute, severe, and progress to glomerulonephritis and pulmonary hemorrhage, referred to as pulmonary renal syndrome. Patient is very ill with constitutional symptoms, fever, renal disease (100% of the time), arthralgias, purpura, pulmonary disease; 1/3 of patients will develop pulmonary disease (beginning with cough, dyspnea, shortness of breath, leading to hemoptysis) (Firestein et al., 2012), neurologic conditions such as mononeuritis multiplex (Fauci & Langford, 2006), and ear, nose, and throat involvement (Firestein et al., 2012).

C. Laboratory findings include anemia, elevated sedimentation rate, thrombocytosis, leukocytosis.

1. ANCA is present in at least 75 % of people with this disease and is associated with MPO antibodies (Fauci & Langford, 2006).

2. Renal: Hematuria, proteinuria (less than 3.6 mg/24 hours), abnormal renal sediment with red cell casts. Presence of red cell casts indicates active glomerulonephritis. Loss of renal function can occur quickly. Dialysis may assist in return of some renal function.

a. Red cells can be present in individuals who have had long term disease. This can be indicative of active disease, damage, or side effects of therapy such as cystitis or bladder cancers that can occur with cyclophosphamide (Firestein et al., 2012).

(1) Pulmonary: Chest X-ray may show alveolar infiltrates (patchy or diffuse), hemorrhage, and effusions.

D. Treatment.

1. Glucocorticoids and cyclophosphamide similar to therapy used in granulomatosis with polyangiitis (Wegener's) (Fauci & Langford, 2006).

2. One third of those treated relapse and treatment is repeated with induction therapy (Fauci & Langford, 2006).

3. Treat chronic diseases such as osteoporosis, hypertension, diabetes, and hyperlipidemia, if present.

4. Encourage smoking cessation.

5. Decrease alcohol consumption if excessive.

6. Recommend daily physical activity, preferably weight bearing.

7. Suggest weight reduction, if appropriate.

4
4.1
4.2
4.3
4.4
4.5
4.6
4.7
4.8
4.9
4.10

IX. Granulomatosis with Polangiitis (GPA) (previously known as Wegener's).

A. Pathology.

1. Affects small arteries and veins, necrotizing vasculitis (Fauci & Langford, 2006).

2. Classic triad: Upper and lower respiratory tract and kidney. However, any organ can be involved with granuloma formation, vasculitis or both (Fauci & Langford, 2006).

3. PR3-ANCA is highly specific for GPA (Firestein et al., 2012).

4. Granuloma formation is present in both extravascular and intravascular areas.

5. Lung involvement: Multiple, bilateral nodulare cavitary infiltrates (Fauci & Langford, 2006).

6. GPA that is limited to the respiratory tract is referred to as "limited GPA."

7. In one study (Firestein et al., 2012), 10% of individuals with limited GPA developed systemic disease with the median time of 6 years.

    a. Upper respiratory (sinuses, nasopharynx) lesions: Inflammation, some necrosis and granuloma formation.

    b. Renal: Begins as a central or sectional glomerulonephritis. May progress into crescentric glomerulonephritis. Formation of granulomas is rarely seen on biopsy (Firestein et al., 2012).

8. Immunopathogenesis unclear. Thought to be an abnormal cell-mediated immune response to exogenous or endogenous antigens. Staphylococcus aureus has been associated with an increased relapse rate in GPA, but no evidence has been found that this organism is the cause of the disease (Firestein et al., 2012).

9. Similar to MPA. Granulomas present as well as vasculitis.

B. Diagnosis.

1. PR-3 ANCA highly specific for GPA (caution, some titers can be false positive).

2. Generally found in the respiratory system (limited GPA). Usually granulomatous, without vasculitis.

3. Presents as upper airway disease in about 70% of people and actually develops in 90%. Can begin as an otitis and loss of hearing can occur. Nasal involvement: Swelling, occurs from the collapse of the nasal septum following perforation (Fauci & Langford, 2006).

4. Sinusitis occurs in about 80% of the cases. May result in deterioration of the bone which can contribute to relapse.

    a. Laryngotracheal disease begins as hoarseness. May progress to stridor and airway obstruction.

    b. Pulmonary involvement affects about 90% of the patients at some time during the disease. May be asymptomatic and detected through imaging.

        (1) Radiographs (X-rays): Will show pulmonary infiltrate. Significant in the cases of pulmonary or hilar lymph nodes that are seen on CT.

        (2) Pulmonary hemorrage cannot be ruled out by chest X-ray. CT of chest can identify early or small amounts of pulmonary hemorrage.

    c. Will experience vasculitis and capillaritis as well as granulomas, nodules with chronic inflammation that imbed centrally.

    d. Important to rule out infections with sputum culture or bronchoscopy if needed.

5. Pulmonary Function Tests (PFTs) can be helpful to show if obstructive or restrictive component is resent. Fibrosis can develop because of multiple episodes of pulmonary hemorrhage and because of therapies such as with cyclophosphamide-induced pneumonitis (Firestein et al., 2012).

6. Biopsy of the lung, nasal mucosa, skin, or kidney. Findings are compatible with the diagnosis but specific features of the disease may not appear on biopsy.

    a. Open lung biopsies more informative than transbronchial.

    b. Renal pathology is similar between MPA and GPA. Granulomas are rarely seen.

    c. Light microscopy is not useful in diagnosis. Immunofluorescence distinguishes between three types: Pauci immune, immune complex, and antiglomerular basement subtypes (Firestein et al., 2012).

    d. Autoimmune mediated. Associated with PR-3 ANCA (Firestein et al., 2012).

4
4.1
4.2
4.3
4.4
4.5
4.6
4.7
4.8
4.9
4.10

C. Treatment.

1. High doses of IV and oral corticosteroids in combination with cyclophosphamide (2 mg/kg/day) for induction therapy. May continue at pulse therapy which is generally 6 months. Dose adjusted based on leukocyte counts (Coblyn et al., 2011).

2. Prednisone is tapered. Cyclophosphamide can be changed to MTX or azothaprine after pulse therapy is completed (Coblyn et al., 2011).

3. Rituximab has been used successfully and is now US Food and Drug Administration (FDA) approved to treat refractory disease; allows for faster reduction in steroid use (Holle, Laudien, & Gross, 2010).

   a. Treat chronic diseases such as osteoporosis, hypertension, diabetes, and hyperlipidemia, if present.

   b. Encourage smoking cessation.

   c. Decrease alcohol consumption if excessive.

   d. Recommend daily physical activity, preferably weight bearing.

   e. Suggest weight reduction, if appropriate.

4. Plasmapheresis (Langford, 2008).

X. Allergic Granulomatosis with Polyangiitis (PGA) (Churg-Strauss).

A. Pathology.

1. Associated with allergy and atopic conditions such as allergic rhinitis, asthma, and nasal polyposis (Firestein et al., 2012).

2. Elevated IgE levels and elevated eosinophils in blood counts and tissue.

3. Most patients are ACNA negative, but if present may be connected to the MPO.

4. If ANCA positive, greater chance for kidney involvement, mononeuritis multiplex, alveolar hemorrhage, and purpura (Firestein et al., 2012).

5. Patient presents with a series of allergic symptoms, followed by a vasulitic phase and then clinical picture of allergic disease (Coblyn et al., 2011).

6. Pulmonary infiltrates, following active asthma, are seen on chest X-ray (Firestein et al., 2012).

7. May be lobar, interstitial, or nodular in appearance.

8. Pulmonary effusions are possible—eosinophils in the pleural fluid.

9. Alveolar hemorrhage. Peripheral neuropathy will affect about 2/3 of patients diagnosed with AGPA. Can be symmetric or asymmetric. Central nervous system disease and cranial nerves may be involved.

10. Renal involvement can occur, but less common than in GPA or MPA. Presentation includes eosinophils, but otherwise is similar.

11. Multiple organs can be involved, cardiovascular, gastrointestinal, and the eye. Skin involvement is characterized by inflammatory skin nodules (Fauci & Langford, 2006).

B. Diagnosis.

1. Often made by biopsy. Affinity for MP3 ANCA, if present (Firestein et al., 2012).

2. Asthma, eosinophils (>1000 cells per microliter), elevated sedimentation rate, fibrinogen, and alpha globulins found in the majority of patients. Other lab results indicate organ involvement (Fauci & Langford, 2006).

C. Treatment.

1. Use Five Factor Score.

2. Good prognosis, can be managed with corticosteroids alone.

3. Relapse common, 35% of patients relapse within four and a half years.

4. Asthma necessitates the use of long term steroids.

5. If one or two factors: Induce with cyclophosphamide and corticosteroids.

6. Relapse common (Firestein et al., 2012).

7. Azothiaprine used as treatment (Coblyn et al., 2011).

8. Survival at 8 years.

D. Those with good prognosis based on Five Factor Score had survival rate of 97%.

E. Those with more significant disease have 92% survival rate.

4
4.1
4.2
4.3
4.4
4.5
4.6
4.7
4.8
4.9
4.10

1. Most required long term corticosteroid therapy for asthma.

2. No specific duration of therapy has been determined.

3. Rituximab being studied in those who do not respond to therapy (Firestein et al., 2012).

F. Treat chronic diseases such as osteoporosis, hypertension, diabetes, and hyperlipidemia, if present.

   1. Encourage smoking cessation.

   2. Decrease alcohol consumption if excessive.

   3. Recommend daily physical activity, preferably weight bearing.

   4. Suggest weight reduction, if appropriate.

G. Diagnosis (summary) of antibody-associated vasculidities (AAVs) (Firestein et al., 2012).

H. Examine by pathology, a sample/biopsy of affected tissue.

   1. MPA: Kidney, lung, skin.

   2. GPA: Nasal, paranasal biopsy (consistent with rather than diagnostic of).

   3. AGPA: Nerve or muscle biopsy.

I. Laboratory.

J. Leukocytosis, anemia (may be normocytic, normochromic), elevated sedimentation rate, increased eosinophils, increased platelets; C-reactive protein may be elevated.

   1. PR-3- and MPO-ANCA associated with specific antigen routinely checked.

   2. Staining: Binding to neutrophils is c-ANCA, usually associated with PR3 ANCA binding to perinuclear pattern is p-ANCA, usually associated with MPO-ANCA.

   3. Use of PR3 and MPO with c-ANCA and p-ANCA increases specificity for diagnosis of disease.

   4. Be wary of false positives.

K. Treatment.

   1. If untreated, progresses rapidly and is fatal.

2. Goals: Induce remission, maintain remission, and prevent relapse.

3. Based on severity of disease and presence of life threatening organ damage.

4. Cyclophosphamide significantly improved survival rates in patients in their 70s.

5. Cyclophosphamide side effects: Nausea, vomiting during and after infusion, flu like symptoms, alopecia, bone marrow suppression, increase in transaminases, changes in renal function, hemorrhagic cystitis and bladder cancers have been documented. Alert patient to report hematuria.

   a. Ovarian failure in females and azoospermia in males (Colbyn, Bermas, Weinblatt, & Helfgott, 2011).

      (1) Prophylaxis for Pneumocystis carii pneumonia with oral trimethoprim 160 mg/sulfamethoxazole 800 mg 3 x week.

      (2) Side effects include diarrhea that is watery or bloody; feeling light-headed, rapid heart rate, trouble concentrating; skin: Easy bruising, unusual bleeding (nose, mouth, vagina, or rectum), purple or red pinpoint spots, nausea, upper stomach pain, itching, loss of appetite, dark urine, clay-colored stools, jaundice (yellowing of the skin or eyes). Steven's Johnson's Syndrome.

   b. Prednisone side effects: Include depression, psychosis, and mood swings, hypertension, congestive heart failure, hyperglycemia, weight gain, peptic ulcer disease, masks infections, slows wound healing, triggers acne, thins the skin which bruises easily, muscle weakness in long term use, osteoporosis. May cause cataracts or will worsen existing cataracts, glaucoma. Contraindications: Active infections (Doherty, 2010).

XI. Rituximab (Rituxan®, Genentech, 2012).

A. Also is used as initial treatment.

B. Rituximab side effects: Side effects around the time of the infusion can include headache, cough, nausea, stomach upset, sweating, nervousness, muscle stiffness, and numbness. Patients can take mild pain medications, such as acetaminophen, for these symptoms, but should call the healthcare provider if the symptoms are

4
4.1
4.2
4.3
4.4
4.5
4.6
4.7
4.8
4.9
4.10

severe or get worse. Sometimes infusion reactions such as hypotension, mild throat tightening, rash, pruitis, dizziness, and back pain occur. These symptoms can be reduced by use of acetaminophen or diphenhydramine, and slowing or stopping the infusion for a short period of time and restarting it at a lower rate. On occasion a steroid injection is required. The healthcare provider may recommend pre-medicating the patient prior to the next infusion. Patients should be instructed to be aware of infections such as colds and sinusitis and call if they are having any difficulty recovering from the infection.

XII. Maintenance of remission.

A. Use of cyclophosphamide to achieve remission and then use a different disease-modifying drug to maintain the remission with fewer side effects. Maintenance therapy should continue for a minimum of 2 years if successful remission is achieved.

1. MTX side effects: Gastric intolerance, oral ulcers, alopecia, increases in liver function tests, bone marrow suppression and possible pulmonary fibrosis. Contraindications: Acute renal failure, use caution in pulmonary disease, use caution in hepatic insufficiency (Doherty, 2010).

2. Leflunomide: Common side effects include: Diarrhea, bone marrow suppression, changes in renal and hepatic function, nausea, rash (Fauci & Langford, 2006).

    a. Azothiaprine; common side effects include: Nausea, hepatic abnormalities, abdominal pain, leukopenia, infections, thrombocytopenia, pancreatitis (Cush & Kavanaugh, 2005). Contraindications: Acute renal failure, use caution in hepatic disease.

    b. Mycophenolate mofetil: Common side effects include alopecia, nausea, diarrhea, headache, hypertension, peripheral edema, rash, infection, and bone marrow suppression (Harrison, 2006). Contraindications: Pregnancy, bone marrow suppression, severe renal disease.

        (1) Treat chronic diseases such as osteoporosis, hypertension, diabetes, and hyperlipidemia, if present.

(2) Encourage smoking cessation.

(3) Decrease alcohol consumption if excessive.

(4) Recommend daily physical activity, preferably weight bearing.

(5) Suggest weight reduction, if appropriate.

B. Outcomes.

1. Most respond to therapy.

2. Therapy improved with the use of different agents for induction and for maintenance.

C. Mortality rate is 2.6 compared with normal population.

1. Poor prognosis contributed to by increased age and existing renal disease.

2. Cardiovascular disease more common in AAV with similar findings of end stage renal disease.

3. Malignancy rates greater, likely due to cyclophosphamide dosing.

4. Unpredictability of relapse.

XIII. Nursing assessment of the patient with ANCA-associated vasculidities.

A. Understand the need to confirm the diagnosis and begin appropriate therapy when life altering disease is present.

B. Implement appropriate laboratory studies and imaging, and interpret the results to verify or rule out a diagnosis of vasculitis.

C. If a biopsy has been performed, assess site and instruct the patient on appropriate wound care.

D. When treatment has begun.

1. Assess for tolerance and compliance with medications.

2. Assess for flares.

    a. Number since last office (if patient is being treated in rheumatologist's office) visit, severity (did it interfere with work, family life?).

    b. What triggered the flare, what relieved symptoms?

c. Specific symptoms associated with the flare.

3. Assess ability to accomplish activities of daily living, manage stress, participate in work, family, and social life activities.

4. Physical assessment with additional focus on systems affected by the disease to determine improvement or worsening of condition.

XIV. Primary Angiitis of the central nervous system (PACNS).

A. Pathology (Firestein et al., 2012).

1. Very rare, 500 cases discussed world-.wide.

2. Affects the brain, meninges, and spinal cord.

3. No support to recommend any genetic connection.

B. Etiology and epidemiology.

1. About 2.4 cases per one million people.

2. More common in middle aged men with onset average at 50 years.

3. Male to female ratio 2:1.

C. Diagnosis.

1. Laboratory—non-specific.

a. Important to rule out other connective tissue disorders and infections.

b. Cerebrospinal fluid (CSF)—findings non-specific for PACNS; however, useful in ruling out other conditions. May have normal glucose levels and elevated protein. Rule out infection (Coblyn et al., 2011).

2. Imaging—MRI provides sensitive information, detects infarcts (cortex and subcortex bilateral) and other lesions (Coblyn et al., 2011; Firestein et al., 2012).

a. Catheter-directed dye angiography—detects areas of dilation and stenosis. More effective in medium vessels, limited in small vessels. Not specific to PACNS.

3. Brain biopsy—important in ruling out other conditions. Considered low morbidity and mortality. Lesions can be in a patchy formation and may give 'false negative' report. Does not rule out infection or tumor (Firestein et al., 2012).

4. PACNS: More common in male population; cerebrospinal fluid has abnormalities so rule out other conditions; angiograms are abnormal in only about 40-50% of patients; headache is chronic, insidious; infarcts are small and scattered; hemorrhage is very rare (Firestein et al., 2012).

5. Reversible cerebral vasoconstriction syndrome: Spinal fluid is normal, headaches described as "thunder clap," abnormal angiogram (Firestein et al., 2012).

D. Mimics PACNS.

E. More common in women than men; CSF is usually normal, unless another condition is present; headache, sudden, thunder clap; angiogram is always abnormal; infarct is like water shed; hemorrhage (lobar or subarachnoid) common (Firestein et al., 2012).

1. Primary systemic vasculidities.

a. Occurs in about 7-11% of patients with GPA.

b. 14% of patients with Behçet's will have inflammation of the meningeal vessels, but not proven on pathology, so not a true PACNS.

2. Connective tissue diseases (Rheumatoid Arthritis, Systemic Lupus Erythematosus (SLE), Sjögren's Syndrome).

a. 14-18% of adults with SLE will develop PACNS, 22-95% in children.

b. Usually occurs late in the primary disease.

3. Infections.

a. Human immunodeficiency virus (HIV), Treponema pallidum infection, varicella zoster, tuberculosis, hepatitis C, West Nile virus, parvovirus B19, rarely herpes simplex virus, Cytomegalovirus.

4. Lymphoproliferative diseases.

a. Lymphomatoid granulomatosis, often present with HIV.

b. CNS lymphoma and inbravascular lymphoma—mimics PACNS (Firestein et al., 2012).

F. Treatment.

1. Usually Cytoxan® and corticosteroids.

2. Based on type of PACNS and severity of injury.

4
4.1
4.2
4.3
4.4
4.5
4.6
4.7
4.8
4.9
4.10

3. Atypical PACNS—treatment depends on neurological damage and symptoms.

4. Remission should not be misinterpreted because of neurological deficits that have occurred. These may be permanent.

5. Series MRI helpful in monitoring progress.

6. Remission is possible, however up to 20% of patients will have functional deficits (Firestein et al., 2012).

   a. Treat chronic diseases such as osteoporosis, hypertension, diabetes, and hyperlipidemia, if present.

      (1) Encourage smoking cessation.

      (2) Decrease alcohol consumption if excessive.

      (3) Recommend daily physical activity, preferably weight bearing.

7. Suggest weight reduction, if appropriate.

G. Nursing assessment.

1. Understand the need to confirm the diagnosis and begin appropriate therapy when life altering disease is present.

2. Implement appropriate laboratory studies and imaging, and interpret the results to verify or rule out a diagnosis of vasculitis.

3. If a biopsy has been performed, assess site and instruct the patient on appropriate wound care.

4. When treatment has begun.

   a. Assess for tolerance and compliance with medications.

   b. Assess for flares.

      (1) Number since last office visit if patient is being treated in rheumatologist's office, severity (did it interfere with work, family life?).

      (2) What triggered the flare, what relieved symptoms?

      (3) Specific symptoms associated with the flare.

5. Assess ability to accomplish activities of daily living, manage stress, participate in work, family, and social life activities.

6. Physical assessment with additional focus on systems affected by the disease to determine improvement or worsening of condition.

XV. Immune complex-mediated small vessel vasculitis.

A. Many small types of small vessel vasculitis are mediated when an antigen combines with an antibody, otherwise known as immune complexes. This inflammation can lead to a cascade of inflammation of the cells, damage to the vascular walls, decreased circulation to and within an organ, and diminished organ function.

B. Hypersensitivity angiitis (another interchangeable term for vasculitis) was seen in the early 1990s with the use of sulfonamides and horse serum to treat disease. Other disorders include Henoch-Schonlein purpura (HSP), mixed cryoglobulinemia, erythema elevatum diutinum, and hypocomplementemic urticarial vasculitis.

C. Certain forms of vasculitis can present in other diseases such as systemic lupus erythematosus (SLE), rheumatoid vasculitis, and Sjögren's syndrome.

D. In small vessels angiitis and vasculitis are interchangeable terms when speaking about capillaries, arterioles, and venules.

E. Immune complex (IC) mediated vasculitis types share areas of pathology, cutaneous lesions, and some overlap with other conditions as listed above; they are generally discussed together (Fauci, 2006; Firestein et al., 2012).

F. Pathology.

1. Arthus reaction.

2. When immune complexes (ICs) form, they initiate compliment activation. This is followed by a flow of inflammatory cells. These cells accumulate causing thrombus formation and hemorrhagic infarction in the areas heavy with inflammation. In most cases the ICs are cleared by the reticuloendothelial system and eliminate the foreign substances. In some cases, some ICs manage to

continue and deposit in bones, skin, joints, or other tissues resulting in illness.

G. Immunogenicity.

1. The path of ICs is regulated by antigen burden, antibody response, blood vessel function, lumen for blood flow, and any blockages and if the ICs are soluble, themselves. The reticuloendothelial system can remove antigen-antibody pairs. When there is antibody excess, small ICs can form and cause no inflammatory reaction. It is when the antigen is in excess that the IC becomes hemmed in to the vascular bed and leads to a series of events that result in tissue injury.

H. Cutaneous manifestations.

1. Small vessels are those less than 50 micrometers in diameter. These are usually located in the papillary dermis. Skin lesions, purpuric, are usually located symmetrically, and in the lower extremities. These lesions are not always palpable, but this alone is not diagnostic for IC mediated vasculitis. There are other vasculidities that affect small vessels such as granulomatosis with polyangiitis (GPA; formerly known as Webener's granulomatosis) (Holle, Laudien, & Gross, 2010), microscopic polyangiitis, and Churg-Strauss syndrome. The difference between the two groups is the pathology of the tissue.

I. Pathologic features.

1. Skin biopsy obtained preferably within 24-48 hours of the lesion and performed from a non-ulcerated area. (Ulcerated lesions, usually associated with medium vessels, should be biopsied along the edge.)

2. Specimens should be studied by both light microscopy and direct. immunofluorescence (DIF). DIF is especially important in small vessel disease and needs to be pre-planned as a fresh skin sample is necessary for evaluation. Specimens for DIF are frozen and incubated with stained human immunoglobulin, (Ig) G, IgM, Ig A, and C3. This assists with pathophysiology of disease and diagnosis (Firestein et al., 2012).

XVI. IC mediated small vessel disorders.

A. Hypersensitivity vasculitis (Cutaneous leukocytoclastic angiitis) (Calabrese et al., 1990).

1. Occurs after the age of 16.

2. Use of a possible offending medication sequential to symptoms.

3. Palpable purpura.

4. Maculopapular rash.

5. Skin biopsy shows neutrophils around an arteriole or venule.

6. Spares the organs.

7. About one half of patients with hypersensitivity vasculitis have no known trigger.

8. Usual presentation.

   a. Symptoms occur about 7-14 days after beginning a new medication.

      (1) Penicillin and the Cephalosporins are the most common triggers, diuretics and anti-hypertensives are also common.

9. Treatment.

   a. Skin usually clears within days of discontinuing the medication or trigger.

   b. Prognosis depends on the cause.

   c. Steroids are used in patients with significant disease, and can be tapered after 1-2 weeks.

XVII. Henoch-Schonlein purpura.

A. Palpable purpura.

B. Age at onset <20 year.

C. Bowel angina.

D. Vessel wall granulocytes on biopsy (Coblyn et al., 2011).

E. Blood vessel walls have depositions of IgA.

F. Common after upper respiratory infection.

G. Unable to determine if viral, bacterial, or other agent is the cause.

H. More common in children, but when an adult develops HSP, the course of disease is longer with increased bouts of purpura.

I. Usual presentation.

1. Follows upper respiratory infection.

4
4.1
4.2
4.3
4.4
4.5
4.6
4.7
4.8
4.9
4.10

2. Purpuric rash.

3. Arthralgias.

4. Abdominal pain, colicky (possible gastrointestinal [GI] vasculitis) is common.

    a. Generally presents about a week following the onset of rash.

    b. May require endoscopy if GI symptoms appear before the rash.

5. Renal disease (circulating ICs can form in the kidneys and other organs).

    a. Very common and usually self-limited; some patients develop end stage renal disease.

J. Treatment (Firestein et al., 2012).

1. Mild cases, no treatment necessary.

2. No evidence that patients with glomerulonephritis benefit from steroid or immunosuppressive therapies.

3. Prudent to begin therapy in individuals with significant renal disease with a combination of high dose steroids and immunosuppressive therapy such as cyclophosphamide, azathioprine, or mycophenolate mofetil.

4. Side effects: Cyclophosphamide.

    a. Nausea, vomiting during and after infusion, flu like symptoms.

    b. Alopecia.

    c. Bone marrow suppression, increase in transaminases, changes in renal function.

    d. Hemorrhagic cystitis and bladder cancers have been documented. Alert patient to report hematuria.

    e. Ovarian failure in females and azoospermia in males (Colbyn, Bermas, Weinblatt, & Helfgott, 2011).

        (1) Prophylaxis for Pneumocystis carii pneumonia with oral trimethoprim 160 mg/sulfamethoxazole 800 mg 3 times per week.

        (2) Side effects include.

           i) Diarrhea that is watery or bloody.

           ii) Feeling light-headed, rapid heart rate, trouble concentrating;

           iii) Skin: Easy bruising, unusual bleeding (nose, mouth, vagina, or rectum), purple or red pinpoint spots.

           iv) Nausea, upper stomach pain, itching, loss of appetite, dark urine, clay-colored stools, jaundice (yellowing of the skin or eyes); Steven's Johnson's Syndrome.

5. Side effects: Azathioprine.

    a. nausea, hepatic abnormalities, abdominal pain, leukopenia, infections, thrombocytopenia, pancreatitis (Cush & Kavanaugh, 2005).

6. Contraindications: Acute renal failure, use with caution in hepatic disease.

    a. Side effects: Mycophenolate mofetil.

        (1) alopecia, nausea, diarrhea, headache, hypertension, peripheral edema, rash, infection, and bone marrow suppression (Fauci & Langford, 2006).

XVIII. Cryoglobulinemic vasculitis.

A. Involves small and medium blood vessels.

B. Cryoglobulins bind to circulating antigen and accumulate in vessel walls (small and medium), causing vasculitis.

C. Common in Hepatitis C. Cryoglobulin attaches to a particle of the Hepatitis virus (the antigen) and activates complement.

D. Skin and glomeruli are often involved: Large cutaneous lesions, digital ischemia, and livedo racemosa (reticularis).

E. Three types of cryoglobulinemias.

1. Type I: Monoclonal gammopathy (IgG or IgM), Waldenstrom's macroglobulinemia or multiple myeloma.

    a. Dizziness, headaches, confusion, stroke.

2. Type II and III: Mixed cryoglobulin (both IgG and Ig M).

    a. Type II: Hepatitis C infections cause more than 90% of the conditions.

    b. Monoclonal IgM and polyclonal IgG.

    c. Type II: Non hepatitis association, no known cause.

    d. Mixed essential cryoglobulinemia.

    e. Type III: Polyclonal IgG and polyclonal IgM.

    f. Seen in chronic forms of inflammation and autoimmune disease.

4
4.1
4.2
4.3
4.4
4.5
4.6
4.7
4.8
4.9
4.10

3. Types II and III.

   a. Purpura, myalgias, and arthralgias.

   b. Purpura: Trunk, upper extremities and face, but most often in lower extremities.

   c. Commonly involve the kidneys and peripheral nerves.

     (1) Vasculitic neuropathy, glomerulonephritis.

   d. Rare: Alveolar hemorrhage.

F. Diagnosis.

1. Skin biopsy: Light microscopy and DIF.

2. C4 is very low and disproportionate to C3.

3. May have highly positive rheumatoid factor.

G. Treatment.

1. Anti-viral therapies: Combination interferon-α and ribavirin.

2. Most recent: Combine antiviral therapy and B cell depletion with Rituximab (Rituxan®, Genentech, 2012).

   a. Plasma cells that produce cryoglobulin are decreased with B lymphocyte depletion.

   b. Begin antiviral therapy followed by rituximab within several weeks.

     (1) Patients with alveolar hemorrhage or hyperviscosity symptoms may benefit from plasma exchange (remove inflammatory ICs as quickly as possible).

       i) Interferon-α Peginterferon alfa-2b: Common side effects/adverse effects include infections; mental illness including depression, mood and behavior problems, or thoughts of suicide or hurting others, angina, myocardial infarct, colitis, joint pain, fever, and autoimmune disorders.

     (2) Ribavirin: Common side effects include cough, upset stomach, vomiting, diarrhea, constipation, heartburn, loss of appetite, weight loss. Changes in ability to taste food, dry mouth, difficulty concentrating, difficulty falling asleep or staying asleep, memory loss, rash, dry, irritated, or itchy skin, sweating, painful or irregular menstruation, muscle or bone pain, hair loss, urticaria, angioedema.

     (3) Rituximab: Side effects around the time of the infusion can include headache, cough, nausea, stomach upset, sweating, nervousness, muscle stiffness, and numbness. Patients can take mild pain medications, such as acetaminophen, for these symptoms but should call the healthcare provider if the symptoms are severe or get worse. Sometimes infusion reactions occur such as hypotension, mild throat tightening, rash, pruitis, dizziness, and back pain. These symptoms can be reduced by use of acetaminophen or diphenhydramine and slowing or stopping the infusion for a short period of time and restarting it at a lower rate. On occasion a steroid injection is required. The healthcare provider may recommend pre-medicating the patient prior to the next infusion. Patients should be instructed to be aware of infections such as colds and sinusitis and call if they are having any difficulty recovering from these infections.

   c. Treat chronic diseases such as osteoporosis, hypertension, diabetes, and hyperlipidemia, if present.

     (1) Encourage smoking cessation.

     (2) Decrease alcohol consumption if excessive.

     (3) Recommend daily physical activity, preferably weight bearing.

     (4) Suggest weight reduction, if appropriate.

H. Prognosis.

1. Depends on cause.

2. Type I correlates to the underlying cause.

3. Type II and III associated with hepatitis C; do well if the patient improves with antiviral therapy.

4. If no response to antiviral therapy, or if this is not tolerated, treatment with steroids may be required.

XIX. Hypocomplementemic urticarial vasculitis (UV).

A. Lesions last more than 48 hours, most of the time, take days to resolve.

1. Common urticaria resolves in 34-48 hours.

B. Do not blanch.

C. Changes in pigmentation because of the inflammation.

D. Worsen without therapy.

E. Three types:

1. Normocomplementemic UV.

    a. Self-limited.

    b. Distinguish from neutrophilic urticaria (a condition that is not associated with vasculitis).

2. Hypocomplementemic UV.

    a. Chronic disorder.

    b. Need to distinguish from systemic lupus erythematosus (SLE). Have similar auto antibodies, complement, and dermatitis.

3. Hypocomplementemic urticarial vasculitis syndrome (HUVS).

    a. Severe form of vasculitis.

    b. Extracutaneous disease, chronic obstructive pulmonary disease, uveitis, and angioedema.

4. Skin lesions.

    a. More common on trunk and proximal extremities.

    b. Painful, burning sensation, no pruitis.

F. Diagnosis.

1. Skin biopsy with microscopic and DIF.

G. Treatment.

1. Hypocomplementemic UV may respond to treatments used in SLE.

    a. Prednisone, Hydroxychloroqine, dapsone or other immunosuppressant medications.

    b. Side effects: Hydroxycholorquine: Retinal damage, agranulocytosis, peripheral neuropathy, aplastic anemia, myopathy, pigmentation of the skin (Fauci & Langford, 2006).

    c. Side effects: Dapsone: Nausea, vomiting, loss of appetite, or blurred vision, dizziness, chest pain, bone marrow suppression (low blood counts), and liver damage may occur.

2. HUVS serious form with organ dysfunction.

    a. High dose steroids.

    b. Anti TNF antagonists.

    c. May need to treat accompanying chronic obstructive pulmonary disease and cardiac valve disease.

XX. Erythema elevatum diutinum.

A. Rare disease.

B. Form of leukocytoclastic vasculitis.

C. Limited to the skin.

1. Located on extensor surfaces of joints.

2. Papules, nodules, plaques.

3. Lesions begin as pink or yellow, turn red or purple.

4. Without treatment, persist for years, doughy or hard as time progresses.

5. Usually located in hands and knees, but can be located on the buttocks.

6. Can be seen in connective tissue disease, rheumatoid arthritis, other forms of vasculitis, human immunodeficiency virus infections, and paraproteinemias (IgA).

D. Diagnosis.

1. Biopsy: Findings similar to leukocytoclastic vasculitis with fibrinoid necrosis.

2. DIF results do not show evidence if IC involvement.

E. Treatment.

1. Dapsone.

    a. Side effects: Nausea, vomiting, loss of appetite, or blurred vision, dizziness, chest pain, bone marrow suppression (low blood counts), and liver damage may occur.

2. Sulfapyridine.

    a. Side effects: Rash, nausea, abdominal pain, bone marrow suppression.

    b. Lesions return when treatment is discontinued.

4
4.1
4.2
4.3
4.4
4.5
4.6
4.7
4.8
4.9
4.10

XXI. Connective tissue disease-associated vasculitis.

A. Include systemic lupus erythematosus, mixed connective tissue disease, Sjögren's Syndrome, and overlap connective tissue disease.

B. Commonly over diagnosed.

C. Confirm by biopsy.

D. Associated with high titers of ANA and hypocomplementemia.

E. Vasculitis in SLE associated with lymphocytic proliferation.

F. Variant of CTD associated vasculitis.

1. Hypergammaglobulinemia for Waldenstrom's: True *lymphocytic* vasculitis.

2. Have anti Ro antibodies.

3. Mild symptoms of Sjögren's Syndrome.

4. Lymphocytic vasculitis is less destructive to the blood vessel, always present in small blood vessels.

XXII. Rheumatoid vasculitis (RV).

A. Distinguish from isolated digital vasculitis.

1. Unless severe, does not necessitate vasculitic therapy.

B. Rheumatoid vasculitis.

1. Bywater's lesions: Splinter-like lesions, periungual region. May involve medium and small vessels.

2. Sometimes unable to differentiate between RV and polyarteritis nodosa.

3. Occurs in patients who have aggressive joint disease, accompanied by nodules that are rheumatoid factor positive.

C. Diagnosis.

1. Purpuric lesions.

2. May or may not have evidence of medium vessel vasculitis.

3. Skin biopsy with DIF examination.

4. Characteristic RV: Deep cutaneous ulcers near the malleoli.

a. Require good wound care and immunosuppression.

D. Treatment.

1. High dose steroids.

a. Side effects: Depression, psychosis, and mood swings, hypertension, congestive heart failure.

b. Hyperglycemia.

c. Weight gain, peptic ulcer disease.

d. Masks infections, slows wound healing, triggers acne, thins the skin which bruises easily.

e. Muscle weakness in long term use, osteoporosis.

f. May cause cataracts or will worsen existing cataracts, glaucoma.

2. Contraindications: Active infections (Doherty, 2010).

a. Rituximab: Side effects around the time of the infusion can include headache, cough, nausea, stomach upset, sweating, nervousness, muscle stiffness, and numbness. Patients can take mild pain medications, such as acetaminophen, for these symptoms, but should call the healthcare provider if the symptoms are severe or get worse. Sometimes infusion reactions occur such as hypotension, mild throat tightening, rash, pruitis, dizziness, and back pain. These symptoms can be reduced by use of acetaminophen or diphenhydramine and slowing or stopping the infusion for a short period of time and restarting it at a lower rate. On occasion a steroid injection is required. The healthcare provider may recommend pre-medicating the patient prior to the next infusion. Patients should be instructed to be aware of infections such as colds and sinusitis and call if they are having any difficulty recovering from the infection.

b. Cyclophosphamide. Side effects include:

(1) Nausea, vomiting during and after infusion, flu like symptoms.

(2) Alopecia.

(3) Bone marrow suppression, increase in transaminases, changes in renal function.

4
4.1
4.2
4.3
4.4
4.5
4.6
4.7
4.8
4.9
4.10

(4) Hemorrhagic cystitis and bladder cancers have been documented. Alert patient to report hematuria.

(5) Ovarian failure in females and azoospermia in males (Colbyn, Bermas, Weinblatt, & Helfgott, 2011).

c. Prophylaxis for Pneumocystis carii pneumonia with oral trimethoprim 160 mg/sulfamethoxazole 800 mg 3 times per week.

d. Side effects include.

(1) Diarrhea that is watery or bloody.

(2) Feeling light-headed, rapid heart rate, trouble concentrating.

(3) Skin: Easy bruising, unusual bleeding (nose, mouth, vagina, or rectum), purple or red pinpoint spots.

(4) Nausea, upper stomach pain, itching, loss of appetite, dark urine, clay-colored stools, jaundice (yellowing of the skin or eyes); Steven's Johnson's Syndrome.

e. Treat chronic diseases such as osteoporosis, hypertension, diabetes, and hyperlipidemia, if present.

f. Encourage smoking cessation.

g. Decrease alcohol consumption if excessive.

h. Recommend daily physical activity, preferably weight bearing.

i. Suggest weight reduction, if appropriate.

E. Nursing assessment.

1. Understand the need to confirm the diagnosis and begin appropriate therapy when life altering disease is present.

2. Implement appropriate laboratory studies and imaging, and interpret the results to verify or rule out a diagnosis of vasculitis.

3. If a biopsy has been performed, assess site and instruct the patient on appropriate wound care.

4. When treatment has begun:

a. Assess for tolerance and compliance with medications.

b. Assess for flares.

(1) Number since last office visit (if patient is being treated in a rheumatologist's office), severity (did it interfere with work, family life?).

(2) What triggered the flare, what relieved symptoms?

(3) Specific symptoms associated with the flare.

5. Assess ability to accomplish activities of daily living, manage stress, participate in work, family, and social life activities.

6. Physical assessment with additional focus on systems affected by the disease to determine improvement or worsening of condition.

7. Arteries and veins of various sizes.

XXIII. Behçet's disease in adults.

A. Pathology.

1. Multi factoral: Heredity, infections, clotting factors, immunologic factors, and inflammatory factors (Firestein et al., 2012).

B. Genetic.

1. Associated with an HLA B51 allo-antigen, disease is more severe if HLA B-51 is positive. Role of the gene is not known as a direct cause (Firestein et al., 2012).

2. First degree relatives are at risk, as are children of someone who has Behçet's and may develop the disease earlier (Firestein et al., 2012).

3. Male to female ratio 1:1, however, males tend to have more severe disease (Fauci & Langford, 2006).

4. Common in Middle East, Mediterranean, and Japan.

5. Common features with the spondyloarthropathies, HLA B27 not associated with Behçet's (Firestein et al., 2012).

C. Immune factors.

1. Cytokines, heat shock proteins, changes in macrophage and neutrophil function, and autoimmune processes have been recognized and studied.

2. Diversity of T lymphocytes is seen in Behçet's. Multiple symptoms seen in Behçet's may be a result of antigen response of the T lymphocytes.

3. Evidence for cytokines and tumor necrosis factor participation.

4
4.1
4.2
4.3
4.4
4.5
4.6
4.7
4.8
4.9
4.10

4. Neutophilic vascular reactions occur because of circulating immune complexes.

5. Lesions of Behçet's are known to contain macrophage activation, neutrophil chemotaxis, and phagocytosis.

6. Others: Endothelial dysfunction, increase in nitric acid in synovial fluid and aqueous humor, and increased homocyteine levels seem to have a role in inflammation or vasculitis (Firestein et al., 2012).

D. Infections.

1. Streptococcus sanguis: May be responsible for oral ulcerations.

2. Escherichia coli and Staphylococcus aureus activate lymphocytes.

3. Mycoplasa fermentans has been present in individuals with Behçet's.

4. Helicobacter pylori can cause endothelial impairment, and if treated, has shown a decrease in symptoms of Behçet's.

5. Herpes simplex virus has been detected in blood and in biopsied tissue from genital and gastrointestinal areas (Coblyn et al., 2011; Fauci & Langford, 2006; Firestein et al., 2012).

E. Diagnosis.

1. Difficult and based on clinical findings.

2. No specific lab test is diagnostic.

3. Criteria plus scoring includes: Oral aphthosis = 1 point, skin aphtosis or pseudofolliculitis = 1point, vascular symptoms (phlebitis, large vein thrombosis, aneurism, arterial thrombosis) = 1 point, positive pathergy test = 1 point, genital aphthosis = 2 points and ocular lesions = 2 points. Diagnosis is made with a score of 3 points (International Team for the Revision of International Criteria for Behçet's disease, 2008). Exclude IBD, SLE, reactive arthritis, and herpetic infections.

   a. Biopsy to exclude inflammatory bowel disease, enteropathic arthritis, and acne.

   b. Biopsy for culture and histologic studies of all inflammatory skin lesions.

4. Thorough ophthalmic examination.

5. Consider specialists for arthralgias, neurological symptoms, or gastrointestinal disease (Firestein et al., 2012).

F. Signs and symptoms.

1. Oral aphthae or canker sores usually first symptom, 3-10 lesions.

2. Can be shallow or deep, usually painful, necrotic base.

3. Generally present for 1-2 weeks.

4. Located anywhere in the mouth, no scarring (Fauci & Langford, 2006).

5. Genital lesions, if present, occur on scrotum and penis in males; vulva or vaginal mucosa in females.

6. Less common. Scarring occurs (Firestein et al., 2012).

7. Cutaneous lesions.

   a. Erythema nodosum-like lesions.

   b. Pyoderma gangrenosum-like.

   c. Sweet's Syndrome-like.

   d. Cutaneous small vessel vasculitis.

   e. Pustular vasculitis lesions.

   f. Pathergy-inflammatory (reddened, possibly raised) skin reaction to scratches (Firestein et al., 2012).

8. Ophthalmic.

   a. Responsible for significant morbidity.

   b. Uveitis posterior and inferior.

   c. Retinal vasculitis.

   d. Hypopyon (pus-like fluid).

      (1) Secondary glaucoma, cataract formation.

      (2) Decreased vision and synechiae (iris adheres to the cornea or the lens) formation (Fauci & Langford, 2006).

9. Arthritis.

   a. Usually one or two joints.

   b. Inflammatory, non-erosive disease.

   c. Symmetrical or asymmetric.

   d. More prevalent in the knees and ankles, wrists, and elbows (Fauci & Langford, 2006).

10. Other.

   a. Isolated headaches, venous sinus thrombosis, aseptic meningitis.

4
4.1
4.2
4.3
4.4
4.5
4.6
4.7
4.8
4.9
4.10

b. Gastrointestinal lesions similar to the oral aphthous.

    (1) Ileocecal region.

    (2) Ascending and transverse colon (perforation can occur).

    (3) Esophagus (Firestein et al., 2012).

G. Nursing assessment.

1. Understand the need to confirm the diagnosis and begin appropriate therapy when life altering disease is present.

2. Implement appropriate laboratory studies and imaging, and interpret the results to verify or rule out a diagnosis of vasculitis.

3. If a biopsy has been performed, assess site and instruct the patient on appropriate wound care.

H. When treatment has begun:

1. Assess for tolerance and compliance with medications.

2. Assess for flares.

3. Number since last office visit (if patient being treated in a rheumatologist's office), severity (did it interfere with work, family life?).

    a. What triggered the flare, what relieved symptoms?

    b. Specific symptoms associated with the flare.

4. Assess ability to accomplish activities of daily living, manage stress, participate in work, family, and social life activities.

5. Physical assessment with additional focus on systems affected by the disease to determine improvement or worsening of condition.

I. Treatment (Firestein et al., 2012).

1. Based on the degree and system involved.

2. Mucocutaneous disease.

    a. Oral and genital ulcers:

        (1) Topical, intra lesion, or spray on corticosteroids.

        (2) Topical Tacrolimus.

        (3) Oral tetracycline solutions, rinses with chlorhexiding gluconate, topical anesthetics.

        (4) Colchicine: Common side effects include nausea, vomiting, diarrhea, stomach cramps or pain. More serious side effects include muscle pain or weakness, numbness in the fingers or toes, unusual bruising or bleeding, sore throat, fever, chills, and other signs of infection, weakness or tiredness, paleness or grayness of the lips, tongue, or palms (National Institutes of Health, 2009).

        (5) Dapsone (Aczone®) common side effects include nausea, vomiting, loss of appetite, or blurred vision, dizziness, chest pain, bone marrow suppression (low blood counts), and liver damage may occur (Doherty, 2010).

        (6) Etanercept (Embrel®): Common side effects include local injection site reactions, risk of infections, bone marrow suppression, allergic reaction such as pruitis, throat tightening, swelling of the lips or tongue. Contraindications: Do not administer during an infection.

3. Severe mucocutaneous disease.

    a. Thalidomide (Thalomid®): Common side effects include birth defects, drowsiness, somnolence, peripheral neuropathy, orthostatic hypotension, dizziness, neutropenia, seizure disorder, bradycardia, and Steven's Johnson's Syndrome.

    b. MTX: Common side effects include gastric intolerance, oral ulcers, alopecia, increase in liver function tests, bone marrow suppression. and possible pulmonary fibrosis. Contraindications: Acute renal failure, use caution in pulmonary disease, use caution in hepatic insufficiency (Doherty, 2010).

    c. Prednisone: Common side effects include depression, psychosis, and mood swings, hypertension, congestive heart failure, hyperglycemia, weight gain, peptic ulcer disease; masks infections, slows wound healing, acne, thins the skin which bruises easily; muscle weakness in long term use, osteoporosis, may cause cataracts or will worsen existing cataracts, glaucoma.

        (1) Contraindications: Active infections (Doherty, 2010).

4. Systemic disease (includes those with cardiovascular disease and eye disease).

4
4.1
4.2
4.3
4.4
4.5
4.6
4.7
4.8
4.9
4.10

a. Systemic corticosteroids as single therapy or in combination.

b. Azothiaprine: Common side effects include nausea, hepatic abnormalities, abdominal pain, leukopenia, infections, thrombocytopenia, pancreatitis (Cush & Kavanaugh, 2005).

   (1) Contraindications: Acute renal failure, use caution in hepatic disease.

c. Interferon-alpha: Common side effects/ adverse effects include infections, mental illness (depression, mood, and behavior problems, or thoughts of suicide or hurting others), angina or myocardial infarction, colitis, joint pain, fever, and autoimmune disorders (National Institutes of Health, 2009).

d. Cyclosporine: Common side effects include infection, sore throat, fever, chills, cough, dysuria, skin lesions night sweats, lymphadenopathy, dyspnea, chest pain, abdominal pain, bloating, hypertension and changes in renal function.

e. Cyclophosphamide: Common side effects include nausea, vomiting during and after infusion, flu like symptoms, alopecia, bone marrow suppression, increase in transaminases, changes in renal function; hemorrhagic cystitis and bladder cancers have been documented. Alert patient to report hematuria. Ovarian failure in females and azoospermia in males (Colbyn, 2011).

f. Prophylaxis for Pneumocystis carii pneumonia with oral trimethoprim 160 mg/sulfamethoxazole 800 mg 3 times per week.

   (1) Side effects include diarrhea that is watery or bloody; feeling light-headed, rapid heart rate, trouble concentrating; easy bruising of skin, unusual bleeding (nose, mouth, vagina, or rectum), purple or red pinpoint spots. Nausea, upper stomach pain, itching, loss of appetite, dark urine, clay-colored stools, jaundice (yellowing of the skin or eyes); Steven's-Johnson's Syndrome.

g. Chlorambucil: Common side effects include nausea, vomiting, sores in the mouth and throat, fatigue, changes in menses, skin rash, hematuria, cough, unusual bleeding, bruising, black tarry stools. Individual may develop cancers.

5. Eye disease:

   a. Prednisone: Common side effects include depression, psychosis, and mood swings, hypertension, congestive heart failure, hyperglycemia, weight gain, peptic ulcer disease; masks infections, slows wound healing, triggers acne, thins the skin which bruises easily; muscle weakness in long term use, osteoporosis, may cause cataracts or will worsen existing cataracts, glaucoma.

      (1) Contraindications: Active infections (Doherty, 2010).

   b. Azothiaprine: Common side effects include nausea, hepatic abnormalities, abdominal pain, leukopenia, infections, thrombocytopenia, pancreatitis (Cush & Kavanaugh, 2005). Contraindications: Acute renal failure, use caution in hepatic disease.

      (1) If no response, change to another disease-modifying antirheumatic drug (DMARD).

   c. Mycophenolate mofetil: Common side effects include alopecia, nausea, diarrhea, headache, hypertension, peripheral edema, rash, infection, and bone marrow suppression (Harrison, 2006).

      (1) Contraindication: Pregnancy, bone marrow suppression, severe renal disease.

   d. Rituximab: Common side effects around the time of the infusion can include headache, cough, nausea, stomach upset, sweating, nervousness, muscle stiffness, and numbness. Patients can take mild pain medications, such as acetaminophen, for these symptoms, but should call the healthcare provider if the symptoms are severe or get worse. Sometimes infusion reactions such as hypotension, mild throat tightening, rash, pruitis, dizziness, and back pain occur. These symptoms can be reduced by use of acetaminophen or diphenhydramine and slowing or stopping the infusion for a short period of time and restarting it at a lower rate. On occasion a steroid injection is required. The healthcare provider may recommend pre-medicating the patient prior to the next infusion. Patients should be instructed to be aware of infections such as colds and sinusitis and call if they are having any difficulty recovering from the infection.

4
4.1
4.2
4.3
4.4
4.5
4.6
4.7
4.8
4.9
4.10

(1) Treat chronic diseases such as osteoporosis, hypertension, diabetes, and hyperlipidemia, if present:

    i) Encourage smoking cessation.

    ii) Decrease alcohol consumption if excessive.

    iii) Recommend daily physical activity, preferably weight bearing,

(2) Suggest weight reduction, if appropriate.

6. Outcome.

    a. Variable pattern of disease.

    b. Exacerbations and remissions.

    c. Difficult to diagnose. Eye and neurological disease can occur after initial diagnosis.

    d. Increased morbidity in those with ocular disease (uveitis, retinal vasculitis), central nervous system disease as well as vascular disease.

    e. Low mortality rates unless there is associated pulmonary or central nervous system involvement or bowel perforation (Firestein et al., 2012).

XXIV. Relapsing polychondritis.

A. Pathology.

1. Cartilage destruction begins at the edges and advances toward the center (Fauci & Langford, 2006).

2. The inflammation is due to infiltrates that consist of mononuclear cells and some plasma cells (Fauci & Langford, 2006).

3. Degeneration of the cells of the cartilage is replaced with granulation tissue, which leads to fibrosis and zones of calcification (Fauci & Langford, 2006).

4. Microscopic exam shows immunoglobulin and complement. Electron microscopic exam shows tissue consisting of immunoglobulin and enzymes or proteoglycans (Fauci & Langford, 2006).

B. Etiology.

1. Occurs in age groups of 40-50 years, but has occurred in children and the aged (Fauci & Langford, 2006).

2. Occurs equally in males and females and in all races (Fauci & Langford, 2006).

3. May be related to the HLA-DR4 gene as this is present more often in individuals with relapsing polychondritis than in the general population (Latinis et al., 2004). There is a negative correlation with HLA-DR6 (Coblyn et al., 2011).

4. Antibodies to Collagen II can be seen in 20 – 50% of patients (Latinis et al., 2004).

5. Patients may present with another type of rheumatoid condition, most generally vasculitis, followed in frequency by rheumatoid arthritis, Systemic Lupus Erythematosus, Sjögren's Syndrome, or Ankylosing Spondylitis (Fauci & Langford, 2006).

6. Individuals with primary biliary cirrhosis, inflammatory bowel disease, or myelodysplastic syndrome may also have relapsing polychondritis (Fauci & Langford, 2006).

C. Nursing diagnosis.

1. Understand the need to confirm the diagnosis and begin appropriate therapy when life altering disease is present.

2. Implement appropriate laboratory studies and imaging, and interpret the results to verify or rule out a diagnosis of vasculitis.

3. If a biopsy has been performed, assess site and instruct the patient on appropriate wound care.

4. When treatment has begun:

    a. Assess for tolerance and compliance with medications.

    b. Assess for flares.

      (1) Number since last office visit (if patient is being seen in a rheumatologist's office), severity (did it interfere with work, family life?).

      (2) What triggered the flare, what relieved symptoms?

      (3) Specific symptoms associated with the flare.

5. Assess ability to accomplish activities of daily living, manage stress, participate in work, family, and social life activities.

4
4.1
4.2
4.3
4.4
4.5
4.6
4.7
4.8
4.9
4.10

6. Physical assessment with additional focus on systems affected by the disease to determine improvement or worsening of condition.

D. Diagnosis.

1. 3 or more of the following present plus a positive biopsy of the ear, nasal, or respiratory cartilage (Fauci & Langford, 2006).

   a. Recurrent chondritis of both auricles; "Cauliflower" deformity may occur (Colbyn, Bermas, Weinblatt, & Helfgott, 2011).

   b. Non-erosive inflammatory arthritis (Fauci & Langford, 2006).

   c. Chondritis of nasal cartilage.

   d. Inflammation of the eye: Conjunctivitis, keratitis, scleritis/spiscleritis and/or uveitis.

   e. Inflamed laryngeal and/ or tracheal cartilages.

   f. Vestibular damage-vertigo, cochlear damage, neurosensory hearing loss or tinnitus.

   g. Biopsy is not always necessary. In some patients with firm cartilage structures, diagnosis is clearly evident. In some circumstances, the diagnosis is made by the patient's response to dapsone or steroids.

   h. First symptoms typically begin with the auricle, either together or sequentially. 85% of patients will develop chondritis at some point in the disease. Swelling of the Eustachian tube can cause infection or loss of hearing. Cochlear branch or vestibular artery inflammation can result in vertigo, hearing loss, nausea, and vomiting. Vertigo almost always leads to hearing loss.

   i. Nasal cartilage can become inflamed during the first episode or thereafter and will affect about 50% of patients with this condition.

   j. Patient presents with stuffy nose, rhinitis, and epistaxis. Bridge of the nose involved; swollen, tender, and may collapse (saddle nose). More common in women and young people.

E. Arthritis.

1. Occurs as first symptom in about 30% of patients.

2. Asymmetric, one or more joints; large and small.

3. No joint deformity, resolves within days to weeks.

4. Can involve the costochondral, sternoclavicular, and sternomanubrial cartilage.

5. Can occur in individuals who already have reactive arthritis, rheumatoid arthritis, ankylosing spondylitis, or psoriatic arthritis.

F. Eye involvement.

1. Seldom the first symptom, but will be present in about 50% of the patients with this condition.

2. Blindness can occur as a result of corneal ulcer or perforation.

3. Retinal vasculitis, optic neuritis, eyelid, and periorbital edema can occur as well.

G. Laryngotracheobronchial.

1. Present in about 50% of patients with hoarseness, non-productive cough.

2. Patient will have tenderness with palpation of the larynx and proximal trachea.

3. Airway obstruction occurs as a result of mucosal edema, strictures, or collapse of the cartilage.

4. Bronchial cartilage collapse can result in pneumonia.

H. Vascular structures.

1. About 5% of people with relapsing polychondritis will develop aortic regurgitation.

2. Occurs because of valve (cusps) or aortic ring damage.

3. Other heart valves less affected. Pericarditis, myocarditis, aneurysms of the aorta are additional complications (Fauci & Langford, 2006).

I. Systemic vasculitis (Fauci & Langford, 2006).

1. Most common: Leukocytoclastic vasculitis, polyarteritis, temporal arteri, and Takayasu's arteritis. Commonly affects the cranial nerves II, III, VI, and VII.

2. Patient presents with stroke, seizure, ataxia.

4
4.1
4.2
4.3
4.4
4.5
4.6
4.7
4.8
4.9
4.10

J. Skin (Fauci & Langford, 2006).

1. Lesions reflect vasculitis, not diagnostic for relapsing polychondritis.

2. Duration of disease varies from days to weeks and ends suddenly. Episodes may reoccur. Some individuals will have continuous chronic disease.

K. Laboratory/Imaging (Fauci & Langford, 2006).

1. Generally elevated sedimentation rate and C reactive protein.

2. Mild anemia, leukocytosis. Occasional low positive rheumatoid factor and ANA C ANCA and P ANCA can be found positive in active disease, but not diagnostic.

3. Kahlear tomography, laryngotracheography CT, and bronchoscopy evaluate presence of disease in upper and lower airways and degree of involvement. Bronchoscopy also assesses airway narrowing.

4. MRI used to evaluate trachea and larynx and aneurism dilation.

5. Pulmonary function tests determine intrathoracic airway obstruction (Coblyn et al., 2011).

6. Chest X-ray used to evaluate the aorta, narrowing of the trachea or main bronchi (Fauci & Langford, 2006).

7. Individuals who present with skin disease, consistent with vasculitis, should also be evaluated for possible malignancy (Coblyn et al., 2011).

L. Treatment.

1. Begin individuals with active disease on Prednisone 40-60 mg/day, and begin tapering when the disease is controlled (Fauci & Langford, 2006).

2. Some patients require 10-15 mg prednisone daily to suppress the disease.

3. Nonsteroidal anti-inflammatory drugs (NSAIDs) and colchicine have been used to treat relapsing polychondritis (Coblyn et al., 2011).

a. Common side effects for NSAIDs: Nausea, heartburn, hypertension, fluid retention/edema.

b. Contraindicated in ulcerative disease, in those on anticoagulant therapy, and in some individuals with cardiovascular disease.

4. Common side effects of colchicine are dose related and include nausea, vomiting, diarrhea, stomach cramps or pain. More serious side effects include muscle pain or weakness, numbness in the fingers or toes, unusual bruising or bleeding, sore throat, fever, chills, and other signs of infection, weakness or tiredness, paleness or grayness of the lips, tongue, or palms.

M. A steroid-sparing drug, dapsone, is often used if long term therapy is necessary (Fauci & Langford, 2006). Common side effects of dapsone include nausea, vomiting, loss of appetite, or blurred vision, dizziness, chest pain. Bone marrow suppression (low blood counts) and liver damage may occur.

N. Disease-modifying antirheumatic drugs (DMARDs) such as MTX, cyclophosphamide, azathioprine, or cyclosporine are reserved for individuals who do not respond to prednisone or if higher doses of medication are needed to control the disease (Fauci & Langford, 2006); however, the effectiveness of these DMARDs has not been established in clinical trials (Coblyn et al., 2011).

1. Eye disease may require intraoccular as well as oral steroids (Fauci & Langford, 2006).

2. Surgery may be indicated for aortic valve replacement or aneurism repair.

3. Tracheostomy may be necessary for airway compromise (Fauci & Langford, 2006).

4
4.1
4.2
4.3
4.4
4.5
4.6
4.7
4.8
4.9
4.10

Summary

I. In all patients with a diagnosis of vasculitis, the rheumatology nurse plays an important part on the management team.

   A. History.

      1. For the new patient, an accurate history including family, social, medical, and surgical will assist in an accurate diagnosis.

         a. Insurance/financial history, enough to assess ability to afford therapy or if assistance needed.

      2. For the established patient, assess:

         a. Adverse effects to prescribed therapies.

II. The patient's ability to perform activities of daily living (ADL) (Health Assessment Questionnaire) (Wolfe, Michaud, & Pincus, 2004).

   A. Disease activity score.

   B. Any changes in medications/has the patient been hospitalized.

   C. Review communications from other healthcare providers.

III. Physical assessment.

   A. Monitor for changes in vital signs, pain level, and disease activity score.

   B. Review lab reports for any signs of increased disease activity, co-morbid conditions or drug toxicity.

   C. Complete the physical exam with focus on specific systems involved.

IV.   Education.

   A. Provide written information for the patient to review at home, including a summary of the office visit, and reputable websites.

   B. Explain the specifics of the disease in terms that the patient can understand and allow for questions.

   C. Discuss symptoms to expect, when to notify the healthcare provider, what is an emergency situation.

   D. Discuss the rationale for the medication prescribed, how it is taken, what to do if a dose is missed, what monitoring is needed such as lab or X-ray, and potential side effects of the medication.

   E. Stress the importance of adequate rest, physical activity, nutrition, and weight management. Counseling for anxiety, stress management, or depression may be necessary.

   F. Competence of the rheumatology nurse.

   G. It is important to maintain a level of expertise related to disease processes and therapies available to treat disease. The rheumatology nurse should be able to thoroughly explain to the patient the actions of medications, typical time frames to expect some improvement of the disease, and side effects that may occur.

      1. Professional nursing societies/organizations offer educational opportunities to members in online as well as professional conference formats.

      2. Offer to teach other nurses, share patient experiences.

References

Amgen. (2012). *Enbrel®: Prescribing information.* Thousand Oaks, CA: Author.

Arend, W.P., Michel, B.A., Bloch, D.A., Hunder, G.G., Calabrese, L.H., Edworthy, S.M.,... Zvaifler, N.J. (1990). The American College of Rheumatology 1990 criteria for the classification of Takayasu arteritis. *Arthritis & Rheumatism, 33*(8), 1129-1134.

Calabrese, L.H., Michel, B.A., Bloch, D.A., Arend, W.P., Edworthy, S.M., Fauci, A.S., ... Zvaifler, N.J. (1990). The American College of Rheumatology 1990 criteria for the classification of hypersensitivity vasculitis. *Arthritis & Rheumatism, 33*(8), 1108-1113.

Colbyn, J.S., Bermas, B., Weinblatt, M., & Helfgott, S. (2011). *Brigham and women's experts' approach to rheumatology.* Sudbury, MA: Jones and Bartlett Learning.

4
4.1
4.2
4.3
4.4
4.5
4.6
4.7
4.8
4.9
4.10

Cush, J.J. & Kavanaugh, A. (2005). *RA: Early diagnosis and treatment.* West Islip, NY: Professional Communications, Inc.

Doherty, M. (2010). *Therapeutic strategies in rheumatology.* Oxford: Atlas Medical Publishing Ltd.

Fauci, A. S., & Langford, C.A. (Eds.). (2006). *Harrison's rheumatology.* New York: McGraw-Hill Medical Publishing Division.

Firestein, G.S., Budd, R.C., Gabreil, S.E., McInnes, I.B., & O'Dell, J.R. (2012). *Kelly's textbook of rheumatology* (9th ed.). Philadelphia: Saunders Elsevier.

Genentech. (2012). *Rituxan®*: Prescribing information. San Francisco, CA: Author.

Holle, J.U., Laudien, M., & Gross, W. L. (2010). Clinical manifestations and treatment of Webener's Granulomatosis. *Rheumatic Disease Clinics of North America, 36*(3), 507-526.

International Team for the Revision of International Criteria for Behçet's disease. Clinical manifestation of Behçet's disease. The ITR-ICBD report. (2008). *Clinical and Experimental Rheumatology, 26*(Suppl 50), S1-S18.

Langford, C. A. (2008, October). Wegener's Granulomatosis Treatment Today. *The Rheumatologist.* Retrieved 10 January 2015, from http://www.the-rheumatologist.org/details/article/967923/Wegenerx27s_Granulomatosis_Treatment_Today.html

Latinis, K.M., Dao, K.H., Gutierrez, E., Shepherd, R.M., Velazquez, C.R. (Eds.). (2004). *The Washington Manual™ Rheumatology Subspecialty Consult.* Philadelphia: Lippincott Williams & Wilkins.

Lightfoot, R.W. Jr., Michel, B.A., Bloch, D.A., Hunder, G.G., Zvaifler, N.J., McShane, D.J., ... Wallace, S.L. (1990). The American College of Rheumatology 1990 criteria for the classification of polyarteritis nodosa. *Arthritis & Rheumatism, 33*(8), 1088-1093.

National Institutes of Health. (2009). *Medlineplus: Drugs, herbs and supplements.* Retrieved from www.nlm.nih.gov/medlineplus/druginformation.html

Wiik, A.S. (2010). Autoantibodies in ANCA-Associated Vasculitis. *Rheumatic Disease Clinics of North America, 36*(3), 479-489.

Wolfe, F., Michaud, K., & Pincus, T. (2004). Development and validation of the health assessment questionnaire II: A revised version of the health assessment questionnaire. *Arthritis & Rheumatism, 50*(10), 3296–3305. DOI: 10.1002/art.20549

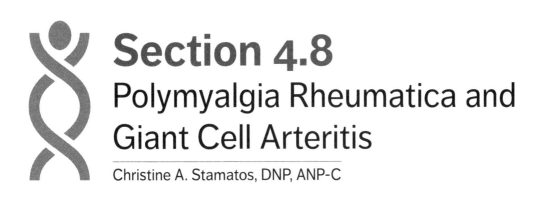

Section 4.8
Polymyalgia Rheumatica and Giant Cell Arteritis

Christine A. Stamatos, DNP, ANP-C

Introduction

This chapter will present a description of and the distinction between two inflammatory conditions often found together in older adults: Polymyalgia Rheumatica and Giant Cell Arteritis. A discussion of the incidence, presentation, and distinction of each will be provided. In both cases, these conditions are characterized by sudden, severe constitutional symptoms and a systemic inflammatory response that can be significant. The basis of treatment for both conditions is long term steroid use. Therefore a comprehensive review of steroid use, complications, and therapeutics currently under investigation to minimize cumulative dose of steroids will be presented.

Learning Objectives

Upon completion of this chapter, the nurse will be able to:

1. Describe the characteristic features of Polymyalgia Rheumatica.

2. State the symptoms unique to Giant Cell Arteritis.

3. Identify the most common adverse events associated with glucocorticoid therapy.

4. State the most serious complications of Giant Cell Arteritis.

5. Develop a plan to minimize the risks of long-term glucocorticoid therapy.

Content Outline

I. Pathophysiology.

A. What is polymyalgia Rheumatica (PMR)?

1. PMR is a musculoskeletal inflammatory syndrome of older adults, characterized by sudden onset of severe and disabling proximal stiffness involving bilateral shoulders, neck, and hips ("the girdle") associated with elevated acute phase reactants and constitutional symptoms. Clinical studies reveal overproduction of pro-inflammatory cytokines associated with disease activity (IL6, IL1, and TNF, IFNy) (Healey & Wilske, 1984; Nissen & Gabay, 2010; Parodi, Garlaschi, Silvestri, & Cimmino, 2006; Pulsatelli et al., 2008; Salvarani, et al., 1995; Salvarani, Cantini, Boiardi, & Hunder, 2004).

2. Imaging of shoulders/ hips reveals normal joint space (or degenerative changes based on age/ lifestyle), occasional effusions, with extensive tendinopathy and bursitis (Parodi et al., 2006).

3. Characterized by a rapid and profound response to low dose steroids.

4. It is a self-limiting disease resolving in most within 1-3 years but is characterized by recurrent flares/ relapses in that period. This is the exception rather than the rule.

5. Corticosteroids (CS) are the cornerstone of treatment. Slow taper over months to years is associated with more successful withdrawal (Dejaco et al., 2011; Kremers et al., 2005a; Salvarani et al., 2005).

B. What is giant cell arteritis (GCA)?

1. Large and medium vessel vasculitis associated with intense inflammation and granulomatous deposits of large "giant" cells – macrophages - along the walls of the arterial system affecting the vessels of the head and neck. Most specifically the internal (ocular system) and external branches of the carotids (temporal/ facial system), subclavian, vertebral arteries, and the aorta (see Figure 1). These changes result in luminal narrowing and end-organ ischemia. The most feared acute complications include blindness, infarcts, and late in the disease process (years later) aortic aneurysms and dissections (5-10 years later).

C. How are PMR and GCA related?

1. PMR is associated with GCA 10% of the time. In fact temporal arteries of patients with PMR have evidence of local inflammatory activity. It is believed that the inflammatory process in PMR and GCA are triggered by activation of vascular dendritic cells which is responsible for establishing vasculitis (inflammation of the vessel walls). Patients with PMR should be monitored for the emergence of vasculitis because GCA may develop years later (Announ & Guerne, 2008; Bernatsky et al., 2009; Healey & Wilske, 1984; Kremers et al., 2005b; Myklebust, Wilsgaard, Jacobsen, & Gran, 2003; Salvarani, Gabriel, O'Fallon, & Hunder, 1995a, 1995b; Schmidt & Gromnica-Ihle, 2002; Smeeth, Cook, & Hall, 2006; Warrington et al., 2009).

    a. Consider GCA if ESR > 80 or acute phase response does not improve with treatment.

    b. Nearly 10% of the time GCA is silent.

2. GCA is associated with PMR 40% of the time: Maintain high index of suspicion if there is/are.

    a. Presence of visual changes: Irreversible vision loss 10-15%

    b. Presence of temporal headache or scalp tenderness.

    c. Jaw claudication: Pain upon chewing.

    d. Symptoms of TIA/stroke: Slurred speech, unilateral weakness, asymmetrical facial expression.

    e. Vascular occlusions present as sudden vision loss, hearing loss, stroke, and ischemia of upper extremities.

Figure 1: Arteries commonly affected in GCA.

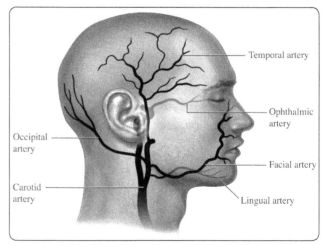

Source: Doctor Stock, Ipswich, MA. Copyright DoctorStock.com

D. Corticosteroids are the cornerstone of treatment for both and are required for long periods owing to much of the morbidity associated with these disease entities.

1. Consider that these diseases present in older adults with multiple comorbidities, many of which (e.g., osteoporosis, hypertension, glaucoma/ cataracts, metabolic disorders, and gastrointestinal problems) they often already have.

2. Long-term corticosteroid use is associated with numerous complications (Caporali, Cimmino, Montecucco, & Cutolo, 2011; Gabriel, Sunku, Salvarani, O'Fallon, & Hunder, 1997; Hernandez-Rodriguez, Cid, Lopez-Soto, Espigol-Frigole, & Bosch, 2009; Weyand, Fulbright, Evans, Hunder, & Goronzy, 1999).

   a. Ideally 50-75% will be off steroids by 2 years.

   b. But 25-50% will require steroids for 2-5 years or more.

   c. 65% will experience at least one steroid-induced side effect.

      (1) Infection (1.3-1.6 infections per 100 cases for low dose/ 2.6- 9.8 per 100 for high dose- 30 mg for more than 6 months).

      (2) Glaucoma/ cataracts.

      (3) Cardiovascular complications: Hypertension, atherosclerosis.

      (4) Metabolic consequences: Diabetes, weight gain, hyperlipidemia. 2-5x higher risk of developing diabetes when compared to age matched controls.

      (5) Osteoporosis and related complications. 2-5x higher risk of developing vertebral or hip fractures than age matched controls.

      (6) Mood disorders (e.g., irritability, psychosis, anxiety), sleep problems.

      (7) Avascular necrosis: Sudden severe joint destruction. There is some evidence that warfarin dosing when high dose steroids are used may prevent this complication.

      (8) Gastrointestinal: Esophageal/ gastric irritation.

      (9) Steroid myopathy: Insidious onset of proximal muscle weakness is the hallmark of this disorder. Associated with moderate to high doses of steroids for several months to years. Muscle enzymes are normal. More common with use of fluorinated steroids (dexamethasone and triamcinolone) than non-fluorinated steroids (prednisone or hydrocortisone). Sedentary lifestyle may increase risk because CS seem to affect less active muscles. Symptoms resolve as steroids are withdrawn (Caporali et al., 2011; Gabriel & Michaud, 2009; Gabriel et al., 1997; Hernandez-Rodriguez et al., 2009; Kremers et al., 2005a; Maradit Kremers et al., 2007; Myklebust et al., 2003; Weyand et al., 1999).

II. Etiology/ Epidemiology.

A. Etiology: PMR and GCA are closely related inflammatory syndromes and often exist together in the same person.

1. In a genetically predisposed individual:

   a. Northern European descent especially noted in the Minnesota region of this country.

   b. Almost exclusively Caucasians; rarely seen in Africans/ Asians.

   c. Age definitely a factor, risk increases markedly with age.

2. Seasonal, cyclical onset suggests possible infection or environmental change as triggering event.

3. Another argument for infection is the intense acute phase response seen in both PMR and GCA; however, specific etiology has yet to be identified (Gabriel & Michaud, 2009; Gonzalez-Gay et al., 2009; Salvarani, et al., 1995a, 1995b; Smeeth et al., 2006; Warrington et al., 2009).

B. Epidemiology.

1. PMR: 2-3x more common than GCA.

   a. Onset nearly always over 50 years of age, peak onset 70-75; Incidence increases with age.

   b. PMR is a common disease with a prevalence rate as high 2.6/100,000 from 50-59 and increases to 44.7/100,000 in the age group 80 years and older.

4
4.1
4.2
4.3
4.4
4.5
4.6
4.7
4.8
4.9
4.10

c. Though the rate of PMR is higher in women 2-3: 1, a relapsing and remitting course is more common in men.

2. GCA.

a. GCA is the most common form of systemic vasculitis in adults.

b. More common in Northern Europeans. As with PMR, Scandinavians have the highest prevalence.

c. Females are affected more often than men.

d. Smoking increases risk 6 fold.

e. In high risk populations: 20/100,000.

f. Onset most often after the age of 60 (80%)

g. Incidence appears to be rising, but is this because of greater awareness (Gabriel & Michaud, 2009; Gonzalez-Gay et al., 2009; Labbe & Hardouin, 1998; Muller et al., 2012; Salvarani, Gabriel, et al., 1995a; Schmidt & Gromnica-Ihle, 2002; Smeeth et al., 2006)?

III. Nursing Assessment.

A. PMR: Initial presentation: Joint stiffness described most significantly as having trouble getting out of bed. "I Need to roll over on my side then fall onto the floor." Slow starting. "I feel 100 years old." Stiffness may last throughout the day in severe cases. Pain and fatigue again overwhelming by the end of the day.

1. Shoulder (70-95%)

2. Hips (50-75%)

3. Distal small joint (50%) looks like onset of RA.

4. Constitutional symptoms (30-50%)

a. Fatigue.

b. Low grade fevers, malaise, anorexia.

c. Weight loss especially significant if time to diagnosis is several months.

5. Critical aspect of diagnosing PMR lies in excluding GCA. A temporal artery biopsy must be done in patients with suspicious vascular symptoms. A positive confirmation of GCA overrides a diagnosis of PMR (Nissen & Gabay, 2010; Schmidt & Gromnica-Ihle, 2002; Soubrier, Dubost, & Ristori, 2006; Stewart, 2003).

B. GCA: Initial presentation: 40% present with similar symptoms to PMR often months before the onset of signs of arterial involvement (see Figure 2).

1. Constitutional symptoms usually significant, often more dramatic then with PMR.

2. Headaches: Different, sometimes "throbbing," often severe, localized in temporal or occipital region.

3. Scalp tenderness, sensitive to light touch with temporal artery thickened or "ropelike," tender, and nodular (not always easy to determine).

4. Visual symptoms.

a. Partial or complete visual loss.

b. Amaurosis fugax (loss of vision in one eye).

c. Blindness is usually permanent.

d. Ophthalmologic examination reveals ischemic optic neuropathy and atrophy later in the disease course.

5. Audiovestibular involvement possible.

a. New onset hearing loss.

b. Vestibular (balance) problems.

6. Facial pain along the side of the face by the ear.

7. Jaw pain especially with chewing "claudication"

8. Tongue fatigue "claudication"

9. Respiratory system/dysphagia: Sore throat, painful swallowing, dry, non-productive cough (Gonzalez-Gay et al., 2009; Healey & Wilske, 1984; Kermani & Warrington, 2012; Nissen & Gabay, 2010).

C. Laboratory assessment.

1. Acute phase reactants:

a. ESR nearly always over 40 but 10-20% will have normal level (less likely to be normal in GCA).

b. CRP more sensitive and less influenced by other metabolic factors. Recommended as a more reliable marker for disease activity and monitoring response to therapy. However, patient report and presentation, not numbers, should guide treatment (Kermani et al., 2012; Nothnagl & Leeb, 2006; Salvarani et al., 2005; Walvick & Walvick, 2011)!

4
4.1
4.2
4.3
4.4
4.5
4.6
4.7
4.8
4.9
4.10

c. Complement levels are normal or slightly elevated.

d. IL6 levels elevated but not routinely available for measurement (Caplanne, Le Parc, & Alexandre, 1996; Hagihara, Kawase, Tanaka, & Kishimoto, 2010; Pulsatelli et al., 2007; Salvarani, Boiardi, et al., 1995; Salvarani et al., 2005).

2. Anemia: Of chronic disease (again if time to diagnosis is protracted). Looks like an iron deficiency anemia. Evaluate entire CBC to assess for other pathology such as infection, thrombocytopenia, or abnormal differential which may indicate alternate pathology.

3. Liver function abnormalities: Mild LFT elevation with 30% increase in aldolase.

4. Muscle enzymes: Extensive tendinopathy, can present like myositis but muscle enzymes and strength are normal. Additionally, EMG and muscle biopsy also without evidence of inflammation.

5. Autoantibodies: The absence of antibodies is essential.

a. Important to rule out other connective tissue diseases.

Figure 2: Clinical Effects Spectrum of Glucocorticoids.

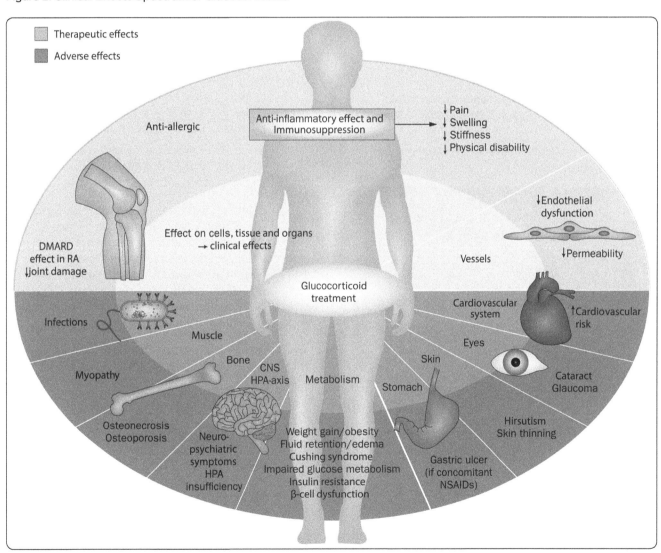

» Clinical Effects Spectrum of Glucocorticoids. Glucocorticoid therapy is associated with both beneficial effects (upper part of figure)—especially relief of symptoms and long-term benefit on radiological progression in RA—and adverse effects (lower part of figure), the incidence and severity of which are dependent on the dose and duration of the glucocorticoid therapy. Abbreviations: CNS, central nervous system; HPA, hypothalamic pituitary adrenal. Adapted from Buttgereit F. et al. Lancet 365, 801-803 (2005) with permission from Elsevier Ltd.70.

Source: Nature Reviews Rheumatology 6, 693-702 (December 2010) doi:10.1038/nrrheum.2010.179

b. Rheumatoid factor (RF): Remember 12% of the general public have positive RF and this percentage rises with age.

c. Anti-CCP sensitive marker for rheumatoid arthritis, Late Onset Rheumatoid Arthritis.

d. Antinuclear antibodies: Any positive studies should prompt additional evaluation. Antineutrophil cytoplasmic antibodies (ANCA- P/ C).

D. Temporal artery biopsy ("gold standard") is essential. Must be done by experienced surgeon (general, vascular, or opthamologic). Important to obtain 2-3 cm in order not to miss "skip lesions." Biopsy should be done as soon as possible. May start treatment immediately to minimize vascular complications and get biopsy within 7-10 days (Taylor-Gjevre, Vo, Shukla, & Resch, 2005; Walvick & Walvick, 2011).

1. Ultrasound imaging studies can be helpful but require highly skilled technicians. May

Figure 3: Remitting Seronegative Synovitis with Pitting Edema (RS3PE): Arm.

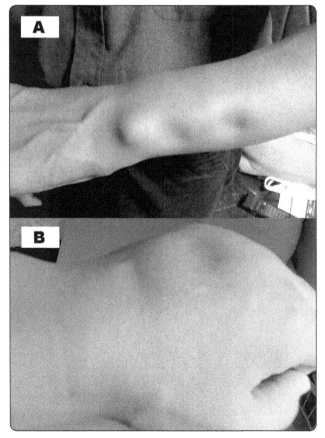

A

B

Source: © 2014 American College of Rheumatology. Used with permission.

be used to identify vascular involvement as well as bursitis and tenosynovitis in PMR.

2. Magnetic resonance imaging (MRI) findings of bursitis, tenosynovitis, and glenohumeral joint synovitis (Kermani et al., 2012; Nothnagl & Leeb, 2006; Parodi et al., 2006; Soubrier et al., 2006; Stewart, 2003).

E. Differential diagnosis: One of the criteria for diagnosis is the absence of other diseases capable of musculoskeletal symptoms.

1. Late Onset Rheumatoid Arthritis (LORA): Very similar presentation.

   a. Distinction can be difficult at onset of symptoms.

   b. Delay in final diagnosis can take months.

   c. Often require higher doses of steroids than other PMR or immediate synovitis returns with lowering of steroids.

   d. Rheumatoid factor (RF) may not be helpful since RF + is present in more than 12% of the general public.

   e. Anti CCP may be a more sensitive marker than RF, but the absence of CCP can be seen with seronegative RA.

2. Remitting Seronegative Symmetrical Synovitis with Pitting Edema (RS3PE) (see Figure 3). A rheumatoid arthritis variant: Synovitis and pitting edema in a symmetrical peripheral pattern associated with pitting edema of the hands/ wrists. May be associated with paraneoplastic syndrome but not necessarily (Okumura, Tanno, Ohhira, & Nozu, 2012).

3. Parkinson's disease: Stiffness in shoulders, neck, and girdle.

4. Hypothyroidism: Overwhelming fatigue and diffuse pain.

5. Statin myopathy.

6. Rotator cuff syndrome.

7. Osteoarthritis of shoulder and hips: May be difficult to differentiate except, OA is slow onset, PMR/ GCA sudden change in condition.

8. Connective tissue disease/ vasculitides.

9. Fibromyalgia (though less likely to present suddenly at an advanced age).

10. Malignancy: Paraneoplastic myalgias.

4
4.1
4.2
4.3
4.4
4.5
4.6
4.7
4.8
4.9
4.10

a. Consider this with incomplete response to steroids.

b. Persistent elevation in ESR/ CRP.

11. Infection: Monitor for fevers, chills, night sweats, change in CBC, lymphadenopathy, follow organ function.

F. Assessing for GCA at every encounter.

1. Always ask about visual changes.

a. Sudden loss or change.

b. Blurred vision.

c. Amaurosis fugax: Loss of vision in one eye.

G. Complications of the disease itself and corticosteroids.

IV. Treatment.

A. Attempts to find a steroid sparing agent have been met with limited success over the years. Methotrexate (MTX) has shown the most promise and is used routinely as a bridge to minimize the overall cummulative dose of steroids. It must be noted, however, that the evidence remains questionable and it is hoped that ongoing research will provide clear guidelines for the future (Caporali et al., 2004; Caporali et al., 2011; Cimmino et al., 2008; G. Ferraccioli, Salaffi, De Vita, Casatta, & Bartoli, 1996; Okumura et al., 2012; Spies, Burmester, & Buttgereit, 2010; van der Veen, Dinant, van Booma-Frankfort, van Albada-Kuipers, & Bijlsma, 1996; Weyand et al., 1999). Others have examined the use of TNF inhibitors as first line agents with disappointing results. There is currently a lack of evidence to support the use of any other treatment and many patients remain steroid dependent for years (Catanoso, Macchioni, Boiardi, Pipitone, & Salvarani, 2007; Salvarani et al., 2007).

B. Treatment of PMR.

1. Low dose steroids.

a. Evidence suggests that starting at levels higher than 20 mg daily are associated with increased adverse events with no benefits over time.

b. Low doses are defined by the international community as prednisone less than 7.5 mg daily. High doses are considered > 30 mg daily (as seen in GCA).

2. Initial dose of 15-20 mg is associated with a dramatic improvement within 48-96 hours. Failure to improve dramatically suggests alternate etiology/ diagnosis. Lower starting doses have actually not been associated with lower cumulative doses of CS.

3. Rate of steroid taper significantly associated with severity and frequency of relapse. Higher rate of relapse is associated with higher initial dose of corticosteroid (> than 20 mg prednisone) and rapid taper (5 mg every 2 weeks is considered fast taper; 1 mg every 4 weeks is a slow taper) (Gonzalez-Gay, Agudo, Martinez-Dubois, Pompei, & Blanco, 2010; Healey, 1984; Kim et al., 2012; Kremers et al., 2005a; Maradit Kremers et al., 2007; Nissen & Gabay, 2010; Nothnagl & Leeb, 2006; Salvarani et al., 2007; Soubrier et al., 2006; Weyand et al., 1999).

C. Treatment of GCA.

1. High dose steroids 1-2 mg/kg starting dose.

2. Should start immediately, do not wait to obtain temporal artery biopsy but biopsy should be done within 7-10 days.

3. Prophylactic doses of aspirin should be started if not contraindicated.

4. Sleep assistance: Not uncommon to need something to help with sleep/ anxiety at these doses. Be sure to obtain adequate psychiatric history; psychosis and severe anxiety disorders can be exacerbated with high dose steroids..

D. Efforts to minimize cumulative dose of steroids.

1. Alternate day dosing: Not effective.

2. Monthly IM injections of steroids: One small study suggested decreased fracture risk and weight gain with similar remission rates. No replication and only 16 patients (Dasgupta, Dolan, Panayi, & Fernandes, 1998).

3. Steroid injections locally again effective, but only 10 patients and more than half went on to require oral dosing with no considerable decrease in cumulative steroid dosing.

4. Chronotherapy: Timing steroid dose to achieve maximum benefit in the early morning when circadian rhythms are associated

4
4.1
4.2
4.3
4.4
4.5
4.6
4.7
4.8
4.9
4.10

with increased inflammatory cytokines. Unfortunately, steroids at bedtime make it difficult to sleep. Currently available in 16 European countries; early studies suggest significant drop in IL6 levels with over 50% improvement in morning stiffness with minimal adverse events (DeVaere, Curtis, & Galante, 2011; Ferraccioli et al., 1996; Ferraccioli, Di Poi, & Damato, 2000; Hagihara et al., 2010; Kim et al., 2012; Nishimoto, Nakahara, Yoshio-Hoshino, & Mima, 2008; Pulsatelli et al., 2008; Salvarani et al., 2005; Salvarani et al., 2007; Spies et al., 2010). In July 2012, Horizon Pharma announced FDA approval of Rayos® (prednisone), delayed-release tablets.

5. Disease modifying agents.

   a. MTX 10-25 mg wkly. Well tolerated but requires careful monitoring of LFTs and renal function.

   b. Infliximab (Remicade®) and other TNF blockers though promising have failed to demonstrate considerable difference in cumulative CS dose.

   c. Hydroxychloroquine and other DMARDs: Research essentially negative for effectiveness.

   d. Anti IL6: Tocilizumab (Actemra®) currently under investigation, case studies promising. Pathophysiology of both PMR/ GCA thought to be mediated throughout excessive IL6.

V. Co-morbid conditions: Related to advanced age and complications of long term CS use.

A. Multiple medical conditions related to aging.

B. Complications of CS therapy.

C. Malignancy: Failure to respond as expected, relapse with immediate taper, or persistently elevated acute phase reactants all suggest consideration of paraneoplastic syndrome, malignancy.

VI. Nursing implications.

A. Teaching.

   1. Discuss potential side effects of corticosteroids (see Table 1). All patients on long term steroids should be carefully screened and monitored, but pay particular

attention to those with GCA and high doses for often several months.

   a. Osteoporosis.

     (1) Baseline DXA and metabolic evaluation for other underlying causes of osteoporosis.

     (2) Follow national guidelines and take appropriate preventive measures.

     (3) GCA: High dose steroids may require prophylactic use of bisphosphonates.

     (4) Be sure to maintain adequate calcium intake of 1200-1500 mg daily.

     (5) Adequate vitamin D levels above 30 mg/dl with 1000-2000 IU daily.

     (6) Weight bearing exercise is important!

   b. Diabetes.

     (1) Baseline fasting glucose with repeat measurements as needed.

     (2) Be aware of need to adjust diabetic medications especially if on high dose steroids.

     (3) Coordinate with primary care providers.

   c. Edema/ HTN/ other cardiovascular: Know the cardiac history.

     (1) Baseline cardiovascular assessment: Check for edema, dysrhythmias, HTN, lipid profile.

     (2) Advise patient to inform provider of changes in cardiopulmonary status: Dyspnea, chest pain, palpitations, peripheral edema, headaches.

   d. Glaucoma/ cataracts: Be aware of history, presence of risk factors, and refer to ophthalmologist for baseline assessment and ongoing evaluation.

   e. Gastrointestinal problems: Increase in GERD symptoms, bloating (mild usually).

   f. Weight gain.

     (1) Minimal risk of weight gain on doses less than 15 mg. However, warn patients of increased desire for high carbohydrate foods; need to make healthy food choices.

     (2) Significant concern if on high dose steroids: Patient will likely see changes such as "moon" face (very upsetting), and central obesity.

     (3) Emphasize that these changes are most often temporary and resolve

4
4.1
4.2
4.3
4.4
4.5
4.6
4.7
4.8
4.9
4.10

as dose is tapered especially once on less than 20 mg daily.

g. Infection: Especially an issue at higher doses.

(1) Importance of vaccinations.

(2) Careful reporting and monitoring especially on higher doses.

(3) Attention to skin: Poor skin turgor, thinning, ecchymosis.

h. Sleep disturbance, anxiety, psychosis: Often number one issue especially on higher doses (usually anything over 15 mg). Most require sleep aids. Important to evaluate for this at every visit. Anxiety is already an issue with use of steroids, but sleep deprivation can exacerbate this. Older patients can experience mental status changes if sleep deprivation is not addressed. Educate the patient

Table 1: Information Card for Patients: Glucocorticoids

Ten important things to know about low-dose glucocorticoid therapy.
Glucocorticoids are medicines, which are commonly called steroids, corticosteroids, or cortisone and include prednisone, prednisolone, methylprednisolone (Medrol®). This leaflet mentions ten important things to know about glucocorticoid therapy. It is applicable for all patients on treatment with low dosages (7.5 mg prednisone or less).
1. Benefits
» Glucocorticoids are effective, simple to use, and they work rapidly.
2. Risks
» The possible side-effects depend on the dose, the duration of use, and the presence of other diseases and medications. The side effects are usually mild on low doses. The most important are osteoporosis, worsening of diabetes, and worsening of glaucoma. Some patients may experience weight gain, skin thinning, bruising, flushing, cataracts, or worsening of hypertension.
3. Monitoring of side effects
» Contact the physician if you are experiencing serious problems with glucocorticoid therapy. Side effects will also be monitored by the rheumatologist.
4. Adjusting the dose and stopping
» The rheumatologist will review individual benefits and risks regularly and will change dosage if needed. The rheumatologist can also advise about the timing of intake. It is important to remember that glucocorticoid therapy should not be stopped suddenly by the patient.
5. Acute illness
» Always mention glucocorticoid therapy. Glucocorticoids should not be stopped suddenly . Actually, extra glucocorticoids may be needed.
6. Surgery
» If surgery is needed inform the physician about glucocorticoid therapy. Extra glucocorticoids may be needed.
7. Pregnancy and lactation
» Low-dose glucocorticoids are relatively safe during pregnancy; never-the-less, patient should notify the rheumatologist if pregnant, planning to get pregnant, or breastfeeding.
8. Bone protection
» Measures to protect bone are often recommended. The rheumatologist will evaluate.
9. General information
» Check out these two websites: » The Arthritis Foundation: http://www.arthritis.org/   » The American College of Rheumatology: http://www.rheumatology.org/
10. Contact Information
» (name, address, and phone number of rheumatology department)

Source: Adapted from Van der Goes, M. C., Jacobs, J. W. G., & Bijlsma, J. W. J. (2011). Toward safer treatment with glucocorticoids: Via patient and rheumatologist perspectives to recommendations on monitoring for adverse events. Clinical and Experimental Rheumatology, 29(Suppl. 68), S116-S120.

4
4.1
4.2
4.3
4.4
4.5
4.6
4.7
4.8
4.9
4.10

and family about these changes and encourage assistance as needed.

2. Important: Be sure patients with PMR are aware of GCA symptom.

   a. Blindness can occur within 24 hours. It is essential that patients and families understand the need to notify the provider of any change in vision: Blurred, double vision, sudden loss of vision in one or both eyes.

   b. Other symptoms of arterial insufficiency: Symptoms of stroke, myocardial infarction.

   c. Other: Hearing loss, jaw pain when chewing, sore throat, neck pain.

B. Psychosocial.

1. Stigma of steroid use:

   a. "I frequently have to defend my use of CS therapy, not only in front of my family and friends but also to physicians such as the general practitioner."

      (1) Provide written materials on use and monitoring of CS therapy.

      (2) May need to do this repeatedly.

      (3) Be sure to emphasize the importance of adherence with regimen and dangers of suddenly stopping steroids: Risk of flare and cortisol insufficiency experienced as severe fatigue, hypotension (dizziness), dramatic increase in symptoms (PMR/ GCA).

   b. "You get really hungry." "I'm going to gain weight."

      (1) Be sure patients understand that they will get really hungry.

      (2) Healthy choices; make sure there is easy access.

2. Mood disorders, personality changes, sleep disturbance.

   a. Mood changes: Patients often describe labile moods, this is normal. Be sure patients understand this.

   b. Anxiety: Very common, presents often as frequent phone calls, numerous questions, non-adherence to treatment regimen, restlessness, agitation, anger.

   c. Sleep disturbance is common, improves as dose is tapered but may not be significantly better until on as little as 5-7.5 mg daily.

      (1) Promote proper sleep hygiene (see Table 2).

      (2) Cautious use of sleep aids as needed because of concerns of the physical, emotional, and safety issues related to sleep deprivation especially in older adults.

3. Resources.

   a. The Arthritis Foundation has information about PMR/ GCA but also about living a balanced life and managing medical conditions. http://www.arthritis.org.

   b. The American College of Rheumatology has excellent materials for patient education and clinician support: Http://www.rheumatology.org/practice/clinical/patients/index.asp.

Summary.

One of the greatest challenges in managing these conditions lies in the monitoring of several co-morbid conditions often associated with aging (PMR and GCA occur in those over 50 years of age) in the presence of chronic steroid use. This chapter covered many of the important considerations and recommendations identified to provide rheumatology nurses with tools to share with patients to minimize complications and optimize function through the 1-3 years or more that are required to treat this usually self-limiting condition.

References.

Announ, N., & Guerne, P. A. (2008). Polymyalgia rheumatica and giant cell arteritis: Recent data and current situation. *Revue Medicale Suisse, 4*(149), 696-698, 701.

Bernatsky, S., Joseph, L., Pineau, C. A., Belisle, P., Lix, L., Banerjee, D., & Clarke, A. E. (2009). Polymyalgia rheumatica prevalence in a population-based sample. *Arthritis and Rheumatism, 61*(9), 1264-1267. doi: 10.1002/art.24793.

Caplanne, D., Le Parc, J. M., & Alexandre, J. A. (1996). Interleukin-6 in clinical relapses of polymyalgia rheumatica and giant cell arteritis. [Letter]. *Annals of the Rheumatic Diseases, 55*(6), 403-404.

Caporali, R., Cimmino, M. A., Ferraccioli, G., Gerli, R., Klersy, C., Salvarani, C., & Montecucco, C. (2004). Prednisone plus methotrexate for polymyalgia rheumatica: a randomized, double-blind, placebo-controlled trial. [Clinical Trial Multicenter Study Randomized Controlled Trial Research Support, Non-U.S. Gov't]. *Annals of Internal Medicine, 141*(7), 493-500.

Caporali, R., Cimmino, M. A., Montecucco, C., & Cutolo, M. (2011). Glucocorticoid treatment of polymyalgia rheumatica. [Review]. *Clinical and Experimental Rheumatology, 29*(5 Suppl 68), S143-147.

Catanoso, M. G., Macchioni, P., Boiardi, L., Pipitone, N., & Salvarani, C. (2007). Treatment of refractory polymyalgia rheumatica with etanercept: an open pilot study. *Arthritis and Rheumatism, 57*(8), 1514-1519. doi: 10.1002/art.23095.

Cimmino, M. A., Salvarani, C., Macchioni, P., Gerli, R., Bartoloni Bocci, E., Montecucco, C., & Caporali, R. (2008). Long-term follow-up of polymyalgia rheumatica patients treated with methotrexate and steroids. *Clinical and Experimental Rheumatology, 26*(3), 395-400. doi: 2324 [pii]

Table 2: Getting A Good Night's Sleep: Do's and Don'ts

Do's	Don't
Keep a neat and comfortable bedroom (change linens regularly, buy good pillows, choose a mattress that doesn't squeak and feels good).	Don't go to bed if not drowsy.
Relax before going to bed; read in living room; listen to soothing music.	No heavy meals before bedtime, caution especially if GERD.
Keep your room at a temperature that will help you sleep.	Have radios, TVs, stereos, computers, and cell phones on in the bedroom.
Make bedroom conducive to sleep (not too much light), minimize irritating sounds.	Eat or drink caffeinated food or beverages after 2-3:00 p.m.
Take pain medication before bedtime if pain wakes you up.	Drink alcohol to help you go to sleep (poor quality sleep).
Have a set time and routine for getting to bed.	Take unscheduled naps during day, and not after 3:00 p.m. Naps should be less than 1 hour, anything more you feel worse.
Wake up at same time as much as possible, even on weekends.	Be too active one day and a slug the next.
Reserve the bedroom for sleep and sex.	Exercise 2-3 hours before bedtime.
Balance activity and rest throughout the day.	Stay out of bed longer than 30 minutes.
Eat balanced or mini meals.	Smoke right before bed, but realize that 2-4 hours after last smoke will have physical symptoms of desire if smoke routinely.
Allow for transition period before bedtime.	Try not to use antihistamines/ hypnotics to help with sleep, poor quality.
Get out of bed if not asleep after 20 minutes; go do something that is not exciting for 30 minutes, then try again.	Don't let children or pets interfere with your sleep.

Source: Author (Stamatos)

Dasgupta, B., Dolan, A. L., Panayi, G. S., & Fernandes, L. (1998). An initially double-blind controlled 96 week trial of depot methylprednisolone against oral prednisolone in the treatment of polymyalgia rheumatica. [Clinical Trial Comparative Study Multicenter Study Randomized Controlled TrialResearch Support, Non-U.S. Gov't]. *British Journal of Rheumatology, 37*(2), 189-195.

Dejaco, C., Duftner, C., Cimmino, M. A., Dasgupta, B., Salvarani, C., Crowson, C. S., . . . Schirmer, M. (2011). Definition of remission and relapse in polymyalgia rheumatica: data from a literature search compared with a Delphi-based expert consensus. *Annals of Rheumatic Disease, 70*(3), 447-453. doi: ard.2010.133850 [pii]10.1136/ard.2010.133850.

DeVaere, R. J., Curtis, G., & Galante, K. (2011). Horizon Pharma announces U.S. Food and Drug Administration acceptance of LODOTRA. New drug application for review for the treatment of rheumatoid arthritis. . Retrieved from Ferraccioli, G., Salaffi, F., De Vita, S., Casatta, L., & Bartoli, E. (1996). Methotrexate in polymyalgia rheumatica: preliminary results of an open, randomized study. *The Journal of Rheumatology, 23*(4), 624-628.

Ferraccioli, G., Salaffi, F., De Vita, S., Casatta, L., & Bartoli, E. (1996). Methotrexate in polymyalgia rheumatica: preliminary results of an open, randomized study. *The Journal of Rheumatology, 23*(4), 624-628.

Ferraccioli, G. F., Di Poi, E., & Damato, R. (2000). Steroid sparing therapeutic approaches to polymyalgia rheumatica-giant cell arteritis. State of the art and perspectives. *Clinical and Experimental Rheumatology, 18*(4 Suppl 20), S58-S60.

Gabriel, S. E., & Michaud, K. (2009). Epidemiological studies in incidence, prevalence, mortality, and comorbidity of the rheumatic diseases. [Review]. *Arthritis Research & Therapy, 11*(3), 229. doi: 10.1186/ar2669.

Gabriel, S. E., Sunku, J., Salvarani, C., O'Fallon, W. M., & Hunder, G. G. (1997). Adverse outcomes of antiinflammatory therapy among patients with polymyalgia rheumatica. *Arthritis and Rheumatism, 40*(10), 1873-1878. doi: 10.1002/1529-0131(199710)40:10<1873::AID-ART22>3.0.CO;2-V.

Gonzalez-Gay, M. A., Agudo, M., Martinez-Dubois, C., Pompei, O., & Blanco, R. (2010). Medical management of polymyalgia rheumatica. *Expert Opinion on Pharmacotherapy, 11*(7), 1077-1087. doi: 10.1517/14656561003724739

Gonzalez-Gay, M. A., Vazquez-Rodriguez, T. R., Lopez-Diaz, M. J., Miranda-Filloy, J. A., Gonzalez-Juanatey, C., Martin, J., & Llorca, J. (2009). Epidemiology of giant cell arteritis and polymyalgia rheumatica. *Arthritis and Rheumatism, 61*(10), 1454-1461. doi: 10.1002/art.24459

Hagihara, K., Kawase, I., Tanaka, T., & Kishimoto, T. (2010). Tocilizumab ameliorates clinical symptoms in polymyalgia rheumatica. *The Journal of Rheumatology, 37*(5), 1075-1076. doi: 37/5/1075 [pii] 10.3899/jrheum.091185

Healey, L. A. (1984). Long-term follow-up of polymyalgia rheumatica: Evidence for synovitis. *Seminars in Arthritis and Rheumatism, 13*(4), 322-328.

Healey, L. A., & Wilske, K. R. (1984). *Polymyalgia rheumatica and giant cell arteritis. The Western Journal of Medicine, 141*(1), 64-67.

Hernandez-Rodriguez, J., Cid, M. C., Lopez-Soto, A., Espigol-Frigole, G., & Bosch, X. (2009). Treatment of polymyalgia rheumatica: A systematic review. *Archives of Internal Medicine, 169*(20), 1839-1850. doi: 169/20/1839 [pii] 10.1001/archinternmed.2009.352

Kermani, T. A., Schmidt, J., Crowson, C. S., Ytterberg, S. R., Hunder, G. G., Matteson, E. L., & Warrington, K. J. (2012). Utility of erythrocyte sedimentation rate and C-reactive protein for the diagnosis of giant cell arteritis. *Seminars in Arthritis and Rheumatism, 41*(6), 866-871. doi: 10.1016/j.semarthrit.2011.10.005

Kermani, T. A., & Warrington, K. J. (2012). Recent advances in diagnostic strategies for giant cell arteritis. [Research Support, N.I.H., Extramural Research Support, Non-U.S. Gov't]. *Current Neurology and Neuroscience Reports, 12*(2), 138-144. doi: 10.1007/s11910-011-0243-6

Kim, H. A., Lee, J., Ha, Y. J., Kim, S. H., Lee, C. H., Choi, H. J., . . . Suh, C. H. (2012). Induction of remission is difficult due to frequent relapse during tapering steroids in Korean patients with polymyalgia rheumatica. [Research Support, Non-U.S. Gov't]. *Journal of Korean Medical Science, 27*(1), 22-26. doi: 10.3346/jkms.2012.27.1.22

Kremers, H. M., Reinalda, M. S., Crowson, C. S., Zinsmeister, A. R., Hunder, G. G., & Gabriel, S. E. (2005a). Relapse in a population based cohort of patients with polymyalgia rheumatica. *The Journal of Rheumatology, 32*(1), 65-73. doi: 0315162X-32-65 [pii]

Kremers, H. M., Reinalda, M. S., Crowson, C. S., Zinsmeister, A. R., Hunder, G. G., & Gabriel, S. E. (2005b). Use of physician services in a population-based cohort of patients with polymyalgia rheumatica over the course of their disease. *Arthritis and Rheumatism, 53*(3), 395-403. doi: 10.1002/art.21160

4
4.1
4.2
4.3
4.4
4.5
4.6
4.7
4.8
4.9
4.10

Labbe, P., & Hardouin, P. (1998). Epidemiology and optimal management of polymyalgia rheumatica. *Drugs and Aging, 13*(2), 109-118.

Maradit Kremers, H., Reinalda, M. S., Crowson, C. S., Davis, J. M., 3rd, Hunder, G. G., & Gabriel, S. E. (2007). Glucocorticoids and cardiovascular and cerebrovascular events in polymyalgia rheumatica. *Arthritis and Rheum,atism 57*(2), 279-286. doi: 10.1002/art.22548

Muller, S., Hider, S. L., Helliwell, T., Bailey, J., Barraclough, K., Cope, L., ... Mallen, C. D. (2012). The epidemiology of polymyalgia rheumatica in primary care: a research protocol. *BMC Musculoskeletal Disorders, 13*(1), 102. doi: 10.1186/1471-2474-13-102

Myklebust, G., Wilsgaard, T., Jacobsen, B. K., & Gran, J. T. (2003). Causes of death in polymyalgia rheumatica. A prospective longitudinal study of 315 cases and matched population controls. *Scandinavian Journal of Rheumatology, 32*(1), 38-41

Nishimoto, N., Nakahara, H., Yoshio-Hoshino, N., & Mima, T. (2008). Successful treatment of a patient with Takayasu arteritis using a humanized anti-interleukin-6 receptor antibody. *Arthritis and Rheumatism, 58*(4), 1197-1200. doi: 10.1002/art.23373

Nissen, M. J., & Gabay, C. (2010). Polymyalgia rheumatica and giant cell arteritis: what's new?. *Revue Medicale Suisse, 6*(240), 575-576, 578, 580.

Nothnagl, T., & Leeb, B. F. (2006). Diagnosis, differential diagnosis and treatment of polymyalgia rheumatica. *Drugs and Aging, 23*(5), 391-402. doi: 2353 [pii]

Okumura, T., Tanno, S., Ohhira, M., & Nozu, T. (2012). The rate of polymyalgia rheumatica (PMR) and remitting seronegative symmetrical synovitis with pitting edema (RS3PE) syndrome in a clinic where primary care physicians are working in Japan. *Rheumatology International, 32*(6), 1695-1699. doi: 10.1007/s00296-011-1849-3

Parodi, M., Garlaschi, G., Silvestri, E., & Cimmino, M. A. (2006). Magnetic resonance imaging in the differential diagnosis between polymyalgia rheumatica and elderly onset rheumatoid arthritis. *Clinical Rheumatology, 25*(3), 402-403. doi: 10.1007/s10067-005-0010-7

Pulsatelli, L., Boiardi, L., Pignotti, E., Dolzani, P., Silvestri, T., Macchioni, P., ... Meliconi, R. (2008). Serum interleukin-6 receptor in polymyalgia rheumatica: a potential marker of relapse/recurrence risk. *Arthritis and Rheumatism, 59*(8), 1147-1154. doi: 10.1002/art.23924

Pulsatelli, L., Dolzani, P., Silvestri, T., Boiardi, L., Salvarani, C., Macchioni, P., ... Meliconi, R. (2007). Circulating RANKL/OPG in polymyalgia rheumatica. *Clinical and Experimental Rheumatology, 25*(4), 621-623. doi: 2105 [pii]

Salvarani, C., Boiardi, L., Macchioni, P., Rossi, F., Tartoni, P., Casadei Maldini, M., ... Portioli, I. (1995). Role of peripheral CD8 lymphocytes and soluble IL-2 receptor in predicting the duration of corticosteroid treatment in polymyalgia rheumatica and giant cell arteritis. *Annals of the Rheumatic Diseases, 54*(8), 640-644.

Salvarani, C., Cantini, F., Boiardi, L., & Hunder, G. G. (2004). Polymyalgia rheumatica. *Best Practices and Resarch. Clinical Rheumatology, 18*(5), 705-722. doi: 10.1016/j.berh.2004.06.003 S1521694204001019 [pii]

Salvarani, C., Cantini, F., Niccoli, L., Macchioni, P., Consonni, D., Bajocchi, G., ... Boiardi, L. (2005). Acute-phase reactants and the risk of relapse/recurrence in polymyalgia rheumatica: a prospective followup study. *Arthritis and Rheumatism, 53*(1), 33-38. doi: 10.1002/art.20901

Salvarani, C., Gabriel, S. E., O'Fallon, W. M., & Hunder, G. G. (1995a). Epidemiology of polymyalgia rheumatica in Olmsted County, Minnesota, 1970-1991. *Arthritis and Rheumatism, 38*(3), 369-373.

Salvarani, C., Gabriel, S. E., O'Fallon, W. M., & Hunder, G. G. (1995b). The incidence of giant cell arteritis in Olmsted County, Minnesota: apparent fluctuations in a cyclic pattern. *Annals of Internal Medicine, 123*(3), 192-194.

Salvarani, C., Macchioni, P., Manzini, C., Paolazzi, G., Trotta, A., Manganelli, P., ... Hunder, G. G. (2007). Infliximab plus prednisone or placebo plus prednisone for the initial treatment of polymyalgia rheumatica: a randomized trial. *Annals of Internal Medicine, 146*(9), 631-639. doi: 146/9/631 [pii].

Schmidt, W. A., & Gromnica-Ihle, E. (2002). Incidence of temporal arteritis in patients with polymyalgia rheumatica: a prospective study using colour Doppler ultrasonography of the temporal arteries. *Rheumatology (Oxford), 41*(1), 46-52.

Smeeth, L., Cook, C., & Hall, A. J. (2006). Incidence of diagnosed polymyalgia rheumatica and temporal arteritis in the United Kingdom, 1990-2001. *Ann Rheum Dis, 65*(8), 1093-1098. doi: ard.2005.046912 [pii] 10.1136/ard.2005.046912.

Soubrier, M., Dubost, J. J., & Ristori, J. M. (2006). Polymyalgia rheumatica: diagnosis and treatment. *Joint Bone Spine, 73*(6), 599-605. doi: S1297-319X(06)00220-X [pii] 10.1016/j.jbspin.2006.09.005.

Spies, C. M., Burmester, G. R., & Buttgereit, F. (2010). Methotrexate treatment in large vessel vasculitis and polymyalgia rheumatica. *Clin Exp Rheumatol, 28*(5 Suppl 61), S172-177. doi: 4323 [pii].

Stewart, P. A. (2003). Polymyalgia rheumatica. The great impressionist. *Adv Nurse Pract, 11*(5), 73-74.

4
4.1
4.2
4.3
4.4
4.5
4.6
4.7
4.8
4.9
4.10

Taylor-Gjevre, R., Vo, M., Shukla, D., & Resch, L. (2005). Temporal artery biopsy for giant cell arteritis. *The Journal of rheumatology, 32*(7), 1279-1282.

van der Veen, M. J., Dinant, H. J., van Booma-Frankfort, C., van Albada-Kuipers, G. A., & Bijlsma, J. W. (1996). Can methotrexate be used as a steroid sparing agent in the treatment of polymyalgia rheumatica and giant cell arteritis? *Ann Rheum Dis, 55*(4), 218-223.

Walvick, M. D., & Walvick, M. P. (2011). Giant cell arteritis: laboratory predictors of a positive temporal artery biopsy. [Comparative Study]. *Ophthalmology, 118*(6), 1201-1204. doi: 10.1016/j.ophtha.2010.10.002.

Warrington, K. J., Jarpa, E. P., Crowson, C. S., Cooper, L. T., Hunder, G. G., Matteson, E. L., & Gabriel, S. E. (2009). Increased risk of peripheral arterial disease in polymyalgia rheumatica: a population-based cohort study. *Arthritis Res Ther, 11*(2), R50. doi: ar2664 [pii]10.1186/ar2664.

Weyand, C. M., Fulbright, J. W., Evans, J. M., Hunder, G. G., & Goronzy, J. J. (1999). Corticosteroid requirements in polymyalgia rheumatica. [Research Support, Non-U.S. Gov't Research Support, U.S. Gov't, P.H.S.]. *Archives of internal medicine, 159*(6), 577-584.

Van der Goes, M. C., Jacobs, J. W. G., & Bijlsma, J. W. J. (2011). Toward safer treatment with glucocorticoids: Via patient and rheumatologist perspectives to recommendations on monitoring for adverse events. *Clinical and Experimental Rheumatology, 29*(Suppl. 68), S116-S120.

Nice review and guidelines for the use of glucocorticoids.

Suggested Readings

Caporali, R., Cimmino, M. A., Montecucco, C., & Cutolo, M. (2011). Glucocorticoid treatment of polymyalgia rheumatica. *Clinical and Experimental Rheumatology, 29*(Suppl. 68), S143-S147.

Broad overview of glucocorticoids for PMR, short, easy to read, informative.

Dixon, W. G., Abrahamowicz, M., Beauchamp, M.E., Ray, D.W., Bernatsky, S., Suissa, S., & Sylvestre, M.P. (2012). Immediate and delayed impact of oral glucocorticoid therapy on risk of serious infection in older patients with rheumatoid arthritis: A nested case-control analysis. *Annals of the Rheumatic Diseases* (Online). doi: 10.1136/annrheumdis-2011-200702

Overview of the evidence regarding the safety of glucocorticoids in rheumatoid arthritis (similar dosing seen in PMR).

Gonzalez-Gay, M. A., Martinez-Dubois, C., Agudo, M., Pompei, O., Blanco, R., & Llorca, J. (2010). Giant cell arteritis: Epidemiology, diagnosis, and management. *Current Rheumatology Reports, 12*(6), 436-442.

Updated review of GCA. Easy to follow.

Section 4.9
Scleroderma and Systemic Sclerosis

Christine A. Stamatos, DNP, ANP-C

Introduction

This purpose of this chapter is to provide an understanding of the definition and classification of the various types and manifestations of scleroderma. Although the pathophysiology of changes in the connective tissue may be similar for all systems, manifestations will vary depending on whether scleroderma is limited or systemic in nature. Treatment options and specific nursing considerations will be addressed to promote improved function and quality of life for those caring for and living with scleroderma.

Learning Objectives

Upon completion of this chapter, the nurse will be able to:

1. Define scleroderma and differentiate between systemic, limited, and mixed.

2. Describe the epidemiology and pathogenesis of scleroderma.

3. Describe the clinical course, prognosis, and risk factors for complications of scleroderma.

4. Discuss treatment options for scleroderma.

5. Identify daily symptoms commonly experienced by patients with scleroderma.

6. Discuss nursing interventions to address fatigue, pain, pruritus, restricted mobility, and change in body image, role, and independence related to scleroderma.

Content Outline

I. Pathophysiology.

A. What is scleroderma? (see Figure 1).

1. Derived from Greek word "sclerosis" meaning hardness and "derma," meaning skin, "scleroderma" literally means hard skin. Defined as a rheumatic and a connective tissue disease.

   a. Rheumatic disease: Inflammation or pain in muscles, joints, or fibrous tissue.

   b. Connective tissue disease: Connective tissue is a fibrous tissue found throughout the body (skin, tendons, muscle, cartilage, bone, adipose, blood, and lymphatic system). The function of connective tissue is energy storage, organ protection, structural integrity, and connection

Figure 1: Scleroderma

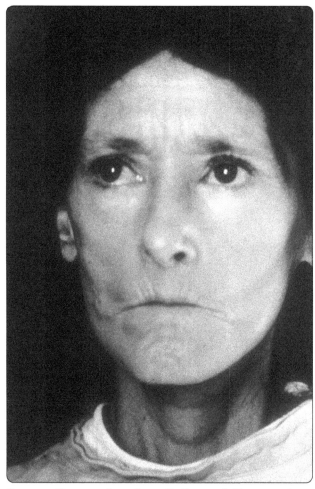

of body tissues. Fibroblasts are the cells responsible for the production of connective tissue (Mayes & Assassi, 2011; Mayes, Varga, Buch, & Seibold, 2008).

B. Group of diseases that involve abnormal growth of connective tissue, which support the vascular system, skin, and internal organs. Often divided into the following classifications:

1. Limited scleroderma.

2. Diffuse scleroderma.

3. Mixed.

C. A "triggering event" (some kind of physical or emotional stressor/ exposure) in a genetically predisposed individual initiates a series of changes activating the immune system resulting in inflammation, vascular damage, and generalized fibrosis. The individual significance of each pathology varies from one person to another.

D. Changes in blood vessels: Widespread small-vessel abnormality (obliterative) due to immune activation from autoimmunity (antibodies formed against self) affecting arteries, arterioles, and capillaries.

1. There is an increased sensitivity to vasoconstriction and structural damage to the lining of blood vessel walls (endothelial cells) resulting in significant tissue ischemia.

2. Physical examples of these changes are Raynaud's phenomenon, telangiectasis, nail fold changes, digital pit formation, ulcerations, scleroderma renal crisis, and pulmonary hypertension.

3. Eventually, endothelial cells are damaged, and fibrotic changes occur in blood vessel walls. Endothelial injury leads to platelet aggregation, further stimulating cellular destruction with perivascular fibrosis and progressive luminal obstruction resulting in chronic tissue hypoxia (ischemia)/reperfusion injury (damage to tissue as a result of cytokines—inflammatory proteins—released during hypoxia), manifesting most significantly with chronic progressive pain and disfigurement.

E. Fibrosis: Excessive activation of fibroblasts throughout the body results in increased

4
4.1
4.2
4.3
4.4
4.5
4.6
4.7
4.8
4.9
4.10

production of collagen substances increasing stiffness of the matrix disrupting tissue architecture and progressive dysfunction with potential to severely affect organ function.

1. Mast cells are activated and contribute to significant swelling and pruritus associated with the formation of fibrotic changes.

2. Physical examples of these changes are thickened skin, gastrointestinal dysmotility, interstitial pulmonary and renal fibrosis, and changes in myocardial function (Chizzolini, Brembilla, Montanari, & Truchetet, 2011; Mayes & Assassi, 2011; Mayes et al., 2008).

F. Organ specific changes:

1. Skin / Joint:

   a. Loss of hair follicles, sweat glands (difficulty maintaining temperature, always cold).

   b. Skin atrophies (shrinks) with nearly complete absence of adipose tissue.

   c. Tendon fibrosis leads to limited mobility and contractures in severe cases.

   d. Digital tip ulcers, gangrene, and acro-osteolysis (absorption of bone, shortening of fingers).

   e. Ulcerations also form over bony prominences of hands because of stretched, tight skin and mechanical trauma.

   f. Firm calcium nodules, calcinosis, form on hands, elbows, forearms, knees, legs, and more. More common in limited scleroderma but can occur in late in diffuse disease.

2. Lungs:

   a. Pulmonary disease is now the leading cause of death in patients with scleroderma ((Steen & Medsger, 2007). Lung injury is common in all forms of scleroderma.

   b. Vascular and fibrotic changes contribute to pulmonary hypertension (PAH). Pulmonary fibrosis leads to poor diffusion capacity because of destruction of alveoli and decreased lung volumes known as interstitial lung disease (ILD).

   c. Early changes in exercise tolerance and dry cough can predict abnormality, but early pulmonary hypertension and fibrosis (when most responsive to intervention) can only be detected through pulmonary

function tests. One of the most significant predictors of risk for pulmonary complications is the degree of skin involvement. While PAH is more common in limited scleroderma (8-12%), and fibrosis is more common in diffuse scleroderma (20%), progressive pulmonary involvement is marked by both (Mayes & Assassi, 2011; Mayes et al., 2008; Robertson et al., 2005).

3. Gastrointestinal (GI):

   a. Ninety percent of all patients with scleroderma experience changes throughout the GI tract, which can occur from ischemia, inflammation, and fibrosis at any level.

   b. The esophagus is nearly always affected, and scar tissue formation throughout affects peristalsis resulting in esophageal reflux/ strictures (causing dysphagia), small bowel dysmotility, pseudo-obstruction, malabsorption, constipation and stool incontinence, and bacterial overgrowth which contributes to persistent activation of the immune system.

   c. There are similar findings in both forms of scleroderma.

   d. Primary biliary cirrhosis occurs more often in patients with scleroderma than in the general population (Chifflot, Fautrel, Sordet, Chatelus, & Sibilia, 2008; Mayes et al., 2008; Shah & Wigley, 2008; Steen, 2008).

4. Kidneys:

   a. Dominated by vascular changes resulting in acute scleroderma renal crisis (SRC) presenting as malignant hypertension (> 150/85 with decreased renal function) 10-20% diffuse scleroderma/ 1-2% limited scleroderma experience SRC.

   b. Poor outcomes are associated with more extensive vascular thrombosis and glomerular collapse.

   c. Mild proteinuria without loss of renal function is the most common manifestation of scleroderma renal disease (Chifflot et al., 2008; Mayes et al., 2008; Shah & Wigley, 2008; Steen, 2008).

5. Heart:

   a. Related to both vascular ischemic and thrombotic changes as well as fibrotic deposition throughout is associated with cardiac hypertrophy.

4
4.1
4.2
4.3
4.4
4.5
4.6
4.7
4.8
4.9
4.10

b. Supraventricular arrhythmias, conduction defects, and pericardial effusions are more common than cardiomyopathies (Mayes et al., 2008; Shah & Wigley, 2008; Steen, 2008).

6. Other:

a. Overlap syndromes are frequently associated with joint inflammation and myositis.

b. Fibrosis of thyroid tissue can cause abnormal thyroid function.

c. Vascular problems can result in erectile dysfunction.

d. Fibrosis of salivary and lacrimal glands may be seen with or without Sjögren's syndrome.

e. Neurologic involvement presents as trigeminal neuralgia, peripheral nerve entrapments (carpal tunnel syndrome), and peripheral neuropathies related to multiple causes of vascular and fibrotic nature.

f. Muscle weakness either as overlap syndrome or secondary to multiple other causes from vasculopathy, fibrosis, disuse myopathy, malnutrition, medications (Mayes et al., 2008; Pope, 2007; Shah & Wigley, 2008; Steen, 2008).

II. Etiology/Epidemiology.

A. Etiology.

1. Precise cause of systemic sclerosis is unknown.

2. Genetic factors play a role in determining susceptibility.

a. Scleroderma is an acquired, noncontagious, rare disease.

b. Families with more than one case of systemic sclerosis have been reported.

c. A family and/ or personal history of other autoimmune disease is common.

3. Triggering event difficult to identify. There is currently no evidence of a specific environmental/or occupational trigger.

a. Presence of antibodies to human parvovirus B19/ or cytomegalovirus have been found.

b. Noninfectious environmental agents such as silica dust have been implicated, but no clear causal statement can be made.

4. As with other autoimmune diseases, the genetic predisposition can be turned on with a certain degree of "stress" to the immune system. Many believe physical or emotional stressors may be responsible but cannot be predicted (Barnabe et al., 2012; Chifflot et al., 2008; Mayes et al., 2008; Schieir et al., 2010).

B. Epidemiology.

1. Incidence: Reported at 15-20 cases per million per year.

2. Prevalence: More than 250 patients per million are affected in the United States (40-165,000 people in the United States)(Barnabe et al., 2012; Chifflot et al., 2008; Mayes et al., 2008; Schieir et al., 2010).

3. Several subtypes: Localized and diffuse (systemic, limited, and mixed).

a. Localized scleroderma: Skin and underlying tissue but not internal organs.

(1) Morphea and linear scleroderma. One to several distinct patches/or lines of thickened skin; often fades over time.

(2) Linear scleroderma more common in children and can affect growth and function of affected extremity/ or face resulting in deformities.

b. Systemic sclerosis (focus of this chapter): Involves skin and tissues, blood vessels, and major organs.

(1) Divided further into different subsets: Limited cutaneous scleroderma, diffuse scleroderma, and mixed.

C. Age, gender, race, and subtype determine prognosis.

1. Scleroderma has one of the highest mortality rates of all connective tissue diseases (CTDs).

2. Rare in children with peak occurrence between ages 35-65.

3. Female predominance 7-12:1 ratio.

4. African Americans are affected at a younger age and have more diffuse scleroderma with more severe lung disease.

5. Progressive pulmonary fibrosis occurs less frequently and survival rates are better for Caucasian patients.

4
4.1
4.2
4.3
4.4
4.5
4.6
4.7
4.8
4.9
4.10

6. African Americans are more likely to have antitopoisomerase I (Scl-70) antibodies, while Caucasians are more likely to have anticentromere (ACA) antibodies.

D. Survival: Has improved over past decade.

1. Limited scleroderma >70% at 10 years (pulmonary hypertension).

2. Diffuse scleroderma 40-60% at 10 years; death often related to lung involvement (pulmonary hypertension and/or pulmonary fibrosis).

3. Mixed survival depends on presentation, often milder (Barnabe et al., 2012; Chifflot et al., 2008; Mayes et al., 2008; Schieir et al., 2010; Steen & Medsger, 2007).

III. Nursing Assessment.

A. Limited cutaneous systemic sclerosis.

1. Occurs gradually, restricted to certain areas, preceded by a long history of Raynaud's, and associated with PAH.

2. Anticentromere antibody (ACA) positive.

3. Limited to skin of fingers, hands, lower arms and legs, and face.

4. Acronym: Limited cutaneous scleroderma is CREST, although accepted term is now limited scleroderma (Avouac et al., 2009).

5. Calcinosis: Hard calcium deposits in the connective tissue anywhere on the body. Frequently found on fingers, hands, face, elbows, or knees. Can break through skin and cause painful ulcerations. May also be painful based on location in joints, forearms/shins, even buttocks (see Figure 2).

B. Raynaud's.

1. Most have Raynaud's phenomenon for years before skin thickening.

2. Small blood vessels of the hands, feet, nose, and ears contract (vasospasm) in response to cold and anxiety.

3. Areas frequently affected: Hands, feet, ears, and nose turn white and cold then blue and are associated with pain, numbness, and tingling. As blood flow returns, extremities become red and painful.

4. Poor perfusion can persist and result in chronic digital ulcerations, gangrene, and loss of skin and bone in severe cases.

C. Esophageal dysfunction.

1. Can be severe with significant gastroesophageal reflux (GERD) which can lead to Barrett's esophagitis (precancerous tissue associated with 30-fold increase in risk of esophageal cancer).

2. Dysphagia (beware of choking), gastroparesis (early satiety- fullness), and constipation are all common. Bacterial overgrowth from changes in the bowel presents as diarrhea.

D. Sclerodactyly (localized thickening and tightness of the skin of the fingers and toes).

1. Early changes include "puffy" non-pitting edema, pruritus (itching-can be profound), and erythema.

2. Eventually thick and tight skin on fingers, may appear shiny, darkened, and without hair.

3. Need to monitor for perfusion problems, pitting, or digital ulcerations (though less prominent in limited scleroderma).

E. Telangiectasis.

1. Swelling of tiny blood vessels, resulting in red spots that appear on face and hands.

2. These are not painful but can be cosmetically bothersome.

Figure 2: Calcinosis

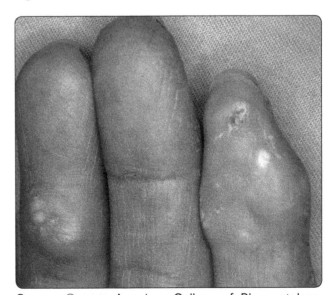

F. Lung Involvement in Limited Scleroderma (12%).

1. PAH occurs late in the course of progression and is initially asymptomatic.

2. Vascular and fibrotic changes in the blood vessels lead to pulmonary hypertension, which can be severe and very debilitating. May remain asymptomatic until quite advanced.

3. PAH is typically discovered during regular pulmonary function test (PFT) monitoring and echocardiography and is associated with normal lung volumes and a decrease in diffusion capacity (DLCO2).

4. It is confirmed by right heart catheterization with evidence of elevated pulmonary pressures (Nihtyanova, Brough, Black, & Denton, 2008; Robertson et al., 2005; Steen et al., 2008).

G. Diffuse cutaneous systemic scleroderma (see Figure 3).

1. Comes on suddenly with recent development of Raynaud's and is associated with antitopoimerase (Scl-70) antibody. Often associated with severe Raynaud's and complications from ischemic changes.

2. Skin thickening quickly (over period of months) affects entire body progressing distally-proximally: Hands, face, upper arms, upper legs, chest, stomach symmetrically. Of note, skin often improves somewhat after the first 2-3 years, though contractures will persist.

3. Greater risk for internal organ involvement early. Maintain high index of suspicion.

4. Internal organ dysfunction.

H. Pulmonary fibrosis (Interstitial Lung Disease - ILD) (20%) is more common in diffuse scleroderma but PAH can also be seen.

1. Early changes are asymptomatic, requiring frequent PFTs.

2. A decrease in lung volumes and a decrease in diffusion capacity (DLCO2) are indicative of restrictive disease due to fibrosis.

3. Computed tomography (CT) scan of the lung is more sensitive than plain radiographs for the detection of early fibrotic changes, seen on CT as "ground glass" appearance, suggesting inflammation or aleveolitis, (Chizzolini et al., 2011; Homer & Herzog, 2010; Veraldi, Hsu, & Feghali-Bostwick, 2010).

I. Scleroderma renal crisis (15-20%)

1. Presents suddenly with malignant hypertension.

2. May precede diagnosis of scleroderma 20% of time.

3. If renal dysfunction occurs with a normal blood pressure need to consider other nonscleroderma-related causes.

4. SRC develops within a year of diagnosis 60% of the time and has been associated with high doses of corticosteroids (if on prednisone,

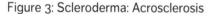

4
4.1
4.2
4.3
4.4
4.5
4.6
4.7
4.8
4.9
4.10

Figure 3: Scleroderma: Acrosclerosis

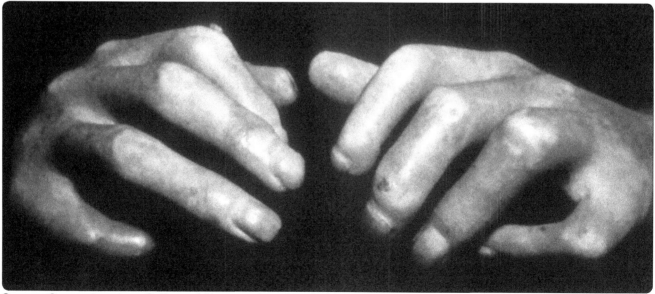

Source: © 2014 American College of Rheumatology. Used with permission.

needs to be maintained < 15 mg/day) (Denton & Steen, 2011; Nihtyanova et al., 2010).

J. Cardiac involvement.

1. Usually a late finding.

2. Myocardial changes are insidious and may be due to ischemic, fibrotic, and inflammatory muscle changes.

3. When present, cardiac changes are related to conduction defects causing arrhythmias, myopathy, and pericarditis.

4. Small to moderate sized pericardial effusions are frequently noted, but large pericardial effusions are associated with poor prognosis (Mayes et al., 2008; Shah & Wigley, 2008).

K. Gastrointestinal tract.

1. Progressive sclerosis of GI tract can lead to diffuse, severe hypomotility, malabsorption, constipation, and/or incontinence with diarrhea (due to bacterial overgrowth).

2. Vascular changes in the stomach can cause GI bleeding.

3. Endoscopic exam reveals a pattern that looks like the stripes of a watermelon, referred to as "watermelon stomach."

4. It can present as frank bleeding or a chronic anemia and could be one of the first

presentations of scleroderma (Di Ciaula et al., 2008; Thoua et al., 2010).

L. Significant constitutional and multisystem symptoms:

1. Fatigue can be overwhelming, significantly affects quality of life (QOL).

2. Loss of appetite, bloating, constipation, incontinence, and weight loss.

3. Joint pain, swelling, tightness, contractures.

4. Severe itchiness (pruritus) especially early in the course but may persist in up to 44% cases for years (El-Baalbaki et al., 2010; Godard, 2011; Mayes et al., 2008; Shah & Wigley, 2008; Thombs, Taillefer, Hudson, & Baron, 2007; Thombs et al., 2010).

M. Overlap syndromes:

1. Mixed connective tissue disease and myositis with scleroderma features.

IV. Diagnosis.

A. Physical exam: Important to determine duration of disease (marked by first non-Raynaud's disease sign or symptom).

1. Skin: Common and major impact on QOL.

    a. Raynaud's (see Figure 4).

4
4.1
4.2
4.3
4.4
4.5
4.6
4.7
4.8
4.9
4.10

Figure 4: Raynaud's Phenomenon: Hands

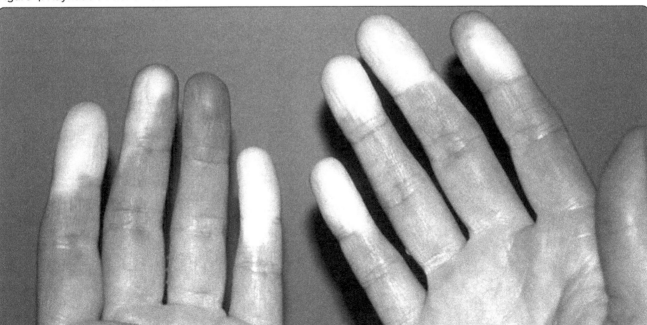

(1) Areas of clear demarcation in response to cold, stress, or anxiety. Digital tip pitting scars, ulcers, and even gangrene if perfusion remains poor.

(2) Monitor for secondary infection due to slow wound healing and recurrent mechanical trauma.

(3) Persistent perfusion defects can lead to digital tip pitting scars, ulcerations, and acro-osteolysis (bone resorption/ shortening, often asymptomatic). Areas of hyper/ hypopigmentation ("salt and pepper" appearance), and telangiectasias on the hands, face, and chest (< 1 mm size, blanch with pressure).

b. Sclerodactyly/skin thickening.

(1) Initially puffy skin changes distally and progressing proximally in diffuse disease replaced with areas of thickened skin in pattern consistent with either localized, limited, or diffuse skin changes. Skin becomes shiny, without hair, and taut.

(2) Degree of thickening predicts morbidity and mortality.

(3) Pruritus and pain are common and often predate overt skin changes (related to mast cell release of histamine).

(4) In diffuse disease, skin thickening may actually improve after 2-3 years.

(5) Loss of adipose tissue and sweat glands results in difficulty maintaining body temperature.

(6) The Modified Rodnan Score (MRSS) is a system of classifying the extent of skin involvement.

c. Calcinosis.

(1) Firm nodules that can erupt through the skin can become infected and difficult to manage especially in presence of poor vasculature.

2. Musculoskeletal.

a. Joint pain and stiffness, swelling, tendon inflammation, and contractures are all possible with extent determined by type of autoantibodies and stage of disease progression.

3. Cardiopulmonary.

a. Blood pressure monitoring for hypertension 3x/wk is important to identify early onset of potential for scleroderma renal crisis.

b. Monitor for breathlessness especially on exertion, dry cough.

c. Exam reveals bilateral inspiratory crackles.

d. Assess for arrhythmias, evidence of bruits/ rubs, murmurs.

4. Gastrointestinal.

a. Very common and major impact on QOL (Thoua et al., 2010).

(1) Oral manifestations: Decreased oral aperture (< 5 cm, making oral hygiene difficult) thinning and retraction of lips, vertical wrinkling around the mouth. 70% also present with xerostomia (dry mouth) contributing to dental caries/gum disease.

(2) Reflux: Heartburn, chest pain.

(3) Dysphagia/Hypomotility: GERD, early satiety (fullness), bloating. In severe cases change in bowel pattern, bloating, diarrhea, fecal incontinence/constipation, foul smelling, pseudo-obstruction.

(4) Malabsorption: Weight loss, poor wound healing, fatigue.

b. Careful monitoring of body weight and body mass index (BMI).

5. Constitutional, non-specific symptoms.

a. Fatigue/malaise, low grade fever in 75% of patients with scleroderma and most closely related to physical function even more than all other symptoms such as pain, disease subtype, and depression (Godard, 2011; Thombs et al., 2007; Thombs et al., 2010).

b. Pain related to ischemic, inflammatory, and fibrotic changes affecting skin, perfusion, and digestion. Pain is experienced by 60-80% of patients with limited or diffuse scleroderma (Schieir et al., 2010).

c. Pruritus especially in diffuse scleroderma during rapid skin thickening phase (69%) although it has been known to persist for many years in some patients (44%) significantly contributing to QOL issues (El-Baalbaki et al., 2010; Jewett et al., 2010; Kowal-Bielecka et al., 2009).

d. Headaches should always be viewed with caution and high index of suspicion for SRC especially with diffuse scleroderma (with + Scl-70 and/ or anti-RNA POL3 antibodies) (Denton & Steen, 2011; Mayes et al., 2008;

4
4.1
4.2
4.3
4.4
4.5
4.6
4.7
4.8
4.9
4.10

Nihtyanova et al., 2008; Nihtyanova & Denton, 2008).

e. Mood disorders from anxiety to depression (Thombs et al., 2010).

(1) Psychosocial dysfunction: Mood disorders related to chronic disease.

(2) Self-esteem significantly affected as result of changes in body image and role capabilities. Ability to maintain work, home, social, and activities of daily living can become challenging (Jewett et al., 2010; Knafo, Jewett, Bassel, & Tahombs, 2010; Mayes et al., 2008; Nihtyanova et al., 2008).

f. Relationships are stressed because of changing body image, role expectations, and challenges with activities of daily living. Vascular problems in men may lead to erectile dysfunction, and in women the thickening of vaginal tissue along with dryness results in painful intercourse. Intimacy is further challenged by pain, fatigue, and depression (Godard, 2011; Knafo, Haythornthwaite, Heinberg, Wigley, & Thombs, 2011; Knafo et al., 2010; Sandusky, McGuire, Smith, Wigley, & Haythornthwaite, 2009).

g. The Pain-Fatigue-Depression triad: Each one affects the other and results in significant challenges in being able to cope with this complex chronic medical condition.

(1) Depression is common with 35-65% reported in epidemiological studies and is associated with emotional suffering, impaired functional outcomes, greater use of health care, and increased comorbidity and mortality (Thombs et al., 2007; Thombs et al., 2010).

(2) Fatigue is common with 76% persons reporting fatigue and 61% listing fatigue as one of the top three distressing features. The exhaustion is often disproportionate to exertion and not improved with rest (Sandusky et al., 2009). Fatigue is one of the most important factors affecting QOL for this and many rheumatologic conditions. It remains an issue throughout the entire course of the disease.

(3) Pain is also a constant feature for many living with scleroderma. Pain is due to inflammatory, vascular, and structural changes that affect nearly every aspect of life. Pain is made worse by fatigue and depression (Knafo et al., 2011; Sandqvist, Scheja, & Hesselstrand, 2010; Sandusky et al., 2009).

V. Laboratory assessment: Auto antibody status can predict disease and direct monitoring and treatment decisions. Each antibody is associated with a different subset of clinical symptoms. Although the antinuclear antibody (ANA) is seen in most disease states of autoimmune nature, the scleroderma-specific antibodies are infrequently seen in other connective tissue diseases (Satoh, Vazquez-Del Mercado, & Chan, 2009).

A. Antinuclear antibody (ANA): Ninety-five percent of all patients with scleroderma have +ANA.

1. Anticentromere (ACA).

   a. Limited scleroderma.

   b. High percentage of women, few African Americans.

   c. Half of patients with ACA who die from scleroderma will die of PAH. Since patients do not develop pulmonary or renal complications early, they usually have more severe GI complaints on a routine basis. Cardiac diseases are uncommon and when present are related to dysrhythmias more than myopathic changes.

B. Anti-Th/To.

1. Associated with limited scleroderma. This is not readily available but is identified by a "nucleolar" pattern on immunofluorescence (ANA will be reported as a "nucleolar" pattern).

2. This particular pattern is more prevalent in males.

3. Most importantly, these patients have increased frequency and severity of lung disease with both PAH and interstitial fibrosis as major factors in decreasing survival when compared to other patients with limited scleroderma.

4. These patients also have a shorter duration of Raynaud's preceding diagnosis, less severe esophageal involvement, but greater small bowel dysfunction.

4
4.1
4.2
4.3
4.4
4.5
4.6
4.7
4.8
4.9
4.10

C. Antitopoimerase (Scl-70).

1. Diffuse scleroderma. The antinuclear pattern is often speckled or homogenous. This is the classic diffuse presentation with Raynaud's usually as the first symptom, progressing quickly, within the first 2 years, into developing diffuse cutaneous symptoms. Ulcerations, gangrene, and acro-osteolysis are more frequent. Extensive joint and tendon involvement early in disease results in significant deformities.

2. Severe interstitial lung disease (fibrosis) is the hallmark of this presentation and occurs early in the disease, with patients dying of lung-related problems within 10 years of diagnosis of scleroderma (Homer & Herzog, 2010; Mayes et al., 2008; Nihtyanova et al., 2010; Steen & Medsger, 2007).

D. Anti-RNA polymerase III (POL3).

1. Recognized by a speckled antibody, negative Scl-70 and anticentromere antibody, prominent skin and tendon involvement, and normal lung volumes.

2. Highest risk of developing SRC (25-33%).

3. Also associated with the highest incidence of skin involvement and presents earlier than other scleroderma cases because of a high frequency of carpal tunnel syndrome, inflammatory joint symptoms, and swollen hands/legs, often without Raynaud's.

4. Very high risk for severe contractures. Less likely to experience severe lung and GI complications.

5. Only recently routinely available to detect a unique subset of diffuse systemic scleroderma (Parker, Burlingame, Webb, & Bunn, 2008).

E. Anti-PM/Scl.

1. Associated with overlap CTD syndrome and presents with acute onset of inflammatory muscle disease and dermatomyositis cutaneous skin changes ("mechanics' hands") along with Raynaud's and sclerodactyly similar to that seen with limited scleroderma (or CREST syndrome) without severe GI or cardiac involvement.

2. However, like other forms of myositis, it is more frequently associated with interstitial fibrosis.

3. Less common in African Americans.

F. Anti-U1-RNP.

1. Associated with classic mixed connective tissue disease (MCTD) associated with inflammatory muscle (27%) and joint disease (94%), Raynaud's, limited cutaneous disease (though 20% develop diffuse).

2. All have manifestations of scleroderma, but complications are less common.

G. Renal function.

1. Estimate creatinine clearance and urinalysis every 3 months. Assess urine for protein, hematuria, and granular casts.

H. CBC.

1. Anemia, thrombocytopenia/thrombocytosis common.

2. Important to monitor disease activity and medication side effects.

I. CMP and LFTs for drug monitoring.

1. Hepatitis B/C testing prior to immunosuppressive therapy.

J. CPK/Aldolase.

1. Elevations noted in myositis associated with overlap syndromes.

VI. **Diagnostic studies.**

A. Pulmonary function tests (PFTs) routinely (baseline and every 3-6 months for first 4 years in both limited and diffuse scleroderma).

1. Reduction in $DLCO_2$ without changes in forced vital capacity (FVC) is associated with pulmonary hypertension.

   a. Decreased lung volumes are associated with interstitial lung disease (fibrosis/restrictive lung disease).

   b. Assessment for evidence of restrictive lung disease is measured by a decrease in diffusion capacity ($DLCO_2$) as well as a decrease in vital capacity and lung volumes often abnormal in asymptomatic patients with normal chest x-ray.

   c. Decreased $DLCO_2$ is the earliest abnormality in scleroderma lung disease; when chest imaging is normal, this is suggestive of pulmonary vascular disease such as PAH seen more frequently in limited

4
4.1
4.2
4.3
4.4
4.5
4.6
4.7
4.8
4.9
4.10

scleroderma but present in both (Avouac et al., 2011; Homer & Herzog, 2010; Nihtyanova & Denton, 2008; Nihtyanova et al., 2010).

B. High resolution CT scan of chest looking for fibrotic changes "ground glass appearance" (inflammation of the alveoli). Should be done at baseline, routinely based on subset of disease (ANA-nucleolar pattern and/or Scl-70), and with changes in pulmonary status/or reduction in PFTs (Mayes et al., 2008; Nihtyanova & Denton, 2008; Nihtyanova et al., 2010).

C. EKG and echocardiogram yearly and right heart catheterization as gold standard if PAH is suspected. Routine monitoring of BP at home and identification of early hypertension is critical to identify early signs of scleroderma renal crisis.

D. If persistent dyspepsia, dysphagia, abdominal discomfort, or weight loss: Endoscopy at baseline and with persistent symptoms. Barium swallow with small bowel follow through, gastric emptying study, and colonoscopy as indicated.

VII. Treatment:

A. To date, no effective treatment that addresses the underlying disease process exists specifically, although numerous biologic targets are currently under investigation. It is important to note that the vascular changes are eminently treatable; inflammatory features are partially treatable; and fibrotic changes have responded with modest efficacy to recent treatments.

B. At this time, treatment is largely symptom driven with attention to specific organ involvement with goal of minimizing complications. Vigilant monitoring with timely intervention is essential to minimize complications from comorbid conditions such as PAH, pulmonary fibrosis, scleroderma renal crisis, gastrointestinal, and musculoskeletal complications. Identification of the most progressive cases (often presenting with the most aggressive skin disease) is essential, and recommendations for consideration in clinical trials is important.

C. Emerging evidence of effective treatments has minimized mortality over the past 10 years, but attention to the overall multisystem disease burden must still be a priority (Distler & Distler, 2008; Homer & Herzog, 2010; Khanna & Denton, 2010; Nihtyanova & Denton, 2008; Nihtyanova et al., 2010; Robertson et al., 2005; Steen & Medsger, 2007; Veraldi et al., 2010).

D. Anti-inflammatory therapy: Immunosuppressive/ disease modifying.

1. High-dose immunosuppressive therapy (HDIT) with autologous stem haematopoietic stem cell transplantation (HSCT).

2. Immune system ablation and replacement with stem cells in effort to decrease autoimmunity.

3. Multicenter randomized trials in Europe and United States underway. Completed phase I and II studies suggest promising results. Dramatic improvement/resolution of dermal fibrosis and stabilization/ improvement of pulmonary dysfunction reported up to eight years.

4. Currently recruiting for phase III trials (Distler & Distler, 2008; Henes et al., 2012; Sullivan, Muraro, & Tyndall, 2010; Walker & Pope, 2012).

E. Disease modifying agents decrease inflammation associated with fibrosis and synovitis:

1. Methotrexate (MTX) up to 25 mg/wk oral or subcutaneous.

   a. Can improve skin scores in early diffuse disease.

   b. Well tolerated although need to monitor for GI intolerance, liver toxicity, cytopenias, teratogenicity, and rare induction of interstitial lung disease.

   c. Side effects can be minimized by adjusting dosing regimens, route of administration, and use of folic acid supplements (Pope, Harding, Khimdas, Bonner, & Baron, 2012; Torok & Arkachaisri, 2012).

2. Mycophenolate mofetil (Cellcept®) up to 2 gm daily (Koutroumpas, Ziogas, Alexiou, Barouta, & Sakkas, 2010).

3. Azathioprine (Imuran®): Few studies (Pope et al., 2012; Walker & Pope, 2012).

4
4.1
4.2
4.3
4.4
4.5
4.6
4.7
4.8
4.9
4.10

4. Cyclophosphamide (CTX) (Cytoxan®) has demonstrated modest evidence of stabilization of lung fibrosis with effects lasting months after completion of therapy, but long term use is not associated with improved outcomes.

   a. Can be given as daily oral dose or monthly intravenous infusions x 6 months.

   b. Potential risks of bone marrow suppression, teratogenicity, gonadal failure, and haemorrhagic cystitis must be considered.

5. Cyclosporin (Neoral®): Few studies.

6. Intravenous immunoglobulin (IVIG) infusions: Few studies.

7. Steroids: Minimize the inflammatory process but have been associated with higher risks of developing SRC in doses over 15 mg/d (Pope et al., 2012; Torok & Arkachaisri, 2012; Walker & Pope, 2012).

F. Vascular therapy: Vasodilators for Raynaud's, PAH, and SRC (Harding, Khimdas, Bonner, Baron, & Pope, 2012; Nihtyanova et al., 2008; Nihtyanova et al., 2010; Pope et al., 2012; Pope, 2007; Walker & Pope, 2012).

   1. Calcium channel blockers (CCB): First-line therapy for symptomatic Raynaud's absolutely shown to decrease frequency and severity of ischemic attacks.

   2. Prostacyclin derivatives.

      a. Prostaglandin is a steroid naturally produced in the body in response to the inflammatory process and is responsible for relaxation of blood vessels to promote improved blood flow.

      b. There are currently three agents available: Epoprostenol (Flolan®), treprostinil (Remodulin®), iloprost (Ventavis®). These agents are considered when oral vasodilators fail to improve the pulmonary situation. These agents are also used for severe peripheral vascular complications as IV/SC infusions in the most severe cases (less effective orally) when CCB have failed. Several studies have demonstrated IV iloprost efficacy in healing digital ulcers (Robertson et al., 2005; Steen et al., 2008).

      c. For severe PAH, permanent continuous infusions are effective but are complicated by several logistics associated with a continuous central intravenous infusion 24/7.

      d. In addition to the inconvenience and problems associated with continuous infusions, there are many uncomfortable side effects: Nausea, jaw pain, joint pain, flushing, and rash.

      e. Avoid sudden withdrawal; acute exacerbations can be life threatening. This can be particularly an issue if the continuous infusion is interrupted for any reason.

      f. Careful hemodynamic monitoring is essential, especially after dosage adjustments (Nihtyanova et al., 2008; Nihtyanova et al., 2010; Pope et al., 2012; Pope, 2007).

   3. Endothelin-1 Receptor antagonists (ERA): Bosentan (Tracleer®) and ambrisentan (Letairis®).

      a. Endothelin is a protein found within the endothelium (layer of cells which line the heart and blood vessels) and is a potent vasoconstrictor contributing to much of the PAH and vasoconstriction of Raynaud's.

      b. There are two different receptors: Endothelin A regulating smooth muscle vasoconstriction and endothelin B which causes vasodilation through the production of nitric oxide which is thought to protect against excessive vasoconstriction.

      c. This class of drugs has confirmed efficacy in preventing digital ulcerations. It should be considered when multiple ulcerations persist despite CCB or other vasodilators.

      d. Treatment with IV iloprost (Ventavis®) is associated with up to 60% reduction in digital ulcerations in diffuse scleroderma, 40% in limited.

      e. Bosentan (Tracleer®) improves exercise tolerance, hemodynamics, functional class, and overall survival in severe PAH.

      f. These drugs are teratogenic and may reduce the efficacy of hormonal contraceptive therapy. Important to exclude pregnancy prior to use and consider at least two forms of contraception because of association with severe birth defects. It has also been found to decrease sperm count in men.

      g. Close monitoring of liver function tests (LFTs) especially monthly in first few months; 11% of patients may experience up to 3 x nl LFTs (Avouac et al., 2012; Nihtyanova et al., 2008; Pope, 2007; Rubin, 2012; Steen et al., 2008).

4. Phosphodiesterase-5 (PDE 5) inhibitors.

   a. Induces smooth muscle relaxation of blood vessels resulting in vasodilation.

   b. Two examples, sildenafil (Revatio®) and tadalifil (Adcirca®), are currently approved for PAH and often are used for peripheral vasoconstriction as well.

   c. Associated with significant improvement in functional and hemodynamic status and are recommended therapy with very few side effects for moderate to severe PAH in those for whom ERAs have been ineffective..

   d. Cannot be given with protease inhibitors (HIV medications) and should be avoided in those requiring nitrates.

   e. As with any vasodilating medication, beware of dizziness and other signs of low blood pressure. Vascular congestion in the upper respiratory tract is common (Harding et al., 2012; Impens, Phillips, & Schiopu, 2011; Nihtyanova et al., 2008; Pope, 2007).

5. Angiotensin converting enzyme (ACE) inhibitors.

   a. Angiotensin is a potent vasoconstrictor; blocking this substance has a marked effect on blood pressure systemically and specifically within the renal arterial system in SRC.

   b. The goal of therapy is to normalize blood pressure which is associated with up to 90% improvement in survival rate and has significantly reduced the need for dialysis.

   c. Additionally, 50% of those who progress to renal failure can be removed from dialysis if maintained on ACE inhibitors.

   d. As with any vasodilating medication, beware of dizziness and other signs of low blood pressure (Denton & Steen, 2011; Harding et al., 2012; Kowal-Bielecka et al., 2009; Nihtyanova et al., 2010; Pope, 2007; Shah & Wigley, 2008).

6. Other supportive therapy: Diuretics, antiplatelet therapy, statins, and other cardiovascular supportive agents such as digoxin and warfarin (when dysrhythmias or cardiomyopathy are present).

G. Anti-fibrotic therapy.

1. Tyrosine kinase inhibitors: Imatinib (Gleevac®).

2. Early studies suggest regression of fibrosis with fairly good tolerability. Although no specific guidelines have been established, avoid prolonged use.

3. Common side effects to monitor include myelosuppression, hepatotoxicity, nausea/vomiting/diarrhea, and edema.

4. Confirm absence of pregnancy prior to use and consider at least two forms of contraception because of association with severe birth defects and other life-threatening complications.

5. Baseline CBC, LFTs, and then monthly (Chizzolini et al., 2011; Gordon & Spiera, 2011; Harding et al., 2012; Homer & Herzog, 2010; Nihtyanova & Denton, 2008; Nihtyanova et al., 2010; Veraldi et al., 2010; Walker & Pope, 2012).

H. Gastrointestinal/skin: Largely symptomatic.

1. GERD.

   a. PPI should be used to prevent GERD, ulcerations and strictures, and dysplasia (Barrett's esophagitis).

   b. Be aware that chronic use of PPI increases risk of aspiration pneumonia and can contribute to osteoporosis related to malabsorption of calcium and vitamin D.

2. Dysphagia/dysmotility.

   a. Prokinetic agents: Octreotide (Sandostatin®).

   b. Long-term use of octreotide (Sandostatin®) requires baseline measure of thyroid function studies and B12 levels along with baseline glucose with periodic assessments routinely.

   c. Another prokinetic agent is metoclopramide (Reglan®) given before meals and at night when necessary.

     (1) Long-term use is associated with tardive dyskinesia, a movement disorder characterized by Parkinsonian like changes. Careful attention to renal function.

I. Bacterial overgrowth: Rotating antibiotics.

J. Malnutrition: Nutritional supplementation and parenteral hyperalimentation in severe cases.

4
4.1
4.2
4.3
4.4
4.5
4.6
4.7
4.8
4.9
4.10

K. Antihistamines for severe pruritus.

L. Psychosocial support needed to address the multifaceted impact on daily living.

   1. Sleep hygiene is critical and assistive devices should be considered as needed.

   2. Numerous cognitive and behavioral strategies are recommended to address the fatigue, pruritus, anxiety, and pain that accompanies scleroderma.

   3. Each of these issues should be evaluated at every encounter.

VIII. Nursing implications.

A. Teaching.

   1. "If the specificities of these treatments were well explained, including adverse effects and drug interactions with other treatments, it would be easier to handle and deal with it for the patient" (Godard, 2010, p. 292).

B. Monitoring for complications of disease.

   1. Monitor blood pressure routinely at home with a well calibrated home blood pressure device; elevations should be reported immediately. It is important for the patient to know what normal blood pressure is; assess for headaches.

   2. Baseline: PFTs, high resolution CT scan, and echocardiogram then at least yearly and more frequently depending on specific subset.

   3. Routine labs depending on specific treatments.

   4. Endoscopy at baseline and yearly with active GERD.

   5. Consider motility evaluation for dysphagia, weight loss, bloating, constipation/or diarrhea. Routine assessment for GI bleeding through CBC and patient awareness.

   6. Close monitoring of skin for ulceration and infection; institute antibiotics as needed. Assess need for more aggressive therapy when multiple ulcerations or persistent lesions occur.

   7. Maintain annual flu vaccination, routine pneumococcal vaccine. Consider shingles vaccination because of high risk

of development in immunocompromised persons (Singh et al., 2012).

   8. Raynaud's: Monitor for ischemic changes, digital ulcerations, and infection; recognize the need for immediate care. Pain related to ischemic changes can be severe. Treat underlying cause when possible, adequate pain management when not.

C. "SSc patients are always cold and they cannot get warm" (Godard, 2010, p. 291).

D. Non-pharmacological.

   1. No smoking.

   2. Maintain core body temperature by using layers, hats, mittens, scarves. Makes a big difference and cannot be emphasized enough.

   3. Treating digital ulcers.

      a. Major impact on function; pain and infection often limit use of hands all together. Important for patient to understand need for proper nail care, monitoring for adequate perfusion, particular attention to distal extremities, as well as protecting ears/nose when exposed to cold, ulcerations/sores with careful attention to infection and prompt intervention as needed.

      b. Consistency with calcium channel blockers (CCB) as prescribed.

      c. Beware of mechanical trauma to hands as well.

   4. Skin care.

      a. Treatment for pruritus can be top priority.

      b. Maintain moisture as much as possible with ointments and skin protection.

      c. Antihistamines can be helpful often at high doses.

   5. Consider using sedating and non-sedating agents to maintain appropriate sleep/wake cycle (El-Baalbaki et al., 2010).

E. Pulmonary.

   1. Monitor for changes in exercise tolerance, frequent PFTs, baseline and routine cardiopulmonary evaluation as mentioned above.

   2. Cough of any nature should be reported. A dry, non-productive cough is indicative of

4
4.1
4.2
4.3
4.4
4.5
4.6
4.7
4.8
4.9
4.10

ILD/PAH, whereas a moist, productive cough may signal infection; common in this patient population (Lim, 2012).

F. Gastrointestinal.

1. Motility studies, endoscopy evaluation important to assess for strictures, dysplasia, and loss of peristalsis.

2. GERD symptom control through PPI and other medications. Many patients require prokinetic agents such as metoclopramide (Reglan®); Sleep with head/chest elevated as much as possible (try a wedge under the mattress); Monitor intake prior to lying down. Concern with aspiration as it contributes to progressive pulmonary disease and infection.

3. Additionally watch for GI bleeding anywhere from GI tract and consider complications of bacterial overgrowth frequently seen with sclerotic changes to GI tract and present with diarrhea, bloating, and abdominal pain (Thoua et al., 2010).

G. Pain: A critical problem throughout.

1. Raynaud's, ulcerations, contractures, profound fatigue, wasted muscles, poor digestion (malabsorption), breathlessness, difficulty walking, eating, sleeping, sitting in one position, and other changes contribute to the ongoing need for adequate pain management.

    a. First priority is to treat the underlying cause: Ischemia, inflammation, infection.

    b. When pain persists despite this, ensure adequate sleep, address depression with antidepressants as needed, and then consider pharmacologic support with narcotic and non-narcotic analgesics and other adjuvant agents such as anticonvulsants.

    c. Non-pharmacologic strategies should also be employed such as teaching self-management techniques: Relaxation, pacing, cognitive restructuring, and distraction (Dures & Hewlett, 2012).

H. All activities are impaired by this disease.

1. Assistive devices are essential: Deformities, Raynaud's, ulcerations make simple tasks challenging. Assist patients to find devices that promote independence and work with families to better understand limitations appropriately.

2. Physical/occupational therapy to maintain flexibility and independence as much as possible.

I. Need of surgery, beware of the following concerns: Circulatory problems, difficult venous access, difficulty/prolonged healing, problems with intubation, malnutrition.

J. Sexual dysfunction: Erectile dysfunction common 81% related to vasculopathies; changes in vaginal thickening with associated pain limits pleasure. Self-image and depression also have significant impact on sexuality (Knafo et al., 2010; Thombs et al., 2010).

K. Psychosocial: From the words of someone living with scleroderma:
"How do we accept this, how to accept that our face is transformed, aging too fast around the mouth, with wrinkles, and with hardening skin? How can we show our hands without gloves, with wounds, bandages, swollen, blue - in a word ugly? We are always explaining. How can we tolerate the eyes of others, family, work colleagues, and friends? The most important thing is that we must learn to live with scleroderma as best we can... To live the best you can, and especially with the least pain possible. And this, with a little medical help, family or friendly assistance, we can do!" (Godard, 2010, p. 293).

1. Psychological support is essential.

    a. "Who am I?" Loss of identity, difficulty with personal care, household chores, work, and leisure activities significantly affect mood.

    b. Disfigurement leads to body image dissatisfaction.

    c. Profound fatigue contributes to mood as well.

    d. Intimacy and relationships become difficult and often lead to changes in family structure.

    e. Depression is common in many chronic diseases but as high as 75% in patients with scleroderma.

4
4.1
4.2
4.3
4.4
4.5
4.6
4.7
4.8
4.9
4.10

IX. Resources:

A. Encourage empowerment, connection.

B. Social network of family, friends, spiritual groups, and specialty organizations.

C. Team of multidisciplinary providers led by a rheumatologist with pulmonologist, cardiologist, dermatologist along with nurses, physical/occupational therapists, nutritionist, psychologist (as needed) knowledgeable about scleroderma.

D. Connection to center of excellence in nurse's area and awareness of clinical trials.

E. Online resource.

1. Scleroderma Foundation http://www. scleroderma.org/. Up-to-date literature from scientists, healthcare providers, and patients.

F. Other resources.

1. National Institute of Arthritis and Musculoskeletal and Skin Diseases (NIAMS) Information Clearinghouse National Institutes of Health 1 AMS Circle Bethesda, MD 20892-3675 Phone: 301-495-4484 Toll Free: 877-22-NIAMS (877-226-4267) TTY: 301-565-2966 Fax: 301-718-6366 Email: NIAMSinfo@mail.nih.gov Website: http://www.niams.nih.gov.

2. For updates and questions about medications: U.S. Food and Drug Administration Toll Free: 888–INFO–FDA (888–463–6332) Website: http://www.fda.gov/

3. For updates and questions about statistics: Centers for Disease Control and Prevention's National Center for Health Statistics. Website: http://www.cdc.gov/nchs

Summary

Through a systems approach this chapter has provided a description of the signs and symptoms of changes associated with scleroderma affecting every system in the body. A critical analysis of existing recommendations to promote optimal outcomes was presented. Through this information, the nurse should be able to provide support for those facing the complex and often daunting diagnosis of scleroderma.

References

Avouac, J., Fransen, J., Walker, U. A., Riccieri, V., Smith, V., Muller, C., . . . Matucci-Cerinic, M. (2011). Preliminary criteria for the very early diagnosis of systemic sclerosis: Results of a Delphi Consensus Study from EULAR Scleroderma Trials and Research Group. [Consensus Development Conference]. *Annals of the Rheumatic Diseases, 70*(3), 476-481. doi: 10.1136/ard.2010.136929

Avouac, J., Kowal-Bielecka, O., Landewe, R., Chwiesko, S., Miniati, I., Czirjak, L., . . . Matucci-Cerinic, M. (2009). European League Against Rheumatism (EULAR) Scleroderma Trial and Research group (EUSTAR) recommendations for the treatment of systemic sclerosis: Methods of elaboration and results of systematic literature research. *Annals of the Rheumatic Diseases, 68*(5), 629-634. doi: 10.1136/ard.2008.095299

Avouac, J., Meune, C., Ruiz, B., Couraud, P. O., Uzan, G., Boileau, C., . . . Allanore, Y. (2012). Angiogenic biomarkers predict the occurrence of digital ulcers in systemic sclerosis. *Annals of the Rheumatic Diseases, 71*(3), 394-399. doi: 10.1136/annrheumdis-2011-200143

Barnabe, C., Joseph, L., Belisle, P., Labrecque, J., Edworthy, S., Barr, S. G., . . . Bernatsky, S. (2012). Prevalence of systemic lupus erythematosus and systemic sclerosis in the First Nations population of Alberta, Canada. *Arthritis Care & Research, 64*(1), 138-143. doi: 10.1002/acr.20656

Chifflot, H., Fautrel, B., Sordet, C., Chatelus, E., & Sibilia, J. (2008). Incidence and prevalence of systemic sclerosis: A systematic literature review. *Seminars in Arthritis and Rheumatism, 37*(4), 223-235. doi: 10.1016/j.semarthrit.2007.05.003

Chizzolini, C., Brembilla, N. C., Montanari, E., & Truchetet, M. E. (2011). Fibrosis and immune dysregulation in systemic sclerosis. *Autoimmunity Reviews, 10*(5), 276-281. doi: 10.1016/j.autrev.2010.09.016

4
4.1
4.2
4.3
4.4
4.5
4.6
4.7
4.8
4.9
4.10

Denton, C. P., & Steen, V. (2011). Scleroderma renal crisis. In J. Varga, C. Denton, & F. Wigley (Eds.), *Scleroderma: From pathogenesis to comprehensive management* (pp. 361-372): Springer.

Di Ciaula, A., Covelli, M., Berardino, M., Wang, D. Q., Lapadula, G., Palasciano, G., & Portincasa, P. (2008). Gastrointestinal symptoms and motility disorders in pastients with systemic scleroderma. *BMC Gastroenterology, 8*(7). doi:10.1186/1471-230X-8-7

Distler, J., & Distler, O. (2008). Novel treatment approaches to fibrosis in scleroderma. *Rheumatic Disease Clinics of North America, 34*(1), 145-159.

Dures, E., & Hewlett, S. (2012). Cognitive-behavioural approaches to self-managment in rheumatic disease. *Nature Reviews Rheumatology, 8*, 553-559. doi: 10.1038/nrrheum.2012.108

El-Baalbaki, G., Razykov, I., Hudson, M., Bassel, M., Baron, M., & Thombs, B. D. (2010). Association of pruritus with quality of life and disability in systemic sclerosis. *Arthritis Care & Research, 62*(10), 1489-1495. doi: 10.1002/acr.20257

Godard, D. (2011). The needs of patients with systemic sclerosis--what are the difficulties encountered? *Autoimmunity Reviews, 10*(5), 291-294. doi: 10.1016/j.autrev.2010.09.009

Gordon, J., & Spiera, R. (2011). Tyrosine kinase inhibitors in the treatment of systemic sclerosis: The difficulty in interpreting proof-of-concept studies. *International Journal of Rheumatology*, ID 842181, 8pp. doi: 10.1155/2011/842181

Harding, S., Khimdas, S., Bonner, A., Baron, M., & Pope, J. (2012). Best practices in scleroderma: An analysis of practice variability in SSc centres within the Canadian Scleroderma Research Group (CSRG). *Clinical and Experimetal Rheumatology, 30*(2 Suppl 71), S38-43.

Henes, J. C., Schmalzing, M., Vogel, W., Riemekasten, G., Fend, F., Kanz, L., & Koetter, I. (2012). Optimization of autologous stem cell transplantation for systemic sclerosis: A single-center longterm experience in 26 patients with severe organ manifestations. *The Journal of Rheumatology, 39*(2), 269-275. doi: 10.3899/jrheum.110868

Homer, R. J., & Herzog, E. L. (2010). Recent advances in pulmonary fibrosis: Implications for scleroderma. *Current Opinions in Rheumatology, 22*(6), 683-689. doi: 10.1097/BOR.0b013e32833ddcc9

Impens, A. J., Phillips, K., & Schiopu, E. (2011). PDE-5 Inhibitors in sleroderma raynaud phenomenon and digital ulcers: Current status of clinical trials. *International Journal of Rheumatology*, ID 392542, 5pp. doi: 10.1155/2011/392542

Jewett, L. R., Hudson, M., Haythornthwaite, J. A., Heinberg, L., Wigley, F. M., Baron, M., & Thombs, B. D. (2010). Development and validation of the brief-satisfaction with appearance scale for systemic sclerosis. *Arthritis Care & Research, 62*(12), 1779-1786. doi: 10.1002/acr.20307

Khanna, D., & Denton, C. P. (2010). Evidence-based management of rapidly progressing systemic sclerosis. [Review]. *Best Practice & Research Clinical Rheumatology, 24*(3), 387-400. doi: 10.1016/j.berh.2009.12.002

Knafo, R., Haythornthwaite, J. A., Heinberg, L., Wigley, F. M., & Thombs, B. D. (2011). The association of body image dissatisfaction and pain with reduced sexual function in women with systemic sclerosis. *Rheumatology, 50*(6), 1125-1130. doi: 10.1093/rheumatology/keq443

Knafo, R., Jewett, L. R., Bassel, M., & Thombs, B. D. (2010). Sexual function in women with systemic sclerosis: Comment on the article by Schouffoer et al. *Arthritis Care & Research, 62*(8), 1200; author reply 1200-1201. doi: 10.1002/acr.20185

Koutroumpas, A., Ziogas, A., Alexiou, I., Barouta, G., & Sakkas, L. I. (2010). Mycophenolate mofetil in systemic sclerosis-associated interstitial lung disease. *Clinical Rheumatology, 29*(10), 1167-1168. doi: 10.1007/s10067-010-1498-z

Kowal-Bielecka, O., Landewe, R., Avouac, J., Chwiesko, S., Miniati, I., Czirjak, L., . . . Matucci-Cerinic, M. (2009). EULAR recommendations for the treatment of systemic sclerosis: A report from the EULAR Scleroderma Trials and Research group (EUSTAR). *Annals of the Rheumatic Diseases, 68*(5), 620-628. doi:10.1136/ard.2008.096677

Lim, K. G. (2012). Scleroderma lung-associated cough: More than meets the eye? *Chest, 142*(3), 556-557. doi: 10.1378/chest.12-0170

Mayes, M., & Assassi, S. (2011). Connective tissue disorders. In A. Hochberg, A. J. Silman, J. S. Smolen, M. E. Weinblatt, & M. H. Weisman (Eds.), *Rheumatology* (5th ed.). [Digital Edition]. New York: Elsevier.

Mayes, M., Varga, J., Buch, M. H., & Seibold, J. (2008). Systemic scleroderma: Clinical features; Epidemiology, pathology, and pathogenesis; Treatment & assessment. In J. H. Klippel, L. S. Stone, L. J. Crofford, & P. H. White (Eds.), *Primer on rheumatic diseases* (13th ed., pp. 343-362). New York: Springer.

Nihtyanova, S. I., Brough, G. M., Black, C. M., & Denton, C. P. (2008). Clinical burden of digital vasculopathy in limited and diffuse cutaneous systemic sclerosis. *Annals of the Rheumatic Diseases, 67*(1), 120-123. doi: 10.1136/ard.2007.072686

4
4.1
4.2
4.3
4.4
4.5
4.6
4.7
4.8
4.9
4.10

Nihtyanova, S. I., & Denton, C. P. (2008). Current approaches to the management of early active diffuse scleroderma skin disease. *Rheumatic Disease Clinics of North America, 34*(1), 161-179; viii. doi: 10.1016/j.rdc.2007.11.005

Nihtyanova, S. I., Tang, E. C., Coghlan, J. G., Wells, A. U., Black, C. M., & Denton, C. P. (2010). Improved survival in systemic sclerosis is associated with better ascertainment of internal organ disease: A retrospective cohort study. *QJM: An International Journal of Medicine, 103*(2), 109-115. doi: 10.1093/qjmed/hcp174

Parker, J. C., Burlingame, R. W., Webb, T. T., & Bunn, C. C. (2008). Anti-RNA polymerase III antibodies in patients with systemic sclerosis detected by indirect immunofluorescence and ELISA. *Rheumatology, 47*(7), 976-979. doi: 10.1093/rheumatology/ken201

Pope, J., Harding, S., Khimdas, S., Bonner, A., & Baron, M. (2012). Agreement with guidelines from a large database for management of systemic sclerosis: Results from the Canadian Scleroderma Research Group. *The Journal of Rheumatology,39*(3), 524-531. doi: 10.3899/jrheum.110121

Pope, J. E. (2007). The diagnosis and treatment of Raynaud's phenomenon: A practical approach. *Drugs, 67*(4), 517-525.

Robertson, L., Pignone, A., Kowal-Bielecka, O., Fiori, G., Denton, C. P., & Matucci-Cerinic, M. (2005). Pulmonary arterial hypertension in systemic sclerosis: Diagnostic pathway and therapeutic approach. *Annals of the Rheum Diseases, 64*(6), 804-807. doi: 10.1136/ard.2004.026427

Rubin, L. J. (2012). Endothelin receptor antagonists for the treatment of pulmonary hypertension. *Life Sciences, 91,* 517-521.

Sandqvist, G., Scheja, A., & Hesselstrand, R. (2010). Pain, fatigue and hand function closely correlated to work ability and employment status in systemic sclerosis. *Rheumatology, 49*(9), 1739-1746. doi: 10.1093/rheumatology/keq145

Sandusky, S. B., McGuire, L., Smith, M. T., Wigley, F. M., & Haythornthwaite, J. A. (2009). Fatigue: An overlooked determinant of physical function in scleroderma. *Rheumatology, 48*(2), 165-169. doi: 10.1093/rheumatology/ken455

Satoh, M., Vazquez-Del Mercado, M., & Chan, E. K. (2009). Clinical interpretation of antinuclear antibody tests in systemic rheumatic diseases. *Modern Rheumatology, 19*(3), 219-228. doi: 10.1007/s10165-009-0155-3

Schier, O., Thombs, B. D., Hudson, M., Boivin, J. F., Steele, R., Bernatsky, S., . . . Baron, M. (2010). Prevalence, severity, and clinical correlates of pain in patients with systemic sclerosis. *Arthritis Care & Research, 62*(3), 409-417. doi: 10.1002/acr.20108

Shah, A. A., & Wigley, F. M. (2008). Often forgotten manifestations of systemic sclerosis. *Rheumatic Disease Clinics of North America, 34*(1), 221-238; ix. doi: 10.1016/j.rdc.2007.10.002

Singh, J. A., Furst, D. E., Bharat, A., Curtis, J. R., Kavanaugh, A. F., Kremer, J. M., . . . Saag, K. G. (2012). 2012 update of the 2008 American College of Rheumatology recommendations for the use of disease-modifying antirheumatic drugs and biologic agents in the treatment of rheumatoid arthritis. *Arthritis Care & Research, 64*(5), 625-639. doi: 10.1002/acr.21641

Steen, V., Chou, M., Shanmugam, V., Mathias, M., Kuru, T., & Morrissey, R. (2008). Exercise-induced pulmonary arterial hypertension in patients with systemic sclerosis. *Chest, 134*(1), 146-151. doi: 10.1378/chest.07-2324

Steen, V. D. (2008). The many faces of scleroderma. *Rheumatic Disease Clinics of North America, 34*(1), 1-15; v. doi: 10.1016/j.rdc.2007.12.001

Steen, V. D., & Medsger, T. A. (2007). Changes in causes of death in systemic sclerosis, 1972-2002. *Annals of the Rheumatic Diseases, 66*(7), 940-944. doi: 10.1136/ard.2006.066068

Sullivan, K. M., Muraro, P., & Tyndall, A. (2010). Hematopoietic cell transplantation for autoimmune disease: Updates from Europe and the United States. *Biology of Blood and Marrow Transplantation, 16*(1 Suppl), S48-56. doi: 10.1016/j.bbmt.2009.10.034

Thombs, B. D., Taillefer, S. S., Hudson, M., & Baron, M. (2007). Depression in patients with \ s y s t e m i c sclerosis: A systematic review of the evidence. *Arthritis & Rheumatism, 57*(6), 1089-1097. doi: 10.1002/art.22910

Thombs, B. D., van Lankveld, W., Bassel, M., Baron, M., Buzza, R., Haslam, S., . . . Worron-Sauve, M. (2010). Psychological health and well-being in systemic sclerosis: State of the science and consensus research agenda. *Arthritis Care & Research, 62*(8), 1181-1189. doi: 10.1002/acr.20187

Thoua, N. M., Bunce, C., Brough, G., Forbes, A., Emmanuel, A. V., & Denton, C. P. (2010). Assessment of gastrointestinal symptoms in patients with systemic sclerosis in a UK tertiary referral centre. *Rheumatology, 49*(9), 1770-1775. doi: 10.1093/rheumatology/keq147

4
4.1
4.2
4.3
4.4
4.5
4.6
4.7
4.8
4.9
4.10

Torok, K. S., & Arkachaisri, T. (2012). Methotrexate and corticosteroids in the treatment of localized scleroderma: A standardized prospective longitudinal single-center study. *The Journal of Rheumatology, 39*(2), 286-294. doi: 10.3899/jrheum.110210

Veraldi, K. L., Hsu, E., & Feghali-Bostwick, C. A. (2010). Pathogenesis of pulmonary fibrosis in systemic sclerosis: Lessons from interstitial lung disease. *Current Rheumatology Reports, 12*(1), 19-25. doi: 10.1007/s11926-009-0071-8

Walker, K. M., & Pope, J. (2012). Treatment of systemic sclerosis complications: What to use when first-line treatment fails--a consensus of systemic sclerosis experts. *Seminars in Arthritis and Rheumatism, 42*(1), 42-55. doi: 10.1016/j.semarthrit.2012.01.003

Suggested Readings

Godard, D. (2010). The needs of patients with systemic sclerosis: What are the difficulties encountered? *Autoimmunity Reviews, 10*(5), 291-294.

Khanna, D., & Penton, C. P. (2010). Evidence-based management of rapidly progressing systemic sclerosis. *Best Practice & Research Clinical Rheumatology, 24*, 387-400.

Steen, V. D. (2008). The many faces of scleroderma. *Rheumatic Disease Clinics of North America, 31*(1), 1-15.

Shah, A. A., & Wigley, F. M. (2008). Often forgotten manifestations of systemic slcerosis. *Rheumatic Disease Clinics of North America*, 34(1), 221-238.

Thombs, B. D., van Lankveld, W., Bassel, M., Baron, M., Buzza, R., Haslam, S., ... Worron-Sauve, M. (2010). Psychological health and well-being in systematic sclerosis: State of the science and consensus research agenda. *Arthritis Care & Research, 62*(8), 1181-1189.

Section 4.10

The Inflammatory Myopathies:

Dermatomyositis, Polymyositis, and Inclusion-body Myositis

Janice L. Cuzzell, MSN, RN

Introduction

Myositis is a term that is often used interchangeably with the idiopathic inflammatory myopathies (IIM), a group of autoimmune diseases that target the proximal skeletal muscle in children and adults. Two major categories of inflammatory myopathy include dermatomyositis (DM) and polymyositis (PM) (Astrin, 2008). Although these two disease states share a similar clinical presentation, DM and PM differ histologically, with skin involvement being the hallmark of a DM diagnosis. A third category, inclusion body myositis (IBM), is distinctive in that it occurs more frequently in men over the age of 50, is often misdiagnosed as polymyositis, and fails to respond to conventional therapy (Solorzano & Phillips, 2011).

The idiopathic inflammatory myopathies are rare, with an estimated incidence in the United States 0.1 to 1.0 per 100,000 person-years and prevalence of 0.55 to 6 per. 100,000 person-years (Furst, Amato, Iorga, Gajria, & Fernandes, 2012). As with many autoimmune diseases, the underlying cause of the immune system's attack on muscle tissue is poorly understood. Diagnosis is based on a myriad of factors that include clinical symptoms, laboratory evaluation, and histology findings. A definitive diagnosis is often difficult, not only because the IIMs as a group share a similar clinical presentation but also because symptoms overlap with other connective tissue disease states.

Management of patients with myositis also presents a unique challenge for the rheumatology nurse. Progressive muscle weakness can significantly impair activities of daily living and quality of life. During the course of disease, dependence on assistive devices is often accelerated, and elderly patients, in particular, are at increased risk for falls. As with many rheumatic conditions, patients must deal with the debilitating side effects of chronic steroid therapy or use of other immunosuppressive agents. Body image concerns along with the economic impact of chronic disease management can quickly take a toll on an individual's mental, spiritual, and social well-being.

4
4.1
4.2
4.3
4.4
4.5
4.6
4.7
4.8
4.9
4.10

Learning Objectives

Upon completion of this chapter, the nurse will be able to:

1. Name the three major categories of idiopathic inflammatory myopathy.

2. Identify common disease characteristics associated with myositis.

3. Describe the pathological mechanisms of disease initiation and progression.

4. Describe the appearance and distribution of five types of skin rash associated with dermatomyositis.

5. Describe clinical symptoms that differentiate dermatomyositis, polymyositis, and inclusion body myositis, including the anatomical distribution of muscle weakness.

6. List the laboratory tests used to establish and document a diagnosis of myositis and monitor disease activity.

7. Recall pharmaceutical and immunosuppressive therapies commonly used to treat myositis.

8. Discuss the nursing implications of caring for a patient with myositis.

Content Outline

I. Pathophysiology of Myositis.

A. Myositis (inflammation of the muscle) is a non-specific term used when referencing the idiopathic inflammatory myopathies (IIM).

B. There are three major subtypes of the idiopathic inflammatory myopathies:

1. Dermatomyositis (DM).

2. Polymyositis (PM).

3. Inclusion body myositis (IBM).

C. Although these diseases are heterogeneous in nature, common pathologic characteristics include.

1. Moderate to severe muscle weakness in the absence of a causative factor.

2. Inflammatory cell infiltration in muscle tissue.

3. Muscle fiber degeneration, muscle fiber necrosis, and replacement of muscle tissue by fat.

4. Fibrosis of interstitial tissue.

5. Skin and internal organ involvement.

6. Association with cancer (adults) and other autoimmune connective tissue diseases.

D. The specific pathological mechanisms of disease initiation and progression are not well understood.

1. Degree of inflammation observed on muscle biopsy does not always correlate with extent of muscle weakness.

2. Both immune and non-immune mechanisms are thought to be involved in disease pathogenesis.

a. Myositis-specific antibodies (MSAs) and myositis-associated (MAAs) autoantibodies directed against cytoplasmic or nuclear components of muscle cells.

b. Abnormal protein synthesis by muscle cells causing activation of the endoplasmic stress response to intercellular stress.

E. Clinical trials in myositis are lacking because of the relative rarity of the disease and small sample sizes.

II. Etiology/Epidemiology.

A. Incidence/prevalence.

1. Occurs in both children and adults.

2. Incidence and prevalence are difficult to determine based on differences in study methodology (Prieto & Grau, 2010).

a. DM is the most common IIM with an estimated 8 cases per million per year of incidence.

b. PM is the least common IIM with an estimated 4 cases per million per year of incidence.

c. IBM has an estimated prevalence of 4.5 to 9.5 cases per million and occurs most frequently in patients over the age of 50 years.

3. Approximately 50% of all patients have myositis-specific or associated serum antibodies present suggesting autoimmune etiology (Nagaraju & Lundberg, 2011).

4. 10-fold increase higher risk of malignancy in DM and PM compared to the general population (Selva-O'Callaghan, Trallero-Arguás, Grau-Junyent, & Labrador-Horillo, 2010).

B. Genetic /environmental factors.

1. Idiopathic – no known cause.

2. Rare familial occurrences.

3. Association with HLA genes suggests a possible genetic predisposition.

4. Infectious agents, drugs, and ultraviolet radiation have been identified as possible disease triggers or associated with disease exacerbation (Miller, 2009).

a. Group A streptococcus and influenza have strongest evidence of association with onset of juvenile myositis.

b. Toxoplasmosis has the strongest evidence of association with adult DM.

4
4.1
4.2
4.3
4.4
4.5
4.6
4.7
4.8
4.9
4.10

c. Adult DM patients tend to have a history of photosensitivity which is often confirmed by an abnormally low minimal erythema UVB dose.

d. Other environmental factors that are postulated to have an association with myositis onset or exacerbation include psychological stress, muscular exertion, collagen implants, medications, and vaccines.

5. Geographical clustering of cases and seasonal patterns of onset suggest a potential connection with environmental triggers.

C. Dermatomyositis (DM).

1. Most commonly diagnosed myopathy in all age groups.

2. Bimodal incidence pattern, peaking during childhood and then again between 50 and 70 years of age.

3. Female to male predominance of approximately 2:1.

4. African Americans to Caucasian predominance of approximately 3:1.

5. Highest risk of IIM subtypes for associated malignancy.

D. Polymyositis (PM).

1. Least commonly diagnosed myopathy in all age groups.

2. Most commonly seen after the age of 20.

3. Very rare in children.

4. Female to male predominance of approximately 2:1.

5. African Americans to Caucasian predominance of approximately 5:1.

E. Inclusion body myositis (IBM).

1. Age of onset ranges from the late second to ninth decades. Mean age of onset is 56-60 years.

2. Most common acquired myopathy in men after the age of 50.

3. Approximately 17-20% of cases present before the age of 50.

III. Nursing assessment.

A. Muscle weakness.

1. Insidious onset with gradual worsening over weeks to months.

2. Acute onset can occur but is rare.

3. Progressive weakness of proximal muscles with a symmetric distribution.

4. Distal muscle involvement affecting fine motor skills rarely causes impairment in DM and PM.

5. Weakness varies from mild to severe and progresses to quadriparesis.

6. Patients report difficulty with everyday tasks involving skeletal muscles:

   a. Rising from chair.

   b. Climbing stairs.

   c. Stepping off curb.

   d. Combing hair.

   e. Holding up head (head-drop).

7. Mild myalgia's and muscle tenderness seen in 30% to 50% of cases.

8. Dysphagia, nasal regurgitation, or aspiration can occur if oropharyngeal muscles or striated muscles of the upper esophagus are involved.

   a. Esophageal weakness can contribute to frequent bacterial pneumonia in elderly patients.

9. Inclusion body myositis (IBM) symptom differentiation:

   a. Male patients over the age of 50.

   b. Asymmetric weakness involving distal muscles.

   c. Fine motor skills are affected early in disease course.

   d. Wrist and index finger flexors weaker than extensors.

   e. Early involvement of quadriceps muscle and ankle dorsiflexors increases fall risk.

   f. Mild facial weakness.

   g. Often misdiagnosed as polymyositis.

   h. Does not respond to therapy.

B. Skin rash (hallmark symptom that differentiates dermatomyositis from polymyositis).

4

4.1
4.2
4.3
4.4
4.5
4.6
4.7
4.8
4.9
4.10

1. Heliotrope rash (see Figure 1).

   a. Rare skin manifestation, but most specific for DM diagnosis.

   b. Confluent, purple-red macular lesions.

   c. Eyelids and periorbital tissue.

   d. Edema is often present.

2. Gottron's papules (see Figure 2).

   a. Most frequently occurring rash.

   b. Symmetric, raised violaceous lesions that may be difficult to recognize in darkly-pigmented skin.

   c. Shiny and scaly appearance when chronic.

   d. Involves the extensor surfaces of metacarpophalangeal and inter phalangeal joints of the fingers.

   e. May involve extensor surfaces of elbows, knees, and ankles mimicking psoriasis.

   f. Exacerbated by sun exposure.

   g. May be pruritic.

   h. Soft tissue calcinosis can occur as the disease progresses.

3. Shawl sign.

   a. Confluent, purple-red macular lesions.

   b. Involves the deltoids and posterior neck and shoulders.

4. V sign (see Figure 3).

   a. Confluent, purple-red macular lesions.

   b. "V" area of anterior neck and upper chest.

5. Mechanics hands (see Figure 4).

   a. Periungal erythema.

   b. Abnormal nail bed capillaries.

   c. Painful roughening and cracking of the skin on the palmar and lateral surfaces of the fingers.

C. Pediatric manifestations of DM.

   1. Resembles adult dermatomyositis with varying degree of proximal weakness.

   2. Symptoms include frequent irritability and discomfort.

   3. Red flush on face.

   4. Child may be fatigued and avoid socialization.

   5. Tiptoe gait due to flexion contracture of the ankles.

IV. Diagnosis.

A. Laboratory analysis.

Figure 2: Gottron's papules

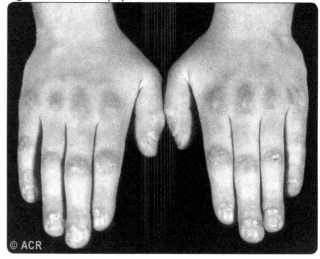

© ACR

» Gottron's papules over the extensor surface of the interphalangeal and metacarpophalangeal joints. Some areas are hypo pigmented with depressions suggestive of atrophic scars. These lesions are typical of dermatomyositis and are distinct from similar lesions found in systemic lupus erythematosus in which the erythema is located between rather than on the joints.

Source: © 2014 American College of Rheumatology. Used with permission.

Figure 1: Heliotrope rash

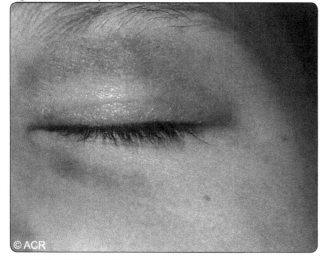

© ACR

» This child with juvenile dermatomyositis demonstrates heliotrope (lilac colored) discoloration and edema of the upper eyelid.

Source: © 2014 American College of Rheumatology. Used with permission.

4
4.1
4.2
4.3
4.4
4.5
4.6
4.7
4.8
4.9
4.10

1. Creatine kinase (CK).

   a. Most reliable muscle enzyme test to use in routine care of adult patients.

   b. Increases of up to 50 times normal are seen in active disease.

   c. CK concentration usually parallels disease activity and can help predict flares.

      (1) Levels rise weeks before overt muscle weakness occurs.

      (2) Levels decrease to normal prior to improvement in muscle strength.

   d. Certain factors can contribute to variation in serum CK reliability:

      (1) Rare occurrences of active biopsy-proven myositis are associated with normal CK levels.

         i) Normal CK levels higher in DM compared to PM.

         ii) Normal CK levels higher in children compared to adults.

      (2) AST and LDH are the best predictors of disease flare in children.

      (3) Persons of Afro-Caribbean descent have an upper limit of normal CK that is higher compared to other ethnicities.

      (4) Factors that can increase the CK level (false positive elevation):

         i) Aerobic and anaerobic exercise.

         ii) Sharp or blunt trauma.

         iii) Medications and drugs (e.g., statins, aspirin, colchicine, alcohol, cocaine).

      (5) Asymptomatic elevations of CK occur in 30% of individuals and have no clinical significance.

2. Aspartate (AST) and alanine aminotransferases (ALT).

3. Lactate dehydrogenase (LDH).

4. Aldolase.

   a. Widely distributed in tissue.

   b. Elevated with liver disease, hematologic disorders, and specimen hemolysis.

   c. Fasting and avoidance of heavy activity recommended for eight hours prior to blood draw.

5. Myoglobin.

B. Needle electromyography (EMG).

1. Non-specific method of evaluating the presence or absence of muscle inflammation.

2. Level of myofibril irritability helps distinguish active myositis from inactive myositis and steroid-induced myopathy.

3. Because of the sensitivity of electromyography, almost all

4
4.1
4.2
4.3
4.4
4.5
4.6
4.7
4.8
4.9
4.10

Figure 3: V-Sign

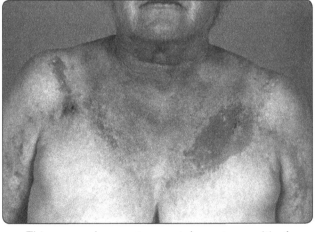

» This woman has acute-onset dermatomyositis. An erythematous eruption is prominent in a mantle distribution over light-exposed areas. Marked inflammatory changes have caused a breakdown in the skin in several areas.

Source: © 2014 American College of Rheumatology. Used with permission.

Figure 4: Mechanic hands

» Cracking (and hyperkeratosis) of the finger pad skin, commonly involving the first, second, and third fingers, is demonstrated in this patient with dermatomyositis.

Source: © 2014 American College of Rheumatology. Used with permission.

patients with active myositis will have an abnormal test result.

4. EMG test site selection:

   a. Unilateral proximal skeletal muscle.

   b. If EMG is abnormal, same muscle on opposite side of body should be used for biopsy.

     (1) Avoid using same muscle for both procedures to rule out inflammation artifact.

C. Muscle biopsy.

1. Gold standard for the diagnosis of myositis.

2. Helps differentiate DM from PM and IBM.

   a. The primary histopathologic features of DM are.

     (1) Microvascular injury mediated by inflammatory immune cell infiltration.

     (2) Perifascicular myofibril atrophy (atrophy of the myofibrils at the edges of muscle fiber bundles).

   b. The primary histopathologic feature of PM (and occasionally IBM) is invasion of healthy (non-necrotic) muscle fibers by cytotoxic T-cells.

D. Skin biopsy.

1. Distinguishes DM from other skin diseases but not from cutaneous lupus.

2. Perivascular inflammation with CD4 positive T-cells in the dermis.

3. Dilatation of superficial capillaries.

E. Radiographic assessment (magnetic resonance imaging [MRI])

1. Allows large masses of muscle to be studied noninvasively.

2. Sensitive detector of anatomical detail and muscle inflammation, increasing the diagnostic yield of muscle biopsy.

3. Indications for MRI include.

   a. Inability to tolerate EMG testing because of pain or fear of needles.

   b. Documentation of disease flare in patients with normal serum enzymes or a normal EMG and muscle biopsy.

   c. Confirmation of DM in a patient where skin lesions are present, but serum enzymes are normal and there is no apparent muscle involvement.

   d. Directing the site of a muscle biopsy.

   e. Distinguishing PM from IBM.

4. Limitations of MRI include.

   a. Expense.

   b. Non-specificity of edema that can be found with other inflammatory processes.

F. Extramuscular organ assessment.

1. Respiratory system.

   a. Pulmonary function testing to determine impact of reduced muscle strength on ventilation.

   b. Radiographic tests to rule out interstitial lung disease.

     (1) High resolution CT scan is much more sensitive than chest x-ray.

2. Cardiac system.

   a. Electrocardiography (EKG) if conduction disturbances are suspected.

   b. Measurement of serum cardiac tropin 1 to rule out myocardial infarct in a patient with myositis.

     (1) The myocardial fraction of CK (CKMB) is elevated in myositis and will produce a false positive for MI.

3. Gastrointestinal system.

   a. Barium swallow in patients with proximal or distal dysphagia.

G. Serum antibodies.

1. Antinuclear or anticytoplasmic antibodies are found in up to 80% of patients with DM and PM (Lundberg & Grundman, 2008).

   a. Anti-Jo-1 is the most common myositis-specific autoantibody (MSA).

     (1) Anti-Jo-1 antibodies are more commonly found in polymyositis, especially in individuals with interstitial lung disease.

   b. Negative antinuclear antibody tests do not exclude the presence of myositis-specific antibodies.

   c. Frequency of antibody positivity is low with IBM.

4
4.1
4.2
4.3
4.4
4.5
4.6
4.7
4.8
4.9
4.10

2. Serum antibody testing helps solidify the diagnosis of myositis in patients with atypical clinical signs and symptoms.

H. Malignancy.

1. Routine cancer screening evaluations of high-risk patients to increase early detection and reduce mortality.

    a. Regular history and physical exams with routine laboratory testing.

    b. Gynecological mammography exams for women.

    c. Age-specific malignancy screening based on risk assessment, including chest, abdominal, and pelvic CT scans.

    d. Colonoscopy.

    e. Serum CA-125 screening for ovarian cancer in women with DM.

V. Treatment.

A. Goals of therapy.

1. Increase muscle strength, thus improving ability to carry out activities of daily living.

2. Prevent muscle atrophy and joint contractures.

3. Improve extramuscular manifestations such as rash, dysphagia, dyspnea, and arthralgia.

B. Pharmacologic therapy.

1. Corticosteroids (Carstens & Schmidt, 2013).

    a. First-line therapy for initial treatment of myositis.

    b. Dose is dependent on disease severity and patient response.

        (1) Methylprednisolone 500 mg to 1 gram IV QD X 3 days followed by oral prednisone taper for severe disease and/or systemic involvement.

        (2) Oral prednisone 1 mg per kg QD for 2 to 4 weeks followed by a steroid taper for mild to moderate weakness.

        (3) Serum CK level is often used as guideline for steroid taper.

        (4) Immunosuppressive agent is added if patient does not improve significantly or fails to maintain a clinical response after 4 to 6 months of prednisone.

2. Immunosuppressive agents (Ernste & Reed, 2013).

    a. Selection of a second line agent depends on assessment of individual patient risk/ benefit and healthcare provider preference.

        (1) Azathioprine - Up to 2.0 to 3.0 mg/kg/day PO.

        (2) Methotrexate (MTX) - Up to 20 mg/ wk PO with folate 1 mg/day PO. (parenteral administration if no response to PO after 1 month).

        (3) Mycophenolate mofetil - Up to 3 g/day PO or IV.

        (4) Cyclosporin – Up to 6 mg/kg/day PO in divided doses to maintain trough serum levels of 50-200 ng/ml.

        (5) Cyclophosphamide - 0.5 to 1.0 g/m2 IV per month or 1.0 to 2.0 mg/kg/day PO.

        (6) Tacrolimus - 2 mg PO twice daily (titrate based on clinical response).

C. Intravenous immune globulin (IVIG).

1. Mechanism of action is unknown, but clinical studies have supported efficacy in DM, PM, and IBM.

2. Often used early in JDM in combination with corticosteroids or another immunosuppressive agent.

3. Administered for two consecutive days per month in conventional doses for a maximum of six months.

4. Useful in infected myositis when immunosuppression is contraindicated.

5. Limitations include availability and expense.

D. Other systemic treatments.

1. Studies support the limited efficacy of plasmapheresis as a treatment option (Aggarwal & Oddis, 2012).

2. Total lymphoid irradiation has proven helpful for some patients but long-term side effects limit its use.

3. Several biologic DMARDs are currently under investigation and target various autoimmune pathways:

    a. Inflammatory cytokine production.

4
4.1
4.2
4.3
4.4
4.5
4.6
4.7
4.8
4.9
4.10

b. T-cell activation.

c. B-cell activation.

E. Rehabilitative therapy.

1. A systematic review of the literature supports the safety and efficacy of exercise in patients with stable IIM (Habers & Takken, 2011).

a. Benefits may be seen in muscle strength, aerobic fitness, and functional measurements.

b. Timing and aggressiveness of physical therapy is controversial because of concern that further muscle damage may result.

c. Monitor patients with concomitant arthritis and osteoporosis for deleterious effects of exercise.

d. Further study is warranted to examine the benefits of exercise training in children.

VI. Co-morbid conditions.

A. Fever and weight loss in severe cases.

B. Contractures.

C. Injuries from falls.

D. Disease state association with occult malignancies.

1. Ten-fold higher increase compared to general population.

2. Highest incidence in dermatomyositis.

3. Most are diagnosed within two years of disease onset.

4. Most common include ovarian, gastrointestinal tract, lung, breast, and non-Hodgkin's lymphoma.

E. Weakened esophageal muscles.

1. Dysphagia.

2. Aspiration.

3. Chronic bacterial pneumonia.

F. Pulmonary abnormalities.

1. Most frequently involved extramuscular organ.

2. Abnormalities include.

a. Respiratory failure due to thoracic muscle weakness.

b. Aspiration pneumonia.

c. Interstitial lung disease.

(1) Significant impact on morbidity and mortality.

(2) Prevalence reported as high as 65% in patients with IIMs (Labirua & Lundberg, 2010).

(3) Often preceded by dyspnea and cough before onset of weakness.

(4) Pulmonary function usually improves with immunosuppressive therapy.

G. Cardiac abnormalities.

1. AV conduction defects.

2. Tachyarrhythmias.

3. Myocarditis.

4. Heart failure due to chronic hypertension from long-term steroid use.

H. Overlap with other connective tissue diseases.

1. Scleroderma.

2. Systemic lupus erythematosus.

3. Rheumatoid arthritis.

4. Sjögren's Syndrome.

VII. Nursing implications.

A. Patient education.

1. Understanding of disease state and prognosis.

2. Diagnostic tests.

3. Prescribed treatment and importance of adherence to treatment regimen.

4. Medication dosing, frequency, and side effects.

5. Infection control.

6. Activity limitations.

7. Use of assistive devices.

8. Energy conservation.

9. Prevention of joint contractures.

10. Prevention of aspiration pneumonia.

11. Fall prevention.

12. Signs and symptoms requiring medical intervention.

B. Psychosocial assessment/intervention.

  1. Assistance with activities of daily living.

    a. Current family support network.

    b. Home healthcare needs.

    c. Handicap parking application.

    d. Assistive device requirements.

  2. Employment status.

    a. Current occupation.

    b. Long-term disability potential.

    c. Financial concerns.

  3. Psychological concerns.

    a. Body image.

    b. Depression.

    c. Access to support groups.

C. Preventive skin care.

  1. Risk of secondary infection if skin barrier is broken (skin rash).

2. Prevention of pressure ulcers due to immobility in severe disease.

D. Additional resources.

  1. American Academy of Dermatology (www.aad.org).

  2. American Academy of Neurology (www.aan.com).

  3. American Autoimmune Related Diseases Association (www.aarda.org).

  4. American College of Rheumatology (www.rheumatology.org).

  5. American Disabilities Act (www.ada.gov)/ Justice Department (www.justice.gov).

  6. Arthritis Foundation (www.arthritis.org).

  7. Assistive Technology Devices (http://mda.org/publications/everyday-life-als/chapter-1).

  8. Clinical Trials (clinicaltrials.gov).

  9. Childhood Arthritis and Rheumatology Research Alliance (www.carragroup.org).

  10. The Myositis Association (www.myositis.org).

4
4.1
4.2
4.3
4.4
4.5
4.6
4.7
4.8
4.9
4.10

Summary

Caring for the patient with myositis presents many challenges for the rheumatology nurse. Knowledge of disease pathophysiology, clinical assessment criteria, and potential impact on quality of life provides a framework for timely patient education and effective intervention. Keeping up to date with the latest evidence, contributing to the body of nursing literature with nursing research, and sharing anecdotal findings is highly needed to fill the gaps in information transfer and education for the rheumatology nurse.

References

Aggarwal, R., & Oddis, C.V. (2011). Therapeutic approaches in myositis. *Current Rheumatology Reports. 13* (3): 182-191.

Astrin, J. (2008). Understanding the idiopathic inflammatory myopathies. *Journal of the American Academy of Physician Assistants, 21*(2), 42-48.

Carstens, P.O. & Schmidt, J. (2014). Diagnosis, pathogenesis and treatment of myositis: Recent advances. *Clinical and Experimental Immunology*, 175 (3). 349-358.

Ernste, F.C. & Reed, A.M. (2013). Idiopathic inflammatory myopathies: Current trends in pathogenesis, clinical features, and up-to-date treatment recommendations. *Mayo Clinic Proceedings. 88* (1), 83-105.

Furst, D.E., Amato, A.A., Iorga, S.R., Gajria, K. & Fernandes, A.W. Epidemiology of idiopathic inflammatory myopathies in a U.S. managed care plan. (2012). *Muscle Nerve. 45* (5). 676-683.

Habers, G.E.A. & Takken, T. (2011). Safety and efficacy of exercise training in patients with an idiopathic inflammatory myopathy – A systematic review. *Rheumatology. (50)* 11. 2113-2124.

Labirua, A., & Lundberg, I.E., (2010). Interstitial lung disease and idiopathic inflammatory myopathies: Progress and pitfalls. *Current Opinions in Rheumatology, 22*(6), 633-638.

Miller, F.W. (2009). Classification of idiopathic inflammatory myopathies. In L. J. Kagan (Ed.), *The Inflammatory Myopathies (pp 15-38)*. New York: Springer Science+Business Media.

References (Continued)

Nagaraju, K., & Lundberg, I.E. (2011). Polymyositis and dermatomyositis: Pathophysiology. *Rheumatic Disease Clinics of North America, 37*(2), 159-171.

Prieto, S., & Grau, JM. (2010).The geoepidemiology of autoimmune muscle disease. *Autoimmunity Reviews. (9). A330-A334.*

Selva-O'Callaghan, A., Trallero-Arguás, E., Grau-Junyent, J.M., & Labrador-Horillo, M. (2010). Malignancy and myositis: Novel autoantibodies and new insights. *Current Opinions in Rheumatology. 22* (6). 627-632

Solorzano, G.E., & Phillips, L.H. (2011). Inclusion body myositis: Diagnosis, pathogenesis, and treatment options. *Rheumatic Disease Clinics of North America, 37*(2), 173-183.

4
4.1
4.2
4.3
4.4
4.5
4.6
4.7
4.8
4.9
4.10

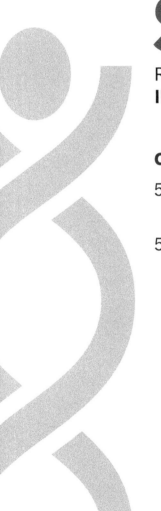

SECTION 5
RHEUMATOLOGY NURSING ACROSS THE LIFESPAN:
INFECTIOUS CONDITIONS

Contents of Section 5

5
5.1
5.2

5
5.1
5.2

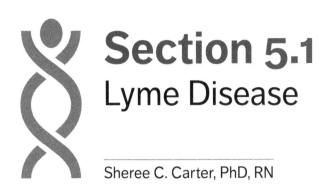

Section 5.1
Lyme Disease

Sheree C. Carter, PhD, RN

Introduction

Lyme disease is a multisystem, multistage inflammatory disease where the diagnosis and treatment continues to remain a challenge. The difficulty to recognize the rash, erythema migrans (aka bulls-eye rash), or the viral-like manifestations of symptoms without a rash can lead to a missed or even a delayed diagnosis, ineffective or no treatment, and the potential for later complications (Lantos, 2011; Meletis, Zabriskie, & Rountree, 2009; Schub & Lawrence, 2012).

The rheumatology office may become involved with the patient who has Lyme disease during these later complications. Differential diagnoses of the patient with Lyme disease in the rheumatology office can range from lupus, fibromyalgia, osteoarthritis, pseudo gout, and even rheumatoid arthritis. This chapter will provide a brief overview of Lyme disease, the incidence and prevalence, stages of the disease, and treatment options.

Learning Objectives

Upon completion of this chapter, the nurse will be able to:

1. Describe the incidence and prevalence of Lyme disease.

2. Identify the stages of Lyme disease.

3. Relate the treatment options for the patient with Lyme disease.

4. Describe the nursing care of patients with Lyme disease.

5. Etiology, Incidence and Prevalence.

I. Lyme disease is:

A. Tickborne infection – Lyme borreliosis – caused by the spirochete bacterium Borrelia burgdorferi sensu lato.

B. The most prevalent tickborne infectious disease in the United States. Prevalent in all 48 contiguous states, the highest concentration is on the coastal northeast, northwest California, and the Great Lakes region. It is the 7th most common reportable disease in the U.S. There are 13 states considered endemic with the highest risk for infection according to the Centers for Disease Control (CDC) as being approximately 35 cases per 100,000 persons (CDC, 2014). The highest ranking state for risk is Connecticut (0.5 cases/1000 persons), followed by and in no particular order; Delaware, Maryland, Maine, Massachusetts, Minnesota, New Jersey, New York, New Hampshire, Pennsylvania, Vermont, Wisconsin, and Virginia. Michigan and Northwest California fell from the previous top 12 states reporting 96% of the reported cases in 2011 (CDC, 2014).

C. Prevalent in some Scandinavian countries, such as Denmark, Austria, and Switzerland and certain parts of Europe such as Germany and the South Downs and New Forest areas of the United Kingdom and Eastern Asia.

II. Pathology.

A. A specific tick, known as a deer tick, is involved in the transmission of Lyme disease. This black-legged tick is known on the East Coast as Ixodes scapularis, and on the West Coast as Ixodes pacificus.

B. There are three life-stage cycles for the Ixodes tick. These are larvae, nymph, and adult. The Ixodes tick takes one blood meal at each stage. They can only become infected by feeding on an infected wild animal carrying the Borrella burgdorferi spirochete during the larval feeding. The infection will remain in the tick for transmission through the nymph and adult phases for transmission to humans. The tick must feed on a human an estimated 24 to 48 hours in order for the transmission of the spirochete bacterium to occur. Because the tick is so small, the likelihood for the tick to remain on the human for transmission is fairly good.

C. Stages of Lyme Disease.

1. Early Localized Infection is the first stage of the disease. This usually begins within 3 to 30 days after the tick bite with the development of a circular rash, erythema migrans. The rash begins in a small area and gradually expands out from the site of the tick bite. This classic-appearing rash does not occur in all patients with Lyme disease. About 75% develop the rash (Meletis, Zabriskie, & Roundtree, 2009). Additionally, the rash is not typically painful nor does it cause puritis. Symptoms seen during this phase are systemic and flulike: Fever, fatigue, arthralgia, and myalgia.

2. The Early Disseminated Disease stage can occur concurrently with the Early Localized Infection stage. Usually within days to weeks after the initial tick bite, the bacteria will spread throughout the body, depositing itself at sites distant from the original lesion. The flulike symptoms of fever, fatigue, chills, headache, swollen lymph nodes, myalgias, and arthralgias will increase. Neurologic, musculoskeletal, and cardiovascular symptoms will begin to appear during this timeframe as well. Additionally, some individuals may develop multiple erythema migrans lesions during this phase. The arthritis symptoms may begin with swelling, stiffness, and pain usually in only one or perhaps a few joints. Interestingly, the most common affected joint in this stage is the knee. The cardiac symptom most commonly seen is heart block; nervous system symptoms include facial nerve palsy or Bell's palsy. The rash from Lyme disease generally will resolve in about one month without treatment.

3. Late Disseminated Infection is the third stage that can occur weeks to years after the initial infection. This stage can occur in patients who did not receive antibiotic treatment for early Lyme disease, or it can be seen in individuals whose antibiotic treatment did not completely eliminate the bacteria causing the infection. According to Meletis, Zabriskie and Roundtree (2009), about 60%

5
5.1
5.2

of the patients with untreated infection will develop monoarticular and oligoarticular arthritis and 10 to 20% of untreated infected patients will develop chronic arthritis. Late disseminated infection also involves the nervous system. Chronic neurologic complaints feature both motor and sensory nerve damage, and in some cases, brain inflammation from months to years after initial infection. The chronic symptoms that may result from late disseminated infection could result in part from an autoimmune response where pro-inflammatory cytokines such as interferon gamma and tumor necrosis factor alpha are affected, although the exact cause of these chronic symptoms is not known.

4. Chronic Lyme disease is a controversial issue. The Infectious Diseases Society of America (IDSA) and the Centers for Disease Control (CDC) do not support the diagnosis of chronic Lyme disease but do refer to Post-treatment Lyme Disease Syndrome. However, many medical experts and scientists disagree with the semantics of the exact definition. Chronic Lyme disease/Post-treatment Lyme Disease Syndrome will not be discussed in this chapter, as more evidence is required for this diagnosis.

III. Prevention.

A. The best prevention for contracting Lyme disease is to avoid the tick bite altogether.

1. Pay particular attention when traveling to the endemic states; be diligent in checking for tick bites, especially during the late spring and early summer.

2. To reduce the chance of tick bites, know that the Ixodes ticks are most commonly found in wooded areas with tall brush or grass, under leaves, and in wood piles.

3. Limiting exposed skin with long pants and long sleeve shirts and tucking pants into the socks can inhibit the tick's ability to find a feeding spot.

4. Insect repellents containing DEET have been shown to reduce tick bites. Clothing commercially impregnated with permethrin can be effective for up to approximately 60 washes. Permethrin can also be sprayed on clothing.

5. Remove ticks as soon as they are found by grasping the tick at the point nearest the attachment with a pair of tweezers and applying gentle, constant pressure for removal. It a minute or two for the tick to fatigue and release its bite from the skin (Quintana, 2012; Schub & Lawrence, 2012).

IV. Treatment.

A. According to Wormser and colleagues (2006), early treatment in the absence of specific neurologic manifestations is recommended as:

1. Doxycycline 100 mg twice a day, amoxicillin 500 mg three times a day, or cefuroxime axetil 500 mg twice a day for 14 days. The range for doxycycline can be 10 to 21 days; the range for amoxicillin or cefuroxime axetil is 14 to 21 days. Refer to product insert for use in children and pregnant women.

2. In the case of Lyme meningitis and other manifestations of neurologic Lyme disease, ceftriaxone 2 g once a day intravenously for 14 days with a range anywhere between 10 to 28 days is recommended for adult patients.

V. Natural supplements.

A. Meletis et al., (2009) reported limited research supporting the use of natural supplements for treating Lyme disease. Suggested supplements include Cats claw, ginger root, stinging nettles, licorice, garlic, Echinacea, probiotics, and Ginkgo biloba.

B. Specific Treatment for Lyme Arthritis.

1. In most cases, Lyme arthritis can be treated successfully with the antimicrobial agents listed above. Doxycycline has been proven to be most successful (Wormser et al., 2006).

2. For patients who have persistent or recurrent joint swelling after a recommended course of oral antibiotic therapy, retreatment with another four-week course of oral antibiotics or the recommended course of ceftriaxone intravenously 2 g once a day between 2 to 4 weeks is recommended (Wormser et al., 2006).

3. Additionally, a second four-week course of oral antibiotic therapy is recommended for patients whose arthritis has substantially improved, but is not yet completely resolved (Wormser et al., 2006).

5
5.1
5.2

4. Symptomatic therapy may include non-steroidal anti-inflammatory drugs (NSAIDs), intra-articular injections of corticosteroids, or disease-modifying antirheumatic drugs such as hydroxychloroquine (Wormser et al., 2006).

5. Expert consultation with the rheumatologist is highly recommended.

6. Persistent synovitis associated with significant pain and limitation of function may require arthroscopic synovectomy to reduce the duration of joint inflammation and discomfort (Wormser et al., 2006).

Summary

Lyme disease is briefly presented because of the related rheumatologic manifestations of diffuse arthralgias, myalgias, or in some cases suspicious fibromyalgias, which are a direct result of a known exposure to a tick bite. The feature of acute or chronic attacks of arthritis in one or more joints is generally not indicative of Lyme disease without the exposure history and signs and symptoms listed within the stages after exposure. Exercising caution and preventive measures when traveling in peak areas of potential exposure and early treatment upon a bite from the Ixodes tick is the best method of avoiding contracting Lyme disease.

References

Centers for Disease Control and Prevention (CDC),National Center for Emerging and Zoonotic Infectious Diseases (NCEZID), Division of Vector-Borne Diseases (DVBD). (2014) Post-treatment Lyme disease syndrome. Retrieved from http://www.cdc.gov/lyme/postLDS/index.html

Centers for Disease Control and Prevention (CDC). (2014). Lyme disease data. Retrieved from http://www.cdc.gov/lyme/stats/

Lantos, P. M. (2011). Chronic Lyme disease: The controversies and the science. *Expert Review of Anti-infective Therapy, 9*(7), 787-797.

Meletis, C. D., Zabriskie, N., & Rountree, R. (2009). Identifying and treating Lyme disease. *Alternative and Complementary Therapies, 15*, 17-23.

Quintana, H. (2012). In the Lyme Light. *Vibrant Life, 28*(4), 28-31.

Schub, T., & Lawrence, P. (2012). Lyme disease. In D. Pravikoff (Ed.), *Quick Lesson About . . .* , (pp. 1-2). Glendale, CA: CINAHL Information Systems.

Wormser, G. P., Dattwyler, R. J., Shapiro, E. D., Halperin, J. J., Steere, A. C., Klempner, M. S., . . . Nadelman, R. B. (2006). The clinical assessment, treatment, and prevention of lyme disease, human granulocytic anaplasmosis, and babesiosis: Clinical practice guidelines by the Infectious Diseases Society of America. *Clinical Infectious Diseases, 43*, 1089-1134. doi: 1058-4838/2006/4309-0001

5
5.1
5.2

Section 5.2
Reactive Arthritis

Deanna L. Owens, MSN, RN

Introduction

Reactive arthritis (ReA) is an unusual disease that often follows a genitourinary or gastrointestinal infection in the body. It is unclear whether these bacterial pathogens infect the synovium in the joint or whether the disease is immune-mediated in response to antigens at the synovial site from infection.

One differentiating factor of ReA in comparison with other rheumatic diseases is the lack of organisms in the synovial fluid of the joint leading to the term sterile arthritis. Treatment options are aimed at treating the underlying infection, decreasing inflammation and managing symptoms of the arthritis.

Learning Objectives

Upon completion of this chapter, the nurse will be able to:

1. Name the most prevalent bacterial pathogens linked to development of reactive arthritis (ReA).

2. List common clinical manifestations of ReA.

3. Define specific symptomatic clinical findings associated with ReA.

4. Name common medications prescribed for the treatment of ReA.

5. Describe patient education opportunities in patients receiving treatment.

6. List necessary laboratory values to be monitored while patients are receiving treatment.

Content Outline

I. Common pathogens leading to development of ReA.

A. Genitourinary.

   1. Chlamydia trachomatis is the most frequently diagnosed sexually transmitted bacterial infection and has been identified in roughly 50% of patients diagnosed with ReA (Owlia & Eley, 2010).

   2. Published data has demonstrated that approximately 4.1% of patients diagnosed with C. trachomatis will develop ReA (Carter & Hudson, 2010).

B. Gastrointestinal.

   1. The frequency of ReA following a gastrointestinal infection is approximately 1-4% (Owlia & Eley, 2010).

   2. The most common enteric related pathogens are Salmonella, Shigella, Yersinia, and Campylobacter (Townes, 2010).

C. Human Immunodeficiency Virus (HIV).

   1. ReA has been reported in approximately 11% of patients infected with HIV (Hamdulay, Glynne, & Keat, 2006).

   2. Healthcare providers should consider HIV screening for patients with ReA whose behaviors put them at risk for HIV infection.

   3. Caucasian patients with HIV related ReA are often Human Leukocyte Antigen B27 (HLA-B27) positive, while non-white patients tend to be negative for the gene (Hamdulay, Glynne, & Keat, 2006).

II. Clinical manifestations.

A. Reactive arthritis (ReA) shares common clinical characteristics with other spondyloarthropathies:

   1. Ankylosing spondylitis.

   2. Psoriatic arthritis.

B. Asymmetric joint involvement predominantly in lower limbs.

   1. Arthritis occurs in approximately 95% of patients (Hamdulay, Glynne, & Keat, 2006).

   2. Presents asymmetrically in the lower limbs specifically affecting the knees, ankles, and metatarsophalangeal joints.

C. Inflammatory back pain (IBP) with symptoms mimicking those seen in ankylosing spondylitis (AS).

   1. No improvement in back pain upon rest.

   2. Pain and stiffness located in one or both buttocks and occasionally in the mid lumbar region (Rudwalet, Metter, A., Listing, Seiper, & Brain, 2006).

   3. Morning stiffness resulting in decreased range of motion (ROM) and immobility.

D. Dactylitis.

   1. Painful inflammation of an entire finger or toe referred to as sausage digits.

E. Conjunctivitis.

   1. Inflammation of membrane lining of eyelids causing pain and discomfort in eye.

   2. Occurs in approximately 30% of patients (Hamdulay, Glynne, & Keat, 2006).

F. Uveitis.

   1. Inflammation of the uvea, the middle layer of the eye containing the iris, choroid, and cilliary body.

G. Urethritis.

   1. Inflammation of the urethra resulting in painful urination.

H. Keratoderma blennorrhagica.

   1. Vesicular pustular skin lesions on hands and soles of feet.

   2. Occurs in approximately 5%-10% of patients (Hamdulay, Glynne, & Keat, 2006).

I. Enthesitis.

   1. Pain, swelling, and tenderness of tendons and ligaments typically in lower extremities.

   2. Most common sites include the achilles and patellar tendons.

5
5.1
5.2

III. Diagnostic criteria.

A. Obtain a thorough medical history.

1. Generally develops 2-6 weeks post genitourinary or gastrointestinal infection.

2. Most cases of ReA last from a few weeks to several months after clinical presentation of symptoms occur with approximately 20% of cases becoming chronic (Schafranski, 2010).

3. Disease state is considered chronic if symptoms persist more than 6 months.

B. Elevated inflammatory markers.

1. Acute-phase reactants, including erythrocyte sedimentation rate (ESR) and C-reactive protein (CRP), are typically elevated but later resolve following adequate treatment, reducing inflammation (Owlia & Eley, 2010).

2. ESR normal range (0-22mm/hr) males, (0-29mm/hr) females.

3. CRP normal range (<0.6 mg/dl).

C. The presence of Human Leukocyte Antigen B27 (HLA-B27) has been linked to the development of ReA and is strongly associated with other spondyloarthropathies.

1. HLA-B27 positive patients typically experience increased severity of symptoms over a longer duration (Owlia & Eley, 2010).

2. The prevalence of HLA-B27 in a healthy general population is around 5-7% (Owlia & Eley, 2010).

3. Although the exact role of HLA-B27 is in need of further research, the following hypothesis gives explanation to the association of the antigen and development of ReA.

   a. HLA-B27 appears to lack the ability to eradicate infected macrophages (white blood cells derived from monocytes) normally, which allows the pathogen to survive (Colmegna, Cuchacovich, & Espinoza, 2004).

4. Patients who are HLA-B27 positive are 50 times more likely to develop ReA, but this disease can also occur in patients who test negative (Owlia & Eley, 2010).

D. X-rays of the affected joints can reveal any damage or abnormalities as a result of inflammation.

IV. Treatment options for ReA (see Table 1).

A. Non-steroidal antinflammatory drugs (NSAIDs).

Table 1: Treatment Options

Medication	Mechanism of Action	Side Effects
Non-steroidal antiflammatory drugs (NSAIDs)	Block prostaglandins in the body that are the cause of fever, pain, and inflammation.	Stomach pain, ulcers, bleeding, reflux, rash, kidney problems, increased blood pressure, and fluid retention.
Corticosteroids	Mimic the hormone cortisol (produced by adrenal glands) to decrease inflammation throughout the body.	Immunosuppression, increased appetite, elevated blood sugar, weight gain, insomnia, poor wound healing, fluid retention, moon face.
Sulfasalazine (SSZ) (DMARD)	Treats pain, swelling, and stiffness associated with arthritis; unclear as to how medication actually works to treat symptoms.	Nausea, abdominal discomfort, immunosuppression, abnormal liver function tests, mouth sores, skin rash, itching.
Methotrexate (MTX) (DMARD)	Blocks enzymes involved in functioning of immune system; unclear as to how medication actually works to treat symptoms.	Nausea, vomiting, immunosuppression, abnormal liver function tests, fatigue, hair loss, mouth sores.
Antibiotic therapy	Used to treat underlying infection, but does not affect the course or duration of the disease.	Side effects vary and are dependent upon type of antibiotic prescribed. Common side effects include gastrointestinal disturbances, rash, headaches.

Source: Author, Deanna L. Owens

5
5.1
5.2

B. Corticosteroids.

   1. Oral prednisone to help treat pain and inflammation.

   2. Steroid injections to affected joints.

C. Disease-modifying antirheumatic drugs (DMARDs).

   1. Sulfasalazine (SSZ) is the only DMARD that has been formally studied in the treatment of ReA (Carter & Hudson, 2010).

   2. Methotrexate (MTX) is a DMARD used to treat pain and inflammation while preventing joint damage from occurring.

D. Antibiotics are prescribed to treat the infection of origin but do not change the progression of the resulting reactive arthritis (Owlia & Eley, 2010).

V. Nursing considerations.

A. Patient education.

   1. Treatment options.

     a. Educate patient regarding medications necessary to treat symptoms of arthritis in addition to antibiotics needed to treat underlying infection.

     b. Instruct patient on importance of adhering to medication regimen and scheduling follow-up appointments.

   2. Drug effectiveness and safety.

     a. Monitor lab values.

     b. Educate about possible side effects.

3. Lifestyle modifications.

     a. Educate about sexual health and preventive measures concerning sexually transmitted diseases.

     b. Elaborate on importance of proper cooking and food storage to avoid getting gastrointestinal infections.

     c. Promote exercise and range of motion (ROM) activities to decrease stiffness and improve flexibility.

B. Monitor lab values based on treatment regimen.

   1. NSAIDs.

     a. Comprehensive metabolic panel (CMP) to monitor kidney function: Serum creatinine, glomerular filtration rate (GFR), and blood urea nitrogen (BUN).

     b. Liver function tests: Alanine aminotransferase (ALT) and aspartate aminotransferase (AST).

     c. Complete blood count (CBC) to monitor blood clotting capabilities: Platelets.

   2. Corticosteroids.

     a. CMP to monitor kidney function and serum glucose levels: Serum creatinine, GFR, BUN, glucose.

     b. Monitor patient's blood pressure because of increased risk of hypertension while being treated with corticosteroids.

   3. DMARDs.

     a. Liver function tests (ALT & AST).

     b. CBC: White blood cells, red blood cells, platelets.

5
5.1
5.2

Summary

Symptoms of reactive arthritis usually present 2-6 weeks following a genitourinary or gastrointestinal infection. Clinical manifestations can often mimic other rheumatologic disorders, so it is imperative to obtain an adequate history from the patient to determine the cause of this particular form of arthritis. The rheumatology nurse plays a critical role in educating the patient on treatment regimens, lifestyle modifications, and prevention methods associated with ReA.

References

Carter, J., & Hudson, A. (2010). The evolving story of chlamydia-induced reactive arthritis. *Current Opinion in Rheumatology, 22*, 424-430.

Colmegna, I., Cuchacovich, R., & Espinoza, L. (2004). HLA-B27-associated reactive arthritis: Pathogenetic and clinical considerations. *Clinical Microbial Reviews, 17*(2), 348-369.

Hamdulay, S., Glynne, S., & Keat, A. (2006) When is arthritis reactive? *Postgraduate Medicine Journal, 82*, 446-453.

Owlia, M., & Eley, A. (2010). Is the role of chlamydia trachomatis underestimated in patients with suspected reactive arthritis? *International Journal of Rheumatic Disease, 13*, 27-38.

Rudwaleit, M., Metter, A., Listing, J., Sieper, J., & Braun, J. (2006). Inflammatory back pain in ankylosing spondylitis: A reassessment of the clinical history for application as classification and diagnostic criteria. *Arthritis and Rheumatism, 54*(2), 569-578.

Schafranski, M., (2010). Infliximab for reactive arthritis secondary to chlamydia trachomatis infection. *Rheumatology International, 30*, 679-680.

Townes J. (2010). Reactive arthritis after enteric infections in the united states: The problem of definition. *Clinical Infectious Diseases, 50*, 247-254.

Suggested Readings

American College of Rheumatology. (2011). Retrieved from http://www.rheumatology.org/

Rohekar, S., & Pope, J. (2009). Epidemiologic approaches to infection and immunity: The case of reactive arthritis. *Current Opinion in Rheumatology, 21*, 386-390.

5
5.1
5.2

5
5.1
5.2

SECTION 6

RHEUMATOLOGY NURSING ACROSS THE LIFESPAN:
PHARMACOLOGIC TREATMENT CONSIDERATIONS

Contents of Section 6

6
6.1
6.2
6.3
6.4
6.5

Section 6.1

Disease-Modifying Antirheumatic Drugs (DMARDs)

Theresa R. Evans, RN

Introduction

Disease-Modifying Antirheumatic Drugs (DMARDs) are a category of drugs that play an essential role in controlling inflammatory diseases by suppressing the autoimmune response, therefore reducing the potential for joint and bone erosions, chronic inflammation, and long-term joint, cartilage, and organ damage. DMARDs have been found to produce symptomatic remission and to delay or halt disease progression and were considered the "gold standard" prior to the introduction of more cell specific biologic response modifiers (BRMs) (Fleischmann, 2011).

Learning Objectives

Upon completion of this chapter, the nurse will be able to:

1. Describe several frequently used DMARDs, including the mechanism of action, dose, side effects, and considerations when prescribing.

2. Identify the nursing considerations for each DMARD.

3. List the Food and Drug Administration (FDA) and non-FDA approved DMARDs for the treatment of rheumatoid arthritis.

Content Outline

I. Commonly used DMARDs in patients with rheumatic conditions.

A. Methotrexate (MTX) – (Trexall™, Rheumatrex®) considered the first-line agent for most patients with rheumatoid arthritis (RA).

1. History (Bahls, 2010; Fleischmann, 2011).

   a. Developed in the late 1940s as a chemotherapeutic agent to treat leukemia.

   b. FDA approved in 1953 as an anti-cancer treatment.

   c. In the 1980s it was shown to improve symptoms in patients with RA.

   d. FDA approved in 1988 as a treatment for RA.

   e. Is now considered a first-line therapy for the treatment of RA and is widely used (off-label) in the treatment of other inflammatory diseases such as psoriatic arthritis, polymyositis, and systemic lupus erythematosus.

   f. Also used in treatment of Juvenile Idiopathic Arthritis (JIA) in children.

2. Mechanism of action (Bahls, 2010; Fleischmann, 2011; and Sadock, 2010).

   a. Methotrexate (MTX) has been shown to have anti-inflammatory effects related to interruption of adenosine and tumor necrosis factor (TNF) pathways and an inhibition of the metabolism of folic acid, resulting in immune system suppression.

3. Dosing (Danesi, Bocci, DiPaolo, Parnham, & Del Tacca, 2011; and Sadock, 2010).

   a. Orally, the standard dosing can range from 7.5 mg to 25 mg taken on the same day, once weekly (Dava, 2010; Duramed, 2005).

   b. Subcutaneous MTX injections such as Otrexup® and Rasuvo® may be given in somewhat higher doses than the oral form; also taken on the same day, once weekly (Antares, 2014; Medac 2014).

   c. Calculated by body weight for children's dose.

4. Side effects:

   a. Most common:

      (1) Gastrointestinal upset including nausea, vomiting, diarrhea, loss of appetite.

      (2) Mouth sores.

      (3) Higher risk of infection.

   b. Less common:

      (1) Headaches, dizziness.

      (2) Fatigue.

      (3) Altered moods.

      (4) Interstitial pneumonitis - lung damage.

      (5) Skin rashes, sun sensitivity.

      (6) Myelosuppression - Blood count abnormalities.

         i) Leukopenia.

         ii) Thrombocytopenia.

         iii) Folate deficiency.

      (7) Lymphomas.

      (8) Hepatotoxicity – Liver damage (Barberio, 2010; and Sadock, 2010).

         i) Increased risk with patients with diabetes.

         ii) Increased risk with hepatitis B or C positive patients.

         iii) Increased risk if on concurrent therapy with certain Nonsteroidal Anti-Inflammatory Drugs (NSAIDs) namely diclofenac sodium/ misoprostol (Arthrotec®) or diclofenac sodium (Voltaren®).

5. Nursing Considerations (Barberio, 2010; Danesi, Bocci, DiPaolo, Parnham, & Del Tacca, 2011; and Sadock, 2010).

   a. Relatively rapid onset of 3-8 weeks.

   b. Ease of administration, oral or subcutaneous injection.

   c. Relatively low cost.

   d. MTX may be taken in combination with other medications.

   e. Requires regular lab monitoring of liver functions and blood counts.

   f. Requires folic acid supplementation while on therapy.

   g. Alcohol avoidance is recommended because of risk of liver toxicity.

h. Pregnancy category X, teratogenic, not for use in pregnancy or while breast feeding.

i. May decrease effects of digoxin. Lab monitoring at regular intervals throughout MTX therapy should be followed.

B. Hydroxychloroquine (HCQ) – (Plaquenil®) - Anti-malarial medication used for its anti-inflammatory properties.

1. History (Alexander, 2011; Moreland, 2012; and Klippel, Stone, Crofford, & White, 2008).

   a. Derived originally from the bark of the Peruvian cinchona tree in the 1820s.

   b. First used during WW II to treat parasitic infections like malaria; it was found also to improve joint pain.

   c. FDA approved in 1955 specifically for the treatment of systemic lupus erythematosus (SLE).

   d. Widely used today for the treatment of SLE, discoid lupus erythematosus (DLE), and (off-label) Sjögren's syndrome.

   e. Long considered one of the safest DMARDs; new dosing guidelines released in 2011 warn of increased risk of developing retinal toxicity with cumulative doses >1000 g.

2. Mechanism of Action (Alexander, 2011; Moreland, 2012; and Klippel, Stone, Crofford, & White, 2008).

   a. Anti-malarial drugs are known to interfere with immune cellular function, altering cell's pH balance. This results in an anti-inflammatory effect. This process also causes blood to thin and platelet aggregation to be altered.

   b. Anti-malarial drugs also affect immune mediator cells called cytokines, causing decreased auto-antibody production, inhibiting lymphocyte activation, which can directly affect deoxyribonucleic acid (DNA). This process is potentially how this class of drug aids in the remission of autoimmune diseases.

3. Dosing (Barberio, 2010; and Sadock, 2010).

   a. In 2011, the American Academy of Ophthalmology updated guidelines for monitoring patients taking antimalarial drugs (Alexander, 2011).

   b. Typical dosing is 200 mg to 400 mg orally per day.

   c. New guidelines recommend that HCQ dosing not exceed > 6.5 mg/kg/day using the patient's ideal weight because of a higher risk of toxicity over time.

4. Side effects (Barberio, 2010; Sadock, 2010; and Shechtman, & Karpecki, 2011).

   a. Most common:

      (1) Gastrointestinal upset (GI) including diarrhea, nausea, vomiting, and loss of appetite.

      (2) Skin rash, hyperpigmentation, and sun sensitivity.

      (3) Changes in hair color, alopecia.

      (4) Tinnitus, loss of hearing.

      (5) Unusual bleeding, bruising.

      (6) Chest pain, palpitations.

      (7) Blurred vision, seeing spots.

   b. Less common:

      (1) Retinal damage due to cumulative medication toxicity.

5. Nursing Considerations (Barberio, 2010; IU School of Optometry Continuing Education, 2011; and Sadock, 2010):

   a. Medication may be taken with food or milk if GI upset occurs.

   b. Patient should have a baseline eye exam by an ophthalmologist prior to starting and every 6-12 months thereafter while on the medication.

   c. Dose may need to be lowered in patients with renal insufficiency.

   d. It may take up to six months for the patient to start to feel a benefit from taking this medication.

   e. HCQ may be taken in combination with other medications.

   f. Pregnancy category C, use with caution if benefits outweigh risks.

   g. Concentrated in breast milk, but compatible with breast feeding.

C. Sulfasalazine (SSZ) - (Azulfidine®).

1. History (Budd, et al., 2004; and Moreland, et al., 2012).

6

6.1

6.2

6.3

6.4

6.5

a. This sulfa-based drug was developed over 70 years ago and FDA approved in 1950 to treat inflammatory diseases such as RA and ulcerative colitis, when it was thought that they were caused by an infectious process.

b. Commonly used in conjunction with MTX and HCQ as triple therapy.

2. Mechanism of action (Bahls, 2010; Fleishmann, 2011; and Sadock, 2010).

a. SSZ has been shown to suppress the immune system by inhibiting various lymphocytic and leukocytic functions which, similarly to MTX, alter cell's adenosine release.

b. SSZ has also been shown to inhibit the body from properly absorbing folic acid.

3. Dosing (Barberio, 2010; and Sadock, 2010).

a. Adult maintenance dose for SSZ is usually 2 grams per day administered orally in divided doses, 2 to 4 times per day, preferably with food.

(1) Azulfidine-EN® tablets are enteric coated to prevent GI upset.

b. Not recommended for patients under the age of two.

4. Side effects (Barberio, 2010; and Sadock, 2010):

a. Most common:

(1) Gastrointestinal upset, nausea, vomiting, diarrhea, and loss of appetite.

(2) Headache.

(3) Skin rash, sun sensitivity.

(4) Decreased sperm count (reversible).

b. Less common:

(1) Fevers.

(2) An orange discoloration of the skin and/or urine.

(3) Myelosuppression – blood count abnormalities:

i) Anemia.

ii) Leukopenia.

(4) Hepatitis.

5. Nursing considerations (Barberio, 2010; and Sadock, 2010).

a. SSZ should not be administered to anyone with a sulfonamide or salicylate allergy.

b. Regular lab monitoring of complete blood count (CBC) is required.

c. Protective clothing should be worn with sun exposure.

d. Proper hydration should be stressed to avoid development of kidney stones.

e. Male patients may need to stop therapy if infertility occurs.

f. Pregnancy category C, use with caution if benefits outweigh risks.

g. Crosses into breast milk, discontinue nursing or the medication.

h. Increases effectiveness of oral anticoagulants and oral hypoglycemic agents.

i. Decreases effectiveness of digoxin, folic acid, and iron.

D. Leflunomide – (Arava®)

1. History.

a. Leflunomide became the first new drug approved for the treatment of active RA in adults in a ten year span when it was FDA approved in 1998 (Bahls, 2010).

2. Mechanism of action.

a. Leflunomide is a pyrimidine synthesis inhibitor with anti-proliferative properties that allow it to reduce joint pain, edema, and structural joint damage (Bahls, 2010).

3. Dosing.

a. Available in 10 mg and 20 mg tablets, either dose taken orally once daily (Barberio, 2010; and Sadock, 2010).

4. Side effects - (Barberio, 2010; and Sadock, 2010).

a. Most common:

(1) Gastrointestinal symptoms including abdominal pain, nausea, and diarrhea.

(2) Higher risk of infections.

(3) Reversible alopecia.

(4) Elevation in liver function tests (LFTs).

b. Less common:

(1) Hepatotoxicity.

5. Nursing considerations (Barberio, 2010; and Sadock, 2010).

a. Regular lab monitoring of liver function is required.

6
6.1
6.2
6.3
6.4
6.5

b. Should not be administered to women of childbearing potential.

c. Women who wish to "wash out" from the drug for pregnancy consideration will need to take an 11 day course of the drug, cholestyramine (Questran®), to remove leflunomide from the system. Blood testing will be required to be certain that the drug has been eliminated from their bodies.

d. Men taking leflunomide who wish to father a child should consider discontinuing the drug and taking an 11 day course of cholestyramine (Questran®) as well to eliminate it from their bodies.

e. Pregnancy category X, teratogenic – not for use during pregnancy.

f. Increases the effectiveness of NSAIDs.

E. Azathioprine (AZA) – (Imuran®)

1. History (Danesi, et al., 2011; and Fleischmann, 2011).

a. Originally FDA approved in 1968 as an immunosuppressant for use in patients who have had a renal transplant.

b. Considered a cytotoxic drug, it has been used for more refractory disease processes such as extra-articular manifestations of RA and off-label for systemic vasculitis diseases such as Behçet's disease.

2. Mechanism of action (Danesi, et al., 2011; Fleischmann, 2011).

a. As indicated on the package insert, the mechanisms of action and properties of immunosuppression on autoimmune diseases are not known.

b. AZA is considered a slow acting drug and effects from it may continue long after the drug itself has been discontinued.

3. Dosing (Barberio, 2010; Sadock, 2010).

a. AZA is available in a 50 mg tablet and recommended initial oral dosing is 3 - 5 mg/kg/day. Once the disease state is relatively controlled, it is recommended that dosing be reduced to a maintenance oral dose of 1 – 2 mg/kg/day.

b. Also available for intravenous (IV) administration in 100 mg/20 ml vials.

4. Side effects (Barberio, 2010; Sadock, 2010):

a. Most common:
   (1) Gastrointestinal upset including nausea, vomiting, and diarrhea.
   (2) Myelosuppression – blood count abnormalities:
   (3) Leukopenia.
   (4) Thrombocytopenia.
   (5) Pancytopenia.
   (6) Macrocytic anemia.
   (7) Unusual bleeding or bruising.
   (8) Higher risk of infection.

b. Less common:
   (1) Hepatotoxicity.
   (2) Rash.
   (3) Fevers.
   (4) Serum sickness.
   (5) Retinopathy.
   (6) Interstitial nephritis.
   (7) Alopecia.
   (8) Rare - hypersensitivity reaction characterized by Raynaud's disease and pulmonary edema.

5. Nursing considerations (Barberio, 2010; and Sadock, 2010):

a. Regular lab monitoring of LFT and CBC required.

b. Numerous drug interactions possible, including with angiotensin-converting-enzyme (ACE) inhibitors, anticonvulsants, and allopurinol (Zyloprim®).

c. If concurrent treatment with allopurinol is necessary, AZA dose should be reduced 50-75%.

d. Pregnancy category D, use in life-threatening emergencies when no safe drug is available.

e. Excreted at low levels in breast milk; therefore, breast feeding is not recommended.

F. Cyclosporine (CsA) (Neoral®, Sandimmune®)

1. History (Heulser, & Pletscher, 2001).

a. The immunosuppressive effects of CsA were discovered in 1972, and it was approved for use in patients who have had an organ transplant in 1983.

b. Since then, it has been approved for use in adult patients with psoriasis and refractory RA; is is also used (off-label) for severe atopic dermatitis, pyoderma gangrenosum, and chronic autoimmune urticaria, among other conditions.

2. Mechanism of action.

a. CsA lowers the activity of T-cells, suppressing their immune response by inhibiting the response of interleukin-2 (Heulser, & Pletscher, 2001).

3. Dosing (Barberio, 2010; and Sadock, 2010).

a. Available in 25 mg, 50 mg, and 100 mg USP modified oral capsules.

b. Neoral® dosing for RA average 2.5 mg / kg / day orally in divided doses twice daily.

c. Maximum dose on all preparations should not exceed 4 mg / kg / day.

d. Neoral® and Sandimmune® are not bioequivalent, and caution should be taken if switching between brands and generics.

e. CsA capsule USP modified should be dosed initially at 1.25 mg / kg divided into 2 doses per day and titrated up if required to a dose not to exceed 4 mg / kg / day.

4. Side effects (Barberio, 2010; and Sadock, 2010):

a. Most common:

(1) Myelosuppression –CBC abnormalities:

   i) Leukopenia.

   ii) Thrombocytopenia.

(2) Hypertension, which may require treatment during CsA therapy.

(3) Tremors.

(4) Renal insufficiency.

(5) Higher risk of infection.

(6) Headache.

(7) Gastrointestinal upset including nausea, abdominal pain, diarrhea, and dyspepsia.

(8) Increased triglycerides.

(9) Photosensitivity.

b. Less common:

(1) Acneiform eruptions.

(2) Convulsions.

(3) Pruritis.

(4) Hyperkalemia and hypomagnesemia.

(5) Pancreatitis.

(6) Hepatotoxicity.

(7) Increased risk of developing lymphomas.

5. Nursing considerations (Barberio, 2010; and Sadock, 2010):

a. Onset of action and therapeutic response may take 4 – 8 weeks in patients with RA.

b. Requires regular lab monitoring of liver functions, blood counts, and chemistries.

c. Can be taken in conjunction with salicylates, NSAIDs, oral corticosteroids, and MTX.

d. Pregnancy category C, use with caution if benefits outweigh risks.

e. Excreted in breast milk. Do not take while breast feeding.

G. Cyclophosphamide (CTX) – (Cytoxan®)

1. History (Appel, et al., 2009; Danesi, et al., 2011; and Meng-Yu & Ming-Fei, 2009).

a. FDAapproved in 1959, cyclophosphamide is a nitrogen mustard alkylating agent used to treat various types of cancers.

b. Although not FDA approved for these indications, it has been shown to decrease the immune system's response, when other DMARDs have been ineffective, in refractory cases of lupus nephritis, severe RA and JIA, as well as vasculopathies, such as granulomatosis with polyangiitis and Behçet's disease.

2. Mechanism of action (Appel, et al., 2009; Danesi, et al., 2011; and Meng-Yu & Ming-Fei, 2009).

a. Forms deoxyribonucleic acid (DNA) cross links between and within DNA strands at certain positions, irreversibly leading to cell death.

b. Through this cell death process, it also induces immunomodulary effects that are not yet fully understood.

3. Dosing (Appel, et al., 2009; Barberio, 2010; Danesi, et al., 2011; and Sadock, 2010).

a. Available for oral administration in 25 mg or 50 mg tablets.

b. Available in powder form for reconstitution at doses of 100 mg, 200 mg, 500 mg, 1 Gram, and 2 Gram.

c. Recommended dose for lupus nephritis is 2 – 3 mg/kg/day daily for up to 12 weeks when corticosteroids have been an ineffective treatment.

d. Recommended dose for RA, JIA, and vasculitis is 10 mg /kg IV every 2 weeks.

4. Side effects (Appel, et al., 2009; Barberio, 2010; Danesi, et al., 2011; and Sadock, 2010):

a. Most common:

(1) Myelosuppression –CBC abnormalities:

(2) Leukopenia.

(3) Thrombocytopenia.

(4) Gastrointestinal upset including nausea, vomiting, diarrhea, abdominal pain.

(5) Lethargy and joint pain.

(6) Alopecia, hair texture and color change.

(7) Hemorrhagic cystitis.

(8) Increased risk of infection and slow wound healing.

(9) Mouth sores.

(10) Hematuria.

(11) Unusual bleeding and / or bruising.

b. Less common:

(1) Sterility.

(2) Acute myeloid leukemia (AML).

(3) Transitional cell carcinoma of the bladder.

5. Nursing Considerations (Appel, et al., 2009; Barberio, 2010; Danesi, et al., 2011; and Sadock, 2010).

a. Requires regular lab monitoring of CBCs and urinalysis.

b. To reduce risk of hemorrhagic cystitis, stress the importance of adequate fluid intake and hydration. An IV detoxifying agent such as Mesna® may be administered to detoxify the bladder in some cases.

c. Pregnancy category D, use in life-threatening emergencies when no safer drug is available.

d. Excreted in breast milk. Do not take while breast feeding.

H. Mycophenolate mofetil – (CellCept®) (Appel, et al., 2009; and Meng-Yu, & Ming-Fei, 2009).

1. History.

a. FDA approved in 1994 as an immunosuppressant to prevent organ transplant rejection.

b. Although not FDA approved for rheumatologic indications, it has been increasingly used to treat lupus nephritis and has been known to be better tolerated than some other DMARDs such as cyclophosphamide, as it has a less severe side effect profile.

2. Mechanism of action.

a. Inhibits the enzyme inosine monophosphate dehydrogenase, which impairs T cell and B cell proliferation, sparing other rapidly dividing cells (Appel, et al., 2009; and Meng-Yu, & Ming-Fei, 2009).

3. Dosing (Barberio, 2010; and Sadock, 2010).

a. Available for oral administration in 250 mg or 500 mg capsules or tablets and 200 mg/ml suspension.

b. Available in 180 mg and 360 mg extended release tablets and 500 mg/vial powder for injection.

c. Used as induction therapy in doses up to 3 g/day and as maintenance therapy of 500 mg to 3 g/day.

4. Side effects (Barberio, 2010; and Sadock, 2010):

a. Most common:

(1) Hyperglycemia.

(2) Hypercholesterolemia.

(3) Hypomagnesemia.

(4) Myelosuppression –CBC abnormalities:

i) Leukopenia.

ii) Anemia.

iii) Dyspnea.

iv) Urinary tract infection (UTI).

v) Pleural effusion.

vi) Gastrointestinal upset including abdominal pain, nausea, and diarrhea.

vii) Higher risk of opportunistic infections such as:

    1) Shingles.

    2) Other herpes infections.

    3) Cytomegalovirus.

    4) BK virus associated neuropathy (Polyomavirus).

viii) Headache.

b. Less common:

    (1) Melanoma and other malignancies.

    (2) GI bleeding.

    (3) Neutropenia.

    (4) Pulmonary fibrosis.

    (5) Progressive multifocal leukoencephalopathy (PML).

5. Nursing Considerations (Barberio, 2010; and Sadock, 2010).

a. Mycophenolate is often more expensive than many other DMARDs.

b. Should not be administered in conjunction with azathioprine as it can cause hematologic toxicity.

c. Requires regular lab monitoring of CBC and blood chemistries.

d. Pregnancy category D, use in life-threatening emergencies when no safer drug is available.

e. Not known if it is excreted in breast milk; therefore, avoid the drug or do not nurse.

I. Tetracycline Derivatives: Minocycline hydrochloride – (Minocin® and Solodyn®) and Doxycycline hyclate – (various brand names).

1. History (Budd, et al., 2004; and Smith, Sayles, Mikuls, & Michaud, 2011).

a. Minocycline was FDA approved in 1972 for the treatment of acne and other skin infections.

b. Doxycycline was clinically developed in the early 1960s and FDA approved in 1967 for the treatment of acne and other inflammatory diseases.

c. Both decrease signs and symptoms of early rheumatoid arthritis but have yet to show prevention of radiographic progression of the disease.

d. Neither minocycline nor doxycycline are FDA approved for treatment of RA.

2. Mechanism of action (Budd, et al., 2004; and Smith, Sayles, Mikuls, & Michaud, 2011).

a. Inhibition of collagenase activity in articular cartilage.

b. Minocycline has been shown to alter the synthesis of the inflammatory cytokine, IL-10 and T-cell proliferation in early RA.

3. Dosing (Barberio, 2010; and Sadock, 2010).

a. Minocycline is available in 50 mg, 75 mg, and 100 mg tablets or capsule. The most common dose for treatment of RA is 100 mg BID or 200 mg QD.

b. Doxycycline is available in 40 mg, 50 mg, 75 mg, 100 mg, and 150 mg capsules. The most common dose for treatment of RA is 100 mg BID or 200 mg QD.

4. Side effects (Barberio, 2010; and Sadock, 2010).

a. Most common:

    (1) Minocycline.

      i) Lightheadedness and dizziness.

      ii) Vertigo.

      iii) Photosensitivity.

      iv) Gastrointestinal symptoms including nausea and diarrhea.

    (2) Doxycycline.

      i) Gastrointestinal symptoms including anorexia, diarrhea.

      ii) Photosensitivity.

b. Less common:

    (1) Minocycline.

      i) Abdominal cramping.

      ii) Myelosuppression –CBC abnormalities:

        1) Eosinophilia.

        2) Hemolytic anemia.

        3) Neutropenia.

        4) Diabetes insipidus.

        5) Skin hyperpigmentation.

        6) Drug rash with eosinophilia and systemic symptoms (DRESS).

        7) Drug induced lupus or hepatitis, usually reversible.

        8) Renal tubular acidosis (Fanconi-like syndrome) in prolonged use.

(2) Doxycycline.

   i) Myelosuppression –CBC abnormalities:

      1) Hemolytic anemia.

      2) Eosinophilia.

      3) Neutropenia.

      4) Thrombocytopenia.

   ii) Exfoliative dermatitis.

   iii) Candidiasis infections.

   iv) Drug induced lupus or hepatitis, usually reversible.

   v) Renal tubular acidosis (Fanconi-like syndrome) in prolonged use.

5. Nursing Considerations (Barberio, 2010; and Sadock, 2010).

  a. Minocycline.

    (1) Avoid with significant renal and/or hepatic impairment.

    (2) Avoid prolonged sun exposure or artificial tanning.

    (3) Not recommended for children 8 and under because of potential to cause permanent tooth discoloration.

    (4) Regular lab and urinalysis monitoring in prolonged use.

    (5) May increase effects of digoxin and oral anticoagulants. Lab monitoring at regular intervals throughout therapy should be followed.

    (6) May decrease effects of antacids, hormones, and contraceptives. Should be taken 1 hour before or 2 hours after antacids and female patients should be advised to use an extra method of contraception while taking it.

    (7) May take with food.

    (8) Pregnancy category D, use in life-threatening emergencies when no safer drug is available.

    (9) Enters breast milk, but in some situations is considered nursing compatible because of calcium chelation of the drug and prevention of its absorption. (Long-term safety of long-term exposure to breastfed children unknown.)

  b. Doxycycline.

    (1) Avoid with significant hepatic impairment.

    (2) Not recommended for children 8 and under because of potential to cause permanent tooth discoloration.

    (3) Avoid prolonged sun exposure or artificial tanning.

    (4) Regular lab and urinalysis monitoring in prolonged use.

    (5) May increase the effects of digoxin and warfarin. Lab monitoring at regular intervals throughout therapy should be followed.

    (6) Decreases the effect of iron, antacids, and barbiturates.

    (7) Pregnancy category D, use in life-threatening emergencies when no safer drug is available.

    (8) Excreted in breast milk. Do not take while breast feeding.

Summary

The use of DMARDS is generally first line for rheumatic diseases. DMARDS are often used in combination. Nurses must be familiar with usual dosages, side effects, and onset of action to effectively counsel patients. Additionally, nurses should be prepared to address adherence with any necessary monitoring (labs, eye exams, etc.).

6
6.1
6.2
6.3
6.4
6.5

References

Alexander, L. (2011). Hydroxychloroquine and chloroquine toxicity: A look at revised guidelines. *An Optometric Retina Society white paper*. Retrieved from http://www.optometricretinasociety.org

Antares Pharma, Inc., (2014) Otrexup®: Prescribing information. Ewing, NJ: Author.

Appel, G.B., Contreras, G., Dooley, M.A., Ginzler, E.M., Isenberg, D., Jayne, D...Aspreva Lupus Management Study Group. (2009). Mycophenolate mofetil versus cyclophosphamide for induction treatment of lupus nephritis. *Journal of the American Society of Nephrology, 20*(5), 1103-1112. doi: 10.1681/ASN.2008101028.

Bahls, C. (2010). The history of DMARDs for RA. *Everyday Health.* Retrieved from http://www.everydayhealth.com/rheumatoid-arthritis/history-of-dmards.aspx.

Barberio, J. (2010). *Nurses pocket drug guide 2010.* Newark, NJ: McGraw-Hill Companies.

Bristol-Myers Squibb Company (2005). Cytoxan®: Prescribing information. Deerfield, IL: Author.

Budd, R., Firestein, G., Genovese, M., Harris, E., Sargent, J., & Sledge, C. (2004). *Kelley's textbook of rheumatology* (7th ed.). Philadelphia: Elsevier Saunders.

Danesi, R., Bocci, G., DiPaolo, A., Parnham, M., & Del Tacca, M. (2011). Cytotoxic drugs. *Principles of immunopharmacology* . F. P. Nijkamp & M. Parnham (Eds.) (3rd ed., pp. 507-524). doi: 10.1007/978-3-0346-0136-8-26.

Dava Pharmaceuticals, Inc., (2010) Rheumatrex®: Prescribing information. Fort Lee, NJ: Author.

Duramed Pharmaceuticals, Inc., (2005) TrexallTM: Prescribing information. Pomona, NY: Author.

Fleischmann, R. (2011). Don't forget traditional DMARDS: Old friends are still useful. *Rheumatology, 50.* doi:10.1093/rheumatology/keq382.

Genentech USA, Inc. (2013). CellCept®: Prescribing Information. South San Francisco, CA: Author.

Heulser, K., & Pletscher, A. (2001). The controversial early history of cyclosporin. *Swiss Medicine Weekly, 131,* 299-302.

IU School of Optometry Continuing Education. (2011). Caring for the plaquenil patient. Retrieved from http://www.opt.indiana.edu/ce/plaq/risks.htm.

Klippel, J.H., Stone, J.H., Crofford, L.J., & White, P.H. (Eds.). (2008). *Primer of the rheumatic diseases* (13th ed.). New York, NY: Springer Science & Business Media, LLC.

Medac Pharma Inc., (2014). Rasuvo®: Prescribing information. Chicago, IL: Author.

Medicis, The Dermatology Company, (2013). Solodyn®: Prescribing information, Scottsdale, AZ.: Author.

Meng-Yu, W., & Ming-Fei, L. (2009). Mycophenolate for treatment of lupus nephritis refractory to cyclophosphamide. *Formosan Journal of Rheumatology, 23,* 8-13.

Moreland, L., et al., (2012). A randomized comparative effectiveness study of oral triple therapy versus etanercept plus methotrexate in early aggressive rheumatoid arthritis: The treatment of early aggressive rheumatoid arthritis trial. *Arthritis & Rheumatism, 64,* pp.2824-2835. doi: 10.1002/art.34498.

Novartis (2013). Neoral®: Prescribing information. East Hanover, NJ: Author.

Novartis (2013). Sandimmune®: Prescribing information. East Hanover, NJ: Author.

Novartis (2014). Votaren®: Prescribing information. North Ryde, NSW: Author.

Onset Dermatologics, LLC, (2014). Minocin®:Prescribing information. Cumberland, RI: Author.

Par Pharmaceutical, Inc., (2012). Questran®: Prescribing information. Spring Valley, NY: Author.

Pfizer, Inc., (2014). Arthrotec®: Prescribing information. New York, NY: Author.

Pfizer, Inc., (2014). Azulfidine®: Prescribing information. New York, NY: Author.

Prometheus Laboratories, Inc. (2011). Imuran®: Prescribing information. San Diego, CA: Author.

Prometheus Laboratories, Inc. (2003). Zyloprim®: Prescribing information. San Diego, CA: Author.

Sadock, B. (2010). Nursing 2011 drug handbook (31st ed.). Philadelphia, PA: Lippincott Williams & Wilkins.

Sagent Pharmaceuticals (2010). Mesna®: Prescribing information. Schaumburg, IL: Author.

Shechtman, D., & Karpecki, P. (2011, April 15). New guidelines. *Review of Optometry,* 105-106.

Sanofi-Aventis (2014) Arava®: Prescribing information. Macquarie Park, NSW: Author.

Sanofi-Aventis Canada Inc. (2014). Plaquenil®: Prescribing information. Laval, Quebec: Author.

Smith, C.J., Sayles, H., & Mikuls, T.R., & Michaud, K. (2011). *Minocycline and doxycycline therapy in community patients with rheumatoid arthritis: Prescribing patterns, patient-level determinants of use, and patient-reported side effects.* Retrieved from http://www.arthritis-research.com/content/13/5/R168.

Warner Chilcott, Inc., (2005). Doxyclcline: Prescribing information. Rockaway, NJ: Author.

6
6.1
6.2
6.3
6.4
6.5

Section 6.2
Glucocorticoids and Potent Immunosuppressant DMARDs

Deborah Hicks, RN

Introduction

Many of the drugs used to treat rheumatic diseases are immunosuppressant by mechanism of action. Conventional immunosuppressive drugs disrupt pathways of the inflammatory cascade, while the newer biologic response modifiers (BRMs) selectively inhibit a pro-inflammatory cytokine and/or block its receptor. The BRMs have become the "go-to" drugs for many of the more well-known rheumatic diseases, such as rheumatoid arthritis, when treatment targets have not been met. At this time BRMs have not been studied extensively in less common conditions that are treated by rheumatologists and therefore are not within the standard of care.

The drugs included in this chapter may be used for conditions that are not generally treated by rheumatologists, and those diseases are not included in this chapter. Only diseases that are generally within the field of rheumatology have been included.

Learning Objectives

Upon completion of this chapter, the nurse will be able to:

1. Identify the mechanisms of action for each medication.
2. Describe the nursing implications for each medication.
3. Relate the indications for each medication.
4. Identify the risks and contraindications of each medication.

Content Outline

I. Glucocorticoids:

A. Short acting:

1. Hydrocortisone (Cortef®)

2. Cortisone (Cortone®).

B. Intermediate acting:

1. Prednisone (Deltasone®)

2. Prednisolone (Delta-Cortef®)

3. Methylprednisolone (Medrol®)

4. Triamcinolone (Kenacort®).

C. Long acting:

1. Dexamethasone (Decadron®)

2. Betamethasone (Celestone®).

D. Mechanism of action.

1. Inhibitory effect on a broad range of specific immune responses mediated by T cells and B cells.

2. Inhibitory effects on both acquired and innate immunologic function.

3. Inhibition of the synthesis of most of the proinflammatory cytokines (Fisher-Betz, Schneider, & Bonbardieri, 2012).

4. Pregnancy risk Category C.

E. Goal of therapy.

1. Induce or maintain remission.

2. Reduce the frequency of flare or relapse.

3. Allow tapering of glucocorticoids while maintaining disease control.

F. Indications/Doses.

1. Conventional terms for glucocorticoid use (See Table 1).

2. Glucocorticoid application.

   a. Infrequent use, for therapy resistant disease, complications, severe flare, major exacerbation, and for bridging the lag-time of recently started therapy (application = 1).

   b. Frequently added to/used as the basic therapeutic strategy (application = 2).

   c. Basic part of the therapeutic strategy. (Fisher-Betz, Schneider, & Bonbardieri) (application = 3).

3. General use of glucocorticoids (reference Table 1 for dose term and *F.2 Glucocorticoid application* for application, i.e., "M2" would be interpreted as "Medium dose + Frequently added to...") (Fisher-Betz, Schneider, & Bonbardieri, 2012).

   a. Arthritides.

      (1) Gouty arthritis, acute (oral M2, H2; intra-articular 2).

      (2) Juvenile idiopathic arthritis (oral M1, H1; intra-articular 2).

      (3) Osteoarthritis (intra-articular 1).

      (4) Pseudogout (intra-articular 2).

      (5) Psoriatic arthritis (oral M1, intra-articular 2).

Table 1: Conventional Terms for Glucocorticoid Use

Term	Glucocorticoid Dose
Low dose (L)	≤7.5 mg prednisone equivalent per day
Medium dose (M)	> 7.5 mg but ≤30 mg prednisone equivalent per day
High dose (H)	>30 mg but ≤100 mg prednisone equivalent per day
Very high dose/or pulse (VH)	>100 mg prednisone equivalent per day
Pulse therapy (P)	≥250 mg prednisone equivalent per day for 1 day or a few days

Source: Adapted from (Fisher-Betz, Schneider, & Bonbardieri; Klippel, Stone, Crofford, & White, 2008).

6
6.1
6.2
6.3
6.4
6.5

(6) Reactive arthritis (intra-articular 1).

(7) Rheumatic fever (oral M1, H1).

(8) Rheumatoid arthritis
(oral L2, M2, H1; IV 1; intra-articular 2).

b. Collagen Disorders.

(1) Dermatomyositis, polymyositis
(oral H3; IV 1).

(2) Mixed connective tissue disease
(oral M1; IV 1; intra-articular 1).

(3) Polymyalgia rheumatica
(PMR) (oral M3; IV 1).

(4) Sjögren's syndrome (oral H3).

(5) Systemic lupus erythematosus
(oral M2, H1; IV 1).

(6) Systemic sclerosis (oral M1).

(7) Systemic vasculitides in
general (oral M3; IV 1).

(8) Intra-articular injections are not
repeated more than 3-4 times per
year because of potential adverse
effects on joint structure such as
tendon weakening (Bartlett, 2006).

G. Adverse events (AEs).

1. Glucocorticoid toxicity is generally
dose and duration dependent. Doses
greater than low-dose (≤7.5 mg/ day)
have an increased number of AEs.

a. Weight gain.

(1) Most common self-reported AE.

b. Hypertension.

c. Hyperglycemia.

(1) Increased difficulty in glycemic
control in patients with diabetes.

d. Hyperlipidemia (unclear if disease or
drug related) (Saag & Furst, 2013).

e. Osteoporosis, vertebral fractures (in
patients with normal bone mineral density).

f. Avascular or ischemic necrosis of bone.

g. Growth impairment in children
on daily therapy.

(1) May be permanent in boys
(Saag & Furst, 2013).

h. Cataracts, glaucoma.

i. Increased incidence of infection.

(1) Dose dependent increase in common
bacterial, viral, and fungal infections.

(2) Early recognition can be impaired
because of reduced inflammatory
and febrile responses.

j. Cushingoid features (dose and
duration dependent).

k. Skin thinning and purpura.

(1) Increased risk of basal cell and
squamous cell skin cancer.

l. Steroid acne.

m. Alopecia.

n. Cardiovascular disease.

(1) Ischemic heart disease.

(2) Heart failure.

(3) Dose dependent and not associated
with low dose glucocorticoid therapy.

(4) These AEs were not seen
in patients with PMR.

(5) Risk of atrial fibrillation and atrial flutter
in new and long-term users but not in
former users (Saag & Furst, 2013).

o. Gastritis, ulcer formation, GI bleeding.

(1) Incidence significantly increased
when used in combination with aspirin
and non-steroidal anti-inflammatory
drugs (NSAIDs) (Saag & Furst, 2013).

p. Fluid retention, particularly in patients with
underlying renal and cardiac disease.

q. Menstrual irregularities, lower
fertility in men and women.

r. Use in pregnancy has an absolute
low risk of cleft palate in offspring.

s. Psychiatric and cognitive symptoms
including mood disturbances,
depression, psychosis, confusion/
disorientation (particularly in the
elderly) (Saag & Furst, 2013).

t. Compromised immune
response to vaccines.

(1) Live virus vaccines should not be
given to patients taking high-dose
glucocorticoids (MMR, Zoster, Varicella).

u. High dose corticosteroids can suppress the
hypothalamic-pituitary-adrenal axis (HPA)
causing adrenal insufficiency/adrenal crisis
upon tapering doses or discontinuation.

H. Limiting adverse events (AEs).

1. Use the lowest dose and shortest
duration possible.

2. Treat pre-existing co-morbid conditions when the use of glucocorticoids is needed.

3. Monitor patients for adverse effects.

I. Nursing implications.

1. Assess for pre-existing co-morbid conditions and educate the patient to observe for AE.

2. Assist the patient in understanding the risks/benefits and how to determine when to taper dose.

3. Encourage exams for ophthalmologic care, skin exam, bone mineral density (DXA), primary care for appropriate adjustments of hyperglycemia, hypertension, cardiac care.

4. Teach patient to observe for infection, seek prompt treatment, avoid infectious exposure.

5. Teach patient signs of GI side effects ; educate on prophylaxis.

6. Draw labs before giving glucocorticoid IV pre-med for infusions (CBC in particular since WBC may be falsely elevated by glucocorticoids).

7. Cardiac monitor for arrhythmias for patients receiving IV pulse therapy.

8. Alert pre-op patients to increased risk of infection with the use of glucocorticoids, especially in moderate to high doses; share that information with surgical staff.

9. Teach patient the signs of adrenal insufficiency when tapering glucocorticoids that have been used for long periods; do not stop glucocorticoids abruptly.

10. Be aware of drugs that look or sound alike.

11. For IV use: Solu-cortef (hydrocortisone sodium succinate), inject directly over 30 seconds to 10 minutes; Solu-Medrol (methylprednisolone sodium succinate), inject directly over at least 1 minute. These drugs are used for premedication when infusing BRMs and other drugs with high risks of infusion reactions.

12. Triamcinolone acetinide/or hexacetonide are for intra-articular injection.

13. Be aware that glucocorticoids are not interchangeable; dosing will vary according to drug.

II. Cyclophosphamide (CTX)(Cytoxan®).

A. Mechanism of action.

1. An alkylating agent that prevents cell division by cross-linking DNA strands and decreasing DNA synthesis.

2. Depletes both B and T cells, affecting both humoral and cellular immunity.

3. Metabolized in the liver.

4. Half-life of 2-10 hours; 95% excreted by the kidney, complete elimination by 48 hours.

5. Pregnancy Category D.

B. Indications.

1. Cyclophosphamide (CTX) (Cytoxan® is one option for some patients with organ- or life-threatening rheumatic disease, unresponsive to standard therapeutic interventions.

2. Newer agents have made the choice of cyclophosphamide less frequent because of this agent's severe side effect profile.

   a. Systemic vasculitis.

      (1) Granulomatosis with polyangiitis (GPA) (Wegener's).

      (2) Microscopic polyangiitis.

      (3) Eosinophilic granulomatosis with polyangiitis.

      (4) Idiopathic Polyarteritis Nodosa.

      (5) Behçet's disease.

      (6) Rheumatoid vasculitis.

      (7) Systemic lupus erythematosus; diffuse proliferative glomerulonephritis (DPGN); Neuropsychiatric systemic lupus erythematosus (NPSLE).

      (8) Inflammatory myopathy (dermatomyositis/polymyositis).

      (9) Scleroderma.

C. Dosing.

1. National Institutes of Health (NIH) protocol for DPGN.

   a. Monthly pulse doses of cyclophosphamide for 6 months with oral prednisone for 4 weeks, with tapering to achieve the lowest dose possible to control disease activity (Fisher-Betz, Schneider, & Bonbardieri, 2012).

6
6.1
6.2
6.3
6.4
6.5

346 CORE CURRICULUM FOR RHEUMATOLOGY NURSING

b. Maintenance pulse cyclophosphamide every 3 months for 2 years or for 1 year after reaching remission (Fisher-Betz, Schneider, & Bonbardieri, 2012).

c. Data support possible efficacy for NPSLE but no clear indication as to which manifestations respond best to cyclophosphamide (Fisher-Betz, Schneider, & Bonbardieri, 2012).

d. No tapering is required at the discontinuation of therapy.

D. Adverse events.

1. Gastrointestinal effects: Nausea and vomiting, anorexia.

2. Alopecia.

3. Mouth sores.

4. Opportunistic infection correlating with degree and duration of neutropenia.

5. Bone marrow suppression: Neutropenia, thrombocytopenia, anemia.

6. Cystitis due to bladder-irritating metabolite.

7. Malignancy: Correlated with overall quantity of CTX received.
   a. Leukemia.
   b. Lymphoma.
   c. Bladder cancer.

8. Infertility for women and men.

9. Hepatitis.

10. Pneumonitis and interstitial pulmonary inflammation and fibrosis (rare).

11. Hypersensitivity reactions are rare but can be confused with underlying disease (fever, "drug rash", liver function test abnormalities, GI symptoms, hypotension).

12. Because of short and long term toxicities, cyclophosphamide should be discontinued in favor of less toxic therapies after 3-6 months, except when used to treat for DPGN in SLE.

E. Nursing implications.

1. Patients must be aware of risks/ benefits of therapy.

2. Laboratory monitoring may be the responsibility of the nurse.

a. WBC no less than every 2 weeks, with borderline WBC more frequently.

b. Dose adjustment with WBC counts outside parameters.

c. Hydration to minimize CTX-induced cystitis due to acrolein (bladder toxic metabolite). 3L orally or IV hydration if given by infusion.

d. Instruct patients taking daily oral CTX to do so in the morning to decrease the likelihood of adverse bladder effects.

e. Antiemetics may be used to control GI symptoms.

f. If patient is given prophylaxis against pneumocystis jirovecii pneumonia, strongly urge adherence with drug regimen.

g. Provide psychosocial support to patient and family.

h. Be ready to respond to infusion/ hypersensitivity reactions.

i. Instruct patient on AE profile and to report AEs promptly.

III. Cyclosporine (CsA).

A. Mechanism of action.

1. Suppresses the immune system by inhibiting the production and release of interleukin (IL)-2 and inhibits IL-2 induced activation of resting T-lymphocytes, specifically targeting calcineurin.

2. Must be metabolized to active metabolites in the liver.

3. Pregnancy category C, but can be continued in pregnant patients with SLE if the benefits outweigh the risks (Klippel, Stoner, Crofford, & White, 2008).

4. Ophthalmic use: Partial immunomodulator, exact mechanism is unknown.

B. Indications and dosing.

1. Supplied as Neoral®, Gengraf®, Sandimmune®
   a. Neoral® and Sandimmune® are not bioequivalent and cannot be interchanged.
   b. Only the micro-emulsion form is FDA approved for treatment of severe RA (Bartlett, 2006).

2. Recommended dosing for RA: 2.5-4 mg/ kg/day divided into 2 equal doses.

a. Higher doses increase the risk of nephropathy.

b. Response should be noted after 8 weeks of treatment.

c. Reserved for severe rheumatoid arthritis unresponsive to other treatment options.

3. Juvenile idiopathic arthritis (JIA).

a. Orally 2.5 mg/kg/day divided q12 hours.

b. Increase by 0.5 mg/kg/day if insufficient response after 8 weeks.

c. Maximum dose 4 mg/kg/day.

4. Doses for SLE range from 2.5-5 mg/kg/day.

a. Generally well tolerated, with reduction of corticosteroid doses and improvement in disease activity.

b. Side effects are dose dependent and reversible.

5. Macrophage Activation Syndrome in Juvenile Idiopathic Arthritis (JIA).

a. The most important complication of JIA.

b. A secondary hemophagocytic histiocytosis occurring in children with active disease.

c. Characterized by sudden development of diffuse intravascular coagulation (DIC) associated with hepatosplenomegaly, pancytopenia, abrupt decrease of ESR, marked elevation of ferritin, and elevated serum levels of liver enzymes and triglycerides.

d. Associated with high morbidity and mortality.

e. Conventional therapeutic approach: Cyclosporine with intermittent IV methylprednisolone pulse therapy (Fisher-Betz, Schneider, & Bonbardieri, 2012).

6. Occular dryness and inflammation; Sjögren's syndrome.

a. Topical collyrium (0.05%) (Restasis®)

b. Use one (1) drop in each eye every 12 hours.

c. With contact lenses: Remove lenses, instill eye drops, wait 15 minutes then reinsert lenses. Most patients will not be contact lens wearers because of the underlying condition.

d. Not tested on patients under age 16.

e. Pregnancy Category C.

C. Box warning(s).

1. May cause hypertension.

2. Increased risk of infection including fatal infections, opportunistic infections.

3. Increased risk of lymphomas and other malignancies, particularly of the skin.

4. Renal impairment including structural kidney damage (when used in high doses).

5. Increased risk of skin cancer, particularly in patients with psoriasis with history of previous treatment with conventional therapy such as methotrexate (MTX), Psoralen plus ultraviolet A (PUVA), or other immunosuppressants.

6. Additional warning: The use of cyclosporine is not recommended in patients with rheumatoid arthritis who are receiving other immunosuppressants.

D. Adverse event profile.

1. Cardiovascular: Hypertension, edema, chest pain, arrhythmia.

2. Central nervous system: Headache, dizziness, pain, convulsions, mood/psychiatric disturbances.

3. Dermatologic: Hirsutism (21%-45%), hypertrichosis, purpura, acne.

4. Endocrine/metabolic: Increased triglycerides, female reproductive disorder, gynecomastia, menstrual disorder.

5. Gastrointestinal: Nausea, diarrhea, gum hyperplasia, abdominal discomfort, dyspepsia, vomiting, flatulence, weight loss/gain, gastric irritation.

6. Neuromuscular and skeletal: Tremor, paresthesia, leg cramps.

7. Renal: Renal dysfunction/nephropathy, creatinine increase, BUN increase, hematuria.

8. Respiratory: Upper respiratory infections, bronchospasm, cough.

9. Miscellaneous: Other infections.

10. Hyperuricemia.

11. Ophthalmic use: Conjunctival hyperemia, discharge, eye pain, foreign body sensation, pruritis, stinging, visual disturbances (blurring).

6
6.1
6.2
6.3
6.4
6.5

E. Nursing implications.

1. Laboratory monitoring may be the responsibility of the nurse.

   a. Serum creatinine levels every 2 weeks.

   b. Monitor hepatic enzymes.

   c. Monitor potassium levels, lipid panel, uric acid as these may be adversely affected by dose.

2. Monitor blood pressure frequently; increase frequency of monitoring with dose increases.

   a. Alert prescriber for sustained hypertension.

   b. Persistent hypertension is an indication for discontinuation.

3. For oral administration, use oral syringe, glass dropper, or glass container (not plastic or styrofoam).

   a. Neoral® may be mixed with orange or apple juice.

   b. Sandimmune® may be diluted with milk, chocolate milk or orange juice.

   c. Mix thoroughly and drink at once.

   d. For pediatric use: To enhance palatability mix with milk, chocolate milk, orange or apple juice at room temperature.

4. Store oral solution in original container, room temperature, protected from light.

5. Be aware of look- and sound-alike drugs to avoid confusion.

6. Use appropriate precautions for handling and disposal.

7. Instruct patient and/or family about side effect profile, especially the increased risk of infection.

8. Serum concentrations may be altered by the use of nutraceuticals such as echinacea, cat's claw and St. John's wort.

   a. Instruct patients to avoid nutraceuticals while taking cyclosporine.

9. NSAIDs alter serum concentrations of cyclosporine as well as enhance the nephrotoxic effect.

   a. Consider alternatives to NSAIDs.

   b. Monitor for evidence of nephrotoxicity (serum cyclosporine concentrations, hypertension).

10. Other concomitant drugs may influence serum concentrations of cyclosporine, review med list often, adjust as necessary.

11. Response to inactivated vaccines may be diminished; live organism and live attenuated vaccines should be avoided.

12. Patients requiring cyclosporine have not responded to conventional treatment, and therefore, are quite ill; they may require additional psychosocial support.

13. Ophthalmic use: Avoid touching conjunctiva with vial.

14. Breastfeeding is contraindicated.

IV. Azathioprine (AZA) (Imuran).

A. Mechanism of action.

1. AZA is a purine analog and a mercaptine immunosuppressant.

2. AZA inhibits nucleic acid synthesis thus affecting both cellular and humoral immunity.

3. Reduces antibody production.

4. Intercellular metabolites are antineoplastic and immune modulating.

B. Indications and dosing.

1. Rheumatic diseases (lupus nephritis, inflammatory myopathies, scleroderma, ANCA associated vasculitis, Behçet's).

   a. Newer more effective agents have made the use of AZA quite limited in rheumatoid arthritis and spondyloarthropathies.

      (1) Patients should be screened for reduced thiopurine methyltransferase (TPMT) activity before starting AZA

      (2) Begin at a dose of 25-50 mg/day for the first week to test for drug hypersensitivity.

      (3) Dose is increased incrementally by 0.5 mg/kg per day for 4-6 weeks until the desired response is seen or a maximal dose of 3 mg/kg/day is reached.

      (4) Lower doses are indicated in patients with renal insufficiency.

      (5) Maintenance dose: Reduce dose by 0.5 mg/kg/day every 4 weeks until the lowest effective dose is reached.

      (6) May be discontinued abruptly.

2. Used as second line therapy for sarcoidosis with progressive disease despite corticosteroid therapy (Bijlisma, 2012).

3. Moderate SLE with serositis (pericarditis and pleuritis), hematologic and cutaneous manifestations.

4. AZA can be used second line/ maintenance for lupus DPGN.

5. AZA has been use in progressive systemic sclerosis but efficacy has not been demonstrated and is not an FDA-approved indication.

6. AZA has been extensively evaluated for eye disease.

   a. Dose 2.5 mg/kg/day (Bijlsma).

   b. AZA was superior to placebo in preventing progression of unilateral to bilateral eye disease.

   c. AZA allowed decreasing dosing of glucocorticoids (GC) in patients with established eye disease (Bijlsma).

7. AZA could have a role in giant cell arteritis (GCA) and polymyalgia rheumatica (PMR) as a corticosteroid sparing agent in longstanding disease in patients unable to use methotrexate (MTX) (Bijlsma).

C. Adverse events profile.

   1. Central nervous system: Fever, malaise.

   2. Gastrointestinal: Nausea, vomiting, diarrhea.

   3. Toxicity including rash, fever, hypotension, liver enzyme elevations; generally reversible upon discontinuation.

   4. Hematologic toxicity: Includes dose-related leukopenia, thrombocytopenia, and anemias

   5. Hepatic: Increased alkaline phosphatase, increased bilirubin, hepatotoxicity, increased transaminases.

   6. Neuromuscular and skeletal: Myalgia.

   7. Infection.

   8. Lymphoma.

D. Box warning(s).

   1. AZA is associated with the development of lymphoma and other malignancies. Hepatocellular T-cell Lymphoma (HTCL), a rare type of T-cell lymphoma, is generally fatal; has occurred predominantly in adolescents and young adults treated for GI diseases (Crohn's disease, ulcerative colitis) and receiving TNF inhibitors, AZA, and/ or other mercaptopurine. These patients were generally treated with combination immunosuppressants, although there have been reports of HTCL in those receiving AZA or mercaptopurine as monotherapy.

E. Nursing implications.

   1. Use special precautions for handling and disposal.

   2. Patients using allopurinol may be sensitive to myelosuppressive effects.

   3. Immune responses to vaccines may be diminished.

   4. Caution should be exercised in patients with hepatic and renal impairment.

   5. Concomitant use of mercaptopurine is contraindicated, emphasize this to patient.

   6. Teach patient signs and symptoms of infections; encourage patient to contact healthcare provider if infection is suspect.

   7. Discuss side effect profile and instruct patient to call healthcare provider with concerns.

   8. Stress importance of keeping follow up appointments, adherence to medication schedule, share medication list with all providers.

   9. Encourage patient to use a single pharmacy for all meds; pharmacist may alert patient and the prescriber of potential drug incompatibilities.

   10. Avoid cat's claw, echinacea.

   11. Women should avoid becoming pregnant while taking AZA.

   12. Breast feeding is not recommended.

   13. AZA is known to sensitize DNA to ultraviolet A radiation, increasing potential for skin cancer; avoid prolonged exposure to sun; use sunscreen daily.

6
6.1
6.2
6.3
6.4
6.5

14. GI side effects may be ameliorated by taking AZA in split doses and with food.

15. Lab monitoring: CBC and liver function tests q 2weeks until stable dose achieved, then q 4-6weeks; emphasize the importance of maintaining monitoring schedule.

V. Mycophenolate mofetil (MMF) (CellCept®, Myfortic®)

A. Mechanism of action.

1. Inhibitor of lymphocyte proliferation.

2. Decreased B- and T-cell proliferation with decreased cytokine production.

3. Pregnancy Category D.

B. Indications and dosing (the following are not FDA approved.)

1. Dosing is 1.5 – 3 g/day.

2. DPLN: MMF is a valuable alternative to cyclophosphamide.

3. Lupus membranous glomerulonephritis: No controlled studies but a small series and a recent report indicate improvement with MMF as first line treatment along with prednisone (Bijlsma, 2012).

4. Moderate to severe SLE (renal, cutaneous, hematologic, and neurologic involvement) resistant to other immunosuppressive drugs (1.5 – 3 g daily).

5. Hematologic manifestations of SLE in those who do not respond to or tolerate AZA (Bijlsma).

6. There are several small series that indicate efficacy with MMF in GPA (ANCA+ vasculitis) and microscopic polyangiitis (MPA).

7. Pediatric dosing for nephrotic syndrome:
   a. 12.5 – 18 mg/kg/dose twice daily; max dose 2 g/day for 1-2 years with a tapering dose of prednisone.
   b. Steroid dependent: 12 – 18 mg/kg/dose or 600 mg/m² twice daily; max dose: 2 g/day.

8. MMF may be a safer alternative to CsA or AZA for immunosuppression (Bartlett, 2006).

C. Box warning(s).

1. Risk of infection is increased.

2. Risk of developing lymphoma and skin malignancy is increased.

3. Should be administered under the supervision of a prescriber experienced in immunosuppressive therapy.

4. Pediatrics:
   a. May result in increased risk of infection.
   b. Increased risk of developing lymphomas and other malignancies, particularly skin.

D. Adverse events.

1. Gastrointestinal: Nausea, diarrhea, abdominal cramping; usually tolerated better with time.

2. Bone marrow suppression: Cytopenias.

3. Infection: May be susceptible to opportunistic infections, possibly due to previous cytotoxic exposure (CsA, CTX).

4. Neoplasia: Lymphoma as a result of immunosuppression.

5. Drug-drug interactions: Antacids, iron supplements, cholestyramine resin decrease the absorption of MMF; chronic administration of rifampin significantly decreases serum levels of MMF; contraceptives may have decreased efficacy when taken with MMF; toxicity may be enhanced by probenecid and AZA.

6. Other side effects were noted during trials for organ rejection.

E. Nursing implications.

1. Lab monitoring: CBC after the first one to two weeks, then once every 6-8 weeks if no cytopenias noted.

2. Adjust dosing to BID to minimize gastrointestinal side effects.

3. Dosing may be started low and rapidly increased to the target dose to improve GI tolerance.

4. Women of childbearing age should have pregnancy test before starting drug and use contraception; a second method of contraception should be considered.

5. Breast feeding is not recommended.

6. Vaccinate with inactivated vaccines; avoid live vaccines.

7. Take on empty stomach (recommended to avoid absorption variability).

8. CellCept® and Myfortic® (delayed release formulation) are not interchangeable.

9. Hazardous agent; use appropriate handling and disposal.

10. Instruct patient to report any neurologic symptoms, consider PML in differential diagnosis.

Summary

Other than glucocorticoids, the immunosuppressant drugs discussed in this chapter tend to be used less frequently and in disease states that are seen less often in many clinical rheumatology settings. It is important for the nurse to be familiar with the use of these medications, to be mindful of the individual drugs' use/adverse event profile, and to have a reference available to review clinically significant information when these drugs are prescribed, if their use is infrequent.

References

Allergan (2013). Restasis®: Prescribing information. Irvine, CA: Author.

Barberio, J. (2010). *Nurses pocket drug guide 2010*. Newark, NJ: McGraw-Hill Companies.

Bijlsma, J.W.J. (Ed.) (2012). EULAR textbook on rheumatic diseases. London: BMJ Group.

Bristol-Myers Squibb Company (2005). Cytoxan®: Prescribing information. Deerfield, IL: Author.

Fisher-Betz, R., Schneider, M., & Bonbardieri, S. (2012). Systemic lupus erythematosis: Treatment. In J.W. J. Biljsma (Ed.), EULAR textbook on rheumatic diseases (pp. 506-519). London: BMJ Group.

Genentech USA, Inc. (2013). CellCept®: Prescribing Information. South San Francisco, CA: Author.

Klippel, J., Stone, J., Crofford, L., & White, P., (Eds.). (2008). Primer on the rheumatic diseases (13th ed.). New York: Springer.

Merck & Co., Inc. (2014) Celestone®: Prescribing information. Whitehouse Station, NJ: Author

Miller, D., & Lee. S. (2006). Pharmacologic interventions: Small molecules. In S. Bartlett (Ed.), Clinical care in the rheumatic diseases (3rd ed., pp. 227-235). Atlanta: Association of Rheumatology Health Professionals.

Novartis (2013). Myfortic®: Prescribing information. East Hanover, NJ: Author.

Novartis (2013). Neoral®: Prescribing information. East Hanover, NJ: Author.

Novartis (2013). Sandimmune®: Prescribing information. East Hanover, NJ: Author.

Pfizer, Inc., (2014). Cortef®: Prescribing information. New York, NY: Author

Prometheus Laboratories, Inc. (2011). Imuran®: Prescribing information. San Diego, CA: Author.

Saag, K., & Furst, D. (2013). Major side effects of systemic glucocorticoids. Retrieved from http:// www. uptodate.com/home

Sadock, B. (2010). *Nursing 2011 drug handbook* (31st ed.). Philadelphia, PA: Lippincott Williams & Wilkins.

6
6.1
6.2
6.3
6.4
6.5

352 CORE CURRICULUM FOR RHEUMATOLOGY NURSING

Section 6.3
Self-Injection Primer

Rebecca L. Gamble, BA, RN

Introduction

The rheumatology nurse must be able to take clinical information and put it in practical, understandable terms for the patient and caregiver. Rheumatic diseases are chronic, resulting in the need for ongoing patient education and encouragement. Rheumatology nurses must appreciate the patient's social, cultural, economic, and educational status in order to effectively communicate with the patient and family. Often the nurse plays a pivotal role in the patient's adherence to the treatment plan. This chapter is designed for the rheumatology nurse to teach proper use of the self-injectable medications and provide nursing considerations when starting self-injections.

Learning Objectives

Upon completion of this chapter, the nurse will be able to:

1. Identify common sites for injection.

2. Describe reasons to avoid certain injection sites.

3. List the side effects from methotrexate (MTX).

4. Identify certain common concerns or contraindications to the Tumor Necrosis Factor (TNF) alpha inhibitors.

Content Outline

I. Adherence.

A. Anxiety: The nurse may encounter multiple sources of fear.

  1. Needle phobia.

    a. Discuss fear with patient to determine extent.

    b. Assess the need to involve a family member or friend.

  2. Fear regarding diagnosis.

    a. Open discussion about fears regarding diagnosis.

    b. Discuss effects of uncontrolled disease.

  3. Fear related to the side effects described in package insert material.

    a. Review the side effects with patient.

    b. Review the difference between disease-related side effect and drug-related side effect.

    c. Discuss the effects of untreated disease:

      (1) Worsening joint damage.

      (2) Cardiovascular compromise.

      (3) Increased pain.

      (4) Decreased mobility.

      (5) Effects of long term stress on the body and its ability to cope.

  4. Concern regarding cost of medication.

    a. Discuss assistance programs.

    b. Complete benefit investigation with patient's insurance provider.

    c. Investigate co-pay assistance.

    d. Consider viable alternatives.

B. Scheduling.

  1. Review with patient the specific schedule of the drug prescribed.

    a. Different injectable medications will have different dosing schedules.

  2. Discuss ways to incorporate the injection into the patient's schedule.

  3. Educate about reasons that injectable

might need to be rescheduled - for example, illness, upcoming surgery or procedure.

C. Lab Considerations.

  1. Baseline lab work.

    a. Lab work needs to be obtained prior to starting injectable medications. Consider the following:

      (1) Hepatitis screening.

        i) Rule out the possibility of reactivation of the hepatitis B virus (HBV) in chronic hepatitis B carriers. Reactivation can be fatal.

      (2) Tuberculosis (TB) screening.

        i) Identify TB carriers as well as reactivation of latent TB.

        ii) Reactivation can occur in the form of systemic TB which may be difficult to identify and to treat.

      (3) Complete Blood Cell Count.

        i) Identify anemia, pancytopenia, leukopenia, neutropenia, thrombocytopenia.

      (4) Comprehensive Metabolic Panel.

        i) Review electrolytes, renal function, and liver function. Monitoring liver function is essential during treatment and may alter the patient's plan of care.

      (5) Sedimentation rate and C-reactive protein - Indicators of non-specific inflammation could be disease related.

      (6) Pregnancy testing - if the patient is of childbearing age.

        i) Rule out the possibility of pregnancy.

        ii) Discuss a plan of reliable birth control.

D. Ongoing lab work.

  1. Routine lab work should be monitored every 3 months at minimum and possibly more frequently if problems arise.

  2. Complete blood count.

  3. Comprehensive metabolic panel.

  4. Sedimentation rate.

  5. C-reactive protein.

E. Vaccines.

1. Instruct patients that it is a good idea to receive the following:

   a. Influenza vaccine yearly - injection only. NOT the nasal mist form (contains live virus).

   b. Pneumonia vaccine.

   c. ILive virus vaccinations are generally contraindicated for patients on biologics; instruct patients to discuss with the provider if they have particular concerns.

   d. Caution patients about being around children who have received recent vaccinations as some of the live vaccine may "shed" (become airborne).

   e. NO LIVE VACCINES FOR CHILDREN while on immunosuppression.

II. Injectable Medication (See Table 1).

A. Mechanism of action.

1. Tumor Necrosis Factor (TNF alpha).

   a. "Is a pro-inflammatory cytokine produced by macrophages and lymphocytes. It is found in large quantities in the rheumatoid joint and is produced locally in the joint synovium. TNF is one of the critical cytokines that mediate joint damage and destruction due to its activities on many cells in the joint as well as effects on other organs and body systems" (Matsumoto, Bathon, & Bingham, 2011, p.10).

Table 1: Injection Guide

Mechanism of Action	Drug	Disease States Treated
Interleukin-1 Receptor Antagonist	Anakinra (Kineret®)	» Rheumatoid Arthritis » Cryopyrin-Associated Periodic Syndromes (CAPS)
Interleukin-6 Inhibitor	Tocilizumab (Actemra®)	» Rheumatoid Arthritis » Juvenile Idiopathic Arthritis
Selective T cell costimulation modulator	Abatacept (Orencia®)	» Adult Rheumatoid Arthritis » Juvenile Idiopathic Arthritis
TNF alpha inhibitor	Etanercept (Enbrel®)	» Rheumatoid Arthritis » Juvenile Idiopathic Arthritis » Psoriatic Arthritis » Ankylosing Spondylitis » Plaque Psoriasis
TNF alpha inhibitor	Adalimumab (Humira®)	» Rheumatoid Arthritis » Juvenile Idiopathic Arthritis » Psoriatic Arthritis » Ankylosing Spondylitis » Plaque Psoriasis » Crohn's disease
TNF alpha inhibitor	Golimunab (Simponi®)	» Rheumatoid Arthritis » Psoriatic Arthritis » Ankylosing Spondylitis » Ulcerative Colitis
TNF alpha inhibitor	Certolizumab pegol (Cimzia®)	» Rheumatoid Arthritis » Crohn's Disease » Psoriatic Arthritis » Ankylosing Spondylitis

Source: Author, Rebecca Gamble

6
6.1
6.2
6.3
6.4
6.5

2. Interleukin-1 Receptor Antagonist.

   a. "Pro-inflammatory cytokine implicated in the pathogenesis of rheumatoid arthritis. Interleukin-1 receptor antagonist is an endogenous blocker of the cytokine. Interleukin -1 has effects on cartilage degradation leading to damage as well as inhibiting repair and is a potent stimulus to osteoclasts leading to bone erosion" (Matsumoto, Bathon, & Bingham, 2011, p. 17).

3. Selective T cell costimulation modulator.

   a. "This agent interferes with the interaction between antigen-presenting cells and T lympocytes and affects early stages in the pathogenic cascade of events in rheumatoid arthritis. T lymphocytes become activated due to an unknown stimulus but likely involving the interaction between antigen presented in the context of the Class II Histocomplexity Complex molecule on the surface of the antigen presenting cells. T cells recognize antigens as foreign and if they receive a second stimulus, will become active, proliferate, traffic to inflamed sites, and secrete pro-inflammatory cytokines including TNF" (Matsumoto, Bathon, & Bingham, 2011, p.14).

4. Interleukin-6 Inhibitor

   a. "Interleukin-6 (IL-6) is a cytokine with effects on numerous cell types, including those involved in the pathogenesis of RA. Interleukin-6 (IL-6) is a pleiotropic cytokine that is abundant in both the synovium and serum of RA patients. IL-6 is known to regulate a diverse array of activities may underlie both systemic as well as local symptoms of RA." (Hennigan & Kavanaugh, 2008).

B. Methotrexate (MTX).

1. Mechanism of action.

   a. Classified a Disease-Modifying Antirheumatic Drug (DMARD). MTX leads to increased adenosine, which has a strong anti-inflammatory effect (Bijlsma, 2012).

2. Usage.

   a. MTX can be used with and is often recommended for use in conjunction with other disease-modifying antirheumatic drugs (DMARDs) and biologic response modifiers (BRMs).

   b. Can be given in an oral or injectable form.

   c. Monitor for side effects.

     (1) Hepatotoxicity - check liver functions.

     (2) Pneumonitis - monitor for chronic cough.

     (3) Bone marrow suppression - monitor CBC.

   d. Make sure that patients have good renal function.

     (1) Because MTX is cleared through the kidneys.

   e. Instruct the patient about appropriate times to stop MTX such as:

     (1) When on antibiotic.

     (2) Scheduled for an upcoming procedure.

     (3) Surgery.

     (4) Call Rheumatologist if uncertainty.

3. Administration.

   a. Oral administration (Oral administration: see Sections 6.1 and 6.2).

   b. Injection

     (1) Instruct the patent to inject medication on the same day weekly. Review aseptic technique, preferred injection sites, storage, and preparation.

4. Contraindications for Administration.

   a. Side effects.

     (1) Such as mouth ulcers and nausea need to be reported to the provider.

   b. Antibiotic use.

     (1) If patient requires an antibiotic for a sinus infection, urinary tract infection, abscess, or other reason, notify provider.

III. Nursing Education.

A. Lab considerations - Monitor lab work according to provider preference. Injectable biologics may cause hematologic changes. Criteria vary with provider.

1. Complete blood cell count - Watch for pancytopenia, neutropenia, anemia, leukopenia, thrombocytopenia. Educate the patient to watch for bruising, fever, pallor, abnormal bleeding.

2. Complete metabolic panel - pay attention to renal function, watch for elevated liver

enzymes; monitor protein and albumin levels which can indicate affected nutritional status.

3. Sedimentation rate and C-reactive protein - These can indicate non-specific inflammation.

4. Screen for tuberculosis before initiating biologic; screening with an Interferon-gamma release assay is preferred.

5. Hepatitis remote profile -- Some biologics may increase the risk of reactivation of hepatitis B in patients who are chronic carriers of this virus. In addition, infection with hepatitis C warrants further workup and clearance by a hepatologist before biologics are initiated.

6. HIV test -- Should also be considered prior to initiating any immunosuppressant, including biologics.

B. Symptoms to Monitor.

1. Watch for and discuss with patient signs of congestive heart failure - increased weight, edema, increased shortness of breath with or without exertion, increase in blood pressure.

2. Monitor for malignancies - watch for swollen lymph nodes, fatigue, changes in bowel patterns as well as new or changing skin lesions.

3. Leukemia- bone pain worse at night, abnormal bruising, fevers, fatigue.

4. Lymphoma - screen for fevers, night sweats and/or unexplained weight loss.

5. Fungal infections - These can be fatal and sometimes hard to diagnose. For patients who travel or have lived in regions where mycoses are endemic fungal infections should be considered. Patients who develop active infection such as pneumonia that is not responsive to standard treatment should be tested for fungal infections such as coccidioidomycosis, histoplasmosis, and blastomycosis.

6. Nervous system disorders - some rare cases of central nervous system demyelinating diseases and infections.

   a. Examples include multiple sclerosis, Guillain-Barrè Syndrome, and progressive multifocal leukoencephalopathy. Ask patients about dizziness, weakness, unsteady gait, headaches, and visual changes at each clinic visit.

IV. Patient Education.

A. Contraindications for injection.

1. Active infections: Fever, chills, persistent cough and/or drainage, urinary symptoms indicating a possible UTI.

2. Reddened or non-healing wounds, draining wounds.

3. Mouth ulcers - especially recurring ulcers.

4. Scheduled surgeries and procedures- instructions will vary depending on provider.

5. Patient should hold injection if currently on an antibiotic.

B. Aseptic technique.

1. Review proper storage of medication.

   a. biologics require refrigeration.

2. Proper hand washing – with soap and water.

3. Proper cleaning of the injection site with an alcohol swab or cotton ball with alcohol applied.

C. Choosing an injection site- refer to package insert, common sites:

1. Lateral thighs.

2. Abdomen- stay away from umbilical area.

3. Posterior arms- may be a difficult area to use if self-injecting.

4. Remember that these are intended to be subcutaneous injections; therefore, the patient needs to select a site that has adequate fat.

   a. Avoid areas that have heavy scarring, bruising or stretch marks, raised areas or psoriasis.

   b. Encourage patient to rotate sites.

D. Auto-injector versus prefilled syringe.

1. Drugs will come in varying forms-most are in easy to use auto injectors. However, sometimes because of insurance coverage, latex allergy, patient preference (usually because of the pain of injection), patient may need to use a prefilled syringe or vial form.

2. Refer to medication package insert and other material such as DVDs and brochures provided by manufacturer to review

administration technique with the patient. Each injectable will have slightly different instructions specific to the product.

E. Reactions.

1. Site reactions.

   a. Can occur immediately following an injection or up to a week later.

   b. Patients can apply ice before and after injection to minimize local reactions.

   c. Patients can apply a topical antihistamine to the site – but instruct them not to massage the area.

   d. Instruct the patient that it may be necessary to also take oral antihistamines as well. However, patient should notify the provider if reaction becomes increasingly worse.

2. Systemic reactions.

   a. These can include but are not limited to.

      (1) Rash.

      (2) Itching.

      (3) Chest tightness.

      (4) Shortness of breath.

      (5) Itchy throat.

   b. Instruct patients with these symptoms to stop the injections and schedule a follow up appointment.

   c. Patients can take an oral antihistamine.

   d. If these symptoms are severe, patient must call 911.

Summary

Patient safety is a priority in self injection training. Nurses should be familiar with methotrexate (MTX) and injectable biologic medications and their side effects. Prescreening is necessary before beginning any patient on biologic medications. Nurses should be prepared to educate their patients on both risks and benefits of therapy as well as potential injection site reactions.

References

Abbott Laboratories. (2011). *Humira®: Prescribing information*. North Chicago, IL: Author.

Amgen Inc. & Pfizer Inc. (2012. *Enbrel®: Prescribing information*. Thousand Oaks, CA: Author.

Bijlsma, J. (Ed.), *EULAR textbook on rheumatic diseases*. London: BMJ Group.

Bristol-Myers Squib Company. (2011). *Orencia®: Prescribing information*. Princeton, NJ: Author.

Centocor Ortho Biotech. (2010). *Simponi®*: Medication Guide. Horsham, PA: Author.

Hennigan, S., & Kavanaugh, A. (2008). Interleukin-6 inhibitors in the treatment of rheumatoid arthritis. Therapeutics and Clinical Risk Management, 4(4), 767–775. Retrieved from http://www.ncbi.nlm.nih.gov/pmc/articles/PMC2621374/

Klippel, J., Stone, J., Crofford, L., & White, P. (2008). *Primer on the rheumatic diseases* (13th ed.). New York: Springer.

Matsumoto, A. K., Bathon, J. & Bingham, C. O. (2011) *Rheumatoid arthritis treatment*. Baltimore, MD: Johns Hopkins.

UCB, Inc. (2012). *Cimzia®*: Prescribing information. Smyrna, GA: Author.

6
6.1
6.2
6.3
6.4
6.5

Section 6.4

Vascular Access and IV Administrations of Pharmacologic Therapies

Diane Gilbert, BSN, RN, CRNI

Introduction

The rheumatology patient often faces frequent blood draws and IV administration of pharmacologic therapies when their disease is refractory to other treatments. Frequent venous access leaves patients with very few options for peripheral vascular access over time, particularly in children and the elderly. Therefore, many patients opt for a more permanent option like a peripherally inserted central catheter (PICC or PIC line), port, or other central line access. With more biologic therapies (including biosimilars) in development, it is more important than ever for the rheumatology nurse to also be an infusion specialist to best meet patients' needs.

6
6.1
6.2
6.3
6.4
6.5

Learning Objectives

Upon completion of this chapter, the nurse will be able to:

1. Identify the three most common types of vascular access devices.

2. Identify the lab test that is the gold standard for identifying latent or active TB infection.

3. List nine facts regarding implanted ports.

4. Identify four common medications and proper dosages used during infusion anaphylaxis and when to call 911.

5. Be able to identify four biologic therapies and their mechanism of action.

Content Outline

I. Peripheral vascular access.

A. Veins that should be considered for peripheral cannulation are those found on the dorsal and ventral surfaces of the upper extremities. Avoid veins on the inner aspect of the wrist as nerves are in close proximity to veins and can be damaged during venous cannulation or medication infusion.

1. Metacarpal veins.

   a. Located on dorsal aspect of hand.

   b. Generally well adapted for intravenous infusions.

2. Cephalic vein.

   a. Formed by convergence of metacarpal veins on the radial aspect of forearm.

3. Basilic vein.

   a. Ascends on the ulnar aspect of the forearm.

4. Median antebrachial vein.

   a. Arises from the venous plexus on palm of the hand and extends upward along ulnar side of front of the forearm.

5. Median cephalic vein.

   a. Large vein located in the antecubital fossa.

   b. Crosses in front of the brachial artery; use with caution.

6. Median basilic vein.

   a. Located outside antecubital fossa on ulnar curve of the arm.

B. Site preparation.

1. Hair removal, if necessary, performed in a manner that preserves skin integrity.

   a. Use scissors or electric clippers.

   b. Use of a razor can cause microabrasions, which increase the risk of infection.

2. Insertion site should be clean prior to application of antiseptic solution.

   a. Antiseptic solution should contain a combination of alcohol (ethyl or isopropyl) and either chlorhexidine or povidone iodine.

   b. Local anesthesia, if necessary, used according to organizational protocols.

3. Catheter placement.

   a. Select the smallest size and shortest length catheter that will accommodate the prescribed therapy.

   b. The nurse placing a catheter should have an understanding of venous anatomy and physiology, vein assessment techniques, and insertion techniques appropriate to the specific device.

   c. A tourniquet is properly applied to promote venous distension and to impede venous but not arterial flow.

   d. Aseptic technique is to be maintained during procedure.

   e. After successful venous cannulation, catheter shall be stabilized according to organizational policies.

      (1) Sterile tapes, surgical tapes, and/or a stabilization device may be used.

   f. A sterile dressing is applied and maintained on access device.

      (1) Gauze or transparent semipermeable membrane dressings may be used.

II. Central venous access devices.

A. Catheter tip in central venous location, generally the superior vena cava (SVC).

1. Preferred when peripheral venous access is unavailable or inappropriate for use.

   a. Monitor chest and ipsilateral upper extremity for complications: Edema, pain, redness, and collateral circulation.

   b. Implanted ports.

      (1) Implantable ports are surgically placed in chest (most common) or upper extremity with attached catheter threaded into venous system. Surgical notes should give the nurse details on how long tubing is (helpful when determining how much solution to flush through) and size/depth of port (important for size selection of a Huber needle , used to access the port under the skin).

      (2) Long-term dwell capacity, can be years if necessary.

      (3) Useful in cyclic therapy.

      (4) Entire device under the skin, no at home care necessary.

(5) Combination lidocaine/prilocaine creams (EMLA® or Oraqix®) to site 1 hour before access in children.

(6) Monthly assessment and maintenance (flushing) required when not in use.

(7) Use only non-coring needle for device access (ie. Huber needle).

(8) No swimming or tub baths for 24 hours after needle removed post-access to prevent infection.

(9) Often used in pediatric patients.

c. Peripherally inserted central catheters (PICC).

(1) Placed in upper extremity by clinically validated health professionals: Nurses, radiologists, physicians, or respiratory therapists.

(2) Catheter follows venous blood flow with tip residing in the SVC.

(3) Although no set dwell time, generally in place several weeks to months.

(4) External portion secured with stabilization device and covered with sterile dressing.

(5) Daily assessment and daily-weekly maintenance necessary (ie. flushes; cap and dressing changes).

d. Tunneled catheters.

(1) Surgically placed for long-term use and frequent venous access.

(2) Catheter cuff located in subcutaneous tunnel helps stabilize device and protect against infection.

(3) Maintenance varies between devices; follow manufacturer instructions.

(4) Not common in children.

e. Non-tunneled catheters.

(1) Generally placed in the inpatient setting for short-term central venous access.

(2) Jugular or subclavian vein used.

(3) Higher risk of infection than other central venous access devices.

(4) Not common in children.

III. Biologic Infusions

(Partial listing for rheumatoid arthritis only. Please see *Section 6.5: Biologics* for full listings).

A. Tumor necrosis factor (TNF) alpha inhibitor: Infliximab (Remicade®) (Jannsen Biotech, Inc, 2013).

1. Neutralizes biologic activity of TNF alpha.

a. Dosage: 3-10 mg/kg.

b. Pre-medicate with anti-pyretic, antihistamine, and corticosteroid as ordered.

c. Administration.

(1) Reconstitute each 100 mg vial of lyophilized powder with 10 ml sterile water using 21 g or smaller needle.

(2) Gently swirl to dissolve; do not shake.

(3) Dilute reconstituted solution in 250 ml normal saline.

(4) Infuse over no less than 2 hours (within 3 hours of reconstituting) using an in-line low protein binding filter.

d. Contraindicated in patients with stage III/IV heart failure and demyelinating disease.

e. Discontinue if lupus-like syndrome develops.

B. Tumor necrosis factor (TNF) alpha inhibitor: Golimumab (Simponi Aria®) (Jannsen Biotech, Inc, 2013b)

1. A human IgG1 kappa monoclonal antibody specific for human TNF-alpha that neutralizes TNF-alpha activity.

2. It binds with both soluble and transmembrane bioactive forms of human TNF-alpha.

3. Dosage.

a. The golimumab dosage regimen is 2 mg per kg given as an intravenous infusion over 30 minutes at weeks 0 and 4, then every 8 weeks thereafter.

4. Startup of golimumab IV Infusion.

a. Calculate the dosage and the number of Golimumab vials needed based on the recommended dosage of 2 mg/kg and the patient's weight. Each 4 mL vial of Golimumab contains 50 mg of golimumab.

b. Check that the solution in each vial is colorless to light yellow and opalescent. The solution may develop a few fine translucent particles, as golimumab is a protein. Do not use if opaque particles, discoloration or other foreign particles are present.

c. Dilute the total volume of the Golimumab solution with 0.9% w/v sodium chloride for infusion to a final volume of 100 ml. Discard any unused solution remaining in the vials.

d. Use only an infusion set with an in-line, sterile, non-pyrogenic, low protein-binding filter (pore size 0.22 micrometer or less).

e. Do not infuse Golimumab concomitantly in the same intravenous line with other agents. No physical biochemical compatibility studies have been conducted to evaluate the use of Golimumab with other intravenous agents in the same intravenous line.

f. Infuse the diluted solution over 30 minutes.

g. Once diluted, the infusion solution can be stored for 4 hours at room temperature.

h. Obtain and record vital signs.

C. T-cell inhibitor: Abatacept (Orencia®) (Bristol-Myers Squib Company, 2013)

1. Inhibits T lymphocyte activation by binding to CD80 and CD86.

2. Dosage: 500-1000 mg based on body weight.

   a. Less than 60 kg: 500 mg.

   b. 60-100 kg: 750 mg.

   c. 100 kg or greater: 1000 mg.

3. Pre-medicate with anti-pyretic and antihistamine as ordered.

4. Administration.

   a. Use only a silicone-free disposable syringe for reconstitution.

   b. Reconstitute each 250 mg vial with 10 ml normal saline.

   c. Gently swirl to dissolve; do not shake.

   d. Dilute reconstituted solution into 100 ml normal saline.

   e. Infuse over 30 min (within 24 hours of reconstitution) using an in-line low protein binding filter.

D. B-cell targeted therapy: Rituximab (Rituxan®) (Biogen Idec, Inc. & Genentech, Inc., 2013)

1. Binds specifically to B-cell antigen CD20 causing rapid depletion of peripheral B cells.

2. Dosage: 2- 1000 mg doses separated by 2 weeks every 24 weeks or by clinical evaluation.

3. Given in combination with methotrexate (MTX).

4. Pre-medicate with methylprednisolone 100 mg or equivalent glucocorticoid 30 minutes prior to infusion.

5. Administration.

   a. Do not administer as intravenous push or bolus.

   b. Available in 100 mg/10 ml and 500 mg/50 ml single-use vials.

   c. Withdraw necessary amount of rituximab from vial(s) and dilute to a final concentration of 1-4 mg/ml in either 0.9% sodium chloride or 5% dextrose in water.

   d. First infusion: Initiate infusion rate at 50 mg/hr, increase by 50 mg/hr every 30 min to a maximum of 400 mg/hr.

   e. Subsequent infusions: Initiate infusion at 100 mg/hr, increase by 100 mg/hr every 30min to a maximum dose of 400 mg/hr.

   f. Cardiac arrhythmias and angina can occur; monitor for these.

   g. Report complaints of abdominal pain as bowel obstruction and perforation can occur.

   h. CBC should be monitored for severe pancytopenia.

E. IL-6 Inhibitor: Tocilizumab (Actemra®) (Genentech, Inc., 2013).

1. Interluekin-6 receptor inhibitor.

2. Dosage:

   a. Adult patients with RA- 4 or 8 mg/kg.

   b. Systemic juvenile idiopathic arthritis- 12 mg/kg if under 30 kg, 8 mg/kg at or above 30 kg.

3. Pre-medicate with antihistamine as ordered.

4. Administration.

   a. Do not administer as intravenous push or bolus.

   b. Available in 80 mg/4 ml, 200 mg/10 ml, and 400 mg/20 ml single-use vials.

   c. Withdraw necessary amount of tocilizumab from vial(s) and dilute with 0.9% sodium chloride for final volume of 50 ml for pediatric and 100 ml for adult patients.

d. May be stored (after dilution) for up to 24 hours refrigerated or at room temperature if protected from light.

e. Infuse over 60 minutes.

f. Use cautiously in patients at risk for gastrointestinal perforation.

g. Potential for changes in neutrophils, platelets, lipids, and liver function tests; monitor lab results accordingly.

IV. Nursing considerations with biologic infusions.

A. Biologics may be used in combination with traditional disease-modifying antirheumatic drugs (DMARDs except for mycophenolate mofetil Cellcept®) but *not* in combination with other biologics due to the degree of immunosuppression that would occur.

B. Biologic therapy puts patients at risk for serious infections.

1. Do not infuse during an active infection.

2. Upper respiratory infection most common adverse reaction.

C. Always use aseptic technique when handling intravenous (IV) equipment.

D. Live vaccines should not be given during therapy.

E. Patient at risk for reactivation of hepatitis B or tuberculosis (TB).

1. Patients should be tested for these prior to initiation of therapy, upon exposure to disease, and periodically throughout course of therapy.

2. Blood tests are available to check for latent hepatitis B and TB. Interferon Gamma Release Assays (IGRAs) (e.g.TB Quantiferon Gold®) have become the gold standard with biologics.

a. Infectious Disease consult if Hep B or IGRA is positive.

b. Antituberculosis therapy should be given for positive test results.

c. Monitor patients for signs and symptoms of both pulmonary and extrapulmonary active disease throughout biologic therapy.

F. Malignancies, gastrointestinal disorders, and cardiac dysfunction have been reported.

G. Monitor for adverse infusion reactions including, but not limited to, headache, blood pressure changes, urticaria, hives, and anaphylaxis.

1. Early intervention can alleviate symptoms and halt progression to a more serious adverse reaction.

2. Stop infusion, notify prescriber, and administer antihistamines and/or corticosteroids as prescribed (additional fluids as warranted).

3. When patient's symptoms stabilize, resume infusion at previously tolerated rate and increase slowly (as ordered if indicated).

4. Have emergency interventions available if patient's condition deteriorates.

5. Best practice is for the RN delivering the infusion therapy to be, at a minimum, Basic Cardiac Life Support (BCLS) certified. Best case scenario is to have at least one Advanced Cardiac Life Support (ACLS) certified practitioner on the premises during the infusions.

H. Laboratory monitoring may include blood counts, inflammatory markers, liver function tests, lipid measurements.

I. Prior to each infusion patients should be assessed for signs and symptoms of active infection (fever, chills, cough, current antibiotic therapy) or developing lymphomas (enlarged lymph glands), open wounds, and upcoming or recent surgeries, (changes in health status).

1. Hold infusion and notify prescriber to determine when it is appropriate to resume biologic.

V. Miscellaneous Infusions.

A. Anti-inflammatory: Methylprednisolone.

1. Exerts a wide variety of physiologic effects including decreasing inflammation by suppression of migration of leukocytes and reversal of increased capillary permeability.

2. Dosage: 15-30 mg/kg; in acute exacerbation of symptoms often ordered 500-1000 mg daily dose for three days (High-dose pulse therapy).

3. Administration:

a. Do not administer high-dose IV push; hypotension, cardiac arrhythmia, and sudden death have been reported.

b. Administer 500 mg over at least 30 minutes.

c. Administer 1000 mg over at least 60 minutes.

B. Intravenous immune globulin (IVIG): Several products available (CSL Behring, 2013).

1. Mechanism of action is not clear, but therapeutic benefits include the suppression of the production of inflammatory cytokines, enhanced production of antiinflammatory mediators, blocking of antigen-presenting cells, stimulation of T cells. Also regulates B cells (suppressing production of autoantibodies).

2. Most often IVIG use in treating rheumatic diseases is considered off label.

3. Used as second line treatment option or in combination with other therapies.

4. Dosage: 300-2000 mg/kg diluted to a 5-10% solution. Higher doses may be spread out over 2 - 5 days.

5. Pre-medicate with steroids, anti-pyretic, and/or antihistamine as ordered.

6. Administration.

   a. Administration rates are generally weight based; follow manufacturer's instructions.

   b. Infusion rates start low and increase slowly as tolerated.

7. Nursing considerations.

   a. IVIG is harvested from donor plasma and is purified and concentrated to a lyophilized state for storage.

   b. No preservative is used so should be infused at as fast a rate as is practical; be aware of adverse reactions from too fast an infusion rate.

   c. Do not combine different brands of IVIG.

   d. IgA-deficient patients with IgA antibodies are at higher risk of adverse reactions.

   e. Use cautiously in patients with renal dysfunction or patients at risk for a thrombotic event.

   f. Make sure patient is adequately hydrated before starting infusion.

   g. Check brand compatibility with diluent; some brands not compatible with 0.9% saline.

   h. Monitor for changes in heart rate and blood pressure; diastolic increases of 30mm or decreases of more than 15mm should be reported to prescriber.

   i. Reduce rate and notify prescriber of backache, chills, chest tightness, headache, dizziness, nausea, sweating.

C. Bisphosphonates: Anti-osteoporosis.

1. Zoledronic acid (Reclast®) (Novartis Pharmaceuticals Corporation, 2014)..

   a. Inhibits osteoclast-mediated bone resorption thereby reducing bone turnover and increasing bone mass.

   b. Dosage: 5 mg in a 100 ml ready to use solution.

   c. Administration:

      (1) Infuse over no less than 15 minutes in separate IV line.

      (2) Generally given once a year.

2. Ibandronate sodium (Boniva®) (Genentech USA, Inc., 2013).

   a. Inhibits osteoclast-mediated bone resorption thereby reducing bone turnover and increasing bone mass.

   b. Dosage: 2-6 mg.

   c. Administration:

      (1) Generally given in 3 mg dose every 3 months.

      (2) Give prefilled syringes of medication over 15-30 seconds.

3. Nursing considerations.

   a. Use cautiously in patients with renal failure.

      (1) Serum creatinine should be assessed prior to administration.

      (2) Make sure patient is well hydrated with infusion.

   b. Transient drops in serum calcium are noted after infusion.

      (1) Supplemental oral calcium and Vitamin D should be used on an ongoing basis.

6
6.1
6.2
6.3
6.4
6.5

(2) Confirm patient is not hypocalcemic prior to infusion.

   c. Jaw osteonecrosis has been reported with bisphosphonate use.

   (1) Have patients report medication use to their dentist.

   (2) Consider a professional oral inspection prior to starting therapy.

   d. Other adverse effects can include muscular pain and digestive upset.

VI. Compounding.

A. Best practice is to have IV solutions prepared by a pharmacist using a laminar flow hood.

B. If pharmacy support is unavailable, nurse may compound medications following manufacturer's instructions.

C. Use aseptic technique throughout procedure.

   1. Wash hands prior to starting process.

   2. Gather all necessary supplies to work area to avoid possible contamination by leaving and returning to work space during procedure.

D. Have a clean dedicated area set up for mixing medications.

E. Keep food and drink away from work area.

F. Equipment: Syringes, needles, vials, tubings, and IV solutions should be single use only.

G. Check for expiration dates; do not use if past expiration date.

H. After removing flip top from vials, clean rubber stopper with an alcohol-containing antiseptic wipe.

I. Reconstitute per manufacturer's instructions. Most products may be gently swirled to mix but not shaken.

J. Dilute to final concentration as instructed.

   1. Best practice is to double check final product with another licensed practitioner if available.

K. Partially used vials should be discarded.

L. Inspect solution for any particulate matter. Gentle mixing of container may be used to complete dissolution of medication.

   1. Do not use if solution is discolored or turbid.

M. Infuse solution within time period specified by manufacturer.

VII. Emergency Measures.
(Always refer to prescriber specific protocols in your area. The following is only an example.)

A. Adverse reactions, including anaphylaxis, may occur at any time. Have emergency equipment available.

B. Medications and dosages for ADULT patients (NOT PEDIATRIC):

   1. Diphenhydramine: Usually 50 mg IV push x1; urticaria, hives.

   2. Acetaminophen: 650-1000 mg po as ordered; fever, backache, headache.

   3. Steroids: Hypersensitivity reaction not responsive to diphenhydramine.

      a. Hydrocortisone: 100 mg IV push.

      b. Methylprednisolone: 125 mg IV push.

   4. A benzodiazepene (several trade names): PO or IV; nausea vomiting, anxiety.

   5. Epinephrine (Epi): 0.1-0.5 mg subcutaneously; may be given for an allergic reaction unresponsive to diphenhydramine and hydrocortisone. MUST CALL 911 IF YOU GIVE EPI. Effects of Epi optimally lasts for about 20 minutes before wearing off. Epi is meant to buy you time to get to the Emergency Department.

C. Medications and dosages for PEDIATRIC patients (NOT ADULTS):

   1. Adverse reactions: Acetaminophen; Diphenhydramine; Methylprednisone; Ondansetron hydrochloride (Zofran®); Many minor adverse reactions can be halted by stopping infusion for 20min. then resuming at 1/2 previous rate.

2. Anaphylaxis: Epi-pen® or Epi-pen Jr.® and every 20min. if needed; Hydrocortisone; Benadryl; MUST CALL 911 IF YOU GIVE EPI.

D. Oxygen.

E. IV solutions for fluid resuscitation in case of severe hypotension or shock.

F. Defibrillator.

G. Emergency transportation to acute care hospital.

Summary

Infusion centers should have a set of evidence-based protocols for each medication they administer to provide patients with the safety precautions they deserve and expect from professional rheumatology nurses. There should also be very clear expectations of how to handle adverse reactions including anaphylaxis. Close observation of patients during and after infusions is crucial. Mock anaphylaxis drills are very helpful to delineate roles of various infusion personnel and review emergency procedures.

References

Biogen Idec, Inc & Genentech, Inc. (2013). Rituxan®: Prescribing information. South San Francisco, CA: Author.

Bristol-Myers Squib Company (2013). Orencia®: Prescribing information. Princeton, NJ: Author.

CSL Behring (2013), Immune Globulin Intravenous. Prescribing information. Bern, Switzerland: Author

Genentech, Inc. (2013). Actemra®: Prescribing information. South San Francisco, CA: Author.

Genentech USA, Inc. [2013] Boniva® Prescribing information. South San Francisco, CA: Author

Jannsen Biotech, Inc (2013a). Remicade®: Prescribing information. Horsham, PA: Author.

Janssen Biotech, Inc. (2013b). Simponi Aria®: Prescribing information. Horsham, PA: Author.

Novartis Pharmaceuticals Corporation (2014). Reclast®. Prescribing Information. East Hanover, NJ: Author.

Suggested Readings

Bayry, J., Negi, V., & Kaveri, S. (2011). Intravenous immunoglobulin therapy in rheumatic diseases. *Nature Reviews/Rheumatology,7*(6), 349-359.

Furfaro, N. (2011). New therapeutic options in rheumatoid arthritis: A focus on interleukin-6 blockade. *Journal of Infusion Nursing, 34*(2), 107-115.

Infusion Nurses Society. (2004). *Core curriculum for infusion nursing* (3rd ed.). Philadelphia, PA: Lippincott Williams & Wilkins.

Infusion Nurses Society. (2011). *Infusion nurses standards of practice.* Norwood, MA: Author.

Mandema, J., Salinger, D., Baumgartner, S., & Gibbs, M. (2011). A dose-response meta-analysis for quantifying relative efficacy of biologics in rheumatoid arthritis. *Clinical Pharmacology and Therapeutics, 90*(6), 828-835. doi: 10.1038.

Nobre, C., Callado, M., Lima, J., Gomes, K, Martiniano, G., & Vieira, W. (2011, August 7). Tuberculosis infection in rheumatic patients with infliximad therapy: Experience with 157 patients. *Rheumatology International* . (E-pub ahead of print).

Tromp, M., Natsch, S., & van Achterberg, T. (2009). The preparation and administration of intravenous drugs before and after protocol implementation. *Pharmacy World & Science, 31*(3) 413-420.

Tuberculosis Testing and Diagnosis. Retrieved from http// www.cdc.gov/tb/testing/default.htm

6
6.1
6.2
6.3
6.4
6.5

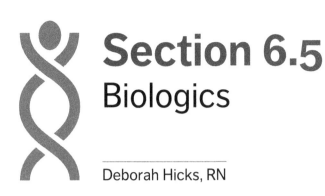

Section 6.5
Biologics

Deborah Hicks, RN

Introduction

Biologic agents have transformed the treatment of rheumatoid arthritis and other common rheumatologic diseases such as ankylosing spondylitis, psoriatic arthritis, osteoporosis, and systemic lupus erythematosus. Advances in the knowledge of the immune system, particularly in autoimmune diseases, has offered prime targets for pharmaceutical research. This has led to the development of agents that target sites along inflammatory pathways, providing effective treatment options. As the knowledge of the immune system expands, additional immune pathways become targets for other biologic response modifiers and increase the treatment armamentarium for healthcare providers of patients with rheumatic conditions.

The complexity of the immune system can be overwhelming and is not the subject of this chapter. But the mechanisms of action for the listed agents are included to allow the reader some insight into the reasons these agents can be used effectively in the treatment of these complex diseases. Only rheumatologic indications are mentioned for each agent even though many of these drugs may have indications for non-rheumatologic conditions.

There remains a need for additional drugs with other mechanisms of action since not all patients will benefit from these agents. This has led to a pipeline that is rich with possible immune targets, different mechanisms of action, other methods of administration, and additional indications. As with all drugs there are safety concerns that must be addressed and monitored, and post marketing surveillance has led to some new concerns with some agents but has reassured prescribers and patients about others. Few new safety signals have emerged.

The rheumatology nurse is in the unique position to provide expert care, to provide learning/teaching opportunities for patients and caregivers that enhance surveillance and adherence, to coordinate care with other healthcare providers, and to assist patients' efforts to obtain expensive medications. The nurse is one of the most trusted members of the healthcare team and as such, must be prepared to guide the patient through decision-making challenges. In order to do that with confidence, being knowledgeable about the biologics is essential.

The drugs discussed in this chapter are current as of this writing (see Table 1). New drugs are already in phase II and III clinical trials. It will be incumbent upon each nurse to keep abreast of new agents as they become FDA approved for use in rheumatology.

Learning Objectives

Upon completion of this chapter, the nurse will be able to:

1. Identify mechanisms of action for biologic agents used in rheumatology.

2. Discuss side effect profiles of each biologic agent.

3. List rheumatologic indications for each agent.

4. Describe dosing and administration specifics for biologic agents used in rheumatology.

Content Outline

I. General guidelines for administering biologic response modifiers (BRMs).

A. Screen patients for infections.

1. Prescreen for tuberculosis/hepatitis B and C, some facilities also screen for other immunodeficiencies such as HIV.

   a. Treat positive findings according to standard guidelines.

   b. Update screening according to facility policy.

2. Update vaccinations according to current guidelines, including consideration of live vaccines such as herpes zoster, before initiation.

   a. Live vaccines are not recommended during treatment with biologics.

3. Screen patients for active infections prior to each dose of IV biologics.

   a. Withhold drug if infection active, complete treatment, symptoms should be resolved before restarting.

   b. Teach patients signs and symptoms of infection, appropriate actions such as seeking medical attention, withholding drug if infection is current or suspected.

4. Concomitant use of immunosuppressants such as glucocorticoids increases the risk of infection.

5. Patients should be cautioned that if they live or they have traveled to areas of endemic tuberculosis or endemic mycoses (coccidioidomycosis, histoplasmosis, blastomycosis), they should share this information with the healthcare provider.

B. Biologics are not recommended for use in combination with other biologics.

1. Small numbers of clinical trials have been done with combinations of BRMs and have not shown additional efficacy beyond that from one biologic alone.

2. The risk of infection is increased with combinations of biologics.

C. Lab monitoring should be done routinely specific to each drug/drug class.

D. Biologics should be stored in refrigerator if indicated in the package insert.

1. Do not freeze.

2. Bring to room temperature before administering.

3. Patients who travel should transport medicine in insulated cooler with an ice pack.

   a. Ice packs should not make contact with medication.

   b. Refrigerate as soon as feasible at destination.

   c. Keep a copy of prescription or prescriber's notes with medication for verification while undergoing security checks.

E. Lyophilized biologics must be reconstituted with sterile water for injection.

1. Dilute using aseptic technique.

2. Direct stream of diluent toward wall of vial.

3. Drugs at room temperature will dissolve more quickly.

4. Do not shake.

5. May be stored for limited time in refrigerator after dilution, protected from light (specific time per drug).

6. Must be used within limited times specific for each drug.

7. Reconstitution is complete when liquid has no visible powdered particulate.

8. Always inspect vial for particulate matter and color.

9. Inject at room temperature, subcutaneously, rotating sites.

10. Infuse at room temperature using in-line, sterile, non-pyrogenic, low-protein-binding filter.

F. Infusible drugs should not be given as bolus or IV push.

G. Unused portions should be discarded.

H. Instruct patient/caregiver in injection technique and proper disposal of used syringes and needles.

I. Prefilled syringes may contain preservative that can cause pain on injection.

 1. Patients may apply cold-pack to injection site prior to injection.

 2. Some sites may be less painful than others, suggest site rotation to determine.

J. Injection site reactions are possible with injectable biologics.

 1. Warn patients about these reactions.

 2. Instruct patient to notify healthcare provider if reaction site increases in size, severity.

K. Immunogenicity is possible with biologics.

 1. Injection site reactions, systemic reactions may occur.

 2. Infusion reactions may occur.
  a. Premedicate with acetaminophen, anti-histamine.
  b. IV methylprednisolone or equivalent should be considered, per facility protocol.

 3. Appropriate patient education, including take home information, should be discussed at each encounter.

 4. Patients should be prepared to manage mild reactions at home and/or post infusion.

 5. Discuss medical emergency measures.

L. Infusible biologics should not be infused concomitantly with other agents in the same IV line.

M. Financial assistance is available through multiple sources for patients unable to afford biologic therapy.

 1. Manufacturers' patient assistance programs.

 2. Foundation-administered assistance.

II. Tumor necrosis factor (TNF) inhibitors.

A. Mechanism of action.

 1. Binds to TNF-alpha (a key cytokine in the inflammatory cascade).

 2. Mediates joint inflammation.

 3. Regulates the production of other inflammatory cytokines.

B. Agents that block TNF (anti-TNF antibodies).

 1. Monoclonal antibodies (mAB) (ending with –mab):

  a. Infliximab (Remicade®, Janssen Biotech, 2013): Binds both soluble and membrane bound forms of TNF.
   (1) It is a human murine chimeric antibody (-ximab).

  b. Adalimumab (Humira®, AbbVie Laboratories, 2013).
   (1) Fully human monoclonal antibody against TNF.

  c. Golimumab (Simponi®, Simponi Aria®, Janssen Biotech, Inc., 2013b).
   (1) A human IgG1 kappa monoclonal antibody specific for human TNF-alpha that neutralizes TNF-alpha activity.
   (2) It binds with both soluble and transmembrane bioactive forms of human TNF-alpha.

  d. Certolizumab pegol (Cimzia®, UCB, Inc., 2013).
   (1) A humanized antibody (-zumab) in which the recombinant Fab fragment that recognizes TNF has been conjugated with a polyethylene glycol chain (pegylated) (increases half life and decreases immunogenicity without affecting affinity and specificity of the antibody) but does not contain an Fc portion.
   (2) It neutralizes membrane associated and soluble TNF-alpha.

 2. Native cytokine receptors coupled with the Fc component of human immunoglobulin (ending with –cept).

  a. Etanercept (Enbrel®, Amgen Inc. & Pfizer Inc., 2013).
   (1) It binds to the target cytokine while it is in serum, thereby inhibiting the cytokine's ability to interact with its cell surface receptors.
   (2) Consists of two p75 TNF receptors bound to the Fc portion of IgG.
    i) Etanercept is bivalent (one etanercept molecule binds with two TNF molecules).

C. Box warning(s).

1. All TNF inhibitors have the same black box warnings.

   a. Increased risk of serious infections may lead to hospitalization or death.

      (1) Tuberculosis (disseminated or extrapulmonary).

      (2) Invasive fungal infections (such as histoplasmosis, candidiasis).

      (3) Bacterial, viral, and other opportunistic infections including Legionella and Listeria.

2. Malignancy.

   a. Lymphoma.

   b. Other malignancies, some fatal, have been reported in children and adolescents.

D. Pregnancy Category B.

1. Nursing mothers.

   a. It is not known if these drugs are excreted in human milk or absorbed systemically.

   b. Because of potential for adverse reactions in nursing infants, a decision must be made regarding discontinuation of breastfeeding or discontinuation of the drug.

E. General Guidelines for the use of TNF Inhibitors.

1. All general guidelines listed in Section I pertain to TNF inhibitors.

2. Patients and healthcare providers must consider less common infections (fungal) when standard of care does not resolve infections.

3. Risk/benefits of treatment with TNF blockers should be considered in patients:

   a. With chronic or recurrent infections.

   b. Who have been exposed to tuberculosis.

   c. With a history of an opportunistic infection.

   d. With underlying conditions that may predispose them to infections.

4. TNF-blockers should be used with caution in patients with congestive heart failure (CHF).

   a. Worsening cases of CHF and new cases have been reported.

   b. These patients should be monitored.

5. Use with caution in patients with pre-existing or recent onset central nervous system demyelinating disorders (e.g., multiple sclerosis, Guillian-Barré syndrome).

6. New onset psoriasis including pustular psoriasis and palmoplantar psoriasis has been reported.

   a. This may resolve with discontinuation of drug.

   b. Recurrence of symptoms may appear when rechallenged with another TNF-blocker.

7. Lupus-like syndrome may occur associated with the formation of autoantibodies.

8. TNF blockers can be used with or without methotrexate (MTX) or other non-biologic disease-modifying anti-rheumatic drugs (DMARDs), specific to each drug.

9. Hematologic abnormalities including medically significant cytopenias (thrombocytopenia, leukocytopenia, pancytopenia) have occurred.

   a. Monitor for signs and symptoms as well as periodic lab monitoring.

10. Many patients have co-morbid conditions and take multiple medications.

    a. Lab monitoring for hematologic, hepatic, and renal abnormalities should be routine.

11. Patients who have an inadequate or fading response to one TNF inhibitor may achieve efficacy with another TNF inhibitor.

F. Indications and dosing for Infliximab (Remicade®, Janssen Biotech, 2013a).

1. Indication: Moderate to severe rheumatoid arthritis (RA).

   a. Reduce signs and symptoms.

   b. Inhibit the progression of structural damage.

   c. Improve physical functioning.

   d. Dosing: 3 mg/kg IV infusion every 8 weeks after induction at 0, 2, 6 weeks.

      (1) Should be given in combination with MTX.

      (2) In patients with incomplete response consideration may be given to increasing dose up to 10 mg/kg as frequent as every 4 weeks.

         i) Risk of serious infections increases at higher doses.

(3) Follow general biologic infusion guidelines.

(4) Infuse over no less than 2 hours.

(5) Observe for infusion reactions.

   i) Risk of infusion reactions is related to timing, not dose.

      1) Infusion reactions are more likely during 3rd and 4th infusion (Management of Infusion-Based Biologic Therapy in Rheumatoid Arthritis, 2008).

      2) Infusion reactions can occur at any time.

   ii) Be prepared to manage infusion reactions.

2. Indication: Ankylosing spondylitis (AS).

  a. Used to reduce signs and symptoms of active AS.

  b. Dosing: 5 mg/kg every 6 weeks after induction at 0, 2, 6 weeks.

  c. Follow infusion guidelines as listed for RA.

3. Indication: Psoriatic arthritis (PsA).

  a. To reduce signs and symptoms of arthritis.

  b. Inhibit the progression of structural damage.

  c. Improve physical functioning.

  d. Dosing: 5 mg/kg every 8 weeks after induction at 0, 2, 6 weeks.

    (1) Can be used with or without MTX.

  e. Follow infusion guidelines as listed for RA.

G. Indications and dosing for Adalimumab (Humira®, AbbVie Inc., 2013).

1. Indication: Moderate to severe RA.

  a. To reduce signs and symptoms.

  b. To induce major clinical response.

  c. To inhibit progression of structural damage in adults.

  d. Dosing: 40 mg subcutaneously (SQ) every other week.

    (1) MTX and other DMARDs, glucocorticoids, non-steroidal anti-inflammatories (NSAIDs) and/or analgesics may be continued with adalimumab.

(2) Patients who are not taking MTX may derive additional benefit from increasing the dosing frequency to every week.

2. Indication: Juvenile idiopathic arthritis (JIA).

  a. To reduce signs and symptoms of moderately to severely active polyarticular JIA in pediatric patients age 2 and older.

  b. Dosing for JIA is weight based:

    (1) 10 kg (22 lbs) to <15 kg (33 lbs): 10 mg SQ every other week.

    (2) 15 kg (33 lbs) to <30 kg (66 lbs): 20 mg SQ every other week.

    (3) ≥30 kg (66 lbs): 40 mg SQ every other week.

3. Indications: Psoriatic arthritis (PsA).

  a. To reduce signs and symptoms.

  b. To inhibit the progression of structural damage.

  c. To improve physical functioning of adults.

  d. Dosing: 40 mg every other week.

    (1) Can be used alone (monotherapy) or in combination with other non-biologic DMARDs.

4. Indication: Ankylosing spondylitis (AS).

  a. To reduce signs and symptoms in adults with active AS.

  b. Dosing: 40 mg SQ every other week.

H. Indications and Dosing for Golimumab (Simponi ®, Janssen Biotech, 2013b; Simponi Aria®, Janssen Biotech, 2013c).

1. Indication: Adults with moderately to severely active rheumatoid arthritis (RA).

  a. Dosing: 50 mg SQ once monthly on the same date of the month (example, the 1st of every month).

    (1) Use in combination with MTX.

    (2) Corticosteroids, non-biologic DMARDs and/or NSAIDs may be continued.

  b. IV (Simponi Aria®): 2 mg per kg, day 0, day 28, then every 8 weeks.

    (1) Used in combination with MTX.

    (2) Corticosteroids, non-biologic DMARDs and/or NSAIDs may be continued.

2. Indication: Adults with active ankylosing spondylitis (AS).

a. Dosing: 50 mg SQ once monthly.

b. Corticosteroids, non-biologic DMARDS and/or NSAIDs may be continued.

3. Indication: Adults with active psoriatic arthritis (PsA).

   a. Dosing: 50 mg SQ once monthly.

   b. May be used alone or in combination with MTX.

I. Indications and dosing for Certolizumab pegol (Cimzia®, UCB Inc., 2013).

1. Indicated for adults with moderate to severely active RA, AS, and PsA.

   a. 400 mg (given in two SQ injections of 200 mg) initially and at weeks 2 and 4, followed by 200 mg SQ every other week.

   b. 400 mg in two injections given every 4 weeks may be considered.

   c. May be used with or without MTX or other DMARDs.

   d. Lyophilized form is administered by a healthcare professional.

   e. Prefilled syringe is self-administered.

   f. May interfere with PTT tests.

J. Indications and dosing for Etanercept (Enbrel®, Amgen Inc. & Pfizer Inc., 2013b).

1. Indicated for rheumatoid arthritis (RA).

   a. Used for reducing signs and symptoms.

   b. For inducing major clinical response.

   c. For inhibiting the progression of structural damage.

   d. For improving physical function in adult patients with moderately to severely active RA.

   e. Dosing: 50 mg SQ once weekly.

     (1) May be initiated with or without MTX.

     (2) MTX, glucocorticoids, salicylates, NSAIDs and/or analgesics may be continued.

2. Indicated for polyarticular juvenile idiopathic arthritis (PJIA).

   a. For reducing signs and symptoms of moderately to severely active JIA in patients age 2 or older.

   b. Dosing: 0.8 mg/kg weekly, with a maximum of 50 mg per week.

3. Indicated for psoriatic arthritis (PsA).

   a. To reduce signs and symptoms.

   b. To inhibit progression of structural damage of active arthritis.

   c. Improve physical function.

   d. Dosing: 50 mg SQ once weekly.

     (1) May be used with or without methotrexate.

     (2) MTX, glucocorticoids, salicylates, NSAIDs and/or analgesics may be continued.

4. Indicated for ankylosing spondylitis (AS).

   a. To reduce signs and symptoms in patients with active AS.

   b. Dosing: 50 mg SQ once weekly.

     (1) MTX, glucocorticoids, salicylates, NSAIDs and/or analgesics may be continued.

K. Dosage Forms and Strengths:

1. Infliximab (Remicade®)

   a. 100 mg, lyophilized powder per vial.

2. Adalimumab (Humira®)

   a. Single-use pen, 40 mg in 0.8 mL.

   b. Single-use prefilled syringe, 40 mg in 0.8 mL.

   c. Single-use prefilled syringe, 20 mg in 0.4 mL.

3. Golimumab (Simponi®)

   a. 50 mg single-use prefilled SmartJect® autoinjector.

   b. 50 mg single-use prefilled syringe.

4. Golimumab (Simponi Aria®)

   a. 50 mg/4 mL vial for IV administration.

5. Certolizumab pegol (Cimzia®)

   a. 200 mg lyophilized powder, with 1 mL of sterile water for injection.

   b. 200 mg/mL single-use prefilled syringe.

6. Etanercept (Enbrel®)

   a. 50 mg single-use prefilled syringe.

   b. 50 mg single-use prefilled SureClick® autoinjector.

   c. 25 mg single-use prefilled syringe.

6
6.1
6.2
6.3
6.4
6.5

d. 25 mg multiple-use vial (lyophilized powder).

III. IL-1 Receptor Antagonist (IL-1Ra).

A. Mechanism of action.

1. Natural antagonists that closely resemble the cytokine structure but deliver no signal when bound by receptor.

   a. Binds the IL-1 receptor and prevents recruitment of the accessory signaling protein.

   b. Greater than 90% of the receptors on the cell surface must be bound in order to be effective, requiring large doses.

B. Anakinra (Kineret®, Amgen, 2001-2003).

1. Recombinant human IL-1Ra (rHuIL-1Ra).

2. Anakinra has modest clinical efficacy compared to anti-TNF agents.

C. Box warning(s): None.

D. Pregnancy Category B.

1. Nursing mothers:

   a. It is not known if anakinra is excreted in human milk.

   b. Caution should be exercised if anakinra is administered to nursing women.

E. General Guidelines.

1. Do not use in combination with TNF blocking agents.

   a. Rates of infections were increased when used in combination with etanercept.

2. Hypersensitivity reactions, including anaphylaxis, have occurred.

3. Live vaccines should not be given concurrently with anakinra.

4. The impact of treatment with anakinra on active and/or chronic infections is not known.

5. The development of malignancies is not known with treatment of anakinra.

6. Dose reduction should be considered in patients with severe renal insufficiency or end stage renal disease (ESRD).

7. Contraindicated in patients with known hypersensitivity to E-coli-derived proteins (anakinra), or any component of the drug.

8. Needle cover of prefilled syringe contains a derivative of latex and should be not be handled by persons with latex sensitivity.

9. Neutrophil counts should be assessed prior to initiating treatment, monthly for 3 months, then every 3 months.

10. The most commonly reported AE was injection site reactions (ISR) (erythema, ecchymosis, pain).

11. Infections were reported in clinical trials and open-label extension studies.

12. Malignancies were reported.

13. In placebo-controlled studies, decreases in total WBCs and neutropenia were observed.

14. Adverse events were similar to other biologics including ISRs, URTI, headache, GI symptoms, flu-like symptoms.

15. Not recommended for pediatric patients with JIA.

16. Toxic drug reactions may be increased in patients with significant renal impairment.

17. Efficacy of anakinra has been shown to be inferior to TNF antagonists.

    a. Anakinra is not used for RA with any frequency at this time.

    b. The need for daily injections has made anakinra less popular than other agents.

F. Indications and Dosing.

1. Indicated for the reduction of signs and symptoms and slowing the progression of structural damage in adults (over 18 years of age) with moderately to severely active rheumatoid arthritis (RA) who have not responded to one or more DMARDs.

   a. Anakinra can be used alone or in combination with non-biologic DMARDs.

   b. 100 mg SQ daily, administered at the same time every day.

G. Supplied form.

1. 100 mg/0.67 mL in single-use preservative free prefilled glass syringe with 27 gauge needle.

2. Trace amounts of small, translucent to white amorphous particles of protein may appear in the solution; if these particles are excessive, do not use.

3. If foreign particulate matter is present and/or the solution is discolored or cloudy, do not use.

IV. Selective B-cell depletor.

A. Mechanism of Action.

1. B-cells are prominent therapeutic targets because they likely play a role in antigen presentation, upregulation of inflammatory cytokines such as IL-6, and autoantibody production.

B. Agent.

1. Rituximab (Rituxan®, Biogen Idec, Inc. and Genentech, Inc. 2013b).

   a. Monoclonal antibody directed against CD-20, a B-cell-specific surface protein present throughout B-cell maturation but not present on mature plasma cells.

   b. Rituximab produces profound depletion of peripheral B-cells with limited effect on total (Matsumoto, 2006).

C. Box warning(s):

1. Infusion reactions:

   a. Administration can result in serious, including fatal, infusion reactions.

   b. Deaths within 24 hours of rituximab infusions have occurred, more often associated with the first infusion.

   c. The vast majority of fatal infusion reactions have occurred in patients receiving rituximab for the treatment of malignancies, not for rheumatologic conditions.

2. Mucocutaneous reactions, some severe (including fatal) have occurred.

3. Progressive multifocal leukoencephalopathy (PML): reactivation of JC virus, resulting in PML and death, has been reported.

D. Pregnancy Category C.

1. Nursing mothers.

   a. It is not known if rituximab is excreted in human milk or absorbed systemically.

   b. Because of potential for adverse reactions in nursing infants, a decision must be made regarding discontinuation of breastfeeding or discontinuation of the drug.

E. General Guidelines.

1. Premedication with acetaminophen and antihistamine, along with pre-treatment with IV methylprednisolone or its equivalent, is recommended.

   a. Reactions typically occur during the first infusion within 30 – 120 minutes.

   b. The incidence of infusion reactions decreases with subsequent infusions.

   c. Symptoms include fever, chills, urticaria/rash, angioedema, sneezing, throat irritation, cough, and/or bronchospasm, with or without associated hypo- or hypertension (package insert).

   d. Early recognition and action/treatment can mitigate severe reactions.

   e. Temporarily or permanently discontinue infusion, depending on the severity of reaction.

   f. After symptoms resolve restart drug at 50% rate reduction.

   g. Monitor patient carefully.

   h. Patients with granulomatosis with polyangiitis (GPA, previously called Wegener's granulomatosis) or microscopic polyangiitis (MPA) may experience different infusion reactions.

      (1) Cytokine release syndrome, flushing, throat irritation and tremor.

      (2) Infusion reaction incidence decreased with subsequent infusions.

2. Serious, including fatal, infections can occur during and up to 1 year after therapy.

   a. Screen for latent hepatitis B, as reactivation has occurred.

   b. Although screening for latent TB is not required, many facilities do screen.

   c. Patients should be made aware of the signs and symptoms of infection and to seek medical attention for any indications of infection (most common infections: Nasopharyngitis, upper respiratory tract infections, urinary tract infections, bronchitis, sinusitis).

6
6.1
6.2
6.3
6.4
6.5

d. Follow infection guidelines in use for all biologics.

e. Concomitant use of immunosuppressants increases the risk of infection.

3. Follow current immunization guidelines and administer non-live vaccines at least 4 weeks prior to a course of rituximab.

a. Responses to vaccines may be diminished in rituximab treated patients.

4. Limited data is available regarding safety and the use of biologics and/or DMARDs other than MTX.

5. Report neurological symptoms.

6. The use of rituximab for RA is not recommended in patients who have not had prior inadequate responses to at least one TNF antagonist.

7. Pneumocystis jiroveci pneumonia prophylaxis is recommended for patients being treated for GPA and MPA.

F. Indications and Dosing.

1. Rheumatoid arthritis (RA).

a. Indicated for the treatment of adult patients with moderately to severely active rheumatoid arthritis, in combination with MTX, who have had an inadequate response to one or more TNF antagonist therapies.

b. 1000 mg IV, 2 weeks apart, may be repeated every 24 weeks or based on clinical evaluation but no sooner than 16 weeks.

(1) Premedicate with acetaminophen and an antihistamine.

(2) Methylprednisolone IV or equivalent is recommended 30 minutes prior to the infusion to reduce the incidence and severity of infusion reactions.

(3) First infusion: Initiate infusion at 50 mg/hour for 30 minutes, increasing 50 mg /hour every 30 minutes to maximum rate of 400 mg/hour.

(4) Second infusion: Start at 100 mg/hour for 30 minutes increasing 100 mg/hour in 30 minute increments to maximum rate of 400 mg/hour.

(5) If infusion reaction occurs during 1st infusion, the subsequent infusion should be administered at the slower rate of the initial infusion (50 mg/hour increments).

2. Granulomatosis with Polyangiitis (GPA) (Wegener's Granulomatosis) and Microscopic Polyangiitis (MPA).

a. In combination with glucocorticoids.

b. 375 mg/m^2 IV infusion weekly for 4 weeks; infusion rate as listed for RA.

(1) Premedicate with acetaminophen and an antihistamine.

(2) IV glucocorticoids bolus prior to infusing is used in most infusion suites.

G. Dose supplied.

1. 100 mg (10 mL) single-use vials; 500 mg (50 mL) single-use vials.

a. Add to 5% Dextrose in Water or 0.9% Sodium Chloride, using aseptic technique.

b. Withdraw amount of infusion solution equivalent to rituximab to yield 1-4 mg/mL.

c. Use of infusion pump may be beneficial.

V. T-cell costimulation modulator.

A. Mechanism of Action.

1. T cell activation occurs when an antigen is presented to the T-cell receptor on the surface of a T-cell antigen presenting cell (APC).

2. For activation to occur, a second T-cell protein (CD28) must bind with the CD80/86 receptor on the APC to activate the costimulatory signaling pathway.

a. Binding the CD80/86 molecules prevents binding of CD28, thus inhibiting the costimulatory pathway and T-cell activation (Matsumoto, 2006).

B. Agent.

1. Abatacept (Orencia®, Bristol-Myers Squibb, 2013).

a. A soluble fusion protein combining the extracellular domains of 2 CTLA-4 molecules with the Fc portion of human IgG1.

6
6.1
6.2
6.3
6.4
6.5

b. Abatacept binds with CD80/86 preventing the binding of CD28, inhibiting the costimulatory pathway and T-cell activation (Matsumoto, 2006).

C. Box warning(s): None.

D. Pregnancy Category C.

 1. Nursing mothers.

  a. It is not known if abatacept is excreted in human milk or absorbed systemically.

  b. Because of potential for adverse reactions in nursing infants, a decision must be made regarding discontinuation of breastfeeding or discontinuation of the drug.

E. General Guidelines.

 1. Concurrent therapy with TNF antagonists or other biologics is not recommended.

  a. Clinical trials demonstrated higher rates of infection with no additional clinical efficacy when abatacept was used in combination with other biologics.

 2. Hypersensitivity reactions can occur, although the incidence in clinical trials was small;

  a. Monitor for signs and symptoms and be prepared to act accordingly.

 3. Immunization response may be blunted.

 4. Patients with Chronic Obstructive Pulmonary Disease (COPD) should be monitored closely for exacerbation of the disease.

  a. These patients developed adverse events including cough, rhonchi, dyspnea.

 5. The IV preparation contains maltose.

  a. May alter blood glucose monitor readings on the day of infusions.

  b. Patients should discuss this with the healthcare provider and use a monitor that does not react with maltose.

 6. Infuse drug over 30 minutes.

F. Indications and dosing.

 1. Adults with moderately to severely active rheumatoid arthritis.

  a. To reduce signs and symptoms.

  b. Induce major clinical response.

  c. Inhibit the progression of structural damage.

  d. Improve physical function.

  e. May be used with or without concomitant DMARDs.

  f. Intravenous dosing:

   (1) Weight- based dose range; initiating at 0, 2, 4 weeks then every 4 weeks thereafter.

    i) Less than 60 kg: 500 mg.

    ii) 60-100 kg: 750 mg.

    iii) More than 100 kg: 1000 mg (maximum dose).

  g. Subcutaneous dosing:

   (1) Following an IV loading dose (weight-based as above), 125 mg SQ given within a day, then 125 mg SQ weekly.

   (2) If unable to receive IV loading dose, initiate weekly injections.

   (3) If making the transition from IV to SQ, administer first SQ dose instead of next scheduled IV dose.

 2. Patients 6 years of age or older with moderately to severely active juvenile idiopathic arthritis.

  a. To reduce signs and symptoms.

  b. May be used concomitantly with MTX or alone as monotherapy.

  c. Intravenous infusion:

   (1) Pediatric patients weighing less than 75 kg: 10 mg/kg.

   (2) Pediatric patients weighing 75 kg or more: Use adult dosing ranges, not to exceed 1000 mg.

  d. Subcutaneous use in pediatric patients less than 18 years old is not FDA approved.

G. Dose forms and strengths.

 1. Intravenous:

  a. Vials supplied as 250 mg lyophilized powder, single-use.

  b. Reconstitute with 10 mL of sterile water using only the silicone-free disposable syringe provided with each vial.

   (1) After reconstitution the concentration of abatacept will be 25 mg/mL.

(2) Subcutaneous: 125 mg single-dose prefilled glass syringe.

H. Guidelines for use.

1. IV use: If silicone free syringe becomes contaminated, use another from stock.

   a. Do not use vial if vacuum is not present.

   b. Vent vial with needle to eliminate foam.

   c. Concentration of abatacept in IV bag should be no more than 10 mg/mL (100 cc bag).

   d. Fully diluted abatacept solution must be infused within 24°, may be stored at room temperature or refrigerated before use.

2. SC use:

   a. Do not allow the pre-filled syringe to freeze.

   b. Store in original container.

   c. Inspect for particulate matter prior to injecting, discard if not clear, colorless or pale yellow.

   d. Instruct patient to inject the entire contents of the syringe.

   e. Rotate injection sites, avoiding areas that are red, bruised, tender or hard.

   f. Injection site reactions can occur but most were mild to moderate in the clinical trials.

VI. IL-6 receptor inhibitor.

A. Mechanism of Action.

1. IL-6 is highly increased in synovial fluid of patients with rheumatoid arthritis.

2. Correlation between serum and synovial IL-6 levels and disease parameters has been identified (McInnes, Vieira-Sousa, & Fonseca, 2012).

3. Inhibition of IL-6 mediated signaling by binding to IL-6 receptors leads to a reduction in cytokine and acute phase reactant production.

B. Agent.

1. Tocilizumab (Actemra®, Genentech, 2013):

   a. Humanized IL-6 receptor inhibitor.

C. Box warning(s).

1. Increased risk of developing serious, sometimes fatal, infections.

   a. Most of these patients were taking concomitant immunosuppressants such as MTX or corticosteroids.

   b. Tuberculosis (disseminated or extrapulmonary); invasive fungal infections (which may present with disseminated rather than localized disease); opportunistic pathogens.

D. Pregnancy Category C.

1. Nursing mothers.

   a. It is not known if tocilizumab is excreted in human milk or absorbed systemically.

   b. Because of potential for adverse reactions in nursing infants, a decision must be made regarding discontinuation of breastfeeding or discontinuation of the drug.

E. General Guidelines:

1. Screen and monitor for infections as noted in general biologic guidelines.

2. Cases of gastrointestinal perforation have been noted in clinical trials.

   a. Use with caution in patients with a history of diverticulitis.

   b. Patients with new onset of abdominal symptoms should be evaluated promptly.

   c. Instruct patients to report abdominal symptoms and seek medical evaluation.

3. Liver enzyme elevations, low neutrophil count, low platelet count, and lipid elevations were noted during treatment with tocilizumab.

   a. Monitor CBC, lipids, and liver enzymes prior to initiation of therapy.

   b. Patients with low platelet and neutrophil counts should not be given tocilizumab.

   c. These parameters should be monitored every 4-8 weeks.

   d. Patients with liver enzyme elevations greater than 1.5x upper limits of normal (ULN) should not be given drug.

      (1) These enzyme elevations were more pronounced when tocilizumab was used in combination with MTX.

      (2) Discontinuation of therapy is recommended if ALT/AST>than 5x ULN.

      (3) Liver enzymes should be monitored every 4-8 weeks.

6
6.1
6.2
6.3
6.4
6.5

e. Lipid parameters should be monitored prior to starting therapy, approximately 4-8 weeks following initiation, then approximately every 6 months.

   (1) Elevations should be monitored and managed appropriately.

4. Follow general biologic immunization guidelines.

5. Doses exceeding 800 mg are not recommended.

6. May be used in combination with DMARDs or as monotherapy.

7. Tocilizumab should not be given in combination with other biologics.

8. Infusion reactions can occur.

   a. Anaphylaxis was noted in 0.1% of patients in clinical trials.

   b. Nursing staff should be prepared to handle these adverse events (AEs).

9. The most frequently reported AE during the infusion was hypertension.

   a. Within 24 hours of completing an infusion the most reported AEs were headache and skin rashes.

10. In the JIA studies, macrophage activation syndrome (MAS) was noted during clinical trials.

    a. Discontinuation of the drug and treatment resulted in resolution of MAS.

11. Infections were reported more frequently in the elderly.

F. Indications and Dosing:

1. Adult patients with RA who have had an inadequate response to at least one DMARD.

   a. May be used as monotherapy or in combination with DMARDs.

   b. IV: 4 mg/kg starting dose and may increase to 8 mg/kg based on clinical response.

      (1) Infused every 4 weeks, starting with 4 mg/kg, increasing to 8 mg/kg based on clinical response (maximum dose 800 mg).

   c. Subcutaneous dosing:

      (1) Less than 100 kg: 162 mg every other week, increasing to weekly based on clinical response.

(2) More than 100 kg: 162 mg every week.

   d. When transitioning from IV to SC, administer the first SC dose instead of the next scheduled IV dose.

   e. Interruption of dose or reduction from weekly to every other week dosing is recommended for management of certain dose-related laboratory changes (elevated liver enzymes, neutropenia, thrombocytopenia).

2. Patients 2 years of age or older with active systemic juvenile idiopathic arthritis (SJIA);

   a. Patients less than 30 kg: 12 mg/kg every 2 weeks.

   b. Patients at or above 30 kg: 8 mg/kg every 2 weeks.

   c. Used alone or in combination with MTX.

   d. Dose should not be based on a single weight as weight can fluctuate.

   e. Subcutaneous use is not approved for SJIA.

3. Patients 2 years of age or older with active polyarticular juvenile idiopathic arthritis (PJIA).

   a. Patients less than 30 kg: 10 mg/kg every 4 weeks IV.

   b. Patients greater than 30 kg: 8 mg/kg every 4 weeks IV.

   c. Used in alone or in combination with MTX.

   d. Dose should not be based on a single weight as weight can fluctuate.

   e. Subcutaneous use is not approved for PJIA.

G. Dose forms and strengths:

1. Tocilizumab is supplied in single-use vials as a preservative free sterile concentrate solution.

   a. (20 mg/mL) for intravenous infusion:

      (1) 80 mg/4 mL vial.

      (2) 200 mg/10 mL vial.

      (3) 400 mg/20 mL vial.

2. Tocilizumab is supplied for subcutaneous use in a 162 mg preservative free pre-filled syringe.

H. Guidelines for use.

1. For patients less than 30 kg: Dose should be added to 50 mL bag of 0.9% Sodium Chloride.

2. For patients weighing 30 kg or more, dose should be added to 100 mL bag of 0.9% Sodium Chloride.

3. Withdraw volume of IV bag equal to volume of tocilizumab, slowly add medication to IV bag to reduce foaming.

4. Infuse over 60 minutes.

5. Fully diluted tocilizumab may be stored for up to 24° at room temp or in refrigerator protected from light.

6. Use general biologic guidelines.

VII. IL-12 and IL-23 inhibitor.

A. IL-12 and IL-23 are naturally occurring cytokines involved in inflammatory and immune responses.

B. Agent.

1. Ustekinumab (Stelara®, Janssen Biotech, Inc., 2014).

   a. Human IgG1κ monoclonal antibody against the p40 subunit of the IL-12 and IL- 23 cytokines.

   b. Ustekinumab was shown to disrupt IL-12 and IL-23 mediated signaling and cytokine cascades by disrupting the interaction of theses cytokines with a shared cell-surface receptor chain, IL-12Rβ1.

C. Box warning(s): None.

D. Pregnancy Category B.

1. Should be used in pregnancy only if the potential benefit justifies the potential risk to the fetus.

2. Nursing women.

   a. Caution should be exercised when administering ustekinumab to nursing women.

   b. The unknown risks of exposure to ustekinumab should be weighed against the known benefits of breast feeding.

   c. It is not known if ustekinumab is absorbed systemically after ingestion.

E. General Guidelines.

1. Serious infections have occurred; previously identified infection guidelines should be considered.

2. Reversible posterior leukoencephalopathy (RPLS) syndrome has been reported.

   a. If suspected, discontinue ustekinumab and treat appropriately.

3. Monitor for therapeutic effect of warfarin, adjust as needed.

4. Monitor drug concentrations of cyclosporine, adjust dose as needed.

5. BCG vaccines should not be given after drug has been initiated or for one year prior to treatment initiation or one year following discontinuation.

6. Immunization recommendations per CDC guidelines for immunosuppressed individuals.

7. Ustekinumab may increase the risk of malignancy.

F. Indications and dosing.

1. Indicated for the treatment of adults (18 years or older) with active psoriatic arthritis.

2. Can be used alone or in combination with MTX.

3. Dosing:

   a. Recommended dose:

      (1) 45 mg initially, then 4 weeks later, followed by 45 mg every 12 weeks.

      (2) For patients with co-existent moderate-to-severe plaque psoriasis weighing >100 kg (220 lbs.), the recommended dose is 90 mg initially and 4 weeks later, followed by 90 mg every 12 weeks.

4. Dose forms:

   a. 45 mg single use prefilled syringe.

   b. 90 mg single use prefilled syringe.

   c. 45 mg single use vial.

   d. 90 mg single use vial.

G. Guidelines for use.

1. Intended for use under the guidance and supervision of a physician.

2. May be self-administered after appropriate training.

   a. Review medication guide with patient/family.

   b. Have patient demonstrate self-injection technique, providing helpful suggestions as needed.

c. Emphasize importance of communicating with the healthcare provider regarding concerns, infections, concurrent/co-existing illnesses, and the need for follow up visits.

3. The needle cover contains dry natural rubber (a derivative of latex). Latex sensitive patients should not handle needle cover.

4. Rotate injection sites.

VIII. B-lymphocyte stimulator (BLyS)-specific inhibitor.

A. "BLyS (B cell activating factor) stimulates B cell survival, development and differentiation into plasma cells" (Fischer-Betz, Schneider, & Bombardieri, 2012, p. 511).

1. Increased levels of BLyS have been observed in patients with systemic lupus erythematosus.

B. Agent.

1. Belimumab (Benlysta®, GlaxoSmithKline, 2014).

a. A fully humanized monoclonal antibody that binds soluble human BLyS.

C. Boxed Warning: None.

D. Pregnancy Category C.

1. Nursing mothers.

a. It is not known if belimumab is excreted in human milk or absorbed systemically.

b. Because of potential for adverse reactions in nursing infants, a decision must be made regarding discontinuation of breastfeeding or discontinuation of the drug.

E. General Guidelines.

1. Previously identified infection guidelines should be considered.

2. In the controlled period during clinical trials more deaths were reported with belimumab than with placebo.

a. No single cause predominated.

b. The deaths were from infection, cardiovascular disease, and suicide.

3. The risk of malignancy may be increased because of the mechanism of action of belimumab, although no increase in malignancy incidence was identified during clinical trials involving belimumab vs. placebo.

4. Hypersensitivity reactions/infusion reactions have been reported.

a. Patients should be informed as to the possibility of hypersensitivity/infusion reactions occurring post infusion.

b. Patients should be prepared to seek medical attention as needed.

c. Because of the overlapping symptoms it was not possible to distinguish between hypersensitivity and infusion reactions.

5. Psychiatric events such as depression, insomnia, and anxiety were observed during clinical trials.

a. Most patients experiencing severe depression or suicidal behavior had a history of depression or psychiatric disorder and were being treated with psychoactive drugs.

b. Patients should be instructed to report worsening depression to the healthcare provider.

6. Live vaccines should not be given for 30 days before or during treatment with belimumab.

7. Belimumab should not be given with other biologics or with IV cyclophosphamide.

8. Not approved for pediatric use.

9. Response rates were lower for African Americans in the clinical trials.

10. During clinical trials of belimumab for patients with systemic lupus erythematosus (SLE) concomitant use of other agents such as corticosteroids, antimalarials, immunomodulatory and immunosuppressive agents (Azathioprine, MTX, Mycophenolate mofetil), statins, and NSAIDs did not affect the pharmacokinetics of belimumab. The reverse has not been evaluated.

11. PML has been identified in users of belimumab. Patients should be made aware of the symptoms and the need to seek medical attention.

F. Dose and indications.

1. Belimumab is indicated for the treatment of adult patients with active, autoantibody positive SLE who are receiving standard therapy.

a. This agent has not been studied in patients with severe active lupus nephritis or severe active central nervous system lupus.

b. 10 mg/kg at 2 week intervals for the first 3 doses then every 4 weeks thereafter.

c. Administer as an IV infusion only in 250 mL of 0.9% Sodium Chloride, over 1 hour.

G. Dose forms and strengths:

1. Lyophilized powder in single-use vials.

   a. 120 mg vial (dilute with 1.5 mL sterile water).

   b. 400 mg vial (dilute with 4.8 mL sterile water).

   c. Diluted drug yields 80 mg/mL.

H. Guidelines for use.

1. Bring to room temp before reconstituting.

2. Reconstitution may take more than 30 minutes to complete.

3. Swirl gently for 60 seconds every 5 minutes after diluting with sterile water.

   a. Do not exceed 500rpm if using a mechanical reconstitution device (swirler).

4. Once added to IV fluid, infuse over 1 hour.

5. Premedication should be considered to lower the risk of infusion reactions (per facility protocol).

6. Belimumab should be infused within 8 hours of reconstitution.

   a. If not used immediately may be stored at room temp or refrigerated.

   b. Protect from light.

7. Do not infuse concomitantly in the same IV line as other agents.

IX. Janus Kinase (JAK) inhibitor.

A. JAKs are intracellular enzymes that transmit signals from cytokine or growth factor-receptor interactions to influence cellular processes of hematopoesis and immune cell function.

1. Within the signaling pathway, JAKs phosphorylate and activate Signal Transducers and Activators of Transcription (STATs) which modulate intracellular activity.

B. Agent.

1. Tofacitinib (Xeljanz®, Pfizer, 2012).

   a. Modulates signaling pathway at the point of JAKs, preventing the phosphorylation and activation of STATs.

C. Box warning(s):

1. Increased risk of serious infections may lead to hospitalization or death.

   a. Tuberculosis (disseminated or extrapulmonary), invasive fungal infections (such as histoplasmosis, candidiasis), bacterial, viral, and other opportunistic infections including Legionella and Listeria.

2. Lymphoma and other malignancies have been observed.

   a. Epstein-Barr Virus-associated post transplant lymphoproliferative disorder has been observed in renal transplant patients being treated with tofacitinib and concomitant immunosuppressive medications.

D. Pregnancy Category C.

1. Nursing mothers.

   a. It is not known if tofacitinib is excreted in human milk or absorbed systemically.

   b. Because of potential for adverse reactions in nursing infants, a decision must be made regarding discontinuation of breastfeeding or discontinuation of the drug.

E. General Guidelines.

1. This is the first oral biologic to receive FDA approval.

2. Should not be used in patients with hepatic impairment.

3. It should not be initiated in patients with low neutrophil or low lymphocyte count, or with hemoglobin level less than 9 g/dl.

4. Patients should be screened for latent tuberculosis (LTB) and for hepatitis B (HBV) and hepatitis C (HCV) prior to initiation of drug, and periodically throughout treatment.

5. Patients should be screened for infection of any kind while on tofacitinib.

a. The most common serious infections reported included pneumonia, cellulitis, herpes zoster, and urinary tract infections.

b. Opportunistic infections noted were tuberculosis and other mycobacterial infections, cryptococcus, esophageal candidiasis, pneumocystosis, multidermatomal herpes zoster, cytomegalovirus, and BK virus.

6. General infection guidelines should be followed.

7. Concomitant use of immunomodulating agents (MTX, corticosteroids) increases the risk of infection.

8. Follow recommended guidelines for current immunizations.

9. Solid cancers and lymphoma have been reported in patients taking tofacitinib.

10. Gastrointestinal perforation has been reported.

a. Caution should be used in patients with diverticulitis or other GI disorders.

b. Patients should report new onset acute abdominal symptoms and seek medical attention.

11. Laboratory monitoring.

a. Lymphocyte count at initiation and every 3 months thereafter.

b. Neutrophils at baseline, after 4-8 weeks of treatment, then every 3 months after.

c. Hemoglobin at baseline, after 4-8 weeks of treatment, then every 3 months.

d. Liver enzymes (elevations have been reported, mostly with background DMARDs (MTX)).

e. Lipid profile at baseline, 4-8 weeks after initiation, then periodically (manage elevations according to guidelines).

f. Serum creatinine.

(1) Dose related elevations were reported.

(2) Clinical significance is unknown.

12. Most common reported adverse events in the clinical trials were diarrhea, nasopharyngitis, upper respiratory tract infections, headache, hypertension.

13. Caution should be used when treating the elderly as they experienced higher rate of infection than those younger than 65 years of age.

14. Dose adjustments may be necessary for moderate hepatic impairment and for moderate to severe renal impairment.

F. Indications and dosing:

1. Indicated for the treatment of adult patients with moderately to severely active rheumatoid arthritis (RA) who have had an inadequate response to or intolerance to MTX.

a. May be used as monotherapy or in combination with MTX or other non- biologic DMARD.

b. 5 mg twice daily, with or without food.

G. Dose forms and strengths:

1. 5 mg tablet; white round, immediate-release film-coated tablet.

a. Embossed with "Pfizer" on one side and "JKI 5" on the other.

X. RANKL inhibitor:

A. Mechanism of Action.

1. RANKL binds to RANK, a receptor on osteoclast membranes, inducing differentiation, activation and survival of osteoclasts.

2. The soluble cytokine osteoprotegerin (OPG) functions as a decoy receptor by competing for binding to RANK.

B. Agent.

1. Denosumab (Prolia®, Amgen, 2010-2012).

a. A fully human monoclonal antibody that inhibits RANKL (receptor activator of nuclear factor κB ligand, a member of the TNF family) (Biver, Costet, & Adami, 2012), a potent stimulator of osteoclasts.

b. It binds selectively and with high affinity to RANKL.

c. Denosumab mimics the effect of OPG on RANKL (Bijlsma).

C. Box warning(s): None.

D. Pregnancy Category X.

6
6.1
6.2
6.3
6.4
6.5

1. Nursing mothers.

    a. It is not known if denosumab is excreted in human milk or absorbed systemically.

    b. Because of potential for adverse reactions in nursing infants, a decision must be made regarding discontinuation of breastfeeding or discontinuation of the drug.

E. General Guidelines.

1. Denosumab is also available as a treatment for bone metastases (oncology) under the brand name Xgeva® (Amgen, 2010-2012). Patients receiving Xgeva® should NOT receive Prolia®.

2. Hypocalcemia must be corrected before initiating denosumab.

    a. Hypocalcemia may worsen in patients with renal impairment.

    b. In patients pre-disposed to hypocalcemia (i.e., with history of hypoparathyroidism, thyroid surgery, parathyroid surgery, malabsorption syndromes, excision of the small intestine, severe renal impairment, and those receiving renal dialysis), clinical monitoring is highly recommended.

3. Serious infections were reported: Skin, abdomen, urinary tract, and the ear.

    a. Endocarditis was reported more often with denosumab than with placebo in clinical trials.

    b. Opportunistic infections were similar in both groups (denosumab/placebo).

    c. Patients on concomitant immunosuppressants or with compromised immune systems may be more at risk for infections.

    d. Patients should seek medical attention for infections and report these to the prescribing healthcare provider.

4. Epidermal and dermal adverse events not specific to injection sites: Dermatitis, eczema, rash.

5. Osteonecrosis of the jaw (ONJ) can occur spontaneously but is generally associated with tooth extraction and/ or local infection with delayed healing.

    a. Patients should have dental screening and preventive dental care prior to initiating denosumab.

    b. Risk factors that may lead to ONJ are tooth extraction, dental implants, oral surgery, poor oral hygiene, cancer, concomitant therapies (chemotherapy, corticosteroids), ill fitting dentures, and preexisting dental disease.

    c. Clinical judgment regarding management of patients requiring invasive dental procedures should include risk/benefit assessment.

6. Atypical femoral fractures (low-energy, low trauma) have been reported.

    a. Causality has not been established.

    b. Patients should report new or unusual thigh (dull, aching thigh pain), hip, or groin pain.

    c. Bilateral fractures have been reported; therefore, consider evaluation of incomplete fracture of the contralateral limb if indicated.

7. Significant suppression of bone remodeling has been noted in clinical trials of postmenopausal women.

    a. The consequences of this finding may contribute to ONJ, atypical femoral fractures, and delayed fracture healing.

    b. Patients should be monitored for this.

F. Indications and Dosing.

1. Postmenopausal women with osteoporosis at high risk for fracture.

    a. High risk is defined as history of osteoporotic fracture, multiple risk factors, those who have not responded to or are intolerant of other available osteoporosis treatments.

    b. Denosumab reduces the incidence of vertebral, non-vertebral, and hip fractures.

2. Men with osteoporosis at high risk of fracture (to increase bone mass).

3. Men receiving androgen deprivation therapy for prostate cancer.

    a. Denosumab reduced the incidence of vertebral fractures at 3 years.

    b. Treatment significantly increased bone mineral density (BMD) at 24 months.

4. Women at high risk of fracture receiving adjunctive aromatase therapy for breast cancer (to increase bone mass).

a. BMD improvement was seen at the lumbar spine, total hip, and femoral neck in the patients treated with denosumab compared to those treated with placebo at 2 years.

5. Doses for all indications.

a. 60 mg sq once every 6 months, administered by a healthcare professional.

b. Treatment duration has not been established.

G. Dose Form.

1. 60 mg/mL in a single-use prefilled syringe.

2. 60 mg/mL in a single-use vial.

H. Guidelines.

1. If using single-use vial, administer 1 mL (60 mg) with 27-gauge needle.

2. The prefilled syringe has a safety guard to prevent accidental needle sticks, activate by sliding over the needle after the injection.

3. Administer missed dose as soon as convenient.

4. Store in refrigerator; bring to room temperature before administering.

5. Visually inspect for particulate/color; discard if discolored, cloudy, or if the solution contains particulate matter.

6. People with latex sensitivity should not handle the gray needle cover on the syringe.

7. Clinical trials in men included 120 men in the placebo group and 120 men in the denosumab group.

a. Reported AEs for the denosumab group > placebo: Back pain, arthralgia, nasopharyngitis.

b. No serious infections were reported.

c. No ONJ was reported.

d. Epidermal and dermal reactions: 4.2% (5 patients).

e. Pancreatitis: 1 patient each group.

f. New malignancies in the denosumab group: (3 prostate CA, 1 basal cell carcinoma); none in the placebo group.

XI. Uricase.

A. Mechanism of Action.

1. Uricase degrades uric acid to allantoin which is soluble and can be disposed of easily.

B. Agent.

1. Pegloticase (Krystexxa®, Savient Pharmaceuticals, 2012).

a. A recombinant uricase.

(1) Pegylated (to reduce immunogenicity and increase the half life of the drug).

(2) Achieves its therapeutic effect by catalyzing the oxidation of uric acid to allantoin, thereby lowering the serum uric acid (SUA).

(3) Allantoin is an inert and water soluble purine metabolite that is readily eliminated primarily by renal excretion.

C. Box warning(s).

1. Anaphylaxis and infusion reactions have occurred during and after administration.

a. Anaphylaxis usually occurs within 2 hours of administration, but delayed hypersensitivity reactions have been reported.

b. Administer in healthcare setting prepared to manage anaphylaxis and infusion reactions.

c. Premedicate with antihistamines and corticosteroids.

d. Monitor for an appropriate amount of time after the administration.

2. Monitor serum uric acid levels (SUA) prior to infusions; consider discontinuing treatment if levels increase to above 6 mg/dL, particularly when 2 consecutive levels above 6 mg/dL are observed.

D. Pregnancy Category C.

1. Nursing mothers.

a. It is not known if pegloticase is excreted in human milk or absorbed systemically.

b. Because of potential for adverse reactions in nursing infants, it is not recommended to administer pegloticase to a nursing mother.

6
6.1
6.2
6.3
6.4
6.5

E. General Guidelines.

1. Do not administer as IV push or bolus.

2. Before starting pegloticase, discontinue and do not restart oral urate-lowering agents while on therapy.

3. Premedicate with antihistamines and corticosteroids.

4. Administer over no less than 120 minutes.

   a. Observe for additional hour post-infusion.

5. If infusion reaction occurs, slow or stop infusion and restart at a slower rate, at the discretion of the physician or the facility protocol.

6. Contraindicated for patients with Glucose-6-phosphate dehydrogenase (G6DP) deficiency due to risk of hemolysis and methemoglobinemia.

   a. Patients at higher risk for G6DP deficiency (African or Mediterranean ancestry) should be screened prior to receiving pegloticase.

7. Because of the risk of delayed hypersensitivity reactions patients should be informed of signs and symptoms and advised to seek immediate medical attention if these occur.

8. Anaphylaxis is increased if SUA levels rise to above 6 mg/dL, particularly for 2 consecutive levels.

9. Reinforce the discontinuation of urate-lowering agents (this may blunt the rise in SUA).

10. Gout flares may occur due to the changing SUA levels resulting in the mobilization of urate from tissue deposits.

    a. Gout flare prophylaxis is recommended with NSAIDs or colchicine at least 1 week prior to initiating pegloticase, and continuing for at least 6 months, unless contraindicated or not tolerated.

    b. The gout flare should be managed concurrently as appropriate for each patient.

11. Use caution in patients with congestive heart failure; monitor carefully.

12. Gout flare and infusion reactions were the most common AEs during the clinical trials.

13. Immunogenicity:

    a. High anti-pegloticase antibody titers were associated with a failure to maintain pegloticase-induced normalization of uric acid.

    b. These patients also had a higher incidence of infusion reactions.

    c. Patients receiving re-treatment after a longer than 4 week interval should be monitored closely for anaphylaxis and infusion reactions.

14. Not recommended for patients less than 18 years of age.

15. No differences were seen in safety or efficacy between younger and older patients.

F. Indications and dosing.

1. Pegloticase is indicated for the treatment of chronic gout in adult patients refractory to conventional therapy (patients whose uric acid levels have failed to normalize and whose signs and symptoms are inadequately controlled with maximum medically appropriate doses of xanthine oxidase inhibitors or for whom these drugs are contraindicated).

2. Not recommended for asymptomatic hyperuricemia.

3. Dose: 8 mg as infusion every 2 weeks; optimal treatment duration has not been established.

G. Drug form.

1. Single-use 2 mL glass vial with a Teflon coated (latex free) rubber injection stopper:

   a. 8 mg pegloticase in 1 mL, discard excess.

H. Guidelines.

1. Infuse using 250 mL of 0.9% or 0.45% Sodium Chloride.

2. Do not mix or dilute with other drugs.

3. Do not shake.

4. Use within 4 hours of dilution; but dilution may be stored in refrigerator, protected from light (use within 4 hours).

5. Never subject pegloticase in the vial or as mixture to artificial heating.

6. Infuse at room temperature.

XII. Phosphodiesterase 4 (PDE4) Inhibitor.

A. Mechanism of Action.

1. Inhibits PDE4 specific for cyclic adenosine monophosphate (cAMP) resulting in increased intracellular cAMP levels.

B. Agent.

1. Apremilast (Otezla®, Celgene Corporation, 2014).

   a. The specific mechanism by which apremilast exerts its therapeutic action is not well defined.

   b. Oral small molecule inhibitor of PDE4.

C. Box warning(s): None.

D. Pregnancy Category C.

1. It is not known if apremilast or its metabolites are present in human milk.

2. Caution should be exercised when administered to a nursing mother.

3. Should be used during pregnancy only if the potential benefit justifies the potential risk to the fetus.

E. General guidelines.

1. Can be administered without regard to meals.

2. Do not crush, split or chew the tablets.

3. Treatment with apremilast has been associated with increase in adverse reactions of depression.

   a. Patients, caregivers should be alert to the signs for the emergence of worsening depression, suicidal thoughts or other mood changes.

   b. Alert healthcare provider if these occur.

4. Weight loss of up to 10% of body weight.

   a. Regularly weigh patients.

   b. Evaluate weight loss. Discontinue apremilast if clinically warranted.

5. The use of cytochrome P450 enzyme inducers (rifampin, phenobarbital, carbamazepine, phenytoin) is not recommended.

   a. Co-administration of these agents may result in loss of efficacy of apremilast.

6. The most commonly reported adverse reactions are diarrhea, nausea, and headache.

   a. These tended to get better over time with continued dosing.

7. The dose should be reduced in patients with severe renal impairment.

8. No dose adjustment is required in patients with moderate to severe hepatic impairment.

9. No significant pharmacokinetic interactions were observed when administered with either oral contraception, ketoconazole, or MTX.

F. Indications and Dosing.

1. Indicated for the treatment of adult patients with active psoriatic arthritis; adults with plaque psoriasis.

2. Oral dosing: (attempt to minimize GI symptoms during initiation of therapy).

   a. Day 1: 10 mg.

   b. Day 2: 10 mg AM and PM.

   c. Day 3: 10 mg AM, 20 mg PM.

   d. Day 4: 20 mg AM and PM.

   e. Day 5: 20 mg AM, 30 mg PM.

   f. Day 6 and thereafter: 30 mg AM and PM.

G. Dose Forms.

1. 2 week starter pack: Contains 10 mg, 20 mg, 30 mg tablets in a blister pack.

   a. 10 mg tablets are pink, engraved with APR on one side, 10 on the other.

   b. 20 mg tablets are brown, engraved with APR on one side, 20 on the other.

   c. 30 mg tablets are beige, engraved with APR on one side, 30 on the other.

   d. Directions are on the package.

2. 30 mg tablets come in a 14 day blister pack (2 packs per carton) or 60 tablet bottle.

Summary

As of the completion of this chapter, several drugs described above are already in clinical trials for additional indications and/or additional methods of administration. This group of biologic agents will continue to grow and add to the ability to treat individuals with these complex rheumatic diseases. It is incumbent upon the rheumatology nurse to keep abreast of new therapeutic options as they become available.

Table 1: Chart for Indications and Dosing

Drug	Mechanism of Action	Indication	Dosing
Infliximab (Remicade®)	TNF inhibitor	Moderate to severely active RA	3 mg/kg q8wks after induction at 0, 2, 6wks. May increase up to 10 mg/kg as often as q4wks depending on response; given with MTX.
		AS	5 mg/kg q6wks after induction at 0, 2, 6 weeks.
		PsA	5 mg/kg q8wks after induction at 0, 2, 6 weeks; with or without MTX.
Adalimumab (Humira®)	TNF inhibitor	Moderate to severely active RA	40 mg SQ every other week. Some patients with RA not receiving MTX may benefit from increasing the frequency to 40 mg every week.
		Moderate to severely active JIA (Pts. 2 yrs or older based on weight)	10 kg (22 lbs) to <15 kg (33 lbs): 10 mg every other week 15 kg (33 lbs) to < 30 kg (66 lbs): 20 mg every other week ≥ 30 kg (66 lbs): 40 mg every other week
		AS	40 mg SQ every other week.
		PsA	40 mg SQ every other week
Golimumab (Simponi®)	TNF inhibitor	Moderate to severely active RA	50 mg SQ monthly on the same date; with MTX. IV: 2 mg per kg day 0, 28, then every 8 weeks thereafter; with MTX.
		AS	50 mg SQ once monthly.
		PsA	50 mg SQ once monthly; (alone or in combination with MTX).
Certolizumab pegol (Cimzia®)	TNF inhibitor	Moderate to severely active RA	400 mg initially and at Weeks 2 and 4, followed by 200 mg every other week; for maintenance dosing, 400 mg every 4 weeks can be considered.
		PsA	400 mg initially and at week 2 and 4, followed by 200 mg every other week; for maintenance dosing, 400 mg every 4 weeks can be considered.
		AS	400 mg (given as 2 subcutaneous injections of 200 mg each) initially and at weeks 2 and 4, followed by 200 mg every other week or 400 mg every 4 weeks.
		Crohn's Disease	400 mg initially and at Weeks 2 and 4. If response occurs, follow with 400 mg every four weeks.

Table 1: Chart for Indications and Dosing (Continued)

Drug	Mechanism of Action	Indication	Dosing
Etanercept (Enbrel®)	TNF inhibitor	Moderate to severely active RA	50 mg SQ once weekly; with or without MTX.
		JIA (patients 2 years or older)	0.8 mg/kg weekly, with a maximum of 50 mg per week.
		PsA	50 mg SQ once weekly; MTX, NSAIDs, glucocorticoids, salicylates may be continued.
		AS	50 mg SQ once weekly; MTX, NSAIDs, glucocorticoids, salicylates may be continued.
Anakinra (Kineret®)	Interleukin-1 receptor antagonist (IL-1Ra)	RA	100 mg SQ daily (at the same time); alone or in combination with DMARDs.
Ritximab (Rituxan®)	Selective B-cell depletor	RA	1000 mg IV, 2 weeks apart; may repeat q 24 weeks or based on clinical evaluation but no sooner than 16 weeks; with MTX.
		Granulomatosis with Polyangiitis (GPA) (Wegener's Granulomatosis) and Microscopic Polyangiitis (MPA)	375 mg/m² IV weekly for 4 weeks; retreatment regimen has not been established.
Abatacept (Orencia®)	T-cell costimulation modulator	RA	Weight based, initiate at 0, 2, 4 weeks followed by every 4 weeks, IV infusion. <60 kg 500 mg 60-100 kg 750 mg >100 kg 1000 mg (maximum dose) use with or without DMARD's. - or - After IV loading dose (weight based), 125 mg SQ within a day, then 125 mg SQ weekly; may be started at time of next infusion if unable to get loading dose.
		JIA ages 6 and older	Weight based, initiate at 0, 2, 4 weeks then every 4 weeks, IV infusion. <75 kg 10 mg/kg ≥75 kg adult dosing ranges not to exceed 1000 mg; with or without MTX
Tocilizumab (Actemra®)	Interleukin 6 (IL6) receptor inhibitor	RA	4 mg/kg infusion starting, increase to 8 mg/kg based on clinical response; used with or without DMARDs. Dose should not exceed 800 mg. SQ injection: <100 kg, 162 mg every other week, may give weekly. >100 mg kg, 162 mg weekly, with or without DMARDs.
		JIA ages 2 or older	Infusions every 2 weeks <30 kg 12 mg/kg ≥30 kg 8 mg/kg Used with or without MTX. Dose should not exceed 800 mg.

6
6.1
6.2
6.3
6.4
6.5

Table 1: Chart for Indications and Dosing (Continued)

Drug	Mechanism of Action	Indication	Dosing
Belimumab (Benlysta®)	B-lymphocyte stimulator (BLyS-specific) inhibitor	Adults with active autoantibody positive systemic lupus erythematosis (SLE)	10 mg/kg IV at 2 week intervals for the 1st 3 doses then every 4 weeks thereafter.
Ustekinumab (Stelara®)	IL-12 and IL-23 inhibitor	Adults with active psoriatic arthritis	45 mg SQ initially and 4 weeks later, then 45 mg every 12 weeks.
		Adults with PSA and co-existent moderate to severe plaque psoriasis >100 kg	90 mg SQ initially and 4 weeks later, then 90 mg every 12 weeks.
		Adults with moderate to severe plaque psoriasis	≤100 kg: 45 mg SQ initially and 4 weeks later, followed by 45 mg SQ every 12 weeks; >100 kg: 90 mg SQ initially and 4 weeks later, followed by 90 mg every 12 weeks.
Tofacitinib (Xeljanz®)	Janus Kinase (JAK) inhibitor	RA	5 mg, po, twice daily; with or without food; may be used with or without MTX/DMARDs.
Denosumab (Prolia®)	RANKL inhibitor	Post menopausal women with osteoporosis	Same dose for all indications: 60 mg SQ, administered by a healthcare professional, every 6 months.
		Men with osteoporosis at high risk of fracture to increase bone mass	
		Men receiving androgen deprivation therapy for prostate cancer	
		Women at high risk of fracture receiving aromatase therapy for breast cancer to increase bone mass	
Pegloticase (Krystexxa®)	Recombinant uricase	Adults with chronic symptomatic gout refractory to conventional therapy	8 mg IV infusion, every 2 weeks. No optimal treatment duration has been established.
Apremilast (Otezla®)	PDE4 inhibitor	Adults with active psoriatic arthritis; adults with plaque psoriasis	30 mg po twice daily after initial upward titration with starter pack.

References

AbbVie Inc.. (2013). Humira®: Prescribing information. North Chicago, IL: Author.

Amgen Inc. and Pfizer Inc. (2013). Enbrel®: Prescribing information. Thousand Oaks, CA: Author.

Amgen Inc. (2001-2003). Kineret®: Prescribing information. Thousand Oaks, CA: Author.

Amgen Inc. (2010-2012). Prolia®: Prescribing information. Thousand Oaks, CA: Author

Amgen Inc. (2010-2012). Xgeva®: Prescribing information. Thousand Oaks, CA: Author.

Biogen Idec, Inc. and Genentech, Inc. (2013). Rituxan®: Prescribing information. South San Francisco, CA: Author.

Biver, E., Costet, B., & Adami, S. (2012). Osteoporosis: Treatment. In J. Bijlsma (Ed.), *EULAR textbook on rheumatic diseases* (pp. 793-807). London: BMJ Group.

Bristol-Myers Squib Company. (2013). Orencia®: Prescribing information. Princeton, NJ: Author.

Celgene Corporation. (2014). Otexla®: Prescribing information. Summit, NJ: Author.

Fischer-Betz, R., Schneider, M., & Bombardieri, S. (2012). Systemic Lupus Erythematosus: Treatment. In J. Bijlsma (Ed.), *EULAR textbook on rheumatic diseases* (pp. 506-521). London: BMJ Group.

Genentech, Inc. (2013). Actemra®: Prescribing information. South San Francisco, CA: Author.

GlaxoSmithKline. (2014). Benlysta®: Prescribing information. Research Triangle Park, NC: Author.

Janssen Biotech, Inc. (2013). Remicade®: Prescribing information. Horsham, PA: Author.

Janssen Biotech, Inc. (2013a). Remicade®: Prescribing information. Horsham, PA: Author.

Janssen Biotech, Inc. (2013b). Simponi®: Prescribing information. Horsham, PA: Author.

Janssen Biotech, Inc. (2013c). Simponi Aria®: Prescribing information. Horsham, PA: Author.

Janssen Biotech, Inc. (2014). Stelara®: Prescribing information. Horsham, PA: Author.

McInnes, I., Vieira-Sousa, E., & Fonseca, J.E. (2012). Rheumatoid Arthritis: Treatment. In J. Bijlsma (Ed.), *EULAR textbook on Rheumatic Diseases* (pp. 232-254). London: BMJ Group.

Management of Infusion-Based Biologic Therapy in Rheumatoid Arthritis. (2008). *Rheumatology Nurse Newsletter*, 1(2). Philadelphia: The Institute for Continuing Healthcare Education.

Matsumo, A. (2006). Pharmacologic Interventions: Biologic Agents. In S. Bartlett (Ed.). *Clinical care in the rheumatic diseases (*3rd ed., pp 237-241*)*. Atlanta, GA: Association of Rheumatology Health Professionals.

Pfizer. (2012). Xeljanz®: Prescribing information. New York: Author.

Savient Pharmaceuticals, Inc. (2012). Krystexxa®: Prescribing information. Bridgewater, NJ: Author.

UCB, Inc. (2013). Cimzia®: Prescribing information. Smyrna, GA: Author.

6
6.1
6.2
6.3
6.4
6.5

390 CORE CURRICULUM FOR RHEUMATOLOGY NURSING

SECTION 7

RHEUMATOLOGY NURSING ACROSS THE LIFESPAN:
SYSTEMIC CONDITIONS IN PEDIATRICS AND ADULTS

Contents of Section 6

7
7.1
7.2
7.3

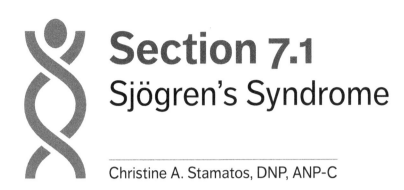

Section 7.1
Sjögren's Syndrome

Christine A. Stamatos, DNP, ANP-C

Introduction

Sjögren's Syndrome is a diverse autoimmune disorder that may exist as a component of systemic lupus or as a disease entity of its own. It is characterized by dysfunction of exocrine glands leading to the classic complaint of dry eyes and dry mouth. However, Sjögren's Syndrome is really a multisystem disorder requiring careful monitoring of each system in order to minimize the daily symptoms and potential complications associated with this condition. In rare instances, Sjögren's Syndrome is associated with a poor prognosis; thus, key characteristics suggesting poor prognosis are presented.

Learning Objectives

Upon completion of this chapter, the nurse will be able to:

1. Describe the pathophysiology associated with Sjögren's syndrome.
2. Distinguish between primary and secondary Sjögren's syndrome.
3. Identify the potential systemic effects seen in primary Sjögren's syndrome.
4. State four clinical findings associated with a poor prognosis.
5. Identify common comorbidities associated with Sjögren's syndrome.
6. List at least three strategies to help patients manage dry eye syndrome.
7. List at least three strategies to help patients manage dry mouth.

7
7.1
7.2
7.3

Content Outline

I. Pathophysiology of Sjögren's Syndrome (pronounced Show-Grins).

A. What is Sjögren's Syndrome?

1. Dr. Henrich Sjögren was the first to describe an association between dry eyes and arthritis. Sjögren's syndrome (SS) refers to a systemic disease in which patients present with dry eyes, dry mouth, and arthritis. Dr. Sjögren also introduced the term "keratoconjunctivitis sicca" to describe the changes characteristic of this syndrome.

2. Key terms:

   a. Keratoconjunctivitis: Term used when inflammation of the cornea and conjunctiva results in dryness of the eye.

   b. Sicca (means dryness): Another term used to describe dry eyes and mouth.

   c. Xeropthalmia: Lacrimal dysfunction results in dry eyes.

   d. Xerostomia: Hyposalivation results in dry mouth.

   e. Dyspareunia: Mucosal dryness causes painful intercourse.

   f. Sialidinitis: Inflammation of salivary glands.

   g. Complement: Proteins produced as a part of the inflammatory process. These proteins increase with acute inflammation but can be low in certain autoimmune conditions when the inflammatory response consumes the proteins.

   h. Cryoglobulins: Proteins found in the blood that precipitate (clump together) in the cold and cause organ damage. Often associated with hepatitis C infection, blood cancers (lymphoma/multiple myeloma), and connective tissue diseases such as lupus.

B. Pathophysiology.

1. A "triggering event" (some kind of physical or emotional stressor/exposure) in a genetically predisposed individual initiates a series of changes activating the immune system which then specifically targets the epithelial cells of the exocrine glands resulting in inflammation, fibrosis, and eventually organ dysfunction. Tissue destruction occurs as lymphocytic infiltration alters organ function. T and B-cell activation triggers numerous inflammatory cytokines: Pro inflammatory (IL1, IL6, TNFα) and anti-inflammatory/ immunosuppressive cytokines (INFy, IL4, IL18). Much of the pathology related to poor outcomes is thought to come from excessive B-cell activation. Through an understanding of these pathological pathways, new treatments are emerging (Mavragani, Voulgarelis, & Moutsopoulos, 2012; Ramos-Casals, Tzioufas, Stone, Siso, & Bosch, 2010).

2. Chronic, slowly progressive, systemic, autoimmune, inflammatory condition characterized by lymphocytic infiltration and eventual dysfunction of the exocrine system. Exocrine glands are responsible primarily for lubrication of eyes and mouth but are also present throughout the gastrointestinal and genitourinary tract. Normal secretory elements are gradually destroyed. Once thought to only affect the exocrine glands, many extraglandular manifestations of SS have been recognized as components of Sjögren's syndrome (Daniels, 2008; Fox, 2011; Tzioufas, Mitsias, & Moutsopoulos, 2011).

II. Primary: Etiology/Epidemiology (remainder of chapter will focus on pSS).

A. Etiology.

1. Precise etiology of Sjögren's syndrome is unknown.

   a. Genetic factors play a role in determining susceptibility. It is an acquired, noncontagious, autoimmune disorder. It is not uncommon to find two or more individuals per family with SS.

   b. There is substantial evidence suggesting a connection with viral infection. Epithelial cells of humans host a variety of viruses which create a chronic local immune response.

   c. Hormonal influence: Reports of as high as 20:1 ratio female to male (Schein et al., 1999). Thought to be related to a drop in estrogen levels with onset between 35-50 years of age.

   d. As with other autoimmune diseases, the genetic predisposition can be turned on with a certain degree of "stress" to the immune system. Many believe physical or emotional stressors may be responsible.

B. Epidemiology.

1. Incidence: One of the most common autoimmune disorders, as frequent as systemic lupus erythematosis (SLE) 1/ 1,000 (Malladi et al., 2012; Mavragani, et al., 2012).

2. Prevalence: 0.5-3% of the population (2-4 million people in the U.S.)(Sanchez-Guerrero et al., 2005). About 60% of all cases are secondary to another connective tissue disease. One study in the US found that out of 2,481 individuals aged 65-84 years, 27% reported either dry eyes or dry mouth (Schein et al., 1999) (note: Sicca symptoms are not always SS). 90% are women between 35-50 years of age, and men generally manifest milder disease (Hernandez-Molina et al., 2010; Malladi et al., 2012; Sanchez-Guerrero et al., 2005; Voulgarelis, Tzioufas, & Moutsopoulos, 2008).

3. Subtypes: Primary (pSS) and Secondary (sSS): The clinical manifestations (see Table 1) of SS are the same in both, but risks of extraglandular involvement is determined by very specific risks associated with pSS and by the underlying connective tissue disease in sSS (Hernandez-Molina et al., 2010).

a. Primary SS is diagnosed in the absence of other connective tissue diseases and is associated with a greater risk of extraglandular involvement described below. Though antibodies are present in both, pSS is more often associated with a positive ANA (70-90%) both anti Ro/ SSA (40-60%), anti La/SSB (20-40%), and a positive rheumatoid factor (60-90%) in the presence of an elevated ESR, hypergammaglobulinemia, and low complement levels (C3, C4), and parotid/salivary gland enlargement (see Figure 1). Because pSS exists in absence of other autoimmune disease, there is often a long delay between onset of initial symptom and diagnosis (average 6.5 years) (Daniels, 2008; Foundation, 2006; Fox, 2011; Hernandez-Molina et al., 2010; Malladi et al., 2012)). Each symptom is individually addressed by different specialists, and the connection is not always appreciated for several years. Patient's with pSS develop non-Hodgkins lymphoma at 40 times the normal rate; nearly 5% of pSS will develop lymphoma (Fox, 2011; Hansen, Lipsky, & Dorner, 2005).

Table 1: Clinical manifestations of primary Sjögren's Syndrome at diagnosis and after a 10-year follow-up

	Prevalence at diagnosis (%)	Prevalence at end of follow-up (%)
Glandular disease		
» Xerostomia	90	92
» Dry eyes	95	95
» Parotid gland enlargement	49	53
Extraglandular disease		
» Arthralgias/arthritis	70	75
» Raynaud phenomenon	41	48
Pulmonary involvement	23	29
Kidney involvement		
» Interstitial nephritis	7	9
» Glomerulonephritis	0.4	2
Liver involvement	4	4
Peripheral neuropathy	1	2
Myositis	1	1
Central nervous system disease	0	0
Lymphoma	2	4

Adapted from M. C. Hochberg, A. J. Silman, J. S. Smolen, M. E. Weinblatt, & M. H. Weisman (Eds.). (2011). *Rheumatology* (5th ed.)[Digital edition]. New York: Elsevier.

7
7.1
7.2
7.3

b. Secondary SS exists in the presence of other connective tissue diseases, most commonly rheumatoid arthritis (50%), Systemic Lupus Erythematosus (SLE) (25%), Polymyositis, Scleroderma (caution, dryness can occur as a result of fibrosis within salivary/lacrimal glands and not actually be a lymphoproliferative process), Thyroiditis, Polyarteritis nodosa, Mixed connective tissue disease, and Primary biliary cirrhosis. Though often less likely to be associated with extraglandular features, neurologic complications appear as frequently in sSS as pSS (Hernandez-Molina et al., 2010).

4. Prognosis:

a. Primary SS: Slowly progresses with serologic findings remaining stable over time. When compared to age matched healthy controls, mortality was only increased in those patients with adverse predictors (Garcia-Carrasco et al., 2002; Hansen et al., 2005; Malladi et al., 2012; Sanchez-Guerrero et al., 2005; Voulgarelis et al., 2008).

b. Presence of both anti-Ro/SSA and La/SSB is associated with earlier disease onset, longer disease duration, recurrent parotid gland enlargement, splenomegaly, lymphadenopathy and vasculitis.

c. Significant adverse predictors:

(1) Elevated ESR.

(2) Anemia and leukopenia.

(3) Hypocomplementemia: Low C4.

(4) Hypergammaglobulinemia.

(5) Recurrent parotid enlargement (90%).

(6) Cyroglobulinemia.

(7) Vasculitis: Palpable purpura (see Figure 2).

III. Nursing assessment: Multisystem involvement *(see Figure 3).*

A. Dry eyes: Often insidious sensation of foreign body "gritty/ sandy," worse at end of day and upon rising with ropelike strands along inside corner; redness, especially toward end of the day; difficulty seeing clearly; inability to tear (strongest association with keratoconjunctivitis sicca-KCS), requiring tear supplements more than 3x daily (see Figure 4).

1. Complications: Corneal abrasions/ ulcerations/ infections.

a. Corneal abrasions.

b. Blepharitis (inflammation of eyelash follicles) common and often chronic. Thick, tenacious secretions, use of thick ophthalmic ointments, and chronic infection itself causes plugging of glands.

2. Pay particular attention to other causes of dry eyes:

a. Medications: Hundreds of agents.

b. Ophthalmologic procedures:

Figure 1: Marked bilateral parotid gland enlargement in a patient with primary Sjögren syndrome. Sicca syndrome is a common clinical finding.

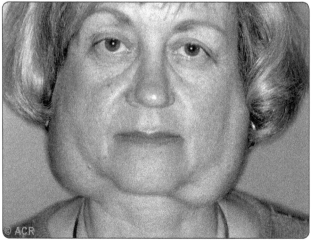

Source: © 2014 American College of Rheumatology. Used with permission.

Figure 2: Palpable purpura: Lukocytoclastic vasculitis.

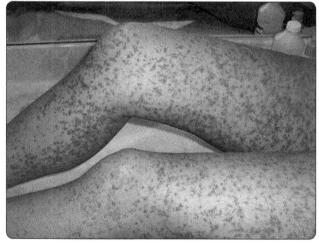

Source: © 2014 American College of Rheumatology. Used with permission.

7
7.1
7.2
7.3

(1) Lasik surgery: Affects nerves responsible for lacrimation.

(2) Botox injections: Directly causes keratoconjunctivitis.

(3) Eyelid "lift": May alter tearing lower lid and creates unprotected zones of the eye at rest.

c. Environment: Pay particular attention when traveling.

B. Dry mouth: Hyposalivation leads to dry mouth, dysphagia, poor taste, burning, painful mouth (decreased volume and increased thickness of saliva).

1. Questions for assessment:

   a. Do you have to drink water at night?

   b. Can you eat a cracker without a drink?

   c. Do you have difficulty swallowing or become easily choked?

   d. Have you had a recent increase in dental decay?

   e. Have you noticed a change in the way food tastes?

Figure 3: Multisystem presentation of "Ways Sjögren's syndrome may affect the body." Source: Sjögren's Syndrome Foundation.

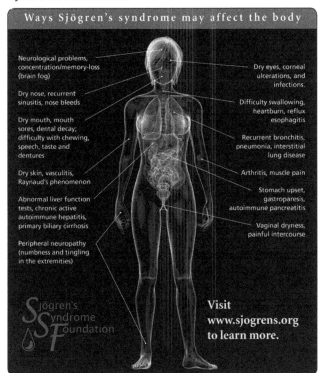

Source: www.Sjogrens.org Reprinted with permission

2. Complications.

   a. Oral candidiasis: (30-70%) especially following use of glucocorticoids and or antibiotics. Presents as diffuse painful erythema (red, beefy tongue), petechiae on hard palate, and cheilitis (dry cracked skin at corners of mouth).

   b. Dental caries at the gingival margins (gumline).

   c. Lichen planus-like changes: White plaque formation on hard palate and buccal recesses.

   d. Parotid/ salivary gland enlargement (can be seen in both primary and secondary but is associated with risk of developing B cell lymphoma pSS) (see Figure 1).

3. Pay particular attention to other causes of dry mouth.

   a. The most common cause is medications. Hundreds of drugs have capacity to cause "dry mouth." (http://www.essology.com/PDF/DryMouthMedications.pdf).

   b. Other diseases: Amyloidosis, sarcoidosis, lipoproteinemias.

      (1) Antibodies will be negative for Ro/La.

      (2) Salivary gland biopsy is essential for differentiation.

   c. Anxiety/ depression.

   d. Mouth breathing.

   e. Head and neck radiation.

C. Other areas of dryness:

   1. Nose: Dry, irritated, congested sensation.

Figure 4: Keratoconjunctivitis with Rose Bengal Staining

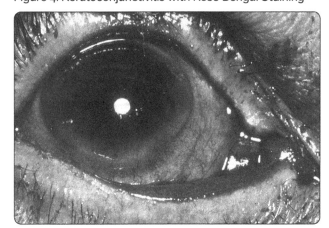

Source: © 2014 American College of Rheumatology. Used with permission.

2. Ears: Increased pressure, dulled hearing, fullness, vertigo, itching.

3. Skin: Dry, pruritic.

4. Vaginal: Can be painful, especially during intercourse.

D. Arthralgias/arthritis (60-70%): Inflammatory, non-erosive arthritis characterized by intermittent bouts of spontaneous swelling which most often resolves on its own. Though it is not erosive, it can lead to hand deformities called Jaccoud's arthropathy (see Figure 5). If erosions are suspected, consider sSS related to Rheumatoid Arthritis.

E. Pulmonary (20-70%):

1. Upper airway (50-70%): Nose bleeds, sneezing, sinus irritation, and posterior pharynx irritation leads to dry persistent/ irritating cough. Bronchial dryness promotes plug formation and recurrent respiratory infections. Caution with acute infections, this is when plugs occur and are made worse with decongestants containing anticholinergics (these should be avoided).

2. Lower airway (9%): Interstitial lung disease is possible but rare; described as "ground glass changes" on CT scan of chest with associated change in diffusion capacity as measured by PFTs.

F. Gastrointestinal (30-35%):

1. Upper: Dysphagia can lead to gastroesophageal reflux (frequent clearing

Figure 5: Jaccoud's arthopathy. Note lack of erosions but significant deformity; on exam these deformities would be reproducible.

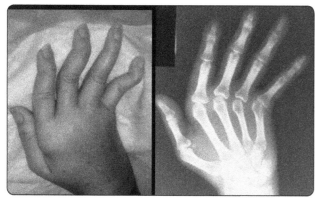

Source: © 2014 American College of Rheumatology. Used with permission.

throat or unexplained hoarseness) resulting in chronic esophagitis/ gastritis.

2. Liver (5-10%): In presence of liver dysfunction:

a. Consider hepatitis C either as the reason for sicca symptoms or as a trigger for SS (both sSS and pSS). Though cryoglobulinemia, hypocomplementemia, and sicca are associated with SS, these same symptoms are found in acute hepatitis C infections.

b. 25% of pSS have hepatomegaly and anti-mitochondrial antibodies (related to Primary Biliary Cirrhosis) with 70% of these patients presenting with elevated liver functions.

3. Pancreatitis (2%): Although asymptomatic, elevated amylase levels can be seen 25% of the time; rarely does this result in acute/ chronic pancreatitis.

G. Endocrine (30-70%):

1. 50% of pSS present with anti-thyroid antibodies and signs of altered thyroid function related to autoimmune thyroid disease (Hashimoto's thyroiditis or Graves disease). Need to be sure thyroid function is normal.

2. Estrogen deficiency: Thought to be a trigger for disease.

3. Cortisol levels low: Contributes to profound fatigue.

H. Genitourinary (10-15%): Can present as any of several renal disorders.

1. Renal tubular acidosis (5-33%): Low serum potassium, high chloride levels, acidic serum/ basic urine; kidney stones common.

2. Interstitial nephritis (rare- early).

3. Glomerulonephritis (rare- late).

4. Suspicious urinalysis:

a. Hematuria.

b. Proteinuria.

c. Casts: Red/white/epithelial cell casts (hyaline casts are usually not a problem).

5. Interstitial cystitis: Lymphoproliferation throughout the bladder leads to sense of urgency, irritation, nocturia, and suprapubic discomfort.

6. Dyspareunia: Painful intercourse due to vaginal dryness (can be severe).

I. Cutaneous: Dry, itchy skin not uncommon.

1. Raynaud's common but not usually associated with ischemic changes.

2. Purpura (see Vasculitis).

3. Subacute cutaneous SLE common with ant-Ro/ SSA antibodies.

   a. Annular/ psoriaform, highly photosensitive rash.

   b. Discoid lupus.

J. Muscle (1-2%): Many patients experience significant myalgias but only rarely are muscle enzymes elevated. Myositis is very rare.

K. Neurologic (10-38%):

1. Peripheral neuropathy (2-38%) "glove & stocking" distribution bilaterally can precede diagnosis by as much as 10 years. Workup for neuropathy otherwise unremarkable.

2. Central nervous system: In addition to chronic asymmetric, paresthesias, numbness, and motor defects; seizures, movement disorders, diffuse brain injury, cognitive dysfunction, dementia, transverse myelopathy has also been seen. Symptoms can mimic Multiple Sclerosis (MS). It is important to note that a + ANA is rarely seen with MS (< 20%) equal to the number of people in the general population with a + ANA (1:5) (Ferreira, D'Cruz, & Hughes, 2005; Tourbah et al., 1998).

3. Sensory deficits may also be accompanied by autonomic neuropathy (a group of symptoms that occur when there is damage to the nerves that manage every day body functions such as blood pressure, heart rate, bowel and bladder emptying, and digestion). This can be very disruptive and significantly influence quality of life.

L. Vascular:

1. Raynaud's (35-40%): Usually precedes sicca symptoms by many years and is mild in nature especially compared to that seen in systemic sclerosis. It is unlikely to be associated with vascular complications and less than 40% require pharmacologic management.

2. Vasculitis (5-10%) presents as palpable purpura (see Figure 2). More common when there is a positive anti-Ro/SSA and La/SSB antibody, Rheumatoid factor, cyroglobulinemia, hypergammablobulinemia, and low complement levels. Lesions may ulcerate and can be painful.

M. Lymphoproliferative disease (5%): 44 x higher relative risk than age, sex, race matched normal controls. Non-Hodgkin's, B-cell origin, lymphoma.

1. Risk factors:

   a. Persistent unilateral or bilateral parotid enlargement.

   b. Splenomegaly and lymphadenopathy.

   c. Low complement levels and cyroglobulinemia.

2. Presentation:

   a. Fever/chills/drenching night sweats.

   b. Fatigue, profound.

   c. Weight loss, decreased appetite.

   d. Lymphadenopathy.

   e. Pancytopenia.

N. Pregnancy: Neonatal Lupus (1-2%) associated with high titer anti-Ro/SSA antibody.

1. Passive acquired autoimmunity.

2. Similar pregnancy outcomes except nearly 4% risk of child experiencing congenital heart block (most often third degree). Should be followed by high risk obstetrician.

3. Mortality rate for the child is 20% with most requiring pacing.

4. Newborn experiences cutaneous manifestations (erythematous, annular lesions affecting eyes, face, and scalp) associated with photosensitivity. Rash resolves within six months as the autoantibodies disappear from the neonatal circulation.

IV. Diagnosis.

A. Dry eye: "Kerotoconjunctivitis Sicca."

1. Symptoms: Red (conjunctival injection), irritated, dry, gritty sensation, itching, photophobia (pain with light exposure).

2. Diagnosis: Assess degree of dryness and presence of corneal irritation.

   a. Schirmer tear test: Strips of filter paper placed in the lid and degree of wetting is measured over 5 minutes (< 5 mm is abnormal).

   b. Rose Bengal Test: Slit lamp exam to detect disruption and devitalized tissue resulting from dryness. Confirms KCS.

3. Differential (53% of dry eye symptoms are associated with isolated ocular symptoms and not SS (primary or secondary).

   a. Medications: Careful assessment.

   b. Ocular cosmetic procedures can exacerbate SS and contribute to dry eye.

     (1) Blepharoplasty (eyelid "lift")

     (2) Lasik surgery.

     (3) Botox injections.

B. Dry mouth.

1. Symptoms: Severe dryness, dysphagia, burning mouth, dental caries.

2. Diagnosis: Symptoms correlate poorly with actual salivary flow rates.

   a. Salivary flow rates (sialometry): Stimulated and unstimulated "spit test" literally measures amount of saliva in 15 minutes (amount varies and abnormal values differ based on test; an abnormal study alone does not confirm SS).

   b. Scintography measures functional activity of salivary glands.

   c. MRI of salivary/parotid glands: Ductal and microvascular changes identified.

   d. Minor salivary gland biopsy: Cornerstone for diagnosis of SS and important to differentiate autoimmune SS from other causes of sicca symptoms (Amyloidosis, Sarcoidosis, infection, malignancy, stones).

3. Differential.

   a. Hundreds of drugs cause "dry mouth." (http://208.109.74.42 /media/ Dry Mouth Medications.pdf).

   b. Other diseases: Amyloidosis, sarcoidosis, lipoproteinemias. Antibodies will be negative for Ro/La.

   c. Anxiety/depression.

   d. Mouth breathing.

e. Head and neck radiation.

C. Laboratory assessment.

1. Autoantibodies.

2. ANA (70-90%) usually in titer at or above 1:320.

3. Anti-Ro/ SSA (40-60%).

4. Anti-La/ SSB (20-40%).

5. Rheumatoid factor (60-90%).

6. Thyroid antibodies: Antithyroglobulin & thyroid peroxidase.

7. Autoimmune liver antibodies:

   a. Antimitochondrial.

   b. Antimicrosomal. (Muratori, Granito, Muratori, Pappas, & Bianchi, 2008).

8. Other:

   a. Anti Sm/RNP/ ribosomal P, dsDNA/ anticardiolipin/ B2 glycoprotien may be seen with SLE.

   b. Anti Scl70 or anticentromere with scleroderma.

   c. Anti-Jo1 with myositis (and more).

9. Hypergammaglobulinemia.

   a. Serum protein electrophoresis.

   b. Quantitative immunoglobulin levels.

10. Changes in CBC.

   a. Anemia: Chronic disease, responds to control of inflammation.

   b. Leukopenia: Poor prognostic finding.

   c. Thrombocytopenia: Rarely seen.

11. Acute phase reactants: ESR vs. CRP.

   a. ESR vs. CRP.

     (1) ESR often elevated.

     (2) CRP rarely elevated unless infection present.

   b. Complement levels: C3 & C4.

     (1) Elevated levels associated with inflammation.

     (2) Low levels associated with poor prognosis.

   c. Thrombocytosis: Rises with acute inflammation.

12. Cryoglobulinemia (30%): Especially with vasculitis and/or lymphoma. Be aware that SS and cryoglobulinemia are also seen in hepatitis C, which can trigger SS (Hansen et al., 2005).

13. Metabolic profile to include urinalysis: Monitor for renal and hepatic involvement.

14. Consider pancreatic enzymes in presence of persistent abdominal complaints: Abdominal pain, nausea/vomiting, early satiety, bloating, change in bowel regimen.

D. Other diagnostic studies dictated by symptom presentation.

  1. Pulmonary evaluation:

    a. Pulmonary function tests as needed.

    b. High resolution chest CT scan: Presents with dry cough, dyspnea at rest, or change in exercise tolerance.

  2. Neurologic studies:

    a. NCS/EMG: Presence of paresthesias, numbness, motor defect.

    b. MRI brain if multiple sclerosis suspected.

    c. Cerebrospinal fluid assessment in rare instances.

  3. Gastrointestinal:

    a. Motility studies.

    b. Endoscopy/colonoscopy.

    c. Abdominal scans as dictated by other findings.

  4. Lymphoproliferative evaluation:

    a. PET scan.

    b. Bone marrow biopsy.

V. Treatment: Important to have "team" of providers based on presentation.

A. Dryness, pain, and fatigue nearly universal, while systemic involvement occurs 20-40% of the time. Treatment is aimed at modifying symptoms and routinely monitoring and treating systemic involvement as needed (Ramos-Casals et al., 2010).

B. Symptomatic.

  1. Topical (Fox, 2011).

    a. Eyes: All patients must be followed closely by ophthalmology.

(1) Natural tears supplements must be preservative free.

(2) Maintain moisture: Even when eyes feel good, consider routine application of natural tears.

(3) Lubricating ointments should be considered but only for night time use.

(4) Be aware of the natural environment and factors that increase dryness Use humidifiers indoors and consider wrap around glasses for windy days.

(5) Caution "screen time" associated with decreased blinking by 90%.

(6) Topical cyclosporine (Restasis®): Several clinical trials support twice daily dosing of topical cyclosporin. May take few days/weeks to work. Keep refrigerated to minimize burning.

(7) Blepharitis (infection of eyelid): Use sterile eyelid cleaners or wash with baby shampoo several times/day. Recommend antibiotics as necessary.

(8) Ophthalmic glucocorticoids/ or non-steroidal anti-inflammatory agents may be effective but caution with long term use given concerns with development of cataracts/ or glaucoma (short term only).

(9) Punctal occlusion will keep moisture on the eye by preventing natural and artificial tears from draining down the nose.

(10) Lubricating pellets (Lacrisert-hydroxypropyl cellulose) fit into lower lids providing (need prescription) (Ramos-Casals et al., 2010).

(11) Autologous serum eye drops: Reserved for severe cases, plasma taken from patients and properly prepared is then applied daily (Michelson & Robert, 2011; Noble et al., 2004).

    b. Mouth: Oral saliva substitutes and stimulants should be used routinely. Remind patients to carry these at all times.

(1) Small frequent meals can stimulate saliva production.

(2) Pills should be coated for easier transit and avoidance of "sticky capsules" that could further irritate esophagus.

(3) Never take NSAIDs on an empty stomach.

7
7.1
7.2
7.3

(4) Moisturizing products such as:

    i) Oral saliva substitutes are available as lozenges, mouth wash, spray, tooth paste, and gum. Most contain sorbitol/ xylitol. Products such as Biotene® and Numoisyn and other products are a must.

    ii) Sugarless gum and hard candy especially containing sorbitol/ xylitol substitutes for sweetening are helpful, especially citrus, cinnamon, or mint flavored.

(5) Try to avoid: Dry food, spicy, salty, acidic foods that can be difficult to swallow and irritating.

(6) Avoid heavy smoking, alcohol, and drugs that have anticholinergic side effects: Many psych medications, muscle relaxants, and cold remedies.

(7) Antifungals: Topical antifungals for oral candidiasis (system antifungals when unresponsive).

(8) Drink water especially after eating to clear material from mouth.

(9) Small sips of water throughout the day increase salivary stimulation.

(10) Strict oral hygiene with routine cleanings every three months. Without natural saliva to wash debris away, increased incidence of dental carries and gum disease.

(11) Do not use mouthwashes with alcohol/or witch hazel.

(12) Particular attention to operative experiences/delayed periods of NPO (Daniels, 2008; Foundation, 2006; Fox, 2011).

  c. Ear: Apply earwax removal/ mineral oils as needed.

  d. Nose: Nasal moisturizers as needed.

  e. Skin:

    (1) Avoid long, hot showers/ baths; warm water is better.

    (2) Pat or naturally dry when coming out of water and apply moisturizer immediately, oil based (kitchen oils are excellent).

    (3) Use sunscreen and protective clothing. Sjögren's, like SLE, can be exacerbated by ultraviolet light exposure.

    (4) Moisturize with Vitamin E.

    (5) Avoid fabric softeners.

  f. Vaginal dryness: Over-the-counter lubricants can be helpful.

2. Systemic (Sialogogue): Stimulation of salivary glands with pilocarpine (Salagen) or cevimeline (Evoxac®) through cholinergic stimulation. Caution with closed angle glaucoma, asthma, bradydysrhythmias, and biliary colic (Minozzi, Galli, Gallottini, Minozzi, & Unfer, 2009; Ramos-Casals et al., 2010).

  a. Pilocarpine: 5-10 mg QID-TID as needed (max 30 mg/d). Flow rates (throughout) improve within 15 minutes and are maintained for 4 hours. Full benefit may not be appreciated for up to 6 weeks.

  b. Cevimeline: 30 mg TID (max 90 mg/d).

  c. Side effects: Sweating, urinary frequency, nausea. Higher doses are associated with more side effects. In one prospective trial as little as 5 mg pilocarpine resulted in greater improvement in subjective symptoms when compared to artificial tears.

C. Immunomodulatory/ Immunosuppressive Drugs: Aim to achieve decreased disease activity and ultimately remission. Understanding that SS is largely driven by lymphocytic infiltration and excessive B-cell activity treatments are emerging but remain largely empirical at this point. Extensive review of the literature suggests that none of the immunomudulatory agents are particularly effective for the sicca symptoms or fatigue associated with SS but may provide some relief for the arthralgias/myalgias and arthropathy frequently experienced. Additionally a number of laboratory assessments are known to improve, suggesting a possible decrease systemic disease activity (Daniels, 2008; Fox, 2011; Hansen et al., 2005; Mavragani et al., 2012; Minozzi et al., 2009; Ramos-Casals et al., 2010).

1. Steroids: Questionable efficacy, conflicting evidence that salivary flow rates have improved. May be helpful with active synovitis and other extraglandular symptoms.

2. Anti-malarial agents: Frequently employed as part of larger SLE picture, specific use

in pSS has not demonstrated significant improvements. Overall, fairly benign, but close attention to visual changes with routine eye exams at appropriate intervals (current recommendations: Baseline within first year, then after 5 years annual examination/testing). There are three agents: Hydroxychloroquin (safest/ best tolerated); chloroquin (more significant eye toxicity- monitoring for toxicity should be more frequent), and quinicrine (not readily available, has to be made at compound pharmacy, minimal eye toxicity).

  a. Remember, response is slow and not evident before 6 weeks, with maximal efficacy noted around 4 months.

  b. Caution: Recent studies have suggested that smoking decreases efficacy of therapy (Daniels, 2008; Fox, 2011; Ramos-Casals et al., 2010).

  c. Anti-malarials may be associated with hyperpigmentation on nails, face, and legs (bluish gray with hydroxychloroquin and yellow with quinicrine).

  d. Hemolytic anemia has been associated with glucose-6-phosphate dehydrogenase (G6PD) deficiency. Monitor CBC.

3. Biologic agents: Most promising B-cell targeted therapy.

  a. Anti-TNF: Small studies without clear recommendations.

  b. B-cell depletion: Most promising targeted therapy.

    (1) Rituximab (Rituxan®) has shown some improvement in glandular as well as extraglandular features. Of note, rituximab is also used in the treatment of B-cell lymphoma.

    (2) Belimumab (Benlysta®): Blocks B-cell activating factor which results in decreased B-cell formation which should ideally decrease disease activity. Preliminary studies are positive (Mavragani et al., 2012).

D. Supportive agents.

  1. Analgesics.

    a. NSAIDs: Caution with use of NSAIDs long term. Close monitoring for hypertension, coronary disease, and gastrointestinal complications. Ideally, the lowest effective dose for the shortest period of time is recommended. Caution when using with aspirin. Only non-selective NSAIDs should be used and must be given at least 2 hours after last dose of aspirin (Bhatt et al., 2008).

    b. Non-opiate pain relievers: Beware of total daily intake of acetaminophen, should not exceed 2,000-3,000 mg routinely.

    c. Opiates: Fibromyalgia is a common co-morbidity. Understand this is a chronic disease and in an effort to minimize dependency on opiates, efforts should be taken to combine self-management strategies for chronic pain with pharmacologic support.

  2. Adjuvant pain medications.

    a. Antidepressants: Can modify pain response and treat co-morbid depression often associated with SS. Caution with agents associated with anticholinergic side effects.

    b. Anticonvulsants for neuropathy/ pain modulation: Can be very effective, but associated with fatigue at least initially. Titrate up slowly to the lowest effective dose.

    c. Sleep aids: Sleep hygiene is critical.

      (1) Muscle relaxants: Caution with side effects profile.

      (2) Anxiolytics: As with opiates, can be addictive.

      (3) Insomnia medications: Do not always promote good quality sleep.

    d. Stimulants may be needed when fatigue is intractable and interferes with quality of life in a profound way.

VI. Co-morbid conditions.

A. Parotid gland enlargement (normal for glands to wax/wane in SS): Not responsive to glucocorticoids. Treatment with warm heat and antibiotics if infection is suspected. Persistent enlargement can be related to lymphoepithelial lesion or MALT Lymphoma (biopsy is required to differentiate). Rapid increase in size with signs of inflammation is most likely acute infectious process, requiring antibiotics. Sudden increase without signs of acute inflammation may signal a transformation to a high-grade lymphoma, diffuse infiltrative lymphoproliferative (DILS) syndrome from human immunodeficiency virus (HIV), or other malignant neoplasm (again, biopsy is necessary).

B. Non-Hodgkins lymphoma: More common with active disease; outcomes are fairly good; clinical course and prognosis is determined by the grade of the lymphoma at the time of diagnosis. Maintaining a high degree of suspicion is helpful.

C. Fibromyalgia (FM): Definitely more prevalent in SLE and SS (Daniels, 2008; Foundation, 2006; Fox, 2011; Tishler, Barak, Paran, & Yaron, 1997; Tzioufas et al., 2011). Additionally, many of symptoms: Fatigue, arthralgias, myalgias, diffuse, migratory neurologic symptoms, memory problems are all part of the constellation of FM. Many patients are given a diagnosis of FM before SS is identified. If diagnosed with SS these patients often benefit from antimalarial therapy. The arthalgias and myalgias often improve, but fatigue, memory and other CNS/ peripheral nervous system symptoms persist. Attention to self management techniques such as routine exercise, pacing, maintaining a meaningful, engaged life is critical for wellbeing.

D. Endocrinopathies.

1. Thyroid (10-70%).
   a. Hashimoto's thyroiditis: Thyroid peroxidase and thyroglobulin antibody.
   b. Graves disease: Thyroid peroxidase antibody and thyroid stimulating hormone receptor antibody.
   c. More common in women.
   d. Caution: Always check thyroid function; this could be a major reason for fatigue.

2. HPA dysfunction results in low cortisol levels which contribute to the overwhelming fatigue and widespread pain often seen with SS.

E. Liver.

1. Primary Biliary Cirrhosis (PBC): Anti mitochondrial antibody + (AMA).
   a. Irritation and swelling of bile ducts causes obstruction. The obstruction damages liver tissue and leads to cirrhosis and eventually liver failure.

b. Presents with sicca syndrome.
c. 5% of those with SS also have PBC. If one is present suspect the other when sicca syndrome exists.
d. Common in women between 35-55.

2. Autoimmune hepatitis: Anti smooth muscle antibody +(ASMA).
   a. Inflammation of liver tissue; this damage can lead to cirrhosis and eventually liver failure.
   b. Responsive to immunosuppressive therapy most of the time.

VII. Nursing implications.

A. Teaching.

1. Eye care: Must have ophthalmologist involved in routine care.
   a. Topical agents.
   b. Avoid the following:
      (1) Botox® eyelid "lift" and Lasik surgery.
      (2) Contact lenses must be prescribed under the care of an ophthalmologist.
      (3) Blepharoplasty "eyelid" lift.
   c. Be sure to alert anesthesiologist of SS. There are several precautions that should be maintained throughout the perioperative and postoperative period to minimize conjunctival irritation.
   d. Monitor for corneal abrasions/infections, maintain high index of suspicion.

2. Oral hygiene: Must have dentist who understands and carefully evaluates.
   a. Schedule dental cleaning and exam at least every three months.
   b. Rinse with water after each meal/ every time patient eats.
   c. Avoid hard/chewy candy/ carbohydrates that stick to teeth.
   d. Use sugarless hard candy/gum that contain sorbitol/ xylitol.
   e. Use Biotene® products and other sialogogues.
   f. Monitor for oral candidiasis: Pain in the mouth should be evaluated.

3. Raynaud's: Rarely associated with ulcerations but can increase pain/discomfort

especially in presence of neuropathies. Important to maintain core body temperature through layers, hats/ scarfs.

4. Neurological/constitutional symptoms: 10-20%.

   a. Fibromyalgia: Symptoms of widespread pain, migratory parethesias/ dyesthesias, overwhelming fatigue, "foggy" mentation.

   b. Neuropathy: Common. Often precedes sicca symptoms.

   c. Multiple sclerosis like symptoms: Migratory sensory and motor abnormalities, balance issues, memory problems.

   d. Fatigue/brain "fog": Overwhelming and debilitating.

   e. Sleep is critical.

      (1) Consistency.

      (2) Pacing activities and exercise (routinely).

   f. Identify and minimize stressors, consider relaxation techniques.

   g. Encourage involvement in care as well as remaining active in work and family life in a balanced way.

5. Joint pain, stiffness:

   a. Remain active but do not over do things.

   b. Communicate change in joint function: More stiffness/ or swelling suggests joint inflammation and usually requires medication to resolve.

B. Psychosocial: Complex and diverse, migratory pains, often long time before clear diagnosis.

   1. See resources below.

   2. Consider support group: Http://www.sjögrens. org/home/get-connected/support-groups

   3. Resources:

      a. Sjögren's Syndrome Foundation: http://www.sjogrens.org/home

      b. Internet resources for Sjögren's syndrome: http://www.dry.org/

      c. Biotene products: http://www. biotene.com/Products/Liquid.aspx

      d. *Pearls and Myths Related to Sjögren's Syndrome*- Google Books: http://books. google.com/books?id=dZ1aJf4DViYC&pg =PA129&lpg=PA129&dq=the+moisture+s eekers++survey+2006&source=bl&ots=7 No8KcHEXq&sig=iGKJHzuvE8gtwp3fJWl 8cxDYFro&hl=en&sa=X&ei=R18lT6HTLa aZoQHqobzWCA&ved=0CCcQ6AEwAQ - v=onepage&q=the moisture seekers survey

      e. *Living Well with Sjögren's Syndrome: Reasonably Well*: http:// reasonablywell-julia.blogspot.com/

Summary

This chapter covered the presentation, pathophysiology, and management guidelines for caring for those living with Sjögren's Syndrome. Subtypes were classified and key characteristics were delineated. Nursing interventions were presented with specific guidelines to minimize dry eyes, dry mouth, and other mucus producing areas of the body. Important recommendations for management and monitoring of neurological, vascular, pulmonary, musculoskeletal, cutaneous, gastrointestinal, renal, and lymphoproliferative complications were presented. Additionally, special considerations for pregnancy and neonatal concerns related to anti-Ro/ SSA antibodies were reviewed.

References

Bhatt, D. L., Scheiman, J., Abraham, N. S., Antman, E. M., Chan, F. K., Furberg, C. D., ... Quigley, F.M. (2008). ACCF/ACG/AHA 2008 expert consensus document on reducing the gastrointestinal risks of antiplatelet therapy and NSAID use: A report of the American College of Cardiology Foundation Task Force on Clinical Expert Consensus Documents. *Journal of the American College of Cardiology, 52*(18), 1502-1517.

Daniels, T. (2008). Sjögren's syndrome. In J. H. Klippel, J. H. Stone, L. J. Crofford & P. H. White (Eds.), *Primer on the rheumatic diseases* (13th ed., pp. 389- 397). New York: Springer.

Ferreira, S., D'Cruz, D., & Hughes, G. R. V. (2005). Multiple sclerosis, neuropsychiatric lupus and antiphospholipid syndrome: Where do we stand? *Rheumatology, 44*(4), 434-442.

Foundation, S. S. (2006). And the survey says... *The Moisture Seekers, 24*, 1-3.

Fox, R. I. (2011). Extraglandular manifestations of Sjögren's Syndrome (SS): Dermatologic, arthritic, endocrine, pulmonary, cardiovascular, gastroenterology, renal, urology, and gynecologic manifestations. In R. I. Fox & C. M. Fox (Eds.), *Sjögren's Syndrome: Practical guidelines to diagnosis and therapy* (pp. 285-316). New York: Springer.

7
7.1
7.2
7.3

Garcia-Carrasco, M., Ramos-Casals, M., Rosas, J., Pallares, L., Calvo-Alen, J., Cervera, R., ... Ingelmo, M. (2002). Primary Sjögren's syndrome: Clinical and immunologic disease patterns in a cohort of 400 patients. *Medicine, 81*(4), 270-280.

Hansen, A., Lipsky, P. E., & Dorner, T. (2005). Immunopathogenesis of primary Sjögren's syndrome: Implications for disease management and therapy. *Current Opinion in Rheumatology, 17*(5), 558-565.

Hernandez-Molina, G., Avila-Casado, C., Cardenas-Valazquez, F., Hernandez-Hernandez, C., Calderillo, M. L., Marroquin, V., Sanchez-Guerrero, J. (2010). Similarities and differences between primary and secondary Sjögren's syndrome. *Journal of Rheumatology, 37*(4), 800-808.

Malladi, A., Sack, K. E., Shiboski, S., Shiboski, C. H., Baer, A. N., Banushree, R., Criswell, L.A. (2012). Primary Sjögren's Syndrome as a systemic disease: A study of participants enrolled in an international Sjögren's Syndrome registry. *Arthritis Care and Research, 64*(6), 911-918.

Mavragani, C. P., Voulgarelis, M., & Moutsopoulos, H. M. (2012). Cytotoxics or biologicals in the treatment of Sjögren's syndrome. *International Journal of Clinical Rheumatology, 7*(1), 63-72.

Michelson, P. E., & Robert, I. F. (2011). Clinical and therapeutic considerations. In R. I. Fox & C. M. Fox (Eds.), *Sjögren's syndrome: Practical guidelines to diagnosis and therapy* (pp. 179-220). London: Springer Verlag.

Minozzi, F., Galli, M., Gallottini, L., Minozzi, M., & Unfer, V. (2009). Stomatological approach to Sjögren's syndrome: diagnosis, management and therapeutical timing. *European Review for Medical and Pharmacological Sciences, 13*(3), 201-216.

Muratori, L., Granito, A., Muratori, P., Pappas, G., & Bianchi, F. B. (2008). Antimitochondrial antibodies and other antibodies in primary biliary cirrhosis: Diagnostic and prognostic value. *Clinics in Liver Disease, 12*(2), 261-276; vii.

Noble, B. A., Loh, R. S., MacLennan, S., Pesudovs, K., Reynolds, A., Bridges, L. R., & Quereshi, S. (2004). Comparison of autologous serum eye drops with conventional therapy in a randomised controlled crossover trial for ocular surface disease. *The British Journal of Ophthalmology, 88*(5), 647-652.

Ramos-Casals, M., Tzioufas, A. G., Stone, J. H., Siso, A., & Bosch, X. (2010). Treatment of primary Sjogren syndrome: A systematic review. *Journal of the American Medical Association, 304*(4), 452-460.

Sanchez-Guerrero, J., Perez-Dosal, M. R., Cardenas-Velazquez, F., Perez-Reguera, A., Celis-Aguilar, E., Soto-Rojas, A. E., ... Avila-Cosada, C. (2005).

Prevalence of Sjögren's syndrome in ambulatory patients according to the American-European Consensus Group criteria. *Rheumatology, 44*(2), 235-240.

Schein, O. D., Hochberg, M. C., Munoz, B., Tielsch, J. M., Bandeen-Roche, K., Provost, T., ... West, S. (1999). Dry eye and dry mouth in the elderly: A population-based assessment. *Archives of Internal Medicine, 159*(12), 1359-1363.

Tishler, M., Barak, Y., Paran, D., & Yaron, M. (1997). Sleep disturbances, fibromyalgia and primary Sjögren's syndrome. *Clinical and Experimental Rheumatology, 15*(1), 71-74.

Tourbah, A., Clapin, A., Gout, O., Fontaine, B., Liblau, R., Batteux, F., & Lyon-Caen, O. (1998). Systemic autoimmune features and multiple sclerosis: A 5-year follow-up study. *Archives of Neurology, 55*(4), 517-521.

Tzioufas, A., Mitsias, D. I., & Moutsopoulos, H. M. (2011). Connective tissue disorders: Sjögren's syndrome. In M. C. Hochberg, A. J. Silman, J. S. Smolen, M. E. Weinblatt, & M. H. Weisman (Eds.), *Rheumatology* (5th ed.)[Digital edition]. New York: Elsevier.

Voulgarelis, M., Tzioufas, A. G., & Moutsopoulos, H. M. (2008). Mortality in Sjögren's syndrome. *Clinical and Experimental Rheumatology, 26*(supplement 51), s66-s71.

Suggested Readings

Malladi, A.S., Sack, K.E., Shiboski, S., Shiboski, C., Baer, A.N., Banushree, R., ...Criswell, L.A. (2012, Jan 11). Primary Sjögren's syndrome as a systemic disease: A study of participants enrolled in an international Sjögren's syndrome registry. *Arthritis Care & Research* [Online]. doi: 10.1002/acr.21610. *Describes the extraglandular features of primary SS in 1,927 persons worldwide. Excellent review of the systemic impact of SS as of 2012.*

Sjögren's Syndrome Foundation website: http://www.sjogrens.org/home *Packed with excellent material for nurses and patients. Explore and enjoy.*

Ramos-Casals, M., & Daniels, T.E. (2009). Sjögren's syndrome. In J. H. Stone (Ed.), *A clinician's pearls and myths in rheumatology* (pp. 107-130). New York: Springer. *Very interesting details about all aspects of SS. Easy to read; available as a Google Book.*

Reasonably Well: Living with Sjögren's Syndrome: a blog: http://reasonablywell-julia.blogspot.com/ *This is a site created and maintained by a nurse living with Sjögren's syndrome. She explains the disease process and the daily efforts it takes to live "reasonably well" despite the disorder. Reference links throughout. Please explore and feel free to e-mail the blogger.*

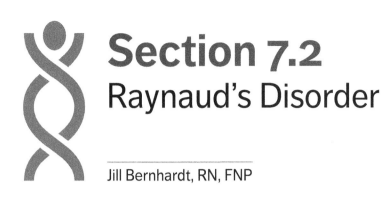

Section 7.2
Raynaud's Disorder

Jill Bernhardt, RN, FNP

Introduction

Raynaud's disorder is rare. It is sometimes referred to as a "disease", a "syndrome", a "phenomenon", or just "Raynaud's". The key feature is marked by brief episodes of vasospasm or constriction of certain arteries. Raynaud's disorder has two distinct types: Primary Raynaud's disease and Secondary Raynaud's phenomenon. In this chapter, each disease will be discussed separately although many of the components are the same for both diseases.

Learning Objectives

Upon completion of this chapter, the nurse will be able to:

1. Distinguish the difference between Primary Raynaud's and Secondary Raynaud's.

2. Describe the three distinct phases of Raynaud's attacks.

3. List the predisposition for Raynaud's according to race, sex, and age.

4. Identify the diagnostic testing used to establish a diagnosis of Raynaud's.

5. List nursing assessments conducted for all patients with the potential diagnosis of Raynaud's.

6. Identify the comorbid conditions associated with Secondary Raynaud's.

7
7.1
7.2
7.3

I. Pathophysiology.

A. Raynaud's (ray-NOHZ) is a condition that causes the constriction of small blood vessels in distal appendages due to vasospasm (National Heart, Lung, and Blood Institute, 2011) (see Figure 1).

B. Color changes with spasm are either blue and/or white. The appendages then turn red with the restoration of blood flow through the vessels (see Figures 2, 3, 4).

C. Areas affected include.

   1. Fingers.

   2. Toes.

   3. Ears.

   4. Nose.

5. Lungs.

6. Nipples (in breast feeding mothers).

7. Often one finger or toe is affected initially, but the rest of the digits and or the nose/ears can be affected with increased exposures to triggers.

D. Patients often describe the changes in three distinct phases:

   1. Vasospasms.

      a. White color to skin.

      b. Cold sensation and decreased feeling in area.

   2. Vasoconstriction.

      a. Blue color to skin.

      b. Numbness/loss of feeling to area.

   3. Rapid refilling of vessels.

      a. Red color to skin.

      b. Intense burning/stinging feeling as blood flow reestablishes.

Figure 1: Acute Raynaud's disorder

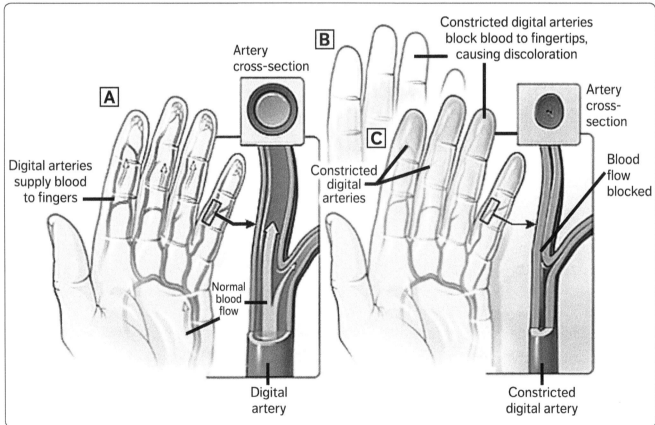

Source: National Heart, Lung, and Blood Institute; National Institutes of Health; U.S. Department of Health and Human Services. What is Raynaud's? Retrieved from http://www.nhlbi.nih.gov/health/dci/Diseases/raynaud/ray_what.html Reprinted with permission.

4. Demarcation is usually a very distinct line between the ischemic area and the unaffected area (see Figure 3).

5. Coughing attacks and or bronchospasm may also occur when breathing in cold air or eating cold food/beverage.

6. An increase in coronary artery disease and stroke has also been seen in patients with Raynaud's (Wigley, 1998).

7. Triggers leading to the presentation of symptoms include (Hansen-Dispenza, 2011).

   a. Cold weather.

   b. Stress.

   c. Medications.

II. Etiology.

A. First discovered in 1862 by Dr. Maurice Raynaud, a French physician, this disorder was described as having a strange presentation:

1. Episodic digital ischemia provoked by cold, cyanosis and emotion. It is classically manifest by pallor of the digits followed by cyanosis and rubor. The pallor reflects vasospasm, cyanosis, the deoxygention of static venous blood, and the rubor reactive hyperemia following the return of blood flow (Belch, 1990, p. 162).

B. Despite many years of research, a full understanding/explanation of the etiology of Raynaud's is not understood.

C. Cause.

1. The cause of Raynaud's is unknown.

   a. Primary Raynaud's is believed to have a genetic component as it is seen in several family members at

Figure 3: Demarcation of Raynaud's Color Change

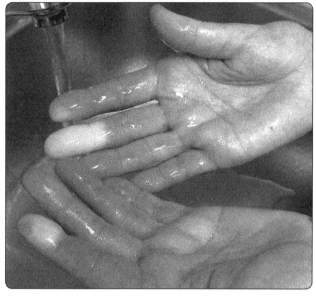

Source: © 2014 American College of Rheumatology. Used with permission.

Figure 2: Blue Color Change Resulting from Vessel Spasm

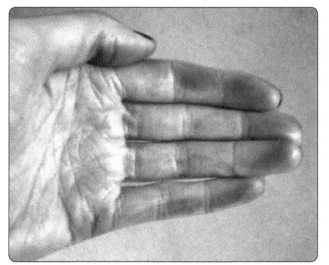

Source: International Scleroderma Network. Retrieved from http://www.sclero.org/medical/symptoms/photos/raynauds/alexandra/a-to-z.html Reprinted with permission.

Figure 4: White Color Change in Vessel Spasm

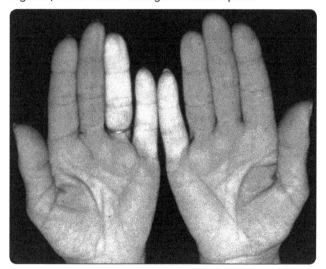

Source: © 2014 American College of Rheumatology. Used with permission.

a time. This may be because of a genetic defect in the construction and flow of small vessels in the affected areas. (Hansen-Dispenza, 2011).

    b. Secondary Raynaud's is also due to micro-vascular structural abnormalities (Hemingway, 2010).

D. Incidence.

    1. A 7-year study of Raynaud's in Caucasians in the United States (Suter, Murabito, Felson, & Fraenkel, 2005) showed baseline prevalence rates of 11% in women and 8% in men, and yearly incidence rates of 2.2% in women and 1.5% in men.

    2. Internationally, the prevalence of Primary Raynaud's varies among different populations, from 4.9%-20.1% in women to 3.8%-13.5% in men.

    3. In both the United States and internationally, the prevalence of Secondary Raynaud's depends on the underlying disorder (Suter, Murabito, Felson, & Fraenkel, 2007).

    4. According to the Raynaud's Association, approximately 28 million Americans are affected by Raynaud's disorder (Anonymous , 2010).

E. Mortality/Morbidity.

    1. Primary Raynaud's is not associated with death or serious morbidity in most cases. Very rarely the ischemia can cause necrosis of the affected areas that may lead to amputation or systemic infections.

    2. Secondary Raynaud's is an important factor in diagnosing other diseases that can lead to serious morbidity or mortality. These underlying diseases or traumas include:

        a. Autoimmune diseases such as scleroderma, lupus, and rheumatoid arthritis.

        b. Hormone imbalances such as hypothyroidism.

        c. Migraines.

        d. Trauma such as frost bite or severe crushing injuries.

        e. Repetitive injuries such as carpel tunnel.

        f. Overuse of vibratory tools (e.g., jackhammers, vibrating saws) (Anonymous, 2011).

F. Race.

    1. There is no predisposition to race in Primary Raynaud's.

    2. Secondary Raynaud's approximates the underlying disease in which it is expressed.

G. Sex.

    1. Primary Raynaud's affects both men and women but is nine times more likely in women than men.

    2. Secondary Raynaud's also affects both men and women; it is seen more often in women, but the prevalence is related to the underlying disease.

H. Age.

    1. Primary Raynaud's usually generally presents between the ages of 15-30.

    2. Secondary Raynaud's usually manifests after age 30 (Anonymous, 2011).

III. Nursing assessment.
(O'Connor, 2001).

A. Take notice and document when and how often episodes occur.

B. Make notations on which extremities are affected.

C. Assess for triggers that bring on episodes or, are associated with episodes.

D. Document family history of Raynaud's disorder or other autoimmune diseases.

E. Gather information in the psychosocial history including; amount of stress in life, how the patient deals with episodes while out in public and in social situations, hobbies/type of work such as repetitive injuries/use of tools that could be bringing on episodes.

F. Document all current medications and herbal supplements.

IV. Diagnosis.

A. Diagnosis of Primary Raynaud's is usually done by a thorough history and absence of other confounding conditions that can cause the symptoms.

1. Observation and/or history from patient.

2. Must have at least one color change (blue to red, white to red).

3. Positive episode with a Cold Stimulation Test.

    a. Performed by placing the patient's hand in ice water for 30 seconds to 1 minute and then watching the resulting color changes.

4. Laboratory tests for underlying diseases causing Secondary Raynaud's.

    a. Usually a standard autoimmune panel is drawn including Antinucular antibody (ANA), erythrocyte sedimentation rate (SED rate, or ESR), C-reactive protein (CRP), rheumatoid factor (RF), Anti SS-A antibody, Anti SS-B antibody, and thyroid levels including a thyroid antibody.

5. Nail-fold Observation.

    a. Observation of the nail folds (the base of the nail where it grows from the finger) of the hands under ophthalmoscope/ microscope with emersion oil can establish underlying disease of scleroderma (Shiel, 2010) (see Figure 5). Section A shows capillaries that are enlarged and starting to become irregular or disorganized. Section B shows hemorrhages and loss of capillaries as the disease progresses. Section C shows late disease including avascular areas where the vessels are completely absent and angiogenesis or new vessels growing out of current vessels. Section D represents what a normal nail fold looks like without the disorder.

Figure 5: Nailfold Changes in Scleroderma

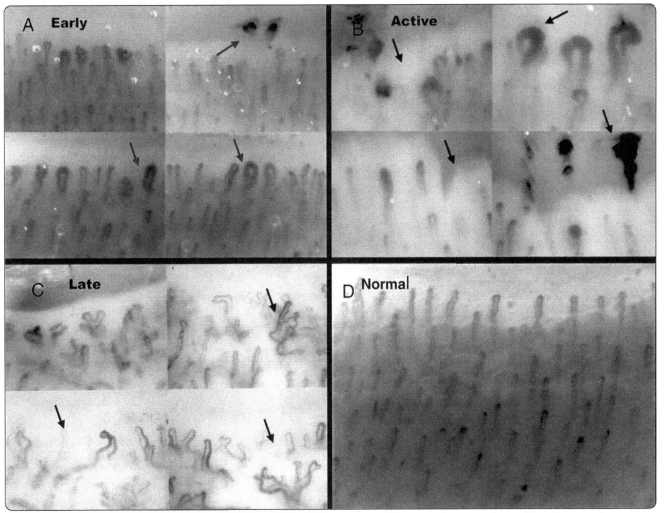

» A, early SSc pattern; B, active SSc pattern; C, late SSc pattern and D, normal pattern (magnification 200×)

Source: Cutolo M et al. Rheumatology 2006;45:iv43-iv46 The Author 2006. Published by Oxford University Press on behalf of the British Society for Rheumatology. All rights reserved.

V. Treatment.

A. According to the Raynaud's Association, only 1 in 5 women seek treatment for their symptoms (Anonymous, 2010).

B. Primary Raynaud's.

   1. Prevention and symptom relief.

      a. Wearing gloves/mittens when touching cold objects. Mittens are recommended more as they allow the fingers to keep in contact, therefore increasing body heat.

      b. Keeping room temperature slightly higher.

      c. Covering feet with socks at all times even in the summer time.

      d. Avoiding tight fitting clothing and jewelry that can cut off or impede circulation.

      e. Decreasing or avoiding caffeine and other medications that increase symptoms.

      f. Medications that can cause vasoconstriction include.

         (1) Decongestants containing pseudoephedrine.

         (2) Over-the-counter weight control medication containing caffeine.

         (3) Beta blockers such as propranolol or metaproprolol.

         (4) Birth control pills.

   2. Steps to take during an episode.

      a. Wiggle fingers and toes.

      b. Place fingers under armpits to warm them up.

      c. Make windmill exercises with arms to increase circulation.

      d. Move in place.

      e. Place hands under warm, not hot, water to rewarm.

C. Secondary Raynaud's.

   1. Prevention and symptom relief as defined above.

   2. Treat infections in affected areas early to avoid systemic complications such as sepsis.

   3. Medications to decrease symptoms:

      a. Nitroglycerin paste.

         (1) Nurses should instruct patient to apply small amount from a toothpick to crease below affected area to avoid possible headache side effect.

      b. Calcium channel blockers that work by relaxing and opening up blood vessels.

         (1) Nifedipine (Procardia®) and verapamil (Covera-HS®) most often used.

      c. Alpha blockers that work by counteracting norepinephrine (a hormone that shrinks blood vessels).

         (1) Prazosin hydrochloride (Minipress®) and doxazosin (Cardura®).

      d. Pentoxifylline (Trental®) is believed to act to make red blood cells more flexible so they can slip through narrowed vessels.

      e. Use of other Over-The-Counter (OTF) medications:

         (1) Low dose aspirin to thin blood.

         (2) Vitamin E to improve circulation.

         (3) Calcium and magnesium to prevent muscle spasms.

         (4) Fish Oil to decrease vessel inflammation.

      f. Prostaglandins to decrease blood pressure and relax the smooth muscle to prevent vasospasm.

         (1) Iloprost (Vextaris®) and alprostadil (Prostin VR Pediatric®).

   4. Surgery in extreme cases.

      a. Sympathectomy—strip nerves near blood vessels in fingers/toes to help them not react to triggers. This is not always effective (Shiel, 2010).

VI. Co-morbidities.

A. There are no comorbidities in Primary Raynaud's as symptoms without any known cause is the definition of the diagnosis. All the comorbidities below are related to Secondary Raynaud's:

   1. Scleroderma.

   2. Systemic Lupus Erythematosis.

   3. Mixed connective tissue disorder.

   4. Rheumatoid arthritis.

   5. Hypothyroidism.

   6. Hashimoto's thyroiditis.

7. Addison disease.

8. Migraines.

9. Trauma such as crushing injuries from falls and car accidents.

10. Smoking.

11. Repetitive injuries such as carpal tunnel.

12. Use of vibratory tools (e.g., jack hammer) (Suter et al., 2007).

VII. Nursing Implications.

A. Patient education.

1. Disease.

2. Treatment options:

   a. Purpose of medications.

   b. Side effects of medications.

3. Outcomes.

B. Lifestyle modifications.

1. Smoking cessation.

   a. Should take caution using nicotine replacement products as it is the nicotine that causes vasoconstriction.

2. Avoiding cold exposure.

   a. Wear gloves or mittens when in a grocery store refrigeration/freezer section.

   b. Place a barrier such as a napkin between hands and a cold beverage.

   c. Avoid very cold foods such as ice cream/popsicles so the core body temperature is not lowered.

   d. Avoid cold pools and bodies of water for swimming.

   e. Keep home/office warmer in winter and summer.

C. Coping techniques.

1. Biofeedback training.

   a. The patient may be able to control his/her body temperature by using his/her mind (biofeedback). This may help to decrease the intensity and/or frequency of attacks. This is accomplished by using several techniques including guided imagery to increase the temperature of hands and feet, deep breathing, and other relaxation exercises. Therapists trained in biofeedback, books, and other media are available on the subject.

D. Spiritual care.

1. Stress relief through prayer or meditation (O'Connor, 2001).

E. Resources.

1. Raynaud's Association (http://www.raynauds.org).

2. The Vascular Disease Foundation (http://www.vdf.org).

3. Local chapters of the Raynaud's Association or Scleroderma Association.

F. Research.

1. Research is always occurring for new medications and techniques to treat Raynaud's. Encouraging patients to seek these alternatives can allow them to obtain treatments not yet available commercially. Most research studies can be found at global research resource Centerwatch (www.centerwatch.com).

Summary

Raynaud's can be a painful and debilitating condition. Patient education on both pharmacologic and non-pharmacologic interventions is paramount to favorable patient outcomes. Nurses must consider medications, comorbid conditions, and lifestyle when counseling patients.

7
7.1
7.2
7.3

References

Anonymous. (2010) The Raynaud's association. Retrieved from http://www.raynauds.org/

Anonymous. (2011) Raynaud's disease. Retrieved from http://www.mayoclinic.com/health/raynauds-disease/DS00433

Belch, J.J.F. (1990). The phenomenon, syndrome and disease of Maurice Raynaud. *British Journal of Rheumatology, 29*(3), 162-165.

Hansen-Dispenza, H. (2011). *Raynaud phenomenon.* Retrieved from http://emedicine.medscape.com/article/331197-overview#a0199

Hemingway, T.J. (2010). *Hyperviscosity syndrome.* Retrieved from http://emedicine.medscape.com/article/780258

O'Connor, C.M. (2001). Raynaud's phenomenon. *Journal of Vascular Nursing, 19*(3), 87-94. doi: 10.1067/mvn.2001.117786

Shiel Jr., W. C. (2010). *Raynaud's phenomenon.* Retrieved from http://www.medicinenet.com/raynauds_phenomenon/article.htm

Suter, L.G., Murabito, J.M., Felson, D.T., & Fraenkel, L. (2005). The incidence and natural history of Raynaud's phenomenon in the community. *Arthritis and Rheumatism, 52*(4), 1259-1263.

Suter, L.G., Murabito, J.M., Felson, D.T., & Fraenkel, L. (2007). Smoking, alcohol consumption, and Raynaud's phenomenon in middle age. *American Journal of Medicine, 120*(3), 264-271.

Wigley, F. M. (1998). *Hopkins: Is Raynaud's a Predictor of Heart Disease?* Aetna InteliHealth.

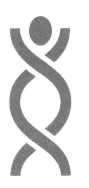

Section 7.3
Antiphospholipid Syndrome

Patricia Weinstein, PhD, ARNP, NP-C, CNE

Introduction

Antiphospholipid syndrome (APS), also known as Hughes Syndrome, is the most common cause of acquired thrombophilia and characterized by detectable antiphospholipid antibodies (aPLs) and vascular thrombosis and/or pregnancy morbidity and mortality. Although considered primarily a coagulopathy, APS is a complex and systemic disease with diverse organ and tissue manifestations. APS may occur as a primary autoimmune disease or secondary to other autoimmune disorders and has a particularly strong association with systemic lupus erythematosus (SLE).

Learning Objectives

Upon completion of this chapter, the nurse will be able to:

1. Explain the pathophysiologic mechanisms of APS that promote thrombosis.

2. Identify the diagnostic criteria for APS.

3. Describe pertinent assessment findings related to APS.

4. Discuss pharmacological therapies used in APS to prevent and manage thrombosis.

5. Formulate a nursing plan of care to reduce the risk of thrombosis in patients with APS.

6. Devise a teaching plan for the patient with APS that addresses thrombotic risk reduction, medication management, and safety.

Content Outline

I. Pathophysiology.

A. aPLs bind to different epitopes of the autoantigen β2glcyoprotein I and interact with other phospholipid-binding proteins, in particular prothrombin, thus mediating procoagulant processes, activating the complement cascade and inducing adverse effects on endothelium, platelets, and neural tissue (Devreese & Hoylaerts, 2010; Mackworth-Young, 2004; Meroni, Borghi, Raschi, & Tedesco, 2011).

B. aPL subtypes.

   1. anticardiolipin (aCL).

   2. anti-β2-glycoprotein I (anti-β2GPI).

   3. Lupus anticoagulant (LA) -– strongest predictor of thrombosis and recurrent miscarriage (Ruffatti, Del Ross, et al., 2011).

   4. Less frequent: Anti-phosphatidylserine, anti-prothrombin, and anti-annexin V (Zigon et al, 2013).

C. aPL–mediated mechanisms of thrombosis (Meroni et al., 2011).

   1. Interfere with natural anticoagulants.

   2. Inhibit factor IX activation.

   3. Interfere with activation of protein C.

   4. Interfere with annexin A5.

   5. Inhibit fibrinolysis.

   6. Activate endothelial cells to express adhesion molecules and inhibit prostacyclin production.

   7. Induce circulating monocytes to express tissue factor.

   8. Activate platelets and complement.

D. aPL–mediated mechanisms of fetal loss (Meroni et al., 2011).

   1. Placental tissue thrombosis.

   2. Acute inflammation.

   3. Inhibition of syncitium-trophoblast differentiation.

   4. Induction of decidual cell inflammatory phenotype.

   5. Activation of complement.

   6. Induction of embryo and/or placental apoptosis.

E. Two hit hypothesis (Shoenfeld, Meroni, & Toubi, 2009).

   1. Explains why thrombotic events occur only occasionally in the presence of persistent aPLs.

   2. Antibody (first hit) causes a thrombogenic state, but clotting occurs only in the presence of another thrombogenic condition (second hit), such as SLE, cardiovascular risk factors, tobacco, estrogens, etc.

F. Risk factors for thrombosis (Danowski, de Azevedo, de Souza Papi, & Petri, 2009; Ruffatti, Del Ross, et al., 2011; Uppal, Stillaert, & Hamdi, 2008).

   1. Hypertension.

   2. Hypertriglyceridemia.

   3. Hyperhomocysteinemia.

   4. Hereditary thrombophilia.

   5. SLE.

   6. Oral contraceptives.

   7. Hormone replacement therapy.

   8. Infection.

   9. Surgery.

   10. Pregnancy.

   11. Malignancy.

   12. Immobilization.

   13. Nephrotic syndrome.

II. Clinical manifestations.
(Alarcon-Segovia, 1992; Cervera et al., 2002; Uthman & Khamashta, 2007; Ruiz-Irastorza, Crowther, Branch, & Khamashta, 2010).

A. Central nervous system.

   1. Stroke – most common arterial event.

7
7.1
7.2
7.3

2. Transient ischemic attack.

3. Headache (migraine-like but not migraine) – common complaint, anticoagulant therapy sometimes provides relief.

4. Mild cognitive impairment, primarily memory loss (~40%) – strongly associated with cerebral white matter lesions (Tektonidou, Varsou, Kotoulas, Antoniou, & Moutsopoulos, 2006).

5. Transverse myelitis.

6. Atypical seizures.

7. Idiopathic intracranial hypertension (Kesler et al., 2010).

8. Chorea.

9. Amaurosis fugax (loss of vision in one eye due to temporary loss of blood flow).

10. Multiple sclerosis-like syndrome.

B. Cardiac.

1. Valvular heart disease.

2. Occlusive arterial disease (atherosclerosis and myocardial infarction [MI]).

3. Intracardiac emboli.

4. Acute/chronic cardiomyopathy secondary to microangiopathy.

C. Pulmonary.

1. Pulmonary microthrombosis.

2. Antiphospholipid lung syndrome.
   a. Pulmonary embolism (PE).
   b. Pulmonary hypertension.
   c. Adult respiratory distress syndrome.
   d. Postpartum syndrome.

3. Diffuse alveolar hemorrhage.

D. Vascular.

1. Venous thromboembolism – most common venous event.

2. Leg ulcers.

3. Hemolytic anemia.

4. Retinal artery or vein thrombosis.

E. Gastrointestinal.

1. Hepatic – Budd-Chiari Syndrome, hepatic-veno occlusion, autoimmune hepatitis.

2. Abdominal "migraine" – intestinal ischemia, infarction.

F. Renal.

1. Antiphospholipid syndrome nephropathy (APSN) – small vessel vaso-occlusive disease.

2. Thrombosis at any location within renal vasculature.

3. Renal artery stenosis and/or malignant hypertension.

4. Renal infarction.

5. Renal vein thrombosis.

6. Glomerulonephritis.

G. Endocrine.

1. Adrenal failure.

2. Adrenal hemorrhage (rare).

H. Cutaneous – often first sign of disease. (Rai, Sekar, & Kumaresan, 2010).

1. Livedo reticularis (15-40%).

2. Necrosis of the extremities.

3. Digital gangrene.

4. Leg ulcers.

5. Superficial thrombophlebitis.

6. Subungal splinter hemorrhage.

7. Raynaud's phenomenon.

I. Hematologic.

1. Thrombocytopenia (25-40%) – platelets <150,000/mm^3.

2. Hemolytic anemia.

3. Bone marrow necrosis.

J. Obstetric.

1. Recurrent miscarriage (before 10 weeks).

2. Fetal loss (after 10 weeks).

3. Pre-eclampsia, eclampsia and HELLP syndrome (hemolysis, elevated liver enzymes, low platelet count).

4. Placental insufficiency.

III. Diagnosis.

A. Revised Sydney classification (Miyakis et al., 2006) Presence of at least one clinical and one laboratory criterion.

1. Clinical criteria.

   a. ≥1 vascular thrombosis, arterial, venous, or small vessel, in any tissue or organ without significant evidence of inflammation of the vessel wall and confirmed by validated criteria (imaging studies or histopathology).

   b. Pregnancy morbidity.

      (1) ≥1 unexplained fetal death at or beyond 10 weeks gestational age with normal fetal morphology documented by ultrasound or direct examination of fetus.

      (2) ≥1 premature birth of morphologically normal neonate before the 34th week of gestation because of eclampsia, severe pre-eclampsia, or placental insufficiency.

      (3) ≥3 unexplained spontaneous abortions on or before the 10th week of gestation excluding maternal anatomic or hormonal abnormalities or paternal/maternal chromosomal causes.

2. Laboratory criteria.

   a. Lupus anticoagulant (LA) present in plasma on ≥2 occasions at least 12 weeks apart and detected according to guidelines of the International Society on Thrombosis and Hemostasis.

   b. Anticardiolipin (aCL) antibody of IgG and/or IgM isotype in serum or plasma present in medium or high titer (>40 GPL or MPL, or >99th percentile) on ≥2 occasions at least 12 weeks apart as measured by a standardized ELISA.

   c. Anti-β2GPI antibody of IgG and/or IgM isotype (>99th percentile) in serum or plasma present on ≥2 occasions at least 12 weeks apart as measured by a standardized ELISA.

B. Diagnostic clues (not classification criteria). (Uppal, Stillaert, & Hamdi, 2008).

1. Cardiac valve disease, livedo reticularis, thrombocytopenia, nephropathy (APSN), neurological manifestations.

2. Non-criteria antibodies –aCL IgA, antithrombin antibody.

3. Other antibodies – antiphosphatidylserine antibodies, antiphosphtidylethanolamine antibodies, phosphtidylserine-prothromin complex antibodies.

C. APS and multiple sclerosis (MS).

1. APS can mimic MS with manifestations such as myelitis, balance problems, and sensory disturbances.

2. MS can occur in association with aPLs.

3. MRI findings of APS difficult to distinguish from those of MS; usually non-traditional diffusion-weighted MRI can discriminate between APS and MS (Stosic et al., 2010).

4. Causes misdiagnose of both disease.

D. Classification of APS (Miyakis et al., 2006; Uppal, Stillaert, & Hamdi, 2008).

1. APS without associated rheumatic disease (ARD) (formerly primary antiphospholipid syndrome).

2. APS with ARD (formerly secondary antiphospholipid syndrome).

3. Catastrophic antiphospholipid syndrome (CAPS).

   a. Accelerated widespread small vessel occlusions.

   b. 1% patients with APS develop CAPS; rare but lethal.

IV. Etiology/Epidemiology.

A. Familial association.

1. aCL and LA occur in families with HLA-DR4, -DR7 and DRw53 haplotypes.

2. HLA-DR4 more important in Anglo-Saxons, DR7 in those of Latin decent (Sebastiani, Galeazzi, Morozzi, & Marcolongo, 1996).

3. aPLs occur in 1-5% healthy individuals, may increase with age.

4. aPLs can occur in adults with infections, malignancy and taking certain drugs but they do not develop APS.

B. APS most likely multifactorial with thrombosis resulting from different pathogenic pathways as well as interplay with environmental factors.

C. Prevalence of APS.

1. Most common cause of acquired venous and arterial thrombosis.

2. 0.3–1% of general population, accounts for 20% of all episodes of deep vein thrombosis (DVT).

3. Occurs most commonly in young to middle-aged adults, mostly women (80%), but also can occur in children and elderly.

   a. APS without ARD constitutes one-half of all individuals with APS.

   b. aPL detected in 20% patients who have had cerebrovascular accident (CVA) at <50 years of age.

   c. 30-40% SLE patients have aPL, 10% of whom will develop APS and 30-40% of those will eventually have thrombotic event.

   d. Cause of 15-20% unexplained recurrent miscarriages.

V. Nursing assessment.

A. History.

1. Thromboembolic events (MI, CVA, transient ischemic attack, DVT, PE).

2. Pregnancy outcomes in female patients.

3. Risk factors for thrombosis – hypertension, hyperlipidemia, activity level, tobacco use.

4. Infections associated with aPLs – skin, human immunodeficiency disease (HIV), pneumonia, hepatitis C, urinary tract.

5. Medications that can induce aPLs – procainamide, quinidine, propranolol, hydralazine, phenytoin, chlorpromazine, interferon alpha, quinine, amoxicillin.

6. Medications associated with thrombotic risk – oral contraceptives, hormone replacement therapy, heparin-induced thrombocytopenia (HIT).

7. Illnesses to be suspected/excluded – SLE, inherited and acquired coagulopathies, malignancies, nephrotic syndrome, thrombotic thrombocytopenia purpura, hemolytic-uremic syndrome, polyarteritis nodosa and other forms of systemic vasculitis; arterial thrombosis – atherosclerosis, atrial fibrillation, endocarditis.

B. Review of systems.

1. Skin – rashes (livedo reticularis), color changes, petecchiae, bruising.

2. Head/Eyes/Ears/Nose/Throat (HEENT) – headaches, visual disturbances, hearing loss.

3. Cardiovascular – murmur, valvular disease, myocardial infarction (MI).

4. Respiratory – PE, pulmonary hypertension, hemoptysis.

5. Gastrointestinal (GI) – ascites, abdominal pain.

6. Renal disease.

7. Neurological – stroke, TIA, hemiparesis, speech difficulties, memory problems.

C. Physical exam.

1. Fundoscopic – retina, optic disk margins.

2. Skin – rashes, color changes.

3. HEENT – facial symmetry, pupillary response.

4. Neurological – mental status, pupils, motor strength, speech pattern.

5. Cardiac – heart sounds, peripheral pulses, skin/temp changes in extremities, symmetry of calves, swelling, Homan's sign.

6. Lungs – breath sounds, respiratory rate and effort, oxygen saturation.

7. Abdomen – distention (ascites in Budd-Chiari).

D. Laboratory.

1. aPLs – LA, aCL IgG and/or IgM, anti-β2GPI.

2. Complete blood count with platelets.

3. Clotting studies if patient on anticoagulant therapy.

E. Formalized risk assessments.

1. Antipospholipid Score (aPL-S) (Otomo et al., 2012) and Global Antiphospholipid Syndrome Score (GAPSS) (Sciascia et al, 2013)– assist in identifying those patients for increased risk of APS complications and initiating appropriate medical management.

VI. Medical treatment.
(Ruiz-Irastorza et al., 2010; Scoble, Wijetilleka, & Khamashta, 2011; Tuthill & Khamashta, 2009).

A. Primary prophylaxis.

1. Low-dose aspirin combined with hydroxychloroquine in patients with SLE with lupus anti-coagulant (LA) or persistently positive anticardiolipin, or both (Wahl, Bounameaux, de Moerloose, & Sarasin, 2000).

2. Hydroxychloroquine.

   a. Reverses platelet aggregation induced by aPLs and restores the annexin A5 shield; safe to use in pregnancy potentially protecting human placental syncytiotrophoblasts from aPLs (Wu, Guller, & Rand, 2011).

   b. Consider as adjuvant to antithrombotic therapy in SLE patients positive for aPLs as well as in patients with APS and recurrent thrombosis who, despite adequate anticoagulation, have difficulty maintaining adequate anticoagulation or are at risk for hemorrhage (Petri, 2011).

B. Management of thromboses.

1. Goal: Decreasing risk of thrombosis while balancing risks of anticoagulant therapy.

2. Prolonged/lifetime anticoagulation (warfarin) after thrombotic event.

   a. Only treatment shown to reduce rate of further thrombosis.

   b. Moderate intensity warfarin (INR 2.0-3.0) as effective as high intensity warfarin (INR 3.0-4.0) (Crowther et al., 2003; Finazzi et al., 2005).

3. Identify and address thrombotic risk factors.

4. Refractory thrombosis.

   a. LMWH (Ruiz-Irastorza et al., 2011).

   b. Risk of heparin-induce thrombocytopenia and osteoporosis on long-term low molecular weight heparin (LMWH) therapy.

C. Pregnancy (ACOG, 2011).

1. Serial ultrasonographic assessment.

2. Antepartal testing in the third trimester.

3. Referral to a physician with expertise in treatment of APS.

4. Daily LMWH plus low-dose aspirin (Ruffatti, Gervasi, et al., 2011).

5. Warfarin potentially teratogenic.

6. Maternal thrombotic risk continues up to 8 weeks postpartum; should remain on anticoagulant therapy for 6-8 weeks postpartum.

D. CAPS (Giles & Rahman, 2009).

1. Early diagnosis and aggressive treatment crucial.

2. Anticoagulation (heparin followed by warfarin derivative), corticosteroids, plasmapheresis, intravenous (IV) gammaglobulin.

3. Intensive care therapy, hemodialysis for renal failure, mechanical ventilation for respiratory failure.

4. Treatment and/or elimination of precipitating factors (infection, tissue necrosis, oral contraceptives, surgical procedures).

E. Preoperative management.

1. Physical anti-thrombotic measures (e.g., sequential compression devices, antiembolic stockings).

2. Periods without anticoagulation should be minimized.

3. Intravascular manipulation should be minimized.

F. Future therapies.

1. Greater use of home management of warfarin therapy with more individualized approach to anticoagulation therapy.

2. Aspirin plus dipyridamole and aspirin plus clopidogrel have shown higher

efficacy than aspirin alone in patients with stroke or atrial fibrillation and might be considered in patients with APS in whom warfarin is not effective or safe.

3. B-cell depletion therapy with the monoclonal antibody rituximab in patients with severe forms of APS showed beneficial clinical effects (Kumar & Roubey, 2010).

4. Fluvastatin has been shown to inhibit procoagulant monocyte activity, which may help prevent thrombosis in patients with APS (Lopez-Pedrera et al., 2011).

5. Direct thrombin inhibitors (dabigatran, rivarobaxan).

    a. Inhibit fibrin formation and platelet aggregation, suppress factors V, VIII, XI, and XIII.

    b. Clinical trials underway in patients with APS.

    c. Dabigatran associated with a higher risk of MI or acute coronary syndrome (Uchino & Hernandez, 2012).

6. Intravenous immunoglobulin (IVIG) – preliminary research shows efficacy when used in addition to conventional therapy (Tenti, Giudelli, Bellisai, Galeazzi & Faioravanti, 2013).

VII. Nursing management.

A. Patient education.

1. Reduction of risk factors for thrombosis.

    a. Increase mobility/exercise.

    b. Avoid sitting in one position for long periods or crossing legs when sitting.

    c. Elevate legs when sitting.

    d. Deep breathing exercises.

    e. Maintain hydration to decrease blood viscosity.

    f. Smoking cessation.

    g. Anti-embolic stockings.

    h. Air travel, long car rides – support stockings, regularly exercise during flight, adequate water, and no alcohol.

    i. Estrogen-free contraception.

2. Notify healthcare provider of symptoms indicating thrombotic event: Pain and/or swelling in calves, sudden onset of shortness of breath and/or chest pain, hemoptysis, pain during inspiration, sudden headache, blurred vision, speech difficulties, or weakness.

3. Anticoagulant therapy.

    a. Monitoring Prothrombin Time and International Normalized Ratio (PT/INR).

    b. Awareness of foods high in vitamin K, medications that interfere with warfarin.

    c. Prevention of bleeding – safety precautions.

    d. Signs of bleeding (dark stools, hematuria, nosebleeds, bleeding gums, bruising, hematomas) and appropriate intervention.

4. Prepregnancy counseling.

B. Hypertension control.

1. Avoidance of high salt foods.

2. Medication adherence.

3. Regular activity.

4. Weight loss if overweight/obese.

C. Hyperlipidemia control.

1. Adherence to anti-lipid therapy.

2. Dietary reduction of saturated fats and simple carbohydrates.

3. Dietary fatty fish and/or fish oil supplements to reduce triglycerides and platelet aggregation.

D. Contraception and pregnancy planning in women.

1. Estrogen-free contraceptives.

2. Non-hormonal birth control methods.

3. Pre-pregnancy counseling regarding APS-associated risk to mother and fetus.

4. Support following pregnancy loss.

E. Menopause.

1. Avoidance of hormone replacement therapy.

2. Non-hormonal control of hot flashes, vaginal dryness.

F. Minimize invasive procedures.

VIII. APS in children:
Most common acquired hypercoagulable autoimmune disorder in children.

A. Neonate (Soares, Castro & Santigao, 2006; Tincani, 2009).

1. ~30% neonates passively acquire maternal aPLs; occurrence of thrombosis rare.

2. Neonatal APS.

a. Rare; neonatal period carries highest risk of thrombosis because of immaturity of hemostatic system and frequent invasive procedures.

b. Cause multifactorial including genetic and acquired risk factors.

B. Pediatric APS (Avcin, 2008).

1. Manifestations.

a. Thrombotic – arterial and vascular occlusions with most presentations lower limb deep vein thrombosis, cerebral vein thrombosis, and ischemic stroke.

b. Non-thrombotic – thrombocytopenia, hemolytic anemia, livedo reticularis, chorea, transverse myelitis, epilepsy, heart valve disease, Reynaud's, digital ulceration (Myones, 2011).

2. Management.

a. No studies on optimal management of pediatric APS, treatments controversial.

b. Must weigh thrombotic risks against risk of anticoagulation therapy (Myones, 2011).

c. High rate of thrombosis recurrence in this population suggests anticoagulation as that used in adult population should be considered with target INR of 2.0–3.0.

C. Catastrophic APS in children.

1. Rare, aggressive microvascular disease affecting kidney, liver, central nervous system (CNS), heart, lung, and skin.

2. Most often precipitated by infection.

IX. Infection-induced APS.

A. Viral (parovirus B19, cytomegalovirus, varicella-zoster) and bacterial (gram-negative, mycoplasma pneumoniae) infections in children.

B. aPL production most often transient and asymptomatic.

Summary

APS is a systemic autoimmune disease characterized by recurrent thromboembolic events and/or pregnancy loss in the presence of persistent antiphospholipid antibodies. APS can occur by itself or in association with a rheumatic disorder and can manifest in almost all systems of the body. Although many health professionals are not familiar with APS, it is not rare. Dr. Graham Hughes, who first described APS, also known as Hughes syndrome, in1983, believes that APS will become the most diagnosed autoimmune disorder of the 21st century (Hughes, 2011). Thus, with knowledge of APS, nurses can timely identify manifestations of a thrombotic event or obstetric complication and decrease the time between symptom onset and treatment. Just as importantly, as patient advocates and educators, nurses can empower patients with APS with self-care tools to decrease their risk for embolic events and poor pregnancy outcomes.

References

Alarcon-Segovia, D. (1992). Clinical manifestations of the antiphospholipid syndrome. The *Journal of Rheumatology, 19*(11), 1778-1781.

Avcin, T. (2008). Antiphospholipid syndrome in children. *Current Opinions in Rheumatology, 20*(5), 595-600.

Cervera, R., Piette, J. C., Font, J., Khamashta, M. A., Shoenfeld, Y., Camps, M. T., ...Euro-Phospholipid Project Group. (2002). Antiphospholipid syndrome: clinical and immunologic manifestations and patterns of disease expression in a cohort of 1,000 patients. *Arthritis and Rheumatism, 46*(4), 1019-1027.

Crowther, M. A., Ginsberg, J. S., Julian, J., Denburg, J., Hirsh, J., Douketis, J., ...Kovacs, M.J. (2003). A comparison of two intensities of warfarin for the prevention of recurrent thrombosis in patients with the antiphospholipid antibody syndrome. *New England Journal of Medicine, 349*(12), 1133-1138.

Danowski, A., de Azevedo, M. N., de Souza Papi, J. A., & Petri, M. (2009). Determinants of risk for venous and arterial thrombosis in primary antiphospholipid syndrome and in antiphospholipid syndrome with systemic lupus erythematosus. The *Journal of Rheumatology, 36*(6), 1195-1199.

Devreese, K., & Hoylaerts, M. F. (2010). Challenges in the diagnosis of the antiphospholipid syndrome. *Clinical Chemistry, 56*(6), 930-940.

Finazzi, G., Marchioli, R., Brancaccio, V., Schinco, P., Wisloff, F., Musial, J., ...Barbui, T. (2005). A randomized clinical trial of high-intensity warfarin vs. conventional antithrombotic therapy for the prevention of recurrent thrombosis in patients with the antiphospholipid syndrome (WAPS). *Journal of Thrombosis and Haemostasis, 3*(5), 848-853.

Giles, I., & Rahman, A. (2009). How to manage patients with systemic lupus erythematosus who are also antiphospholipid antibody positive. *Best Practice & Research. Clinical Rheumatology, 23*(4), 525-537.

Kesler, A., Kliper, E., Assayag, E. B., Zwang, E., Deutsch, V., Martinowitz, U., ...Berliner, S. (2010). Thrombophilic factors in idiopathic intracranial hypertension: A report of 51 patients and a meta-analysis. *Blood Coagulation & Fibrinolysis, 21*(4), 328-333.

Kumar, D., & Roubey, R. A. (2010). Use of rituximab in the antiphospholipid syndrome. *Current Rheumatology Reports, 12*(1), 40-44.

Lopez-Pedrera, C., Ruiz-Limon, P., Aguirre, M. A., Barbarroja, N., Perez-Sanchez, C., Buendia, P., ...Cuadrado, M.J. (2011). Global effects of fluvastatin on the prothrombotic status of patients with antiphospholipid syndrome. *Annals of Rheumtic Diseases, 70*(4), 675-682.

Mackworth-Young, C. G. (2004). Antiphospholipid syndrome: Multiple mechanisms. *Clinical and Experimental Immunology, 136*(3), 393-401.

Meroni, P. L., Borghi, M. O., Raschi, E., & Tedesco, F. (2011). Pathogenesis of antiphospholipid syndrome: Understanding the antibodies. *Nature Reviews: Rheumatology, 7*(6), 330-339.

Miyakis, S., Lockshin, M. D., Atsumi, T., Branch, D. W., Brey, R. L., Cervera, R., ...Krilis, S.A. (2006). International consensus statement on an update of the classification criteria for definite antiphospholipid syndrome (APS). *Journal of Thrombosis and Haemostasis, 4*(2), 295-306.

Myones, B. L. (2011). Update on antiphospholipid syndrome in children. *Current Rheumatology Reports, 13*(1), 86-89.

Otomo, K., Atsumi, T., Amengual, O., Fujieda, Y., ...Koike, T. (2012). Efficacy of the antiphospholipid score for the diagnosis of antiphospholipid syndrome and its predictive value for thrombotic events. *Arthritis & Rheumatism, 64*(2), 504-12.

Petri, M. (2011). Use of hydroxychloroquine to prevent thrombosis in systemic lupus erythematosus and in antiphospholipid antibody-positive patients. *Current Rheumatology Reports, 13*(1), 77-80.

Rai, R., Sekar, C. S., & Kumaresan, M. (2010). Antiphospholipid syndrome in dermatology: An update. *Indian Journal of Dermatology Venereology and Leprology, 76*(2), 116-124.

Ruffatti, A., Del Ross, T., Ciprian, M., Bertero, M. T., Sciascia, S., Scarpato, S., ...Antiphospholipid Syndrome Study Group of Italian Society of Rheumatology. (2011). Risk factors for a first thrombotic event in antiphospholipid antibody carriers: A prospective multicentre follow-up study. *Ann Rheum Dis, 70*(6), 1083-1086.

Ruffatti, A., Gervasi, M. T., Favaro, M., Ruffatti, A. T., Hoxha, A., & Punzi, L. (2011). Adjusted prophylactic doses of nadroparin plus low dose aspirin therapy in obstetric antiphospholipid syndrome. A prospective cohort management study. *Clinical and Experimental Rheumatology, 29*(3), 551-554.

Ruiz-Irastorza, G., Crowther, M., Branch, W., & Khamashta, M. A. (2010). Antiphospholipid syndrome. *Lancet, 376*(9751), 1498-1509.

Ruiz-Irastorza, G., Cuadrado, M. J., Ruiz-Arruza, I., Brey, R., Crowther, M., Derksen, R., ...Khamashta, M. (2011). Evidence-based recommendations for the prevention and long-term management of thrombosis in antiphospholipid antibody-positive patients: Report of a task force at the 13th International Congress on antiphospholipid antibodies. *Lupus, 20*(2), 206-218.

Sciascia, S., Sanna, G., Murru, V., Roccatello, D., Khamashta, M.A. & Bertolaccini, M.L. (2013). GAPSS: the Global Anti-Phospholipid Syndromw Score. Rheumatology, 52(8), 1397-403.

Scoble, T., Wijetilleka, S., & Khamashta, M. A. (2011). Management of refractory anti-phospholipid syndrome. *Autoimmunity Reviews, 10*(11), 669-673.

Sebastiani, G. D., Galeazzi, M., Morozzi, G., & Marcolongo, R. (1996). The immunogenetics of the antiphospholipid syndrome, anticardiolipin antibodies, and lupus anticoagulant. *Seminars in Arthritis and Rheumatism, 25*(6), 414-420.

Shoenfeld, Y., Meroni, P. L., & Toubi, E. (2009). Antiphospholipid syndrome and systemic lupus erythematosus: Are they separate entities or just clinical presentations on the same scale? *Current Opinion in Rheumatology, 21*(5), 495-500.

Soares, R., Casro, M. & Santiago, M.B. (2006). Neonatal antiphospholipid syndrome. *Lupus, 15*(5), 301-3.

Stosic, M., Ambrus, J., Garg, N., Weinstock-Guttman, B., Ramanathan, M., Kalman, B., ...Zivadinov, R. (2010). MRI characteristics of patients with antiphospholipid syndrome and multiple sclerosis. *Journal of Neurology, 257*(1), 63-71.

Tenti, S., Guidelli, G.M., Bellisai, F., Galeazzi, M. & Fioravanti, A. (2013). Long-term treatment of anti-phospholipid syndrome with intravenous immunoglobulin in additionto conventional therapy. *Clinical & Experimental Rheumatology*, 31(6), 877-82.

Tincani, A. (2009). Neonatal effects of antiphospholipid syndrome. *Current Rheumatology Reports, 11*(1), 70-6.

Tektonidou, M. G., Varsou, N., Kotoulas, G., Antoniou, A., & Moutsopoulos, H. M. (2006). Cognitive deficits in patients with antiphospholipid syndrome: Association with clinical, laboratory, and brain magnetic resonance imaging findings. *Archives of Internal Medicine, 166*(20), 2278-2284.

Tuthill, J. I., & Khamashta, M. A. (2009). Management of antiphospholipid syndrome. *Journal of Autoimmunity, 33*(2), 92-98.

Uchino, K., & Hernandez, A. V. (2012). Dabigatran association with higher risk of acute coronary events: Meta-analysis of noninferiority randomized controlled trials. *Archives of Internal Medicine.*

Uthman, I. &Khamashta, M. (2007). The abdominal manifestations of the antiphospholipid syndrome. *Rheumatology, 46*(11), 1641-7.

Uppal RS, Stillaert FB, Hamdi M. (2008). Antiphospholipid syndrome—a rare cause of free flap thrombosis in perforator flap breast reconstruction. *Journal of Plastic, Reconstructive & Aesthetic Surgery*, 61(3):347–8.

Wahl, D. G., Bounameaux, H., de Moerloose, P., & Sarasin, F. P. (2000). Prophylactic antithrombotic therapy for patients with systemic lupus erythematosus with or without antiphospholipid antibodies: Do the benefits outweigh the risks? A decision analysis. *Archives of Internal Medicine, 160*(13), 2042-2048.

Wu, X. X., Guller, S., & Rand, J. H. (2011). Hydroxychloroquine reduces binding of antiphospholipid antibodies to syncytiotrophoblasts and restores annexin A5 expression. *American Journal of Obstetrics and Gynecology, 205*(6), 576 e577-514.

Zigon P, Cucnik S, Ambrozic A, et al. (2013). Detection of antiphosphatidylserine/prothrombin antibodies and their potential diagnostic value. *Clinical and Developmental Immunology*, 2013:724592.

7

7.1

7.2

7.3

SECTION 8

RHEUMATOLOGY NURSING ACROSS THE LIFESPAN:
OLDER ADULT

Contents of Section 8

8
8.1
8.2

8
8.1
8.2

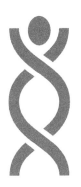

Section 8.1
Nursing Management of Patients with Osteoporosis

Ina Radziunas, MEd, BScN, RN, Victoria Ruffing, RN, CCRP, and Sheree C. Carter, PhD, RN

Introduction

Osteoporosis literally means "porous bone." The World Health Organization (WHO) defined osteoporosis as "a systematic skeletal disease characterized by low bone density and microarchitectural deterioration of bone tissue" (2003, p. 27) that can lead to increased bone fragility and fracture risk. Osteoporosis is a condition in which bone mass and bone quality may decrease to the point of increasing the fracture risk for individuals. These fragility fractures, or low-trauma fractures, related to osteoporosis, put individuals at risk for increased morbidity and mortality. Fortunately, osteoporosis is a largely preventable and treatable condition in which lifestyle modifications and medical treatment, as may be required, provide individuals with protection from these low-trauma fractures. Even if such fractures have already occurred, it is possible to decrease the risk of further fractures.

A few short decades ago osteoporosis was a little known concept in the clinical setting. It was customary for a nurse working on an orthopedic unit to provide care to elderly women and men who had experienced hip and other fractures. As individuals aged, they became more frail or fragile, and fractures were considered a natural consequence of aging.

In the 21st century individuals are living fuller, longer lives. The face of aging is changing rapidly. The advances in knowledge about osteoporosis have significantly changed how bone health and fracture risk are viewed. Hip and other fractures are no longer a simple consequence of 'aging.' Fracture risk can be assessed and monitored from middle age. Implementation of prevention strategies, such as lifestyle changes and appropriate medical treatment if required, are significant in protecting individuals against osteoporosis-related fractures, and the potential alteration of the quality of life – including morbidity and mortality. Ideally, prevention of osteoporosis should begin early in life through bone healthy living strategies.

There have also been many advances and changes in the field of osteoporosis. The focus has moved away from treating only low bone mineral density results to the prevention of fragility fractures and their potential consequences. Osteopenia, the decrease in bone mass zone between normal and osteoporosis, is now an outdated term – now more often and more correctly referred to as low bone mass (International Society of Clinical Densitometry [ISCD], 2007). Individuals are no longer being told that they "have the bones of an 80 or 90 year old." The severity of osteoporosis is no longer based solely on bone mineral density T-score results but on multifactorial fracture risk assessments. Osteoporosis is not simply a condition experienced only

Learning Objectives

Upon completion of this chapter, the nurse will be able to:

1. Describe the pathophysiology of osteoporosis.
2. Discuss fracture risk as it relates to osteoporosis.
3. Identify tools / tests to accurately assess fracture risk in patients.
4. Describe bone health, screening, treatment, and prevention of osteoporosis.
5. Identify three interventions to support bone health.

8
8.1
8.2

Introduction (continued)

by middle-aged post-menopausal women. Even HRT (hormone replacement therapy), formerly a first line treatment for osteoporosis, has been replaced by many other pharmacological treatments.

Osteoporosis is a chronic disease – often the first one that healthy individuals are diagnosed with. Commonly referred to as a "silent condition," the individual with osteoporosis may be completely without symptoms until a low-trauma fracture occurs; thus, presenting various challenges for both patients and healthcare providers. The psychological adjustment to a condition without any symptoms tests adherence to treatment and plans of care. Osteoporosis lends itself to the principles of self-management and health coaching – both significant opportunities and roles for nurses.

Nurses working with patients in many clinical settings can benefit from knowing about the risk factors for bone loss and increased fracture risk. Various disease processes and related treatments may have negative consequences on bone health, placing patients at increased fracture risk.

This chapter focuses on bone health and potential increased fracture risk related to osteoporosis. It addresses prevention strategies, including lifestyle changes, and the diagnosis and management of osteoporosis to decrease fracture risk for patients.

Content Outline

I. Pathophysiology.

A. Basic bone biology (International Osteoporosis Foundation, 2011).

1. Major functions of bone are to provide:

   a. Structural support for the body.

   b. Protection of vital organs.

   c. Environment for marrow.

   d. Mineral reservoir for calcium homeostasis within the body.

2. Bone composition:

   a. Support cells - osteoblasts and osteocytes.

   b. Remodelling cells – osteoclasts.

   c. Non-mineral matrix of collagen and non-collagenous proteins – osteoid.

   d. Inorganic mineral salts deposited within the matrix.

3. Bone cells involved in the production, maintenance, and modeling of osteoid.

   a. Osteoblasts: Derived from mesenchymal stem cells. Responsible for bone matrix synthesis and mineralization. The "bone building" cells.

   b. Osteocytes: Osteoblasts that become incorporated within the newly formed osteoid which eventually becomes calcified bone.

   c. Osteoclasts: Large multinucleated cells that function in the resorption of mineralized tissue. Found attached to the bone surface at sites of active bone resorption. The "bone removal" cells.

4. Bone matrix is made of protein that is saturated with minerals.

   a. Proteins make up 10% of bone matrix (Cummings, Cosman, & Jamal. 2002).

      (1) 90% of the proteins in bone matrix are collagen, type 1. Same type that is contained in skin, tendon, dentin, sclera, cornea.

      (2) Manufactured and secreted by osteoblasts.

      (3) Collagen chains form fibrils which line up in a parallel manner. They are held together by the formation of protein cross-links. When osteoclasts resorb the collagen it releases these protein cross-links. These cross-links can be measured in the blood as markers of the rate of bone-resorption (bone turnover markers).

      (4) Remaining 10% of bone proteins are of various types (e.g. osteocalcin) – binds calcium in the bone matrix.

   b. Minerals make up 90% of bone by weight (Cummings, Cosman, & Jamal, 2002).

      (1) Primary mineral salt (70%), calcium hydroxyapatite (calcium and phosphate) that forms the crystals that bind to the bone proteins in the osteoid matrix.

      (2) Makes the bone hard and provides stiffness to bone.

      (3) Also contains magnesium carbonate and other impurities that make the calcium hydroxyapatite crystals in bone smaller and easier to dissolve.

   c. Mineralization of bone (Cummings, Cosman, & Jamal, 2002).

      (1) Mineralization of the proteins in the bone is primarily controlled by

osteoblasts. These osteoblasts actively transport calcium, phosphate, and hydroxyl ions into and out of the extracellular fluid that surrounds newly formed bone.

(2) Calcium salts in the extracellular fluid continue to precipitate, contributing to bone mineralization. Known as passive mineralization.

5. Bone structure.

a. Cortical – outer rigid shell of tightly packed bone that resists deformation. Built from osteons – microscopic layered cylinders of bone that surrounds a vascular canal (Cummings, Cosman, & Jamal, 2002).

b. Trabecular – inner spongelike network of columns, bridges, and plates that provides strength. Bone marrow fills spaces between structures.

c. Periosteum – dense fibrous membrane that covers the surface of bones providing an attachment for tendons and muscles; contains nerves and blood vessels that provide nutrients for the bone.

d. Endosteum – thin layer of vascular connective tissue that lines the marrow cavity.

6. Bone development and growth – bone modeling / reshaping.

a. Rapid bone growth (increase in both length, diameter) from birth through childhood and adolescence to early adulthood.

b. Responsible for increase in skeletal mass and changes in skeletal form.

c. During this phase of bone growth, bone resorption and bone formation are separate processes. They occur on different surfaces at the same time, and are not joined ("coupled") processes.

7. Bone maintenance and repair - Bone remodeling / bone turnover.

a. Bone replacement in adulthood to maintain bone mass. Bone that is damaged (microfractures) through the normal processes of the "wear and tear" of everyday life, and old bone, is constantly being replaced by new bone.

(1) During this phase of bone maintenance and repair, bone resorption and bone formation are linked processes. They occur sequentially on the same surface, and are joined ("coupled") processes.

(2) Six phases (see Figure 1).

Figure 1: The Bone Remodeling Process

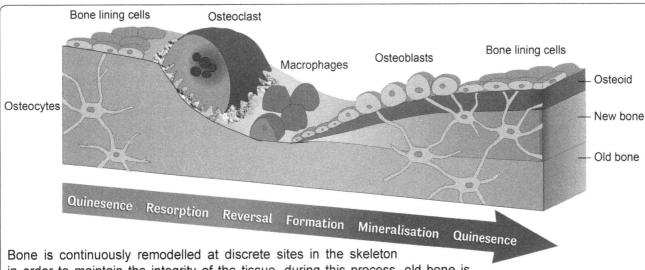

Quinesence   Resorption   Reversal   Formation   Mineralisation   Quinesence

Bone is continuously remodelled at discrete sites in the skeleton in order to maintain the integrity of the tissue. during this process, old bone is resorbed by osteoclasts and replaced with new osteoid, secreted by osteoblasts. First osteoclasts are activated, and the resorption phase takes approximately 10 days. Followin resorption, unclassified macrophage-like cells are found at the remodelling site in the intermediate, or reversal phase. Osteoblast precursors are then recruited, which proliferate and differentiate into mature osteoblasts, before secreting new bone matrix. the matrix then mineralises to generate new bone and this completes the remodelling process.

© Biomedical Tissue Research, University of York

Source: © Biomedical Tissue Research Group, Department of Biology, University of York. Reprinted with permission.

i) Activation of bone remodeling.

   1) Preosteoclasts are stimulated and differentiate into mature active osteoclasts.

   2) Surface of the bone is exposed to allow osteoclasts to resorb bone.

ii) Resorption of bone.

   1) Osteoclasts digest old bone, eroding it and causing resorption pits.

iii) Reversal.

   1) End of resorption by osteoclasts; they leave resorption pits.

iv) Formation of new bone.

   1) New bone matrix is synthesized by osteoblasts.

v) Mineralization.

   1) The new bone, layers of osteoid, are mineralized.

vi) Quiescence / Inactive phase of bone remodeling.

   1) Osteoblasts become resting bone lining cells.

b. Pathophysiology of bone remodeling (International Osteoporosis Foundation, 2011).

   (1) Peak bone mass (Lu, Cowell, Lloyd-Jones, Brody, & Howman-Giles, 1996).

      i) Achieved in early adulthood (mid 20s).

      ii) Natural gradual decrease with age (begins after age 30).

   (2) Long bone architecture (Parfitt, 2001).

      i) Long, tubular shape.

      ii) Outer layer – cortical bone.

      iii) Inner core – trabecular bone.

      iv) Strong, light, flexible, absorb stress.

   (3) Vertebral bone architecture.

      i) Cube shape.

      ii) Outer layer – cortical bone.

      iii) Inner core – trabecular bone.

      iv) Compress when temporarily loaded and return to original shape.

   (4) Bone remodelling.

      i) Believed to be genetically based.

      ii) Bone is living tissue that is constantly undergoing changes to ensure maintenance of bone health.

      iii) Bone preservation and strength are maintained through an ongoing fine balance between resorption by the osteoclasts (the removal of small amounts of old or damaged bone) and deposition by the osteoblasts (laying down of new mineralized bone).

         1) Bone remodelling cycle takes approximately 5-6 months at each remodeling site called bone remodeling unit or Basic Multicellular Unit (BMU).

         2) Activation of osteoclasts = bone resorption.

         3) Brief reversal phase with osteoblast precursors in resorption pit.

      iv) Short resorption phase followed by longer formation phase. Estimated that 2-3 million remodelling sites are at work at any given time (Orwoll, 2003).

      v) Balance between these two cell types determines whether bone is built, maintained, or lost. When the balance tips in favor of excess resorption by osteoclasts, both bone mass and bone quality decrease, resulting in an increased osteoporosis-related fracture risk.

      vi) Bone strength = bone quality (architecture and bone turnover) + bone quantity (bone mineral density) (National Institutes of Health, 2000).

   (5) Factors influencing activity of osteoclasts and osteoblasts:

      i) Age-related factors (Access Medicine, 2012):

         1) A slow process of bone loss that begins after age 30.

         2) In the elderly, it is thought that the balance between osteoclastic and osteoblastic activity is altered, with a reduced osteoblast response to continued osteoclast resorption. This may result in decreased filling of the resorption cavities by new bone formation leading to the imbalance and resulting decrease in bone mass.

3) Capacity of the digestive system to absorb calcium decreases with age. As renal losses of calcium are part of the body's normal physiology, this decreased efficiency of calcium absorption necessitates increased calcium intake in the elderly to prevent a negative calcium balance. If this does not occur, the calcium reservoir of the skeleton is triggered to release calcium into the bloodstream to maintain homeostasis, negatively affecting the bones.

4) Hyperparathyroidism of aging.

5) Endogenous factors – hormones are thought to be most crucial modulators of bone formation, depending on how they alter the activity of the osteoclasts and osteoblasts.

   (a) Estrogen - has the most direct effect on bone cells by interacting with specific receptors on the surfaces of osteoblasts and osteoclasts (Zallone, 2006).

   (b) Parathyroid hormone (and vitamin D).

   (c) Testosterone.

6) Exogenous factors – lifestyle factors such as diet and exercise.

7) Release of various "signalling" molecules (Raisz, 2005).

   (a) RANK / RANKL (RANK ligand).

8) Genetics.

9) Environmental factors.

II. Fracture Risk (see Figure 2).

Osteoporosis is defined as "low bone mass" – the bone itself is normal; however the amount is decreased and the quality may be affected – increasing the risk for a fracture. The most common osteoporosis-related fractures are in the spine, hip, or wrist. The bones that are not considered to be included are those in the hands, feet, face/skull. These fractures occur following minor incidents or accidents or circumstances under which normal bone would not break (e.g.. falls from a standing height, activities such as lifting, twisting), or even without any evident injury.

The importance of focusing on fracture risk (National Osteoporosis Foundation (NOF), 2010): Characteristic pattern of age-specific incidence of osteoporotic fractures.

A. Colles' fracture (wrist)– rises until 65 years, then plateaus.

Figure 2: Micrographs of Normal vs. Osteoporotic Bone

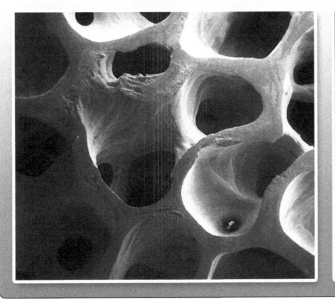
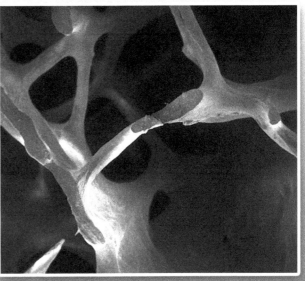

Normal Bone **Osteoporotic Bone**

Source: Dempster, DW et al. *Journal of Bone and Mineral Research.* 1986,1:15 21.
   Printed with permission from The American Society for Bone and Mineral Research (ASBMR).

B. Hip fracture – uncommon until 70 years, then incidence increases sharply (NOF, 2010).

1. Most serious of all osteoporosis-related fractures.

2. 10-20% excess mortality following hip fracture in the first year following fracture in those 50+ years. Mortality rates for men 31%, women 17%.

3. Up to 30% of patients post hip fracture require long-term nursing home care.

4. Only 15% of patients post hip fracture can ambulate unaided 6 months post fracture.

5. <20% of hospitalized patients recover their pre-fracture level of activities of daily living.

C. Vertebral fracture – increases in a linear fashion from age 40 years, reflecting increased trabecular bone at this site (NOF, 2010).

1. Majority are "silent" fracture – no symptoms until diagnosed on spine x-ray. Only 25-30% present with acute pain as a clinical symptom.

2. Prior vertebral fracture increases vertebral fracture risk 5-fold and hip fracture risk 2-fold (Lindsay et al., 2001).

3. 50% of all who fracture will fracture again within 3 years, and many fracture again within the first year.

4. Up to 20% excess mortality following vertebral fractures, comparable to that seen following hip fracture.

5. Clinical consequences:
   a. Acute back pain, which can lead to chronic back pain.
   b. Kyphosis.
   c. Respiratory and abdominal symptoms (shortness of breath).
   d. With multiple vertebral fractures:
      (1) Height loss.
      (2) Abdominal organ compression (decreased appetite, indigestion, constipation).
      (3) Restricted mobility and loss of independence.
      (4) Limited physical function.

(5) Low self-esteem, body image, and mood.

III. Prevention.

During childhood and adolescence, bone mass is accumulated at a very rapid rate, estimated to peak ("peak bone mass") by the mid-20s. Unless there are other risk factors affecting bone health, bone mass remains stable until later in life, when both women and men lose very small amounts of bone mass as a natural part of aging. Women experience a more dramatic period of loss of bone mass during the first few years of menopause, the rate of which levels off.

A. During childhood and adolescence many factors contribute to the achievement of maximum peak bone mass, including - nutrition (well-balanced nutrition including adequate amounts of the two key building blocks of bone – calcium and Vitamin D), exercise and physical activity, and general good health.

B. Peak bone mass is also significantly linked to heredity and genetics. Through process of elimination, all other risk factors may be excluded – often leaving a family history of osteoporosis or osteoporosis-related fractures as the main risk factor.

C. It is a well-known fact that African-Americans have higher peak bone mass as compared to Caucasians and Asians, and as a result, African-Americans are not affected by osteoporosis at the same rate.

D. Two of the most significant risk factors for the development of osteoporosis and increased fracture risk are sex hormone deficiency and exposure to glucocorticoid therapy.

1. Sex hormone deficiency- For both genders, the sex hormones of estrogen and testosterone are very protective of bone mass, and deficiency of either of these hormones takes away that protection and results in accelerated loss of bone mass.
   a. Estrogen deficiency: Menopause – natural, chemical (chemotherapy), surgical.
      (1) Trabecular bone is remodelled most rapidly; therefore, bone loss is most evident in this type of bone structure.

(2) Up to 20% bone loss during first 5-7 years of menopause (3-5% annual loss) (NOF, 2010).

(3) Bone loss slows by years 6-8 following menopause.

b. Amenorrhea – female athlete triad (over exercising), eating disorders.

c. Testosterone deficiency:

(1) Hypogonadism.

(2) Adrogen deprivation therapy for prostate cancer.

2. Glucocorticoid (corticosteroid)-induced osteoporosis.

a. Chronic therapy with medications from this category have a significant effect on reducing bone mass, and is the most common of the secondary causes of osteoporosis.

b. Use of corticosteroids for a period of a minimum of 3 months at doses of 5 to 7.5 mg per day, at any point in a patient's life, can have significant effect on bone – increasing the risk of osteoporosis and potential fracture.

c. Corticosteroids' effect on bone is to decrease bone formation and increase bone resorption, as a result of direct effects on osteoblasts, inhibition of production of insulin-like growth factor IGF-I, and testosterone and increased osteoblast and osteocyte apoptosis (NOF, 2010).

d. These medications also increase bone resorption because of increased secretion of PTH (parathyroid hormone) and decreased secretion of androgens and estrogens which stimulate the activity of osteoclasts (NOF, 2010).

e. Because of the direct effects on the kidneys, glucocorticoids increase renal calcium excretion, decrease intestinal absorption of calcium, and increase the release of calcium from the bone to ensure calcium homeostasis (NOF, 2010).

E. Osteoporosis can be classified as:

1. Primary – caused by natural aging, menopause, and genetic factors.

2. Secondary – caused by other health conditions/diseases, medications used with other health conditions.

3. Idiopathic – despite thorough assessment, no direct or modifiable causes are identified..

F. Causation/contribution to osteoporosis and fracture risk (see Tables 1, 2).

IV. Nursing Assessment.

A. According to the Surgeon General's report (U.S. Department of Health and Human Services, 2004), and experience from clinical practice situations, healthcare professionals, including nurses, have a critical role to play in assisting patients to maintain their bone health by:

1. Being aware of and recognizing risk factors that put patients at risk of osteoporosis, and facilitating proper testing, interpretation of results, and action based on results.

2. Assessing patient's nutritional status, activity and exercise, fall and fracture prevention, and other lifestyle issues related to bone health and bone healthy living.

3. Advising patients to take steps to ensure good health (smoking cessation, moderating alcohol consumption, being active).

4. Being aware of possible secondary causes of osteoporosis and facilitating investigation of these causes.

5. Being familiar with treatment options. Counseling patients and following-up to maximize compliance and adherence.

V. Bone Mineral Density Measurement and Classification (see Table 3).

A. Contraindications for bone mineral densitometry (ISCD, 2007).

1. Pregnancy.

2. Recent gastrointestinal contrast studies and nuclear medicine tests (wait at least 72 hours, or for gallium – 7 days before having a dual-energy x-ray absorptiometry [DXA aka DEXA] scan) (see Figure 3).

B. Dual-energy x-ray absorptiometry (DXA) measurement of the hip and spine (and when required the forearm) is the gold standard technology used world-wide to establish or to verify a diagnosis of osteoporosis, as

Table 1: Osteoporosis Risk Factors

GENETIC FACTORS	» Cystic fibrosis » Gaucher's disease » Glycogen storage diseases » Hemochromatosis » Hypophosphatasia » Idiopathic hypercalciuria	» Menkes steely hair syndrome » Parental history of osteoporosis or hip fracture » Porphyria » Riley-Day syndrome
GENETIC FACTORS Connective Tissue Diseases	» Ehlers-Danlos » Homocystinuria	» Marfan syndrome » Osteogenesis imperfect
LIFESTYLE FACTORS (mostly modifiable)	» Calcium – low intake » Vitamin D insufficiency » Caffeine – excess intake > 3 cups per day. Caffeine is a diuretic and increases calcium loss through the urine. » Alcohol – excess intake > 1 beverage per day for women. Interferes with calcium absorption and excretion.	» Vitamin A – excess intake » Salt – excess intake » Aluminum (in antacids) » Smoking (active or passive) » Physical activity – inadequate » Immobility » Propensity to fall » Underweight
MEDICATIONS	» Anticoagulants » Anticonvulsants » Aromatase inhibitors » Barbiturates » Cancer chemotherapeutic medications » Immunosuppresants » Depo-medroxyprogesterone	» Glucocorticoids (Corticosteroids » Gondadotropin releasing hormone agonists (GnRH-a) » Thyroid hormone » Possible: PPIs (proton pump inhibitors); SSRIs (antidepressants); TXHs (thiazolidiniediones)

ENDOCRINE	» Adrenal insufficiency
	» Hypogonadism:
	  › Amenorrhea – menopausal
	  › Amenorrhea – non-menopausal: female athlete triad (over exercising), anorexia nervosa / bulimia, medications
	  › Android insensitivity
	  › Hyperprolactinemia
	  › Panhypopituitarism
		» Hypogonadism (continued):
		  › Premature ovarian failure
		  › Turner's syndrome
		  › Klinefelter's syndrome
		» Hypercortisolism
		» Hyperthyroidism
		» Hyperparathyroidism
		» Type 1 diabetes

GASTROINTESTINAL FACTORS	» Celiac disease » Gastric bypass / Bariatric surgery » GI surgery – subtotal gastrectomy » Inflammatory bowel disease	» Malabsorption syndromes » Pancreatic disease » Primary biliary cirrhosis
HEMATOLOGICAL FACTORS	» Hemophilia » Leukemia and lymphomas » Multiple myeloma	» Sickle cell disease » Systemic mastocytosis » Thalassemia
RHEUMATIC and AUTOIMMUNE FACTORS	» Ankylosing spondylitis » Lupus	» Rheumatoid arthritis
OTHER FACTORS	» Alcoholism » Amyloidosis » Chronic metabolic acidosis » Congestive heart failure » Depression » Emphysema » End stage renal disease » Epilepsy	» Idiopathic scoliosis » Multiple sclerosis » Muscular dystrophy » Total parenteral nutrition (TPN) » Post-transplant bone disease » Prior fragility fracture at >40 years of age » Sarcoidosis

Source: Adapted from National Osteoporosis Foundation. (2010). *Clinician's guidelines for prevention and treatment of osteoporosis.* Washington, DC: Author. http://nof.org/files/nof/public/content/file/344/upload/159.pdf and Papaioannou, A., Morin, S., Cheung, A. M., Atkinson, S., Brown, J. P., Feldman, S.,.. .Leslie, W.D. (2010). 2010 clinical practice guidelines for the diagnosis and management of osteoporosis in Canada: *Summary. Canadian Medical Association Journal,* 182(17),1864-1873. doi:10.1503/cmaj.100771.

a parameter to be included to assist in the prediction of future fracture risk, and to monitor patient progress by performing serial assessments (NOF, 2010). Referred to as *central DXA*.

C. Bone mineral density (BMD) measurement through DXA is an essential component in the diagnosis and ongoing management of osteoporosis, demonstrating the correlation with bone strength, a strongly predictive future fracture risk for the individual. As BMD decreases, fracture risk increases (NOF, 2010).

D. People with low bone mass or density are not necessarily at high fracture risk (ISCD, 2007). Alternate technology to measure BMD is *peripheral DXA* which measures the heel or finger using x-ray or ultrasound. The results from *central* DXA may not be compared to *peripheral* DXA.

E. The WHO (1994) diagnostic T-Score criteria, which indicate normal bone mass, low bone mass, and osteoporosis, are applied to BMD measurement by central DXA at the lumbar spine, total hip, and femoral neck in postmenopausal women and men aged

≥50 yrs (NOF, 2010). The T-score expresses the comparison between postmenopausal women and men aged ≥50 yrs to the expected young healthy norms (i.e., young adults at peak bone mass) – the huge database that is stored in the computer software of the DXA technology. The difference is expressed as a standard

Figure 3: Example of bone mineral density (BMD) measurement by dual-energy x-ray absorptiometry (DXA aka DEXA)

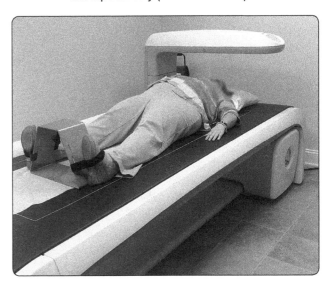

Source: Author (D. Hicks)

Table 2: Evaluation of Risk Factors for Falling

Environmental Factors	» No assistive devices available or assistive devices not being used by the individual. » Loose throw rugs. » Inadequate or low level lighting. » Obstacles (e.g., clutter, pets) in the way.	» Inappropriate footwear or clothing. » Slippery surfaces (indoors/outdoors). » Changes in texture on walking surfaces (e.g., from carpeting to tiled or hardwood flooring)
Health Factors	» Advancing age. » Cardiac arrhythmias. » Cognitive decline. » Dehydration, malnutrition. » History of previous falls. » Female gender. » Hypotension – orthostatic. » Mental health – anxiety, agitation, depression. » Oversedation by medications - narcotic analgesics, anticonvulsants, psychotropics, sleeping pills.	» Polypharmacy. » Transfer and mobility impairment (e.g., muscle weakness, stroke). » Urinary urgency or frequency. » Vertigo. » Visual impairment, use of bifocals or old eyeglasses. » Vitamin D insufficiency - vitamin D 25(OH) <30ng/ml (75nmol/L).
Neurological and Musculoskeletal Factors	» Balance – impaired. » Kyphosis.	» Muscle weakness. » Proprioception – reduced.
Other Factors	» Fear of falling.	» Slow walking velocity.

Source: Adapted from the National Osteoporosis Foundation. (2013). *Clinician's Guide to Prevention and Treatment of Osteoporosis.* Washington, DC: Author. http://nof.org/files/nof/public/content/resource/913/files/580.pdf

deviation (SD) above or below the young adult reference mean: 1 SD = 10-15% of the bone density value (see Table 4).

1. According to the ISCD (2007), the BMD at the following skeletal sites should be measured with DXA:

    a. All patients: Posterior-anterior spine and hip.

    b. Forearm should be measured in the following circumstances:

        (1) Hip and/or spine cannot be measured or interpreted (e.g,. previous surgery, joint replacement).

        (2) Hyperparathyroidism.

        (3) Very obese patients who are over the weight limit of the DXA exam table for the machine.

    c. Spine:

        (1) Use L1 to L4 vertebrae – must have a comparison of a minimum of two vertebrae for accurate assessment. If only one evaluable vertebra exists need to look at other valid skeletal sites.

        (2) Vertebrae that are affected by significant structural changes or degenerative changes should be excluded.

    d. Femoral neck is used for fracture risk scoring in Canada. If the femoral neck T-score is not at or lower than -2.5, then the alternate sites of the total hip, lumbar spine, or forearm may be used for assessment if either site is lower than T-score -2.5.

    e. Forearm:

        (1) Use if spine or hip are unsuitable for assessment.

        (2) Use 33% radius (the middle 1/3 of the radius) on the non-dominant forearm.

F. The criteria are not to be applied to premenopausal women and men aged <50 yrs, as well as to children. For these particular individuals, the diagnosis of osteoporosis should not be made based on BMD alone. According to the International Society of Clinical Densitometry (ISCD, 2007), ethnic or race-adjusted Z-scores should be used (see Table 5).

Table 3: Indications for measuring Bone Mineral Density in the U.S. (NOF, 2010; ISCD, 2007)

Older Adults (age ≥ 50 years)	Younger Adults
Age ≥ 65 years - All women.	Younger postmenopausal women <65 years with risk factors for osteoporosis-related fractures.
Age ≥ 70 years - All men.	Men 50-69 years with clinical risk factors for osteoporosis-related fractures.
» Fragility fracture after age 50 yrs. » Disease or condition associated with low bone mass or bone loss. » Taking a medication associated with low bone mass or bone loss. » Being considered for pharmacological therapy for osteoporosis. » Being treated for osteoporosis - to monitor the effectiveness of treatment. » Those not currently receiving treatment, in whom evidence of bone loss would lead to treatment. » Postmenopausal women who are discontinuing estrogen therapy.	» Fragility fracture after age 50 yrs. » Women in menopausal transition with clinical risk factors for fracture (low body weight, previous fracture, or use of high-risk medication). » Disease or condition associated with low bone mass or bone loss. » Taking a medication associated with low bone mass or bone loss. » Being considered for pharmacological therapy for osteoporosis. » Being treated for osteoporosis - to monitor effectiveness of treatment. » Those not currently receiving treatment, in whom evidence of bone loss would lead to treatment. » Postmenopausal women who are discontinuing estrogen therapy.

Source: Adapted from National Osteoporosis Foundation. (2010). *Clinician's guidelines for prevention and treatment of osteoporosis.* Washington, DC: Author.

VI. Bone mineral density (BMD).

A. The site and reference technology is DXA at the femoral neck. T-scores are based on the NHANES reference values for women aged 20-29 years (Papaioannou et al., 2010). The same absolute values are used in men.

VII. Treatment - Prevention and Management of Osteoporosis.

A. Lifestyle factors.

1. It is commonly known and accepted that lifestyle factors, which are modifiable, are central to the effective prevention and management of osteoporosis. These make up the foundation that must be in place before pharmacotherapy, if it becomes necessary, is added to the plan of care.

   a. Calcium.

   b. Vitamin D.

   c. Exercise: Weight-bearing and muscle-strengthening.

   d. Falls: Assessment of risk and prevention strategies.

   e. Avoidance of smoking.

   f. Moderation of other dietary factors: Consumption of caffeine, alcohol, salt, protein.

2. Calcium (NOF, 2010; Papaioannou et al., 2010):

   a. A crucial mineral involved in the regulation of the functioning of many of the body's organ systems.

   b. Skeleton is the body's reservoir for calcium, and plays a significant role in the homeostasis of serum calcium. When serum calcium levels are detected to be low, bone is resorbed, releasing calcium into the bloodstream.

   c. One of the key building blocks of bone.

   d. Adequate daily intake is an effective way to decrease fracture risk.

Table 4: BMD Measurement and Classification: Postmenopausal Women and Men aged ≥50 yrs (NOF, 2010)

Classification	T-Score (the number of standard deviations below the mean for young women or men at peak bone mass)
Normal bone mass (bone mass in the normal range)	T-Score - 1.0 or higher
Low bone mass (formerly referred to as "Osteopenia")	T-Score - 1.0 to -2.5
Osteoporosis	T-score -2.5 or lower at the femoral neck (if femoral neck is above -2.5 then consider lumbar spine or total hip if either is -2.5 or lower)
Severe or established osteoporosis	T-score -2.5 or lower with one or more osteoporosis-related fragility fractures

Source: Adapted from National Osteoporosis Foundation. (2010). *Clinician's guidelines for prevention and treatment of osteoporosis*. Washington, DC: Author.

Table 5: BMD Measurement and Classification: Premenopausal Women and Men aged <50 yrs (ISCD, 2007)

Classification	Z-Score (the number of standard deviations below the mean for age-matched women or men)
Within the expected range for age.	Z-Score - 2.0 or higher
Low BMD for chronological age, or, below the expected range for age.	Z-Score - 2.0 or lower

» Osteoporosis cannot be diagnosed in men under age 50 on the basis of BMD alone (ISCD, 2007)

Source: Adapted from International Society of Clinical Densitometry. (2007). *ISCD Official Positions 2007*. www.ISCD.org..

e. Lifelong requirement – throughout childhood and adolescence during the bone acquisition phase (attainment of peak bone mass), and throughout life for the ongoing maintenance of bone health.

f. Ideally, calcium is best consumed from a diet that contains foods rich in calcium, in its natural state, for maximum bioavailability and absorption. When daily intake through diet is not achieved, only then are calcium supplements a suitable alternative to augment dietary intake. Patients should be encouraged to strive for diet first, supplements as secondary.

g. The National Academy of Sciences (NAS) (NOF, 2010) recommends that women ≥ 50 years have an intake of 1200 mg per day of elemental calcium (the calcium that is available to be absorbed by the body). This is the total from all sources. It is a common misconception by patients that they are to take in dietary calcium (without regard for the total amount) and to also take the full supplement amount of 1200 mg in addition to diet. Excessive intake of calcium has limited potential benefit and may actually result in calcium deposits within the body, namely the cardiovascular system. In susceptible individuals it may result in the formation of renal stones.

h. Calcium intake from both dietary and supplement sources should be spread out over the day (every few hours), as the body is able to absorb and use approximately 500 mg at a time. Excess amounts are excreted by the kidneys. For example – if a calcium rich meal contains 500 mg of calcium, then additional calcium sources should be deferred until a later meal or time of day.

i. Many "calcium-calculator"-type teaching tools are available for use. Patients can access such tools on the Internet.

3. Vitamin D (NOF, 2010; Papaioannou et al., 2010):

a. The other key building block of bone that plays a significant role in calcium absorption.

b. Also involved in muscle performance and risk of falling and in the prevention of many cancers and other chronic diseases.

c. Endogenous vitamin D is produced through exposure to the sun (sunscreens and sunblocks block production and skin production of vitamin D from sunlight declines with age). Sunlight is absorbed by 7-dehydrocholesterol in the skin, where is it is transformed to previtamin D3. This is then converted to vitamin D3. The vitamin D3 is then metabolized in the liver to vitamin D3 25(OH). From there it is metabolized in the kidney to its active form of vitamin D3 1,25 (OH)2 – calcitriol.

d. NOF (2010) recommendation is a daily intake of vitamin D3 of 800-1000 international units (IU or 'units') for individuals ≥ 50 years.

e. Aside from fish sources of vitamin D3, few foods have adequate amounts of the vitamin to enable individuals to attain the recommended daily intake levels from their diet alone. Cod liver oil is very high in vitamin D, however, its use is discouraged due to the high levels of vitamin A that it contains. High intake of vitamin A is believed to be linked to increased fracture risk.

f. Factors associated with high risk for vitamin D deficiency: Malabsorption syndromes (e.g., celiac disease), chronic renal insufficiency, chronic illnesses, limited sun exposure.

4. Exercise: Weight-bearing and muscle-strengthening:

a. Improvement in muscle strength and balance, and improved quality of life related to physical function and pain have been found to result from exercise (Papaioannou et al., 2010).

b. Benefits of exercise related to osteoporosis (NOF, 2010):

(1) Improved muscle strength.

(2) Improved balance, flexibility, posture.

(3) Decreased risk of falling.

(4) Improved bone mass and bone strength.

5. Actions (Papaioannou et al., 2010).

a. Consultation with physical therapist or certified fitness trainer with experience in working with individuals who have osteoporosis.

b. Resistance training exercises – muscle strengthening exercises (e.g., weight training).

c. Weight-bearing aerobic exercises – bones and muscles work against gravity with the feet and legs bearing the body's weight, (e.g.. walking, jogging, stair climbing, dancing, tennis).

d. Core stability exercises for those who have already had vertebral compression fractures.

e. Balance exercises (e.g., Tai Chi).

f. Balance and gait training for those at risk for falls.

6. Precautions (NOF, 2010) – avoid:

a. Forward flexion of the spine.

b. Forward bending from the waist.

c. Exercises that twist or jerk the spine.

B. Exercise Advice (Papaioannou et al., 2010).

1. General Exercise Tips.

a. To avoid injury and excessive muscle soreness, exercise should be introduced gradually. Start with shorter durations and/or lower intensities, and gradually work up.

b. Comfortable, properly fitting clothing and footwear should be worn.

c. Stretching of major muscle groups is recommended after exercise (not before). Hold each stretch for 15 - 30 seconds in a position of mild discomfort. It should not be painful.

d. Seek out trained professionals, such as physiotherapists or kinesiologists, to help with the design of an osteoporosis-specific exercise program.

2. Endurance Exercise.

a. Endurance exercises are activities that are performed continuously that increase heart rate and breathing, such as biking, walking, dancing, climbing stairs or aerobics.

b. Endurance exercises should be performed 4 - 7 days per week for 20 to 60 minutes, where the time needed depends on effort. High intensity exercises like jogging, stair-climbing or fast dancing can be performed for 20-30 minutes, whereas moderate intensity exercises like walking or water aerobics should be performed for 30-60 minutes.

c. Perform several shorter exercise bouts throughout the day if the required amount of time cannot be achieved all at once.

d. Choose weight-bearing exercises, such as brisk walking, dancing, or land aerobics more often than non-weight bearing exercises such as swimming or biking.

e. Individuals with moderate or high risk of fracture should avoid high-impact activities, such as skipping, or activities with a high fall risk.

f. Strength training exercises are activities where muscles are used against something that provides resistance, such as dumbbells or body weight.

g. Strength training exercises should be performed 2-4 days per week.

h. Choose exercises for all of the major muscle groups. At minimum, include exercises for the legs (hip and knee extensors and flexors), chest, back extensors, abdominal muscles, and muscles that pull the shoulders back (scapular retractors). Exercises for the arms, shoulders, and lower leg muscles can also be added. Ideally, 8-10 exercises should be performed.

i. Eight to12 repetitions of each exercise should be performed. The weight chosen should be such that the intensity of each exercise (how hard it feels at the end of 8-12 repetitions) should be moderate to high (5-8 on a scale of 0-10). It is best to start with one set of each exercise and progress to 2-3 sets.

j. Individuals with moderate or high risk of fracture should avoid exercises that involve bending, twisting or holding weights overhead. Since many exercises for the abdominal muscles involve bending and twisting, it may be better to choose isometric exercises (where a position is held but there is no joint movement) or pelvic tilts.

k. Strength training exercises can modified to standing, seated or lying positions.

l. Exercises for correcting posture and posture awareness training are recommended for individuals with a curved spine.

3. Balance Training.

a. Balance training activities are those that challenge stability, and they should be performed two or more times per week.

b. Start with simple exercises and progress to more challenging ones, depending on ability.

(1) An example progression:

i) Stand behind a chair holding on with both hands then remove one hand; remove the other hand.

ii) Stand on one leg (with or without hands on chair); repeat these steps with eyes closed.

iii) Progress to more dynamic exercises like sidestepping or walking heel to toe.

4. Actions to decrease the risk of falls.

a. Review fall risks.

b. Assessment by an occupational therapist.

c. Home safety assessment.

d. Assessment by geriatric assessment program.

e. Education through falls prevention programs.

f. Use of hip protectors.

g. Regular, suitable weight-bearing and muscle strengthening exercises.

h. Balance exercises (e.g., Tai Chi).

i. Balance and gait training for those at risk for falls.

j. Vitamin D sufficiency (vitamin D 25 (OH) > 30ng/ml (75 nmol/L)).

VIII. Pharmacotherapy.

A. According to the NOF (2010), initiation of osteoporosis medication therapy is recommended in order to reduce fracture risk in postmenopausal women and men ≥50 years as follows:

1. If the individual has had a hip or vertebral fracture.

2. If the T-score is:

a. ≤ -2.5 in the spine, total hip, or femoral neck after appropriate evaluation to exclude secondary causes.

b. Low bone mass (T-score between -1.0 and -2.5 at the femoral neck, total hip or spine) with a 10 year probability of hip fracture ≥ 3%, or a 10 year probability of any major

osteoporosis-related fracture ≥ 20% based on the U.S.-adapted fracture risk assessment tool (FRAX) tool.

B. Classification of approved medications for the treatment of osteoporosis. Nurses are encouraged to familiarize themselves with these medications (see Table 6).

1. Antiresorptives (bone retaining) – inhibit osteoclast activity and resorption of bone which may lead to increase in bone mass. Reduce fracture risk.

2. Bisphosphonates:

a. Alendronate (Fosamax®), oral.

b. Alendronate (Fosamax Plus D®) with vitamin D added, oral.

c. Ibandronate sodium (Boniva®), oral and IV.

d. Risedronate sodium (Actonel®), oral.

e. Zoledronic acid (Reclast®), IV.

3. Calcitonin, nasal spray or subcutaneous (Fortical® or Miacalcin®).

4. Estrogen agonists/antagonists selective estrogen-receptor modulators (SERMS):

a. Raloxifene hydrochloride (Evista®), oral.

5. Anabolic (bone forming):

a. Teriparatide (PTH 1-34 - parathyroid hormone) (Forteo®).

6. Human monoclonal antibody to RANK-ligand:

a. Denosumab (Prolia®).

IX. Co-morbid Conditions.

A. Excess calcium intake (NOF, 2010):

1. Intake of calcium in excess of the recommended upper limit of 1200 mg of elemental calcium per day has limited benefit, and may increase an individual's risk of developing kidney stones or cardiovascular disease.

B. Bisphosphonates and osteonecrosis of the jaw (ONJ) (Papaioannou et al., 2010).

1. Defined as the presence of exposed bone in the maxillofacial region that did not heal within eight weeks after identification by a healthcare provider, typically following a dental extraction or some other trauma.

2. Incidence.

   a. Occurs most often in patients with cancer who are receiving high doses of IV bisphosphonates.

   b. Oral bisphosphonates: Between 1 in 10,000 & <1 in 100,000 patient-treatment years.

   c. IV bisphosphonates: Two cases reported in randomized controlled trials (RTCs) in postmenopausal osteoporosis (one in placebo group).

   d. Information on incidence of ONJ is rapidly evolving: The true incidence may be higher.

3. In patients receiving bisphosphonates after being properly put on these medications, the benefits of bisphosphonate therapy significantly outweigh the risks of developing ONJ.

C. Bisphosphonates and atypical fracture (Papaioannou et al., 2010).

   1. Rare type of fracture with a distinctive fracture pattern.

   2. Pain in thigh typically precedes the fracture and requires investigation.

   3. Case series reported an increased incidence of atypical subtrochanteric fractures with long-term (>5 yr) use of bisphosphonates.

   4. Found more commonly in patients on steroids or other medications that affect bone metabolism.

X. Nursing implications (e.g., teaching, psychosocial, medications, side-effects, resources, spiritual care).

A. Universal counselling strategies for all patients at risk for developing osteoporosis or those already identified with osteoporosis (NOF, 2010).

   1. Counsel on risk reduction (e.g., awareness of current medications that may decrease BMD or increase patients' risk of falling).

   2. Instruct regarding adequate intake of the two key building blocks of bone: Calcium and vitamin D.

   3. Encourage and provide guidelines for regular participation in weight-bearing and muscle-strengthening exercises to reduce risk of falls and fractures.

   4. Review risks and provide strategies for fall prevention.

   5. Counsel regarding lifestyle factors known to negatively affect bone health: Avoidance of smoking and excessive alcohol intake.

B. Patient counselling regarding osteoporosis medications:

   1. Proper administration guidelines for oral bisphosphonates.

   2. Possible side effects for all bisphosphonates.

   3. Possible side effects for oral bisphosphonates.

   4. Possible side effects for IV bisphosphonates.

   5. Nurse to be aware of requirement for adequate renal status of patients on bisphosphonates.

C. Adherence to bone health plan (Papaioannou et al., 2010).

   1. The expectation is that treated patients will experience anti-fracture benefits similar to those reported in clinical trials.

   2. Suboptimal adherence to medication treatment reduces or eliminates anti-fracture benefits.

   3. Poor adherence leaves patients at higher risk of fracture.

   4. 50% adherence leaves patients at approximately the same fracture risk as no therapy.

   5. Types of non-adherence:

      a. Frequently missed doses.

      b. Failing to take the medication correctly to optimize absorption and action.

      c. Discontinuation of therapy.

      d. Reported one-year adherence rates: 25% –50%.

      e. Marginally better with less frequent dosing regimens.

   6. Patient education and support is crucial for the success of treatment with a plan that may include:

Table 6: FDA approved medication for Osteoporosis

Medication (Generic)	Medication (Trade)	Indication for: Postmenopausal Osteoporosis	Indication for: Glucocorticoid Osteoporosis	Indication for: Increase bone mass in men with Osteoporosis	Dosing	Frequency	Black Box Warning(s)	Selected Nursing Considerations and Potential Drug Interactions
Category Ia: Antiresorptives- Bisphosphonates								In all bisphosphonates – severe bone, joint, and/or muscle pain may occur, gastric disturbances, atypical fractures, and osteonecrosis of the jaw have been reported.
Alendronate sodium	Fosamax® Fosamax D®	Yes	Yes	Yes	70 mg	Daily or Weekly Dose varies on indication	None	Correct hypocalcemia prior to use. Aspirin/Nonsteroidal anti-inflammatory drugs may worsen gastric upset. Calcium supplements and other medications with multivalent cations interfere with absorption. Must swallow tablets whole with 6-8 ounces of water at least 30 minutes before first food/drink/ medications of the day. Do not lie down for at least 30 minutes after taking medication.
Risedronate	Actonel® Actonel Combi®, Actonel Combi D®	Yes	Yes	N/A	5 mg, 35 mg, 75 mg or 150 mg tablet	Daily, weekly, twice monthly or monthly	None	Correct hypocalcemia, and other bone mineral metabolism dysfunctions prior to use. Supplemental calcium and vitamin D is advantageous. Protect against potential gastric upset.
Ibandronate	Boniva®	Yes	N/A	N/A	3 mg every 3 months intravenously (over a period of 15 to 30 seconds)	Monthly Every 3 months (provided in a kit)	None	Do not mix with any other intravenous solutions. Check for severe renal impairment.
Zoledronic Acid	Reclast®	Yes	Yes	Yes	5 mg in a 100 mL ready-to –infuse solution over no less than 15 minutes	IV infusion yearly or for prevention of postmenopaus- al osteoporosis 5 mg infusion once every 2 years	None	Hydrate well before infusion. Administration of acetaminophen following Reclast® administration may reduce the incidence of acute-phase reaction symptoms. Monitor calcium levels.

8
8.1
8.2

Table 6 (continued): FDA approved medication for Osteoporosis

Category Ib – Antiresorptives - Other

Drug	Trade name			Form	Dose	Risk	Comments
Estrogen (hormone)	Various trade names	Hormone Replacement Therapy (HRT) for postmeno-pausal women	No	Transdermal skin patch or pill	Varies	None	No longer widely used as HRT has been connected to increased risks of uterine cancer, breast cancer, stroke, heart attacks, blood clots, and even mental decline.
Calcitocinin (hormone)	Fortical® Miacalcin®	Yes	No	Nasal Spray daily	200 IU, one spray per day (alternate nostrils)	None	Concomitant use of calcitonin and lithium may lead to a reduction in plasma lithium concentrations due to increased urinary clearance of lithium. The dose of lithium may need to be adjusted. Periodic nasal examinations with visualization of the nasal mucosa, turbinates, septum and mucosal blood vessel status are recommended.
Raloxifine (estrogen agonist/ antagonist	Evista®	Yes	No	60 mg	Daily	Increased risk of venous thromboembo-lism and death from stroke	Do not use with Cholestyramine (Questran®). Monitor prothrombin time if on warfarin. Caution with highly protein-bound drugs.
Denosumab (RANK ligand (RANKL) inhibitor)	Prolia®	Yes	Yes	60 mg	Subcutaneously every 6 months	None	Pre-existing hypocalcemia must be corrected prior to initiating therapy. Take calcium 1000 mg daily and at least 400 IU vitamin D daily. Patients receiving Prolia® should not receive Xgeva®. Dermatitis, rash, and eczema may be seen.

Category II - Anabolic

Drug	Trade name			Form	Dose	Risk	Comments
Teraparatide (recombinant human parathyroid hormone analog)	Forteo®	Yes	Yes	20 mcg	Subcutaneously Daily	Potential risk for osteosarcoma	Use of the drug for more than 2 years during a patient's lifetime is not recommended. Use with caution in patients receiving digoxin. Transient hypercalcemia may predispose patients to digitalis toxicity. Transient orthostatic hypotension may occur with initial doses.

Sources: Amgen, Inc. (2014), Prolia®: Prescribing information. Thousand Oaks, CA: Author.;Eli Lilly and Company. (2012). Forteo®: Prescribing information. Indianapolis, IN: Author.;Eli Lilly and Company. (2011). Evista®: Prescribing information. Indianapolis, IN: Author.; Genentech, Inc., (2013). Boniva®: Prescribing information. South San Francisco, CA: Author.; Merck & Co., Inc., (2010). Fosamax Plus D®: Prescribing information. Whitehouse Station, NJ: Author.; Merck, Sharp & Dohme. (2012). Fosamax®: Prescribing information. Whitehouse Station, NJ: Author.; Novartis (2014a). Reclast®: Prescribing information. East Hanover, NJ: Author.; Novartis (2014b). Miacalcin®: Prescribing information. East Hanover, NJ: Author.; Par Pharmaceuticals Companies, Inc., (2012). Questran®: Prescribing information. Spring Valley, NY: Author.; Sanofi-Aventis. (2011). Actonel Combi®, Actonel Combi D®: Prescribing information. Macquarie Park, NSW: Author.; Upsher-Smith Laboratories, Inc., (2012). Fortical®: Prescribing information. Minneapolis, MN: Author

a. Reminders.

b. Patient information.

c. Counselling.

d. Simplification of the dosing regimen.

e. Self-monitoring.

D. Patient education/counseling to prevent ONJ:

1. Maintain good oral hygiene.

2. Encourage regular dental check-ups.

3. Patients to inform dental professionals that they are taking bisphosphonates.

E. Other clinical considerations for bone health.

1. A review of the risk factors for loss of bone mass and potential fracture risk demonstrate that many patients in many different care areas may be affected. The following list is only a small sampling of areas for consideration:

a. Any prolonged immobility or bed rest.

b. Insufficient calcium and vitamin D intake – question the need to add supplementation.

c. Treatment with medications for other health conditions that may affect bone health (e.g.. glucocorticoids/corticosteroids [e.g., prednisone]).

d. Patients with eating disorders, or suboptimal nutritional intake (hospitalized or institutionalized elderly).

e. Transplant patients (treatment medications).

f. Patients experiencing impaired renal function, renal failure/dialysis, renal transplant.

g. Patients with seizure disorders on chronic anticonvulsant therapy.

h. Patients with malabsorptive disorders (e.g., Crohn's disease, ulcerative colitis, irritable bowel disease [IBD]).

Summary

The field of osteoporosis is constantly changing and evolving. As with all other health conditions, healthcare providers must keep themselves informed about updates, new guidelines, patient management, and treatment options. Osteoporosis is a clinical specialty that relies on the significant role that nurses play in supporting and educating individuals who face the challenging task of being requested to follow recommendations for a symptomless, "silent" condition.

This chapter has incorporated the best practice guidelines for osteoporosis current at the time of writing. In this ever-changing field, healthcare providers should frequently consult with the national osteoporosis organizations for updated best practice guidelines.

References

Access Medicine McGraw Hill www.accessmedicine.com

Amgen, Inc. (2014). Prolia®: Prescribing information. Thousand Oaks, CA: Author.

Burge, R., Dawson-Hughes, B., Solomon, D.H., Wong, J.B., King, A. &, Toteson, A. (2007).

Cummings, S.R., Cosman, F., & Jamal, S.A.(EdsO (2002). *Osteoporosis an evidence-based guide to prevention and management.* Philadelphia: American College of Physicians – American Society of Internal Medicine.

Eli Lilly and Company. (2012). Forteo®: Prescribing information. Indianapolis, IN: Author.

Eli Lilly and Company. (2011). Evista®: Prescribing information. Indianapolis, IN: Author.

Genant, H.K. (1999). Interim report and recommendations of the World Health Organization Task-Force for Osteoporosis. *Osteoporosis International, 10(4),* 259-64.

Genentech, Inc., (2013). Boniva®: Prescribing information. South San Francisco, CA: Author.

International Osteoporosis Foundation. (2011). www. iofbonehealth.org

International Society of Clinical Densitometry. (2007). ISCD Official Positions 2007. Retrieved from www. ISCD.org.

Lindsay, R., Silverman S. L., Cooper, C., Hanley, D.A., Barton, I., Seeman, E. (2001). Risk of new vertebral fracture in the year following a fracture. *Journal of the American Medical Association, Jan 17: 285(3),* 320-323.

Lu, P.W., Cowell C.T., Lloyd-Jones, S.A., Brody, J.N., & Howman-Giles, R. (1996). Volumetric bone mineral density in normal subjects aged 5-27 years. *Journal of Clinical Endocrinology & Metabolism, 81,* 1586-1590.

Merck & Co., Inc., (2010). Fosamax Plus D®: Prescribing information. Whitehouse Station, NJ: Author.

Merck, Sharp & Dohme. (2012). Fosamax®: Prescribing information. Whitehouse Station, NJ: Author.

National Institutes of Health. (2000). *Osteoporosis prevention, diagnosis and therapy.* NIH Consensus Conference, March 27-29, 17, 1-36.

National Osteoporosis Foundation. (2010). *Clinician's guide to prevention and treatment of osteoporosis.* Washington, DC: Author.

National Osteoporosis Foundation. (2010). *National Osteoporosis Foundation presents osteoporosis: What healthcare professionals need to know (slides).* Washington, DC: Author.

Novartis (2014a). Reclast®: Prescribing information. East Hanover, NJ: Author.

Novartis (2014b). Miacalcin®: Prescribing information. East Hanover, NJ: Author.

Orwoll, E.S. (2003). Toward an expanded understanding of the role of the periosteum in skeletal health. *Journal of Bone Mineral Research, 18,* 949-54.

Papaioannou, A., Morin, S., Cheung, A.M., Atkinson, S., Brown, J.P., Feldman, S., & the Scientific Advisory Council of Osteoporosis Canada. (2010). 2010 clinical practice guidelines for the diagnosis and management of osteoporosis in Canada: Summary. *Canadian Medical Association Journal, 182(17),* 1864-1873.

Par Pharmaceuticals Companies, Inc., (2012). Questran®: Prescribing information. Spring Valley, NY: Author.

Parfitt, A.M. (2001). Skeletal heterogeneity and the purposes of bone remodelling: implications for the understanding of osteoporosis. In R. Marcus., D. Zfeldman, & J. Kelsey (Eds.), *Osteoporosis* (pp. 433-434). San Diego: Academic Press.

Raisz, L.G. (2005). Pathogenesis of osteoporosis: Concepts, conflicts, and prospects. *Journal of Clinical Investigation, 115(12),* 3318-3325.

Sanofi-Aventis. (2011). Actonel®, Actonel Combi®, Actonel Combi D®: Prescribing information. Macquarie Park, NSW: Author.

U.S. Department of Health and Human Services. (2004). *Bone health and osteoporosis: A report of the surgeon general.* Rockville, MD: U.S. Department of Health and Human Services, Office of the Surgeon General.

Upsher-Smith Laboratories, Inc., (2012). Fortical®: Prescribing information. Minneapolis, MN: Author.

World Health Organization. (1994) *Assessment of fracture risk and its application to screening for postmenopausal osteoporosis.* Report of a World Health Organization Study Group. World Health Organization Technical Report Series 1994;843:1-129.

World Health Organization. (2003). *The burden of musculoskeletal conditions at the start of the new millennium.* WHO Technical Report Series 919. Geneva, Switzerland: Author.

Zallone, A. (2006). Direct and indirect estrogen actions on osteoblasts and osteoclasts. *Annals of the New York Academy of Science, 1068,* 173-9.

8
8.1
8.2

Resources

Osteoporosis Canada www.osteoporosis.ca

National Osteoporosis Foundation www.nof.org

International Osteoporosis Foundation www.iof.org

Roush, K. (2011). Prevention and treatment of osteoporosis in postmenopausal women: A review. *American Journal of Nursing, 111(8),* 26-35.

World Health Organization. (2003). *Assessment of fracture risk and its application to screening for postmenopausal osteoporosis.* Geneva, Switzerland: Author

Section 8.2
Osteoarthritis

Victor Mo, MSN, RN

Introduction

Osteoarthritis (OA) is the most common form of articular disease. OA is considered to be the end result of different factors creating cartlidge damage. OA is now classified as being either primary or secondary. It is a progressive joint disorder of the gradual loss of cartilage. Three Greek words comprise ostoearthritis: Osteo for bone, arthron for joint, and the suffix itis which denotes inflammation. OA is commonly known as degenerative joint disease (DJD) or osteoarthrosis. The deterioration of cartlidge causes pain, swelling, and reduced motion mainly in weight-bearing joints such as the hands, knees, hips, and spine.

Learning Objectives

Upon completion of this chapter, the nurse will be able to:

1. Describe osteoarthritis (OA) and the common joints that are affected.

2. Describe the differences between primary OA and secondary OA.

3. Discuss the controversies and limitations of primary OA and secondary OA.

4. Identify the common joints affected by OA.

5. Discuss the prevalence of OA and its significant costs to society.

6. Explain how OA is commonly diagnosed.

7. Describe the realistic OA treatments and goals.

8. Describe the commonly used medications for OA to alleviate pain and symptoms.

Content Outline

I. Pathophysiology.

A. Healthy cartilage absorbs the shock of movement. When the cartilage is lost or weakened, the bones rub together. Over time, this rubbing can permanently damage the joint.

B. Secondary nonspecific inflammatory changes may also contribute to osteoarthritis (OA).

1. The term degenerative joint disease (DJD) may no longer be appropriate when referring to OA.

2. Some believe that mechanical stress on joints underlies all OA, including misalignments of bones caused by congenital or pathogenic causes, mechanical injury, overweight, loss of strength in muscles supporting joints, and impairment of peripheral nerves, leading to sudden or uncoordinated movements that overstress joints.

C. Historically, OA has been divided into primary and secondary forms, although this division is somewhat artificial (McCance & Huether, 2006).

II. Primary OA.

A. Primary OA is a chronic degenerative disorder related to aging and typically occurs in older individuals.

B. It is an idiopathic phenomenon, occurring in previously intact joints and having no apparent initiating factor.

C. As a person ages, the water content of the cartilage decreases as a result of a reduced proteoglycan content, thus causing the cartilage to be less resilient.

D. Without the protective effects of the proteoglycans, the collagen fibers of the cartilage can become susceptible to degradation and thus exacerbate the degeneration.

E. Inflammation of the surrounding joint capsule can also occur, though often milder compared to what occurs in rheumatoid arthritis (RA).

F. This can happen as breakdown products from the cartilage are released into the synovial space, and the cells lining the joint attempt to remove them.

G. New bone outgrowths, called "spurs" or osteophytes, can form on the margins of the joints, possibly in an attempt to improve the congruence of the articular cartilage surfaces.

H. These bone changes, together with the inflammation, can be both painful and debilitating.

I. Up to 60% of OA cases are thought to result from genetic factors (Shiel, n.d.).

III. Secondary OA.

A. Secondary OA refers to degenerative disease of the synovial joints that result from some predisposing condition, usually trauma, which has adversely altered the articular cartilage and/or sub-chondral bone of the affected joints (McCance & Huether, 2006).

B. Secondary OA often occurs in relatively young individuals.

C. This type of OA is caused by other factors, but the resulting pathology is the same as for primary OA:

1. Congenital disorders of joints.

2. Diabetes.

3. Inflammatory diseases (such as Perthes' disease), Lyme disease, and all chronic forms of arthritis (e.g., costochondritis, gout, and rheumatoid arthritis). In gout, uric acid crystals cause the cartilage to degenerate at a faster pace.

4. Injury to joints, as a result of an accident or orthodontic operations.

5. Septic arthritis (infection of a joint).

6. Ligamentous deterioration or instability may be a factor.

7. Marfan's syndrome.

8. Obesity.

9. Alkaptonuria.

10. Hemochromatosis and Wilson's disease.

11. Ehlers-Danlos Syndrome.

D. Although OA was traditionally thought to affect primarily the articular cartilage of synovial joints, pathophysiologic changes also occur in the synovial fluid, as well as in the underlying (sub-chondral) bone and in the overlying joint capsule (Lozada, n.d.).

IV. Etiology.

A. The daily stresses applied to the joints, especially the weight-bearing joints (e.g., ankle, knee, hip), play an important role in the development of OA.

1. It is most commonly believed that degenerative alterations in OA primarily begin in the articular cartilage, as a result of either excessive loading of a healthy joint or relatively normal loading of a previously disturbed joint (Lozada, n.d.).

B. External forces accelerate the catabolic effects of the chondrocytes and disrupt the cartilaginous matrix.

C. Risk factors for OA include the following:

1. Advancing age - With advancing age, cartilage volume, proteoglycan content, cartilage vascularization, and cartilage perfusion are reduced and may result in certain characteristic radiologic features, including narrowed joint space and the presence of marginal osteophytes. However, biochemical and pathophysiologic findings support the notion that age alone is an insufficient cause of OA.

2. Obesity - increases the mechanical stress in a weight-bearing joint, especially of the knees and the hips.

3. Trauma - to the articular cartilage, ligaments, or menisci lead to abnormal biomechanics in the joints and enhance their premature degeneration.

4. Menopause (sex hormones) - increases the progression of OA; however, estrogen replacement therapy lowers the expected rate of radiographic and clinical findings in the knees and hips.

5. Muscle dysfunction - compromises the body's neuromuscular protective mechanisms, leading to increased joint motion resulting in OA.

6. Genetics - particularly in generalized OA; a specific gene for OA has been identified.

7. Repetitive use (e.g., jobs requiring heavy labor and bending).

8. Infection.

9. Crystal deposition.

10. Acromegaly.

11. Concomitant rheumatoid arthritis (a chronic inflammatory arthritis).

12. Heritable metabolic causes (e.g., alkaptonuria, hemochromatosis, Wilson's disease).

13. Hemoglobinopathies (e.g., sickle cell disease, thalassemia).

14. Neuropathic disorder leading to a Charcot joint (e.g., syringomyelia, tabes dorsalis, diabetes).

15. Underlying orthopedic disorders (e.g., congenital hip dislocation, slipped femoral capital epiphysis).

16. Disorders of bone (e.g., Pagent's disease, avascular necrosis).

V. Epidemiology.

A. United States statistics.

1. OA affects nearly 27 million people in the United States (Hunter, 2007).

2. About 25% of visits to primary care physicians, and half of all non-steroidal anti-inflammatory drugs (NSAID) prescriptions (Lozada, n.d.).

3. It is estimated that 80% of the population have radiographic evidence of OA by age 65, although only 60% of those will have symptoms (Bijlsma, Berenbaum, & Lafeber, 2011).

B. International statistics.

1. OA is the most common articular disease (Lozada, n.d.).

2. The prevalence of OA differs among various ethnic groups (Felson, 2008).

3. OA is more prevalent in Native Americans than in the general population (Lozada, n.d.).

4. Disease of the hip is seen less frequently in Chinese patients from Hong Kong than in age-matched white populations (Felson, 2008).

5. In persons older than 65 years, OA is more common in whites than in blacks (Lozada, n.d.).

6. Knee OA appears to be more common in black women than in other groups (Felson, 2006).

C. Age and sex-related prevalence.

1. The prevalence of the disease increases dramatically among persons over age 50 (Bijlsma, Berenbaum, & Lafeber, 2011; and Hunter, 2007).

2. Approximately 80-90% of individuals older than 65 years have evidence of primary OA (Felson, 2006).

3. Patients with symptoms usually do not notice them until after age 50 years (Bijlsma, Berenbaum, & Lafeber, 2011; and Hunter, 2007).

4. In individuals older than age 55 years, the prevalence of OA is higher among women than men (Bijlsma, Berenbaum, & Lafeber, 2011; Hunter, 2007; and Lozada, n.d.).

5. Women are especially susceptible to OA in the proximal interphalangeal (PIP) and distal interphalangeal (DIP) joints of the fingers (Lozada, n.d.).

6. Women also have OA of the knee joints more frequently than do men, with a female-to-male incidence ratio of 1.7:1 (Felson, 2008).

7. Women are also more prone to erosive OA of the hand, familial studies suggest genetic factors (Ehrich, 2001).

VI. Nursing Assessment.

A. Detailed history to identify other potential causes. The typical joints involved with OA include the DIP, PIP, and carpometacarpal (CMC) joint at the base of the thumb, knees, hips, and cervical and lumbar spine. The age of onset is typically after the age of 50, unless there has been significant prior trauma, joint deformity, or superimposed inflammatory arthritis (RA, lupus, etc).

Morning stiffness with OA varies with the individual but generally is of short duration (5-30 minutes). The pain worsens with activity and improves with rest. By contrast, inflammatory arthritis has significant amounts of morning stiffness (>30 minutes), improves with activity and worsens with inactivity.

B. Physical examination findings.

1. A deep, achy joint pain is the main presenting symptom of OA.

2. Reduced range of motion and crepitus (a grating sound) are frequently present.

3. Malalignment with a bony enlargement may be visible.

4. Some cases of OA do not involve erythema or warmth over the affected joint(s); however an effusion may be present. The effusion is typically non-inflammatory, meaning that the total white blood cell (WBC) count from the joint aspiration is less than 200/mL. An inflammatory joint fluid, like in rheumatoid arthritis, gout or septic arthritis, typically has an inflammatory effusion with WBC counts in the 2,000 – 100,000/mL range (McCance & Heuther, 2006).

VII. Diagnosis.

A. OA usually is diagnosed by having history of symptoms and physical examination.

1. There is no blood test for the diagnosis of OA. Blood tests are performed to exclude diseases that can cause secondary OA, as well as to exclude other arthritis conditions that can mimic OA.

2. Comprehensive analysis of the location, duration, and character of the joint symptoms and the appearance of the joints helps the providers in diagnosing OA.

3. Bony enlargement of the joints from spur formations is characteristic of OA. Therefore, the presence of Heberden's nodes, Bouchard's nodes, and bunions of the feet can indicate to the provider a diagnosis of OA (Hunter & Lo, 2009).

B. Imaging techniques.

1. X-ray of the affected joints can be used to diagnose OA or to help rule out other joint problems. The common X-ray findings of OA include loss of joint cartilage, narrowing of the joint space between adjacent bones, and bone spur formation. Simple X-ray testing can also be very helpful to exclude other causes of pain in a particular joint as well as assisting the decision-making as to when surgical intervention might be considered (Hunter & Lo, 2009).

2. Ultrasound of the PIP or not of DIP joints can be beneficial to evaluate for superimposed inflammatory arthritis (like RA, gout, or psoriatic arthritis) in patients with OA. Ultrasound can be used in the evaluation and management of the hip OA as well, allowing for more accurate joint aspiration and injection.

3. Ultrasound is also useful in people who have a pacemaker or those who cannot undergo MRI. MRI should be considered prior to arthroscopy of a knee but is dependent on the skill of the technician.

C. Arthrocentesis is a procedure to remove joint fluid for analysis.

1. Joint fluid analysis is useful in excluding gout, infection, and other causes of arthritis.

2. The joint fluid of an osteoarthritic joint is "non-inflammatory"; the total WBC count should be less than 200 (McCance & Huether, 2006).

3. There should be no crystals or micro-organisms in the OA fluid.

D. Arthroscopy is a surgical technique in which a surgeon inserts a viewing tube into the joint space.

1. Abnormalities of and damage to the cartilage and ligaments can be detected and sometimes repaired during this procedure.

2. The long-term efficacy of arthroscopy has come under scrutiny after Kirkely and colleagues (2008) found that arthroscopic surgery for osteoarthritis of the knee provided no additional benefit to optimized physical and medical therapy.

VIII. Treatment.

A. Presently, OA cannot be cured. It will most likely get worse over time; nevertheless, the OA symptoms can be controlled. Patient education is helpful in the self-management of arthritis, which decreases pain, improving function, reducing stiffness and fatigue, and reducing medication use.

B. Lifestyle Changes.

1. Exercise.

   a. Staying active and exercising helps maintain joint and overall movement (e.g., swimming and aquatic exercises are especially helpful).

   b. Moderate exercise leads to improved functioning and decreased pain in people with OA of the knee.

   c. For most people, graded exercise should be the mainstay of self-management.

   d. Functional, gait, and balance training has been recommended to address impairments of proprioception, balance, and strength in individuals with lower extremity arthritis.

   e. Splinting of the thumb for OA of the base of the thumb leads to improvements after one year. Use ring splints for OA of the PIP joints.

2. Physical Therapy (PT) / Occupational Therapy (OT).

   a. PT can help improve muscle strength and the motion of stiff joints, as well as sense of balance.

   b. Likeliness of improvement with therapy may be seen within 6-8 weeks.

   c. OT can help splinting of erosive OA of hands to improve function for activities of daily living (ADLs).

   d. OT can also recommend certain gadgets to use and help with ADLs.

3. Weight Loss.

   a. Weight loss may be an important factor for overweight people.

   b. A meta-analysis has shown patient education can provide on average 20% more pain relief when compared to NSAIDs alone in patients with hip OA (Lane, 2007).

4. Other lifestyle recommendations include the following:

a. Applying heat and cold.

b. Getting enough rest.

c. Protecting the joints; braces and splints can sometimes support weakened joints. Some prevent the joint from moving; others allow some movement.

d. Note: Using a brace the wrong way can cause more joint damage, stiffness, and pain.

C. Medications.

1. Oral medications.

a. Acetaminophen is the first-line treatment for OA. New total daily dose limit is 3000 mgs acetaminophen (Felson, 2006; Hunter, 2007; and Lozada, n.d.).

b. For mild to moderate OA symptoms, over-the-counter (OTC) medications NSAIDs, such as ibuprofen, aspirin, naproxen, may be effective; however, NSAIDs are associated with greater side effects such as gastrointestinal bleeding, increased blood pressure, and increased risk for heart attack and renal impairment (Lane, 2007).

c. Another class of NSAIDs, COX-2 selective inhibitors (such as Celebrex®), is equally effective to NSAIDs but no safer in terms of side effects, and drugs in this class are generally more expensive.

d. Opioid analgesics, such as morphine and fentanyl, improve pain greatly, but at times this benefit does not outweigh adverse events; opioids should serve as the last option and should not routinely be used, especially in the elderly who are at risk for falling and fractures.

e. Oral steroids are not recommended in the treatment of OA because of their modest benefit and high rate of adverse effects. At times oral steroids are used in OA of spine with spinal stenosis.

2. Topical cream.

a. Such as Ingredients such as diclofenac (several Trade names), has fewer systemic side-effects, offers a good alternative for oral NSAIDs.

b. The ingredient derived from chili peppers, capsaicin (several trade names), skin cream can also help relieve pain. Use caution as this can cause burns.

3. Injection medicine.

a. Glucocorticoids (such as hydrocortisone) can be directly injected into the joint to reduce swelling and pain. Length of effectiveness varies by individual. Typically limited to no more than 3-4 times in the same joint per year. Each injection carries a risk of introducing an infection into the joint space, but fortunately as opposed to systemically administered steroids (orally, IV), the risk for the development of other side effects like impairment of blood glucose or avascular necrosis (dead bone) is much less.

b. Hyaluronic acid preparations (several trade names) can also be injected into the knee to relieve pain. Length of effectiveness varies by individual. Insurance will only allow for an injection every 6 months.

c. Epidural steroid injections are sometimes used in the treatment of lumbar spinal stenosis; however, the long term efficacy has not been confirmed by clinical trials (Radcliff et al., 2013).

D. Alternative medicine.

1. Many alternative medicines purport to decrease pain associated with arthritis. However, there is no evidence supporting benefits for most alternative treatments including vitamin A, C, and E, ginger, turmeric, omega-3 fatty acids, chondroitin sulfate, and glucosamine (Bijlsma, Berenbaum, & Lafeber, 2011).

2. Glucosamine was once believed to be effective, but a recent analysis has found that it is no better than placebo. S-Adenosyl methionine may relieve pain similar to nonsteroidal anti-inflammatory medications (Sawitzke, et al., 2010).

3. The OA Research Society International (OARSI) recommends that glucosamine be discontinued if no effect is observed after six months (Bijlsma, Berenbaum, & Lafeber, 2011).

4. The structure-modifying effects of chondroitin sulfate have been described in recent meta-analyses (Hochberg, Chevalier, Henrotin, Hunter, & Uebelhart, 2013). There appears to be a small but significant reduction in the rate of decline in joint space width in patients with knee OA. The quality of

chondroitin sulfate has been poor, and thus, it is recommended that pharmaceutical-grade chondroitin sulfate be used rather than food supplements in the treatment of OA. Other hypotheses as the lack of more robust evidence supporting the beneficial structural effects of chondroitin have to do with the timing (start taking before knee OA develops symptomatically or radiographically) and the duration of treatment (longer is better).

5. S-adenosylmethionine (SAMe, pronounced "Sammy") is a man-made form of a natural byproduct of the amino acid methionine. It has been marketed as a remedy for arthritis, but scientific evidence to support these claims is lacking (Gregory, Sperry, & Wilson, 2008).

E. Alternative treatment.

1. Acupuncture.

   a. It is a treatment based on Chinese medicine. How it works is not entirely clear.

   b. Acupuncture leads to a statistically significant improvement in pain; this improvement is small and may be of questionable clinical significance. Acupuncture does not seem to produce much long-term benefits (Wang, Kain, & White, 2008).

2. Mud pack therapy has been suggested to temporarily relieve pain in patients with OA of the knees. It uses compresses of mineral-rich mud such as that extracted from the Dead Sea. The effectiveness of this therapy varies greatly.

3. Massage therapy may also help provide short-term pain relief. It may be beneficial to work with an experienced massage therapist who understands how to work with sensitive joint areas.

4. While transcutaneous electrical nerve stimulation (TENS) has been used for a long time, there is no evidence to show that it reduces pain or disability (Hunter & Lo, 2009).

F. Surgery.

1. Patients with severe cases of OA might need surgery as an option to replace or repair damaged joints.

2. Arthroscopic surgery - trim torn and damaged cartilage, but arthroscopic surgical intervention for OA of the knee has been found to be no better than placebo at relieving symptoms (Kirkley, et al., 2008).

3. Osteotomy - changing the alignment of a bone to relieve stress on the bone or joint.

4. Arthrodesis - surgical fusion of bones, usually in the spine.

5. Total or partial replacement of the damaged joint with an artificial joint (e.g., knee replacement, hip replacement, shoulder replacement, ankle replacement, elbow replacement) (Felson, 2006).

6. Surgery for CMC OA of the thumb can also be performed to reduce severe pain, but frequently leads to decreased range of motion (thumb opposition) (Beatus & Beatus, 2008).

IX. Nursing implications.

A. Educate patients on the natural history of and management options for OA.

B. Explain the differences between OA and other types of arthritis, such as rheumatoid arthritis and gout.

C. Provide resources and offer support groups (e.g., Arthritis Foundation). Remind patients to use lifestyle management to cope with OA symptoms, for instance, giving proper positioning and support to the neck and back during sitting or sleeping; adjusting furniture, such as raising a chair or toilet seat; and avoiding trauma and repetitive motions of the joint, especially frequent bending.

D. Emphasize the need for follow-up visits and how to take pain medication appropriately and monitor for side effects.

E. Encourage regular exercise to improve muscle strength and weight loss in overweight people (e.g., Exercises that increase strength of the quadriceps muscles also can help decrease knee pain).

F. Physical and occupational therapy can provide additional pain relief and improvement of function through exercises aimed at improving muscle strength, proprioception and joint protection and the use of braces, splints and assistive devices.

Summary

OA is the most common form of articular disease and can occur together with other types of arthritis. It causes pain, swelling, and reduced motion mainly in weight-bearing joints – hands, knees, hips, or spine. The goal of treatment in OA is to reduce pain and improve function. Exercise is an important part of OA treatment because it can help to decrease joint pain and improve function. To date, there is no treatment that can reverse the damage of OA in the joints.

References

Beatus, J., & Beatus, R. A. (2008). Management of the basal joint of the thumb following interposition arthroplasty for pain and instability. *Physiotherapy Theory and Practice*, 24(4), 299-309. doi: 10.1080/09593980701738665.

Bijlsma, J. W, Berenbaum, F, & Lafeber, F. P. (2011). Osteoarthritis: An update with relevance for clinical practice. *The Lancet*, 377, 2115-2126.

Ehrich, G. E. (2001). Erosive osteoarthritis: presentation, clinical pearls, and therapy. *Current Rheumatology Reports*, 3(6), 484-488.

Felson, D. T. (2006). Osteoarthritis of the knee. *The New England Journal of Medicine*, 354(8), 841-848.

Felson, D. T. (2008). Comparing the prevalence of rheumatic diseases in China with the rest of the world. *Arthritis Research & Therapy*, 10(1), 106.

Gregory, P. J, Sperry, M., & Wilson, A. F. (2008). Dietary supplements for osteoarthritis. *American Family Physician*, 77, 177-184.

Hochberg, M., Chevalier, X., Henrotin, Y., Hunter, D.J., & Uebelhart, D. (2013). Symptom and structure modification in osteoarthritis with pharmaceutical-grade chondroitin sulfate: What's the evidence? *Current Medical Research and Opinion*, 29(3), 259-267. doi: 10.1185/03007995.2012.753430.

Hunter, D.J. (2007) In the clinic: Osteoarthritis. *Annals of Internal Medicine*, 147(3), 8-16.

Hunter, D.J., & Lo, G. H. (2009). The management of osteoarthritis: An overview and call to appropriate conservative treatment. *Medical Clinics of North America*, 93(127), 43-49.

Kirkley, A., Birmingham, T., Litchfield, R. B., Giffin, J. R., Willits, K. R., Wong, C. J., Feagan, G., Donner, A., Griffin, S. H., D'Ascanio, L. M., Pope, J. E., & Fowler, P. J. (2008). A randomized trial of arthroscopic surgery for osteoarthritis of the knee. *The New England Journal of Medicine*, 359(11), 1097-1107. doi: 10.1056/NEJMoa0708333

Lane, N. E. (2007). Osteoarthritis of the hip. *The New England Journal of Medicine*, 357 (14), 1413-1421.

Lozada, C. J. (n.d.). *Osteoarthritis*. Retrieved from http://emedicine.medscape.com/article/330487-overview

McCance, K. L., & Huether, S. E. (2006). Alterations of musculoskeletal function. In L. Crowthier, & K. L. McCance (Eds.), *Pathophysiology: The biologic basis of disease in adults and children* (pp. 1529-1531). Saint Louis, MO: Elsevier Mosby.

Radcliff, K., Kepler, C., Hilibrand, A., Rihn, J., Zhao, W., Lurie, J., Tosteson, T., . . . ,Weinstein, J. (2013). Epidural steroid injections are associated with less improvement in patients with lumbar spinal stenosis: A subgroup analysis of the spine patient outcomes research trial. *Spine*, 38(4), 279-291. doi: 10.1097/BRS.0b013e31827ec51f.

Sawitzke, A. D., Shi, H., Finco, M. F., Dunlop, D. D., Harris, C. L., Singer, N. G., . . . Clegg, D. O. (2010). Clinical efficacy and safety of glucosamine, chondroitin sulphate, their combination, celecoxib or placebo taken to treat osteoarthritis of the knee: 2-year results from GAIT. Annals of Rheumatic Disease, 69(8), 1459-1464. doi: 10.1136/ard.2009.120469

Shiel, W. C. (n.d.). *Osteoarthritis*. Retrieved from http://www.medicinenet.com/osteoarthritis/article.htm

Wang, S., Kain, Z. N., & White, P. F. (2008). Acupuncture analgesia II. Clinical considerations. *Anesthesia & Analgesia*, 106(2), 611–621. doi:10.1213/ane.0b013e318160644d

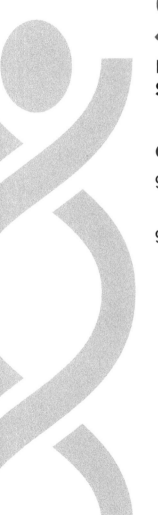

SECTION 9
RHEUMATOLOGY NURSING ACROSS THE LIFESPAN:
SPECIAL CONDITIONS

Contents of Section 9

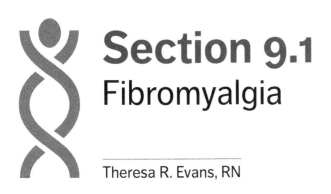

Section 9.1
Fibromyalgia

Theresa R. Evans, RN

Introduction

Fibromyalgia is the most common chronic, widespread pain syndrome diagnosed worldwide. This chapter will touch on key points including proposed causes, symptoms, diagnosis, treatments, and nursing considerations regarding this challenging condition.

Learning Objectives

Upon completion of this chapter, the nurse will be able to:

1. Identify factors that can make diagnosing fibromyalgia a challenge.

2. Identify criteria used to base a diagnosis of fibromyalgia.

3. List nursing assessments when caring for a patient with fibromyalgia.

4. Describe pharmacologic management of fibromyalgia.

5. Discuss non-pharmacologic management of fibromyalgia.

Content Outline

I. Pathophysiology.

A. Fibromyalgia (FM) has scientific debate surrounding whether it should be recognized as a disease or a condition. FM is defined by chronic widespread musculoskeletal pain felt symmetrically in all four quadrants (above and below the waist and both sides) of the body for at least 3 months. This symmetric pain pattern helps to distinguish FM from other pain syndromes. Other symptoms that can commonly occur with FM include:

1. Fatigue.

2. Sleep disturbances and dysfunction.

3. Musculoskeletal stiffness and painful tender points.

4. Cognitive and memory problems (often termed "Fibro-fog")

5. Depression and anxiety.

6. Heightened sensitivity to stimuli such as light, odors, and sound.

7. Increased sensitivity to painful stimuli (hyperalgesia).

B. FM often co-exists with other pain-related disorders such as:

1. Irritable bowel syndrome (IBS).

2. Migraine and tension or cluster headaches.

3. Temporomandibular joint dysfunction (TMJ).

4. Irritable bladder syndrome.

5. Pelvic pain syndromes.

C. FM may occur by itself (primary) or in conjunction with other diseases (secondary), many times inflammatory, autoimmune, and /or viral in nature, such as:

1. Rheumatoid arthritis.

2. Systemic lupus erythematosus.

3. Lyme disease.

4. Epstein-Barr virus.

5. Viral hepatitis.

D. FM affects 2 – 4 % of the population, including:

1. Men.

2. Women (diagnosed three times more prevalently in women than men and children).

3. Children.

II. Etiology.

A. Fibromyalgia (also previously referred to as muscular rheumatism, hysterical paroxysm, and fibrositis) has been studied since the 1800s. As time has passed, it has been thought that FM was strictly a muscle disease, as muscle pain is the primary symptom. It was also thought to be an autoimmune disease; however, research has revealed no specific muscle etiology or consistent immune system abnormalities to bear weight to either of those diagnoses. The term fibromyalgia was first used in 1976 in a more conclusive effort to describe the primary symptom of pain (fibro – meaning fibrous tissue, my – meaning muscle, and algia – meaning pain). In 1990, the American College of Rheumatology (ACR) developed diagnostic criteria for research purposes, and since then, the term fibromyalgia has been the terminology of choice (Richards, 2009).

B. Scientific and clinical studies support the possibility of genetic predisposition for FM. In addition to a genetic link, the following external factors have been known to also play a role in the development of FM (Smith, Harris, & Clauw, 2011):

1. Physical stress such as trauma.

2. Emotional and psychological stress.

3. Chronic sleep deprivation and disorders.

III. Diagnosis.

A. There are no specific imaging or laboratory tests approved to diagnose FM. Diagnosis is routinely based on a thorough history, subjective patient complaints (see Figure 1), and healthcare provider's physical exam in combination with ruling out other disease processes and conditions that FM could mimic, such as:

1. Chronic fatigue syndrome.

2. Autoimmune diseases such as rheumatoid arthritis.

3. Endocrine and thyroid disorders.

4. Hepatitis C.

5. Polymyalgia rheumatica (PMR).

6. Degenerative spinal disease.

7. Lyme disease.

8. Malignancies and cancers.

9. Human immunodeficiency virus (HIV).

B. The physical exam for a patient with widespread pain may include a tender point examination, although this is no longer required for diagnosis. This is performed by the healthcare provider's palpating 18 specific areas of the body, applying pressure enough to blanche the provider's fingertips (an estimated 4 kg of pressure) (Klippel, Stone, Crofford, & White, 2008). A total of 9 or more tender points upon palpation used to be the accepted criterion to consider a FM diagnosis, as opposed to original criteria of 11 out of 18. FM tends to be cyclical in nature (see Figure 2).

C. In 2010, the ACR proposed 3 Key Element Criteria as the basis of diagnosing FM. The proposed 3 Key Element Criteria include the following (Wolfe, et al, 2010):

1. Presentation of widespread pain and symptoms of three months or more.

2. A Widespread Pain Index (WPI) that assesses the number of painful body areas. This is a healthcare provider-administered questionnaire.

3. A Symptom Severity Scale (SSS), another healthcare provider-administered questionnaire that assesses the severity of fatigue, waking un-refreshed, and cognitive symptoms, as well as the extent of other possible somatic symptoms.

D. 21st century research is promising, and studies have shown that FM may be caused by abnormal pain and sensory processing in the central nervous system (CNS), causing symptoms that can affect the entire body. The exact mechanisms of action to cause this widespread pain

Figure 1: Symptons of Fibromyalgia

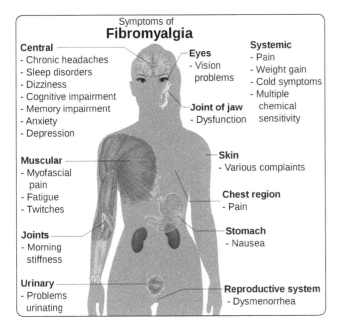

Source: Common signs and symptoms of fibromyalgia. (See Wikipedia: Fibromyalgia #Signs and symptoms). Model: Mikael Häggström (http://commons.wikimedia.org/wiki/File:Symptoms_of_fibromyalgia.png)

Figure 2: Fibromyalgia Tender Points

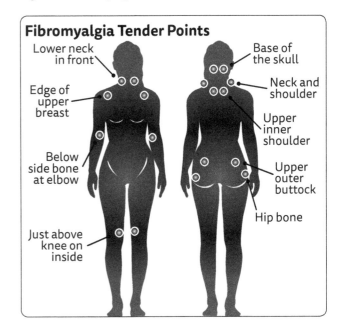

Source: Adapted from: Mind, Body, and Soul Rehab... Symptoms>> Fibromyalgia Tender Points. http://mindbodyandsoulrehab.wordpress.com/symptoms/fibromyalgia-tender-points/

condition are yet to be known; however, it has been seen that cerebrospinal fluid (CSF) in those with FM can contain three times as much of the neuropeptide Substance P and up to four times as much nerve growth factor in comparison with those studied without FM (FitzGibbons, 2007).

E. Research also has shown that patients with FM have decreased stage 4, deep -sleep patterns, which prevents restorative slumber. Chronic sleep dysfunction has consistently been shown to perpetuate pain (FitzGibbons, 2007).

IV. Nursing Assessment.

A. Rheumatology nurses conducting a health assessment of an individual suspected of having FM should ask the following questions:

1. What is the patient's pain level using a universal pain scale (or the WPI as proposed above)?

2. What is the description of the pain (e.g., burning, aching, stiffness, soreness)?

3. What is the patient's psychosocial history including current stress level, mood, history of depression and/or anxiety?

4. What is patient's fatigue level (or the SSS as proposed above)?

5. Is the patient experiencing restorative sleep (or the SSS as proposed above)?

6. Is the patient complaining of or showing signs of cognitive dysfunction (or the SSS as proposed above)?

7. Is the patient displaying impaired physical mobility or range of motion (ROM)?

8. What are the patient's current medications, treatments, or therapies?

V. Treatment.

A. FM is a manageable condition treated therapeutically on an individual basis. Symptoms will vary from person to person. A combination of pharmacologic and non-pharmacologic therapies is usually most beneficial.

1. Prevention.

2. Development of advantageous sleep patterns.
   a. Regular bedtime and wake up time.
   b. No caffeinated beverages after lunchtime.
   c. Regular aerobic exercise in the morning, not evening.

3. Stress management.
   a. Relaxation techniques.
   b. Meditation.
   c. Massage therapy.
   d. Acupuncture.

B. Non-pharmacologic therapies.

1. Stress management, as noted above.

2. Cognitive behavioral therapy.

3. Regular aerobic exercise (pool-based programs help with stiffness, flexibility, and pain management)

4. Physical therapy.

5. Massage and acupuncture therapies.

6. Biofeedback therapy.

C. Pharmacologic therapies.

1. Medications that alter levels of neurotransmitters in the brain are used most often. Medications followed by the + are FDA approved for the treatment of FM.
   a. Tricyclic antidepressants – which may diminish pain by improving sleep.
      (1) Amitriptyline.
      (2) Nortriptyline.

D. Muscle relaxants.

1. Cyclobenzaprine (Flexeril®).

E. SNRIs – Seratonin Norepinephrine Reuptake Inhibitors.

1. Venlafaxine (Effexor®).

2. Duloxetine (Cymbalta®)+.

3. Milnacipran (Savella®)+.

F. SSRIs – Selective Seratonin Reuptake Inhibitors help relieve pain by improving individuals' mood.

1. Fluoxetine (Prozac®).

2. Paroxetine (Paxil®).

3. Sertraline (Zoloft®).

G. Alpha 2-delta ligands (anticonvulsants) – Regulates neurotransmitters such as glutamate and Substance P.

1. Gabapentin (Neurontin®).

2. Pregabalin (Lyrica®)+.

H. Others.

1. Sodium oxybate (Xyrem®) – approved for narcolepsy.

2. Tramadol (Ultram®) – opioid analgesic that affects serotonin and norepinephrine pathways.

VI. Co-morbidities.

A. There are no co-morbidities in primary FM. All co-morbidities listed below are related to secondary FM:

1. Myofacial pain syndrome (MPS).

2. Chronic fatigue syndrome (CFS).

3. Gulf War syndrome.

4. Restless leg syndrome.

5. Periodic limb movement disorder.

6. Irritable bowel syndrome (IBS).

7. Interstitial cystitis (IC).

8. Depression.

9. Sleep disturbances such as insomnia and sleep apnea.

VII. Nursing implications.

A. Patient education.

1. Nature of the syndrome.

a. Chronic, yet manageable.

b. Patient -specific symptom targeted treatments.

2. Preventive measures.

a. Patient education.

b. Lifestyle modification.

(1) Sleep etiquette.

(2) Stress management.

(3) Low impact exercise.

3. Treatment options.

a. Pharmacologic (purpose of medication).

b. Non-pharmacologic.

c. Medication side effects.

d. Low impact exercise.

4. Desired outcomes.

a. Improved and restorative sleep.

b. Improvement in or elimination of pain.

c. Patient verbalization, understanding.

(1) Chronic, yet manageable, syndrome.

(2) Potential medication side effects.

(3) Preventive measures.

(4) Treatment options.

5. Additional resources.

a. Arthritis Foundation - http://www.arthritis.org/

b. National Fibromyalgia Association - http://www.fmaware.org/

c. The American Fibromyalgia Syndrome Association - http://www.afsafund.org/

d. Local chapters of the Arthritis Foundation and Fibromyalgia Associations.

6. Research.

a. FM research is continuously ongoing in centers all around the world. Encouraging patients to explore these centers may allow them to obtain treatments that might otherwise not be available to the public. It also may offer a free alternative if patients are uninsured or cannot afford prescribed therapies. Centers participating in clinical trials for the treatment of fibromyalgia maybe found at the following websites:

(1) http://search.centerwatch.com/default.aspx?SearchQuery=fibromyalgia

(2) http://www.clinicalconnection.com/Default.aspx

Summary

Fibromyalgia is associated with chronic pain. Research continues to better understand the pathophysiology, causes and treatment of fibromyalgia. Nursing support should include a mixture of pharmacologic and non-pharmacologic measures. Nurses should be familiar with community resources such as yoga classes, tai chi, low impact aerobics, massage therapists, and support groups.

References

FitzGibbons, J. (2007, September). Be a myth-buster: Stop the misconceptions about fibromyalgia. *American Nurse Today, 2*(9), 40-45.

Klippel, J.H., Stone, J.H., Crofford, L.J., & White, P.H. (Eds.). (2008). *Primer of the rheumatic diseases* (13th ed.). New York: Springer Science + Business Media, LLC.

Richards, K. (2009). History of fibromyalgia. *Health Central.* Retrieved from http://www.healthcentral.com/chronic-pain/fibromyalgia-287647-5.html

Smith, H.S., Harris, R., & Clauw, D. (2011). Fibromyalgia: An afferent processing disorder leading to a complex pain generalized syndrome. *Pain Physician, 14,* E217-E245.

Wolfe, F., Clauw, D.J., Fitzcharles, M.A., Goldenberg, D.L., Katz, R.S., Mease, P., ...Yunus, M.B.(2010). The American College of Rheumatology preliminary diagnostic criteria for fibromyalgia and measurement of symptom severity. *Arthritis Care & Research, 62*(5), 600-610.

Suggested Readings

Bigatti, S.M., Hernandez, A.M., Cronan, T.A., & Rand, K.L. (2008). Sleep disturbances in fibromyalgia syndrome: Relationship to pain and depression. *Arthritis & Rheumatism, 59*(7), 961-967

Rao, S., Gendreau, J., & Kranzler, J. (2008). Understanding the fibromyalgia syndrome. *Psychopharmacology Bulletin, 40*(4), 24-56.

Rush University Medical Center. (2010, May). New criteria proposed for diagnosing fibromyalgia. *Science Daily.* Retrieved from http://www.sciencedaily.com/releases/2010/05/100524143427.htm

Valdes, M., Collado, A., Bargallo, N., Vazquez, M., Rami, L., Gomez, E., & Salamero, M. (2010). Increased glutamate-glutamine compounds in the brains of patients with fibromyalgia: A magnetic resonance spectroscopy study. *Arthritis & Rheumatism, 62*(6), 1829-1836

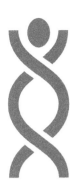

Section 9.2
Human Immunodeficiency Virus (HIV) and Rheumatic Disease

Iris Zink, MSN, RN, ANP-BC and Elizabeth Kirchner, CNP

Introduction

The human immunodeficiency virus (HIV) creates complex interactions with rheumatologic disease, and the patient with HIV is at high risk for several rheumatologic conditions. An understanding of these conditions and interactions is critical to the proper care of patients with HIV.

Since its emergence in 1981, human immunodeficiency virus (HIV) has been classified as a pandemic by the World Health Organization (WHO). HIV and acquired immunodeficiency syndrome (AIDS) have killed more than 25 million people in the past two decades. More than 40 million people are infected worldwide. In 2012, > 1.2 million people were living with HIV in the United States. The Centers for Disease Control and Prevention (CDC) estimates that 50,000 people are infected in the United States annually (http://www.cdc.gov/hiv/statistics/basics/ataglance.html).

Despite the fact that combination antiretroviral therapy (cART) has improved the mortality risk of the disease, the persistent prevalence of HIV infection necessitates that the healthcare provider recognize the disease symptoms and the associated rheumatologic sequelae.

Learning Objectives

Upon completion of this chapter, the nurse will be able to:

1. Describe the importance of human immunodeficiency virus (HIV) testing in rheumatology and identify false positive lab results in patients with HIV.

2. Define diffuse infiltrative lymphocytosis syndrome (DILS) and immune reconstitution inflammatory syndrome (IRIS).

3. Discuss how active antiretroviral (ARV) medications affect the immune system.

4. Identify two of the most common types of arthritis in the patient with HIV.

5. Identify at least two of the sequelae of treatment with ARV medications.

Content Outline

I. Human Immunodeficiency Virus (HIV).

A. AIDS is a syndrome caused by a retrovirus that has its principal effect on the immune system. The CD4 T lymphocytes are destroyed by multiple mechanisms:

   1. Action of cytotoxic T lymphocytes.

   2. Mechanism of apoptosis.

   3. Killing by natural killer (NK) cells.

   4. Cytopathic effect (i.e., syncytia formation) (Azeroual et al., 2008).

B. As the CD4 T cell numbers decline below a critical level, cell-mediated immunity is no longer effective, and the patient becomes increasingly susceptible to opportunistic infections.

C. The stage of HIV infection can be determined in part by measuring the patient's CD4 T cell count and viral load; stages include:

   1. Acute infection.
      a. The acute infection stage lasts for several weeks and may include symptoms such as fever, lymphadenopathy, pharyngitis, rash, myalgia, malaise, and mouth and esophageal sores.

   2. Latency.
      a. The latency stage involves few or no symptoms and can last from a few weeks to more than 20 years depending on the individual.

   3. AIDS.
      a. AIDS is defined by either absolute CD4 T cell counts less than 200 or CD4 percent < 15%, or specific AIDS-related infection or other condition.

   4. cART treatment.
      a. In the treatment phase, regardless of CD4 count, cART is initiated.

D. Prevention.

   1. HIV is typically spread by having sexual contact and/or sharing needles with someone who is HIV+. Educating sexually active patients about the importance of safer sex practices in order to decrease risk of transmission is extremely important. Patients at risk for HIV transmission via non-sexual routes such as drug-related needle sharing should be encouraged to avoid such risky behaviors and referred to appropriate social services when possible.

E. The rheumatology nurse and HIV.

   1. Although staging of HIV is useful, rheumatology-related signs and symptoms may occur at any stage (Patel, Patel, & Espinoza, 2009). The role of the rheumatology nurse is to educate the patient about signs and symptoms of disease progression as well as secondary infections and provide access to resources about the disease state and treatment options. The diagnosis of HIV also necessitates collaboration with infectious disease specialists especially if any antiretroviral treatment is considered. The advanced practice rheumatology nurse (APRN) and the rheumatology registered nurse (RN) function as liaisons between the patient and other specialists within the multi-disciplinary team in making sure the needs of the patient are met.

II. Rheumatology and HIV.

A. Since the first description of AIDS, direct and indirect involvement of every human organ system has been reported, and rheumatologic involvement is no exception (Mody, Parke, & Reveille, 2003). With treatment advances, HIV mortality rates have dropped, and more patients are living with chronic HIV infections and the associated complications. HIV antigens immunologically resemble some host antigens; this molecular mimicry may result in autoimmune responses such as reactive or psoriatic arthritis, diffuse infiltrative lymphocytosis syndrome (DILS), myopathy, vasculitis, or other conditions (Patel, Patel, & Espinoza, 2009). This mimicry can make diagnosis of the autoimmune disease much more complex. Prognosis is worse in those with advanced AIDS.

B. A wide array of arthropathies can occur with HIV infection; presentation can vary (see Table 1).

1. Patients with HIV have been found to have positive rheumatoid factor and anti-cyclic citrullinated antibody (CCP) which may not be prognostic of the rheumatology symptomatology. Anticardiolipin and antiphospholipid antibodies have also been reported but do not seem to be significant risk factors for bleeding or clotting except in those individuals who are also positive for hepatitis C. HIV-infected patients with rheumatologic symptoms require a thorough diagnostic workup to identify underlying causation.

C. HIV in rheumatology.

1. In 2006, the Centers for Disease Control (CDC) recommended that all persons age 13-64 be tested for HIV regardless of perceived risk (Ouedraogo & Meyer, 2012). Given the myriad of rheumatologic clinical presentations related to HIV infection, screening all patients with rheumatic diseases is imperative, as the implications of undiagnosed HIV infection are enormous (Angarone, 2012). HIV exerts potential effects on lab results, is associated with rheumatologic symptoms, and may complicate rheumatologic disease modifying therapy.

2. HIV-induced arthropathy and arthralgias improve with more aggressive HIV treatment; however, cART has created a new generation of secondary autoimmune disease flares because of a phenomenon called immune reconstitution inflammatory syndrome (IRIS).

3. About 5% of patients with HIV report diffuse arthralgias. As the treatment of HIV has improved, the incidence of arthralgias has decreased. The pathophysiology of these arthralgias remains enigmatic, with possible contributions from HIV itself, circulating viral and host immune complexes, and concomitant autoimmunity; the arthralgias may also be related to secondary infections such as hepatitis C, or a bacterial source (Reveille & Williams, 2006). Typically, these arthralgias are characterized by oligo-arthritis, affecting the lower extremities with short (fewer than 6 weeks) duration of symptoms and culture-negative synovial fluid (Maganti, Reveille, & Williams, 2008). Although all varieties of presentations have been noted, most patients do not have radiographic changes and do not progress to inflammatory arthritis.

Table 1: Arthropathies by Distribution, Duration, and Treatment

Arthropathy	Distribution	Duration	Treatment
Arthralgias	Oligoarticular large joints (e.g., knees, shoulders, elbows)	4-6 week average	Non-Steroidal Anti-Inflammatory Drugs (NSAIDs)
Reactive arthritis	Asymmetric axial and polyarticular	Chronic	NSAIDs consider DMARDs/ and or Biologics
Undifferentiated spondyloarthropathy	Asymmetric axial and polyarticular	Chronic	NSAIDs, consider DMARDs/ and or Biologics
Painful articular syndrome	Knees, elbows, and shoulder common	2-24 hours	Analgesics
Gout	Oligoarticular (e.g., feet, hands, wrists)	Acute to chronic	Changing treatment for HIV, uric acid lowering agents, NSAIDs and steroids
Rheumatoid arthritis	Symmetrical, polyarticular	Chronic	NSAIDs, steroids, consider DMARDs and/or Biologics

Source: Adapted from Allroggen, A., Frese, A., Rahmann, A., Gaubitz, M., Hussted, I. & Evers, S. (2005). HIV associated arthritis: Case report and review of the literature. European Journal of Medical Research, 10, 305-308.

III. HIV in Rheumatologic Disease.

A. Painful Articular Syndrome.

1. Painful articular syndrome is characterized by acute onset of severe, sharp, self-limiting joint or bone pain which can last as long as 48 hours. Acute intermittent pain can last up to two weeks. The prevalence of painful articular syndrome is approximately 5-25% of patients and is frequently associated with acute HIV infection (Restrepo et al., 2004). Patients frequently seek hospital care because of the severity of the symptoms. Most patients have spontaneous relief of symptoms, but treatment with opiates during the acute phase is often necessary. Radiographs and synovial fluid cell counts are normal. The knees are most often affected, but case reports document involvement of the shoulder and elbows. Patients with painful articular syndrome need reassurance that the acute pain will be of short duration and adequately addressed.

B. Systemic Lupus Erythematosus (SLE).

1. The diagnosis of systemic lupus erythematosus (SLE) can be complex in patients who are not infected with HIV; however, the diagnosis becomes even more difficult in those with HIV. Patients early in the SLE disease state may have rash, fever, myalgia, oral and nasal sores, and malaise; these symptoms may directly overlap with those of acute HIV infection. To further complicate the diagnosis, patients with HIV often exhibit false positive anti-nuclear antibody rheumatologic lab markers. Case studies concerning patients with SLE pre-dating acquisition of HIV are illustrative. Following the onset of HIV, some patients have gone into SLE remission presumably related to low CD4 T cell counts. Subsequent cART can lead to restoration of the immune system and resultant SLE flare (Nguyen & Reveille, 2009). The rheumatology nurse must educate the patient about the importance of adherence to the treatment regimen and the need for routine follow up.

C. Rheumatoid Arthritis (RA).

1. Cytokine production is central in HIV pathogenesis and appears to foster autoimmune complications. Rheumatoid arthritis (RA) develops from an autoimmune B- and T-cell dysfunction leading to increased TNF alpha and IL1 production via macrophage activity. HIV infection has also been shown to increase serum concentrations of TNF alpha. As HIV infection decreases the body's defense mechanisms by impairing T-lymphocyte response, patients with pre-existing RA may go into remission (Cepeda, Williams, Ishimori, Weisman, & Reveille, 2008). However, following an initiation of cART regimen, patients again may flare because of IRIS, and *de novo* case reports of RA have been seen. Disease-modifying treatment of RA is further complicated because of concerns of immunosuppression-related increased viral load or secondary opportunistic infections. Patients with RA need reassurance that their symptoms will be addressed; adherence with the treatment regimen is essential to enhance positive outcomes.

2. Patients with HIV and arthralgia present difficult diagnostic challenges. RA may be the prime consideration for presentation with symmetric polyarthritis worse in the small joints with radiographic osteopenia, soft tissue swelling, joint effusions, joint space narrowing, marginal erosions, periosteal reaction, and joint deformities such as flexion contractures, ulnar deviation, and swan neck deformities. Nonetheless, the clinician should be mindful that such a presentation with a negative rheumatoid factor, and proliferative bone formation with periostitis should prompt consideration of other entities such as inflammatory arthritis (Restrepo et al., 2004).

D. Immune Reconstitution Inflammatory Syndrome (IRIS).

1. Immune reconstitution inflammatory syndrome (IRIS) in HIV was described after cART availability. IRIS is common after initiation of cART because of rapidly increasing CD4 counts. IRIS has been implicated in highly inflammatory reactions to occult infections such as mycobacterium avium, tuberculosis, and cytomegalovirus, as well as the *de novo* appearance of a new autoimmune process, inflammatory condition, or flare of pre-existing disease (Nguyen & Reveille, 2009). Most autoimmune diseases arise *de novo* during IRIS, with approximately 20% from previous quiescent premorbid diseases (Nguyen & Reveille). Case reports document exacerbations of RA, SLE, and sarcoidosis, as well as the emergence of new conditions such as Graves' autoimmune thyroiditis, adult-onset Still's disease,

Sjögren's syndrome, diabetes mellitus, reactive arthritis, cutaneous lupus, gout, and polymyositis related to IRIS. In most cases, IRIS occurred 3 to 27 months after initiation of cART (Patel, Patel, & Espinoza, 2009). Because of the wide variety of presentations and potential for misdiagnosis, the exact prevalence of IRIS is unknown. Management of IRIS includes the continuation of cART and consideration of corticosteroids if life threatening or vital organ involvement occurs or uncontrolled inflammation intervenes. Most individuals with IRIS have a favorable prognosis with little reported mortality. The rheumatology nurse needs to reassure the patient that this syndrome is well-described and that appropriate monitoring and treatment will be provided.

E. Diffuse Infiltrative Lymphocytosis Syndrome (DILS).

1. Diffuse infiltrative lymphocytosis syndrome (DILS) is an HIV-associated condition that may mimic Sjögren's syndrome in patients presenting with swelling of the parotid and lacrimal glands plus sicca symptoms (see Table 2). The incidence of DILS ranges from 3-50% depending on region, genetics, and cART treatment (Vitali, 2011). Since the availability of cART, the occurrence of DILS has decreased. There is an increased incidence in African patients, which may be due to delay in treatment and genetic predisposition. DILS is characterized by proliferation and increased circulating CD8 cells in direct contrast to those with

Sjögren's syndrome who have increased CD4 proliferation. Patients who are not on antiviral therapy are more likely to have extra-glandular symptoms with DILS; these may include lymphocytic interstitial pneumonitis (LIP), cranial nerve VII palsy, peripheral neuropathy, renal tubular acidosis, polymyositis, and lymphocytic hepatitis (Reveille & Williams, 2006). The pathophysiology of DILS involves T-cell and lymphocytic infiltration of the muscles, nerves, and lungs. Because of associated risk of lymphoma with DILS, it is suggested that patients with parotid swelling undergo computed tomography (CT) scan and salivary or lacrimal gland biopsy to confirm lymphocytic infiltration in the absence of granulomatous or neoplastic involvement. Although the symptoms of DILS generally resolve spontaneously, some individuals with extra-glandular symptoms require corticosteroids, with higher doses needed for LIP (Reveille & Williams, 2006). The rheumatology nurse must educate the patient to reinforce the absolute need for adherence to the treatment regimen and good oral hygiene to prevent complications that occur secondary to dryness.

F. Reactive Arthritis and Psoriatic Arthritis.

1. Prior to the African HIV pandemic, there was an extremely low incidence of psoriatic arthritis in the African population. Spondyloarthritis is associated with HLA-B27 positivity, which is common in Caucasians but rare in black Africans. HIV in Africa has changed the incidence and prevalence of

Table 2: Targets, Symptoms, and Pathophysiology of Sjögren's, Hepatitis C, and DILS

VARIABLE	Sjögren's Syndrome	Hepatitis C	DILS
Sicca symptoms	Present	Present	Present
Extra-glandular	Pulmonary, gastrointestinal, renal, and neurological involvement	Gastrointestinal and musculoskeletal	Musculoskeletal, pulmonary, gastrointestinal, and neurological
Infiltrate character	CD4 T-cells	CD4 T-cells	CD8 T-cells
Autoantibodies	RF, ANA, anti-Ro/ SSA and anti-La/SSB	RF, rare ANA, anti-Ro/SSA and anti-La/SSB	RF, ANA
Parotid swelling	Moderate to severe	Mild to moderate	Moderate to severe

» RF – rheumatoid factor; ANA – antinuclear antibody; DILS – diffuse infiltrative lymphocytosis syndrome.

Source: Adapted from Vitali, C. (2011). Immunopathologic differences of Sjögren's syndrome versus sicca syndrome in HCV and HIV infection. *Arthritis Research & Therapy, 13*, p. 233. http://arthritis-research.com/content/13/4/233

rheumatologic diseases; psoriatic and reactive arthritis are now common manifestations in HIV-infected individuals. Psoriatic arthritis is 40 times more common in HIV-affected individual and reactive arthritis is 100-200 times more common in the patient with HIV compared to non- infected individuals (Takhar & Hendey, 2010). Reactive arthritis can still be activated by both gastrointestinal and sexually transmitted infections such as chlamydia trachomatis, Campylobacter jejuni, Shigella flexneri, Neisseria gonorrhoeae, Mycoplasma species, Ureaplasma urealyticum, Salmonella species, and Yersinia species.

2. HLA markers.

   a. Since the onset of HIV, the genetic marker HLA B*5703 has been identified as a risk factor for the development of spondyloarthropathy in the patient with HIV. In Thailand, spondyloarthropathy is also common and occurs in 55% of the HIV-infected population (Louthrenoo, 2008). HIV-associated reactive arthritis and psoriatic arthritis symptoms often overlap, and some investigators have suggested that the two diagnoses may exist on a continuum; therefore, the term undifferentiated spondyloarthropathy is used.

3. Clinical.

   a. The severity of the HIV directly correlates with the severity of the associated psoriasis. In advanced AIDS, psoriatic arthritis is more common, and the arthritis is rapidly progressive with erosions and deformities developing quickly. The most typical presentation is a sero-negative peripheral arthritis that predominantly affects the lower extremities and is usually accompanied by enthesitis. Enthesopathy and uveitis are prevalent; sacroiliitis and axial disease occur less commonly (Patel, Patel, & Espinoza, 2009). Mucocutaneous disease features are also common especially keratoderma blennorrhagicum and circinate balanitis. Extra articular symptoms of conjunctivitis, urethritis, onycholysis, and psoriasiform skin rashes are frequent (Walker, Tyndall, & Daikeler, 2008). Different forms of psoriasis can exist including vulgaris, inverse, guttate, palmo-plantar, erythrodermic, and pustular in conjunction with both reactive and psoriatic arthritis (Patel, Patel, & Espinoza, 2009). Because of the

known association between depression and psoriasis, the rheumatology nurse must monitor patients for symptoms as well as form an open, therapeutic relationship with the patient in order for symptoms to be reported.

4. Pathophysiology and Treatment.

   a. Cytotoxic CD8 cells are proliferative in HIV-positive reactive arthritis and patients with psoriatic arthritis. T-reg cells are initially deficient in psoriasis but expand when patients are placed on cART (Patel, Patel, & Espinoza, 2009). Cytokines such as tumor necrosis factor alpha play a significant role in stimulation of the autoimmune process in HIV replication and psoriasis; this response can be diminished by the use of cART. Despite the theoretical concerns regarding immunosuppression in the HIV population, there are numerous reports documenting successful treatment of psoriatic and reactive arthritis in patients with HIV using agents which include sulfasalazine (SSZ), cyclosporine, methotrexate (MTX), mycophenolate mofetil, etanercept, infliximab, adalimumab, steroids, or hydroxyurea (Menon et al., 2009).

G. HIV-associated Vasculitis.

   1. Small, medium, and large vessel vasculitis has been reported in the patient who is infected with HIV, with an incidence of approximately 1%. The pathophysiology is unclear but may be related to secondary comorbid infections such as hepatitis B, hepatitis C, cytomegalovirus, herpes simplex virus, or toxoplasmosis; alternatively, the HIV itself may induce the vasculitis because of the presence of viral particles in the vessel wall (Angarone, 2012).

   2. Polyarteritis Nodosa.

      a. Polyarteritis nodosa is one type of vasculitis that commonly targets young males. The symptoms include myalgias, muscle atrophy, mononeuritis, and sensory motor neuropathy, among others. Polyarteritis nodosa is frequently associated with IV drug use and co-morbid hepatitis C (Patel, Patel, & Espinoza, 2009). In Asia, the occurrence of Behçet's-like disease is common as hepatitis C as a co-morbid condition is widespread (Patel, Patel, & Espinoza). Orogenital ulcers are found in 60-70% of these patients (Patel, Patel, & Espinoza).

3. Therapy.

   a. Treatment of vasculitis often involves corticosteroids and other immunosuppressive medications. Nursing considerations include monitoring for secondary infections, patient education, and pain evaluation and management.

H. Myopathies.

1. Polymyositis is the most common muscular presentation in HIV-infected patients occurring in 2-7% of the population (Walker, Tyndall, & Daikeler, 2008). Polymyositis usually occurs in the early stage of HIV infection. Myositis in patients with HIV infection may result from host immune response to viral infection, may be related to medications such as azidothymidine (AZT), or may occur secondary to opportunistic infections such as toxoplasmosis (Restrepo et al., 2004).

2. Bilateral, symmetrical, proximal muscle weakness in polymyositis is due to muscle infiltration by CD8 T lymphocytes; additional features may involve cardiac and esophageal sequelae. Approximately 50% of patients with DILS present with polymyositis features (Hamdulay, Glynn, & Keat, 2006). Other forms of myopathy have been reported (see Table 3). A suspected case of myopathy in the patient who is HIV-infected should be thoroughly evaluated with laboratory muscle enzymes and consideration of biopsy. An MRI of the muscle can also be diagnostically helpful. Electromyographic (EMG) findings are identical to idiopathic polymyositis. The prognosis is generally good with excellent response to immunosuppressive medications. The rheumatology nurse must continually assess the patient for fall risk and ensure there is no issue with completion of activities of daily living because of muscle weakness.

IV. HIV and Rheumatology-related Opportunistic Infections.

A. Septic arthritis and osteomyelitis occur in the patient with HIV at .3 to 3.6 % prevalence (Zalavras, Dellamaggiora, Patzakis, Brava, & Holtom, 2006). Staphylococcus aureus is the most common pathogen isolated in septic arthritis in the patient with HIV, comprising 30-60% of patients with HIV-related septic arthritis (Zalavras et al.). The incidence of HIV-associated septic arthritis is higher in intravenous drug users. These patients present with classic septic arthritis symptoms of fever, joint pain, decreased range of motion, erythema, and warmth of the joint with elevated sedimentation rate and possibly low white blood count. Tuberculosis infections of the bone can also occur. The thoracolumbar spine is the most frequent site of osteomyelitis seen in those with co-morbid HIV (Restrepo et al., 2004). HIV infection is also the largest risk factor in progression from latent TB to active disease (Takhar & Hendey, 2010). Bone biopsy and synovial aspiration are essential to diagnosis and treatment.

V. Other Issues of Potential Rheumatologic Concern.

A. Avascular necrosis (AVN) and osteoporosis occur with an increased prevalence in those who have been on cART. Osteonecrosis affects approximately 4% of patients with HIV which is higher than in the general population (Zalavras et al., 2006). AVN most frequently affects the femoral head but can also affect other bony processes. Theories concerning the increased incidence

Table 3 Myopathies That Can Occur in HIV

HIV polymyositis	Diffuse infiltrative lymphocytosis syndrome	Myasthenia gravis
Inclusion body myositis	HIV wasting syndrome	IRIS related to cART
Nemaline myopathy	Vasculitis (many types)	Rhabdomyolysis

Source: Maganti, R.M., Reveille, J. S., & Williams, F. M. (2008).Therapy Insight: The changing spectrum of rheumatic disease in HIV infection. *Nature Clinical Practice Rheumatology*, 4(8), 428-438. doi:10.1038/ncprheum0836

of AVN include its relationship to treatment with radiation or steroids, and possibly higher alcohol intake in individuals who are HIV-positive. Patients who carry the anticardiolipin antibody may be at further risk because of both venous and arterial thromboses leading to bone necrosis. MRI is the most sensitive method to detect early AVN. Patients often present with deep bone pain that can occur even at rest. Because of the frequency of hip involvement, groin pain is common. Treatment is dependent on the extent of the findings. Patients on cART need to have bone mineral density screening and MUST report any bone pain that persists for greater than two weeks to ensure no secondary malignant process is occurring.

VI. Treatment of HIV-associated Rheumatologic Conditions.

A. The first step in treatment of rheumatic conditions associated with HIV is controlling the underlying HIV infection. Pharmacologic therapies for rheumatic conditions must be assessed on an individual risk-benefit basis. Ideally, before any immunomodulating rheumatic medication is added the CD4 count would be >200 cells/µL and the HIV viral load be below 40 copies/mL; however, in general, rheumatologic directed immunosuppression can often be successfully employed in the HIV population.

B. Hydroxychloroquine (HCQ).

1. Has been successfully used and has been found to decrease the viral replication of HIV (Mody, Parke, & Reveille, 2003).

C. Indomethacin.

1. Has also been found to have antiviral properties and is an excellent choice for symptomatic pain relief (Walker, Tyndall, & Daikeler, 2008). Since NSAIDs are often prescribed along with a PPI (which may interact with certain antiretrovirals) education regarding drug-drug interactions is essential.

D. Methotrexate (MTX).

1. Can be judiciously used.

E. Sulfasalazine (SSZ).

1. Has been effectively used in reactive arthritis, works by inhibiting lymphocyte proliferation.

F. Case reports have also identified the successful use of gold, mycophenolate mofetil, steroids, and hydroxyurea, as well as the use of all available TNF inhibitors. More research concerning the safest and most effective treatments is necessary and ongoing. Diligence is required when combining any immunosuppressive medications in this population and surveillance is needed for falling CD4 counts, increasing viral loads, and secondary opportunistic infections.

G. Rheumatology nurses must educate the patient on the need for adherence to treatment regimens, side effects, and the absolute need for ongoing medical surveillance.

VII. The Future: HIV as a Chronic Disease.

A. As mortality rates of the treated patient with HIV have decreased, HIV has turned into a chronic disease state for many patients. Because of this change, the rheumatology nurse must be aware of long-term associated risks in the HIV-infected individual. Bone pain in any patient is a red flag; in patients with HIV, bone pain may be musculoskeletal manifestations related to one of two common neoplasms: Kaposi sarcoma (KS), and non-Hodgkin lymphoma (NHL). NHL is 60 times more frequent in patients with AIDS compared to the general population (Restrepo et al., 2004). Unlike most other entities, the introduction of cART has seemingly increased the prevalence of NHL in the AIDS population (Restrepo et al.). NHL frequently occurs in late stage of the disease when the CD4 counts are less than 200 cells per micro liter and tends to be more aggressive with a poorer prognosis in patients who are HIV-infected. Extra nodal sites are more common and can occur in 60-95% of patients with AIDS-associated NHL. Patients frequently have bone and muscle involvement and present with fever, painful unilateral limb swelling, anorexia, cachexia, and pathologic fracture.

B. Kaposi sarcoma is a disease in which malignant cancer cells invade the tissue lining the lymph vessels under the skin or in mucus membranes and occurs in 20% of patients with AIDS (Restrepo et al., 2004). Musculoskeletal involvement is rare and more often the vascular neoplasm involves mucocutaneous tissues, lymph nodes, and visceral organs. Because Kaposi sarcoma can affect any organ, close monitoring for any new skin lesion or the occurrence of hemoptysis in the HIV-affected individual is imperative. When musculoskeletal evaluation is necessary, radiography can identify lesions that may be secondary to local extension of the disease and may show cortical lesions including bone erosions and osseous destruction, as well as periosteal reaction. Biopsy is essential for definitive diagnosis (Restrepo et al.).Treatment depends on the location and extent of the tumor.

Summary

Rheumatologic symptoms and disease are common in those with HIV and AIDS. A careful evaluation is required to properly diagnose these conditions. Treatment typically begins with cART. Immunomodulatory therapy can usually be successfully employed in these individuals when required; however, this treatment requires extra vigilance to decrease the risk of complications.

Acknowledgment

The author thanks Eric Eggenberger, DO, for assistance in editing this chapter.

References

Angarone, M. P. (2012, April). Lecture. *HIV and rheumatology. State of the art clinical symposium.* American College of Rheumatology meeting. Chicago, IL,

Azeroual, A., Harmouche, H., Benjilali, L., Mezalek, Z., Adnaoui, M., Aouni, M., & Maaouni, A. (2008). Rheumatoid arthritis associated to HIV infection. *European Journal of Internal Medicine, 19,* e34-e35.Cepeda, E., Williams, F., Ishimori, M., Weisman, M., & Reveille, J. (2008). The use of anti-tumor necrosis factor therapy in HIV-positive individuals with rheumatic disease. *Annals of Rheumatic Disease, 67, 710-712.* doi: 10.1136/ard.2007.081513

Hamdulay, S., Glynn, S., & Keat, A. (2006). When is arthritis reactive? *Post Graduate Medicine Journal, 82,* 446-453. doi: 10.1136/pgmj.2005.044057

Louthrenoo, W. (2008). Rheumatic manifestations of human immunodeficiency virus infection. *Current Opinion in Rheumatology, 20,* 92-99.

Maganti, R., Reveille, J., & Williams, F. (2008). Therapy insight: The changing spectrum of rheumatic disease. *Nature Clinical Practice Rheumatology, 4*(8), 428-438. doi: www.nature.com/clinical practice/rheum

Menon, K., Voorhees, V., Bebo, B., Gladman, D., Hsu, S., & Kalb, R. (2009). Psoriasis in patients with HIV infection: From the medical board of the National Psoriasis Foundation. *American Academy of Dermatology, 62,*(2), 291-299. doi:10.1016/j.jaad.2009.03.047

Mody, G., Parke, F., & Reveille, J. (2003). Articular manifestations of human immunodeficiency virus infection. *Best Practice & Research: Clinical Rheumatology, 17*(2), 265-287. doi: 10.1016/s1521-6942 (03) 00003

Nguyen, B., & Reveille, J. (2009). Rheumatic manifestations associated with HIV in the highly active antiretroviral therapy era. *Current Opinion in Rheumatology, 21*(4), 404-410.

Ouedraogo, D., & Meyer, O. (2012). Psoriatic arthritis in sub-Saharan Africa. *Joint Bone and Spine, 79,* 17-19. doi:10.1016/j.jbspin.2011.06.007

Patel, N., Patel, N., & Espinoza, L. (2009). HIV infection and rheumatic diseases: The changing spectrum of clinical enigma. *Rheumatic Disease Clinics of North America, 35,* 139-161. doi: rheumatic.theclinics.com

Restrepo, C., Lemos, D., Gordillo, H., Odero, R., Varghese, T., Tiemann, W.... Moncada, R. (2004). Imaging findings in musculoskeletal complications of AIDS. *Education Exhibit, 24,* 1029-1049. doi: 10.1148/rg.244035151

Reveille, J., & Williams, F. (2006). Rheumatic complications of HIV infection. *Best Practice & Research: Clinical Rheumatology, 20*(6), 1159-1179. doi:10.1016/j.berh.2006.08.015

Takhar, S., & Hendey, G. (2010). Orthopedic illnesses in patients with HIV. *Emergency Medicine Clinics of North America, 28*, 335-342. doi:10.1016/j.emc.2010.01.009

Vitali, C. (2011). Immunopathic differences of Sjögren's syndrome versus sicca syndrome in HCV and HIV. *Arthritis Research and Therapy, 13*(4), 233. doi:10.1186/ar3361

Walker, U., Tyndall, A., & Daikeler, T. (2008). Rheumatic conditions in human immunodeficiency virus infection. *Rheumatology, 47*, 952-959. doi:10.1093/rheumatology/ken13

Zalavras, C., Dellamaggiora, R., Patzakis, M., Brava, E., & Holtom, P. (2006). Septic arthritis in patients with human immunodeficiency virus. *Clinical Orthopedics and Related Research, 451*, 46-49.

Suggested Readings

Allroggen, A., Frese, A., Rahmann, A., Guabitz, M., Husstedt, I., & Evers, S. (2005). HIV associated arthritis: Case report and review of the literature. *European Journal of Medical Research, 10*, 305-308.

Shah, D., Flanigan, T., & Lally, E. (2011). Routine screening for HIV in rheumatology practice. *Journal of Clinical Rheumatology, 17*(3), 154-156. doi:10.1097/RhU.